TS

The
COMPLETE
GUIDE TO PILLS

THE SPECIALISTS:

Dr. Andrew J. Buda
Chief of Cardiology Section
TULANE UNIVERSITY

Dr. Joseph Caprioli
Director of Ophthalmology
YALE UNIVERSITY

Dr. Paula J. Clayton
Head of Psychiatry
UNIVERSITY OF MINNESOTA

Dr. Michael M. Frank
Chairman of Pediatrics
DUKE UNIVERSITY

Dr. Ernesto Gonzalez
Professor of Dermatology
HARVARD MEDICAL SCHOOL

Dr. Linda C. Giudice
Professor of Ob-Gyn
STANFORD UNIVERSITY

Dr. Steven Rosen
Director of Cancer Center
NORTHWESTERN UNIVERSITY

Dr. Richard S. Shader
Professor of Pharmacology
TUFTS UNIVERSITY

Dr. E. Darracott Vaughan
Chairman of Urology
CORNELL UNIVERSITY

Another Book by Affinity Communications

Edited and compiled by Brenda Adderly

BALLANTINE BOOKS•NEW YORK

New prescription drugs, drug side effects, and drug interactions are discovered all the time, and while this book
provides the most current, up-to-date information that was
available at the time of publication, readers should *always*
consult their physicians if they have any questions, concerns, or problems with their prescriptions.

"An Affinity Communications Book"

Copyright © 1996 by Affinity Communications Corporation

All rights reserved under International and Pan-American Copyright
Conventions. Published in the United States by Ballantine Books, a
division of Random House, Inc., New York, and simultaneously in
Canada by Random House of Canada Limited, Toronto.

http://www.randomhouse.com

ISBN 0-345-40215-4

Manufactured in the United States of America

First Edition: December 1996

10 9 8 7 6 5 4 3 2 1

To Mom, Dad, Veryl, Donna, Michael,
Kathy, Gina, and the Kids—*much* thanks
and love for your eternal support.

ACKNOWLEDGEMENTS

I wish to recognize and express much appreciation to those who have assisted me in the development of this book, especially:

- Dana L. Graves, my "coach," supporter, and reality check;
- Sirkly Dennis for her tireless and precise efforts at fact-checking;
- Laura Dail for keeping the ball rolling;
- Wendy Loreen for her creativity in designing this book;
- Nancy McKinley for ensuring that everything makes sense.

I would also like to thank Neelam Sekhri and Patty Mintz for encouraging me to take the next step.

PUBLISHER'S NOTE

This book is intended to be used only as a reference tool for consumers who want more information about the drugs their physicians may prescribe for them. It is not meant to replace the professional advice and expertise of your physician, or to encourage a patient to evaluate the risks and benefits of using certain medications without consulting their health care providers. Only a physician can prescribe these drugs, advise on their exact dosages and possible drug interactions, and monitor and evaluate the patient's response and reaction to prescription medications.

The publisher does not advocate use of any of the drugs in this book, nor warrant the safety or efficacy of any medication listed in this book that your individual physician may prescribe.

Table of Contents

FOREWORD

"Despite the benefits that [today's] drugs bring..., public health experts are increasingly concerned about a growing problem: people not using medications as they are prescribed."

—Sandy Rovner, *"Improper Drug Use a Cause for Concern,"*
The Washington Post (April 11, 1995)

This growing concern about the use and misuse of prescription drugs can only be met by making more information available to patients. Luckily, in the field of prescription drug books, *The Complete Guide to Pills* is a standout. It provides the important answers to all consumers' needs for useful, easy-to-understand information about prescription pills.

Although interested readers can locate several books in this field, *The Complete Guide to Pills* is the one publication which goes the extra step to present technical medical information in a way that consumers can easily understand. A very important feature of this new book is its visually-oriented, easy-to-follow layout. By using icons as eye-catching "flags" for the reader, important information that consumers need to know can be quickly located and understood. In addition, the entries are written in plain English, which is both quite refreshing and an incredible accomplishment.

The distinguished panel of medical specialists for this book—all of whom represent the top medical schools in the United States—have endorsed the book as being both consumer friendly and very easy to use. As a representative of the pharmaceutical industry, I am in complete agreement with these medical experts' judgment.

I commend the publisher, Ballantine Books, and the book's author, Brenda Adderly (in association with Affinity Communications), on creating a well-thought out and useful book on prescription drugs.

—Fred Tarter
Chairman, The Pharmacy Fund

INTRODUCTION

> *"Medicines are nothing in themselves, if not properly used, but the very hands of the gods, if employed with reason and prudence."*
>
> —Herophilus, Greek Physician, 300 B.C.

You have just received a prescription for a new medication from your doctor. Or perhaps you have been taking a particular prescription for a while. Maybe your child has started taking drugs for an illness. In any case, you definitely want accurate, easy-to-understand, and up-to-date facts about the medications you and your family are taking.

Information You Need to Know

To get the most out of your medicine, you should know the following important facts:

1. What is the name of the medicine?

2. What is the medicine supposed to do? (Make the pain go away? Get to the cause of the pain? Reduce fever? Lower blood pressure? Cure infection?)

3. What side effects might occur?

4. How should you take the medicine? Should you take the drug before meals, with meals, or after meals? If the directions say "every six hours" do you have to get up during the night to take the medicine on time?

5. How long should you take the medicine? If you stop just because you feel good, the symptoms and the disease may recur.

6. Are there other medicines you should not take while you are taking this one?

7. Are there any foods or beverages you should avoid?

8. Should you avoid alcoholic beverages while taking the drug?

The Complete Guide to Pills summarizes all this information—the most important facts—about the most commonly prescribed medications. It provides up-to-date, clear, and precise descriptions of each drug, and lists over 1,700 pills and other commonly prescribed medications.

Brand Drugs and Generic Drugs

To make it easy to find the information you need, we have listed each prescription drug by its Brand Name. This is the drug manufacturer's registered trademark name for a generic drug. You can also find cross-references to all Generic Names for drugs.

Every drug has a "generic"—or chemical—name which is assigned to it when the new drug is being developed. The manufacturer also assigns a shorter, easier-to-remember brand name, which is used to advertise and market the product. After the patent expires on a new drug, other drug companies can produce the same product, either using their own brand name or selling the drug under its generic name.

Generic drugs generally cost from 30 to 50 percent less than their brand-name equivalents, but in some cases the gap is much greater. The Federal Trade Commission has estimated that consumers can save more than $100 million per year by using generics instead of their brand-name equivalents.

All drugs—brand-name and generic—must meet the same U.S. Food and Drug Administration (FDA) standards for purity, strength and quality in order to stay on the market. It has found no difference in the rates of adverse events between generic drugs and brand-name equivalents.

Supplemental Information

This book is meant to supplement the information your doctor and pharmacist have provided. It should not be used to substitute a doctor's care and medical advice, or for self-help or self-medication purposes.

Always remember, use *The Complete Guide to Pills* with caution and lots of common sense!

MEDICAL SPECIALISTS ADVISORY PANEL

HOW TO USE THIS BOOK

If you're about to reach into the medicine cabinet for a prescribed medication, here is some important consumer information from the Food and Drug Administration that you should know before you start taking any medication.

You will find information about all these important issues in *The Complete Guide to Pills*. In addition, the section of this book titled "How to Find the Information You Need" provides detailed guidance on locating key pieces of information using the icon symbols. A very important feature of this new book is its visually-oriented, easy-to-follow layout. Using these icons as eye-catching "flags," readers can quickly locate the important information they need to know.

Adverse Reactions (Side Effects)

Some drugs can cause side effects (adverse reactions). Usually these are mild—a slight rash, mild headache, nausea or drowsiness. Sometimes adverse reactions are much more severe—prolonged vomiting, bleeding, marked weakness or impaired vision or hearing.

Not everyone reacts the same way to medication. One person may experience a reaction to a certain drug while another person may have no problems at all. When a reaction is unexpected or severe, a doctor should be consulted immediately.

Drug-Drug Interactions

Taken at the same time, two or more drugs can interact and affect the way one or the other behaves in your body. For example, an antacid will cause a blood-thinning (anti-coagulant) drug to be absorbed too slowly, while aspirin greatly increases the blood-thinning effect of such drugs.

Two drugs with the same effect when taken together can sometimes have an impact greater than would be expected. This can be helpful, but it can also be dangerous, particularly when several central nervous system depressing drugs are involved.

Even non-prescription drugs—such as antihistamines that are often used to fight colds—can increase the sedative ef-fects of anesthetics, barbiturates, tranquilizers and some pain killers.

Food and Drug Interactions

Food can interact with some drugs, making the drugs work faster or slower, or even preventing them from working at all. Here are some examples:

1. Calcium in dairy products impairs absorption of tetracycline, a widely used antibiotic.

2. Citrus fruits or juices containing ascorbic acid can speed the absorption of iron from iron supplements.

3. Soft drinks, fruit and vegetable juices with high acid contents (such as grape, apple, orange or tomato), cause some drugs to dissolve in the stomach instead of the intestines where they can be more readily absorbed.

4. Eating large amounts of liver and leafy vegetables may hinder the effectiveness of anti-coagulants because the vitamin K found in these foods promotes blood clotting.

The most hazardous food-drug interaction, however, is found with drugs that are sometimes prescribed for severe depression or high blood pressure and foods containing the substance tyramine. Mixing the following foods with such drugs can raise the blood pressure to dangerous levels: aged cheese, Chianti wine, pickled herring, fermented sausages, yogurt, sour cream, chicken liver, broad beans, canned figs, bananas, avocados and foods prepared with tenderizers.

The food-drug interaction effect can also go the other way. Oral contraceptives, for instance, are known to lower blood levels of folic acid. Women who take birth control pills would be wise to include dark green leafy vegetables in their diets.

Drugs and Alcohol

Chronic use of alcohol can cause changes in the liver that speed up the metabolism of some drugs, such as anti-convulsant, anti-coagulants and diabetes drugs. They become less effective because they do not stay in the body long enough.

Prolonged alcohol abuse can also damage the liver so that it is less able to metabolize or process certain drugs. In that case, the drugs stay in the system too long. This is particularly serious when the drugs are phenothiazines (anti-psychotic drugs), which can cause further liver damage.

Alcohol is a central nervous system (CNS) depressant. Alcohol taken along with another CNS depressant drug can affect performance skills, judgment and alertness. If the mixture includes overdoses of barbiturates, diazepam (Valium) or pro-poxyphene (Darvon), the result can be fatal.

Drugs and Smoking

Women who use birth control pills and also smoke cigarettes have an in creased risk of heart attack, stroke and other circulatory diseases.

Nicotine and other tobacco products speed up the metabolism of theophylline, an asthma drug, and pentazocine, a pain-killer, and to a lesser extent, will also affect certain tranquilizers, analgesics and antidepressants.

Thus, smokers may need larger than normal doses of these drugs. When they stop smoking, dosage of these drugs may have to be changed. Smoking also can affect certain diagnostic tests, such as red and white blood cell counts and blood clotting time determinations.

What You Should Tell Your Doctor

Because of these side effects and drug interactions, it is important that you tell your doctor if you:

1. Have had allergic reactions to drugs or foods, such as rashes or headaches.

2. Are taking any medications on a regular basis, such as contraceptives or insulin, or if you use any non-prescription drugs on a routine basis.

3. Are being treated for a different condition by another doctor.

4. Are pregnant or breastfeeding.

5. Have diabetes, kidney or liver disease.

6. Are on a special diet or are taking vitamin and mineral supplements.

7. Use alcohol or tobacco.

General Information for Patients

It's always a good idea to check the prescription before you leave the doctor's office. If there is anything you don't understand, ask about it then before you start taking the drug.

Detailed information for patients does not always accompany most prescription drugs. But for a few, such as contraceptives and estrogens, the Food and Drug Administration does require a leaflet or brochure that tells about the benefits and risks of these products.

If there is such a brochure with a drug prescribed for you, be sure to read it carefully and if you have questions, ask your doctor or pharmacist. Many physicians and pharmacists offer additional written information for patients about the drugs being prescribed. Ask them for this information.

Non-prescription (over-the-counter) drugs must include on their labels information about when and how to take the product, possible side effects or prescription drug interactions. Always read these labels before taking the medicine.

Drug Costs: Brand vs. Generic

When a new drug is discovered, it is patented and given a brand, or trade, name. The drug, company has exclusive rights to that product for 17 years. When the patent expires, other companies may manufacture that drug under another brand name or under the drug's generic, or common, name. These drugs often are less expensive than the original drug.

Almost all states now permit pharmacists to dispense a generic drug instead of a brand name product if the doctor approves. However, not all drugs are available from more than one company, and not all multi-source drugs are "therapeutically equivalent" (that is, they behave in the same way in the body). FDA publishes lists of drugs that identify which ones can be substituted safely. The next time your doctor writes you a prescription, ask if there is an approved generic version of the drug.

Get the Best Results From Prescription Drugs

Here are some tips to help you use prescription drugs safely and effectively:

1. If a drug is not doing what it is supposed to do for you, check with your doctor. You may need a different dosage or a different drug.

2. If you have an unexpected symptom (rash, nausea, dizziness, headache) report it to your doctor immediately.

3. Don't stop taking your medicine just because you're feeling better. You may prevent the drug from doing its work completely.

4. Check drug labels for specific instructions or warnings, such as "do not take on an empty stomach" or "do not take with milk."

5. Check the label, or ask the pharmacist, for storing instructions. Some drugs should be refrigerated; others must be protected from light.

6. Always keep medicines out of the reach of children. Even though most prescription medicines come in childproof containers, children sometimes can open these bottles and swallow the contents.

7. Never let another person use your medicine and never take medicine prescribed for anyone else. Your symptoms may look the same, but you may be suffering from an entirely different problem.

8. Never take medicines without checking the label first. Don't take medicine at night without turning on the light to make sure you're taking the correct one.

9. Don't transfer medicines from the original container. These containers are designed to protect the drugs.

10. Do not keep prescription drugs that are no longer needed. Destroy any leftover medicines by flushing them down the toilet and dispose of containers carefully so children can't get them.

11. Keep a list of all drugs you are taking to show to your doctor and your pharmacist.

12. If you are taking several different drugs and have trouble remembering when and how to take them, your pharmacist may be able to provide you with a handy checklist.

13. If you have a bad experience with a drug (either due to side effects or it didn't work well for you), write down your observations for future reference and discuss with your physician and/or pharmacist.

14. **Immediately seek medical attention when an overdose is suspected.**

15. **Always consult with your doctor before combining medications.**

Check the Drug Photo

To assist you in confirming that the medication you are taking is the correct one your doctor has prescribed, we have included numerous photographs of the most commonly prescribed pills, and at different dosage levels. If you have questions about why your particular medication varies from a picture, check with your pharmacist or doctor for clarification.

Note that the size or color of the pill photo may differ slightly from the actual pill as a result of the book's printing process, so you should rely on your doctor or pharmacist if you have questions. When you are looking for a particular drug photo, be sure not to confuse Brand Name with Generic Name.

Purpose of this Book

This book is meant to supplement the information your doctor and pharmacist have provided. It should not be used to substitute a doctor's care and medical advice, or for self-help or self-medication purposes.

Always remember, use *The Complete Guide to Pills* with caution and lots of common sense!

HOW TO FIND THE INFORMATION YOU NEED

The Compete Guide to Pills has developed an easy-to-use and easy-to-understand format for finding the facts about the most commonly prescribed medications. Each detailed medication entry provides the same level of information on a wide range of drug use issues.

A very important feature of this new book is its visually-oriented, easy-to-follow layout. Using icons as eye-catching "flags" for the reader, important information that consumers need to know can be quickly located and understood. These icon symbols and their meanings are detailed below:

Purpose

 Tells you the conditions and/or symptoms the medication is most often prescribed or used for. If available, we have also included less standard usages for the medication.

Dosage

 How to Take. Gives information on how the medication should be taken, and other tips related to taking the medication. For example, your doctor may suggest taking a pill with food to avoid stomach upset.

 Usual Adult Dose. Guidelines for the usual adult dosages prescribed by a doctor. This is a guideline only; doses are frequently individualized according to your particular needs.

 Usual Child Dose. Guidelines for the usual child dosages prescribed by a doctor. This is a guideline only; doses are frequently individualized according to a child's particular needs.

Missed Dose. Tells you what to do if you miss a dose.

Side Effects

 Overdose Symptoms. Tells you the signs of medication overdose and instructs you to contact medical help if an overdose occurs.

 More Common Side Effects. Side effects that are more often experienced when using the medication.

 Less Common or Rare Side Effects. Side effects that are less often or rarely experienced when using the medication.

Interactions

 Drug Interactions. Lists the medications that interact with your prescribed medication, as well as medications to avoid when using a prescribed medication.

 Food and Other Substance Interactions. Tells you what foods and other substances such as alcohol interact with your prescribed medication.

Special Cautions

 Cautions for Pregnancy and Breastfeeding. Gives important information about the prescribed medication to pregnant women, women planning to become pregnant, and nursing mothers.

 Cautions for Seniors. Tells seniors of any special precautions for using the prescribed medication.

Cautions for Children. Gives special precautions or advice for administering the prescribed medication to children.

 Special Warnings. Provides important information about the prescribed medication that does not fit neatly into any of the categories listed above. It gives you the special, specific information about a pre- scribed medication.

Remember!
- *Seek medical attention when an overdose is suspected.*
- *Consult with your doctor before combining medications.*

Cautions for Children. Gives special precautions or advice for administering the prescribed medication to children.

Special Warnings. Provides important information about the prescribed medication that does not fit the health concerns or the categories listed above. It gives you the most specific information about a prescribed medication.

Overdose.
* Seek medical attention when an overdose is suspected.
* Consult with your doctor before combining medication.

Accupril

Generic name: Quinapril hydrochloride

Accupril is known as an angiotensin-converting enzyme (ACE) inhibitor. It prevents angiotensin I, a blood chemical, from developing into angiotensin II, a stronger form that increases salt and water levels in the body.

℞ QUICK FACTS

Purpose

Used to treat high blood pressure. Also prescribed to treat congestive heart failure.

Dosage

Take with or without meals as directed by your doctor. Follow prescription carefully. Must take regularly for Accupril to be effective. *Do not stop drug without consulting doctor.*

Usual adult dose: *initially*—10 milligrams per day, taken once a day. Doctor may increase up to 80 milligrams per day, taken once a day or divided into 2 doses.

Usual child dose: not generally prescribed for children.

Missed dose: take as soon as possible, unless almost time for next dose. In that case, do not take missed dose; go back to regular schedule. *Do not double doses.*

Side Effects

Overdose symptom: a severe drop in blood pressure. If you suspect an overdose, immediately seek medical attention.

More common side effects: dizziness, headache.

Less common side effects: abdominal pain, coughing, fatigue, nausea, vomiting. Rare side effects: angina (chest pain), back pain, bleeding in the stomach or intestines, bronchitis, changes in heart rhythm, constipation, depression, dimmed vision, dizziness when first standing up, dry mouth or throat, extremely low blood pressure, fainting, heart attack, heart failure, high potassium, increased sweating, inflammation of the pancreas, inflammation of the sinuses, itching, kidney failure, nervousness, palpitations, rapid heartbeat, sensitivity to light, skin peeling, sleepiness, sore throat, stroke, swelling of the mouth and throat, vague feeling of illness, vertigo.

Interactions

Inform your doctor before combining Accupril with: diuretics such as Lasix; Lithium (Eskalith or Lithobid); potassium-sparing diuretics such as Aldactone, Dyazide, and Moduretic; potassium supplements such as Slow-K and K-Dur; salt substitutes containing potassium; Tetracycline (Achromycin V or Sumycin).

Alcohol may increase sedative effects and cause dizziness and fainting; *do not drink alcohol when taking this medication.*

Special Cautions

Accupril can cause injury and death to a fetus when used during the 2nd and 3rd trimesters. If pregnant or planning to become pregnant, inform your doctor immediately. May appear in breast milk; could affect a nursing infant.

Accupril may cause a dramatic decrease in blood pressure after the first dose in seniors.

Not generally prescribed for children.

If swelling of the face, lips, tongue, throat, arms, or legs, or difficulty breathing, occurs, contact your doctor immediately; this may be an emergency situation.

Light-headedness may occur in first days of therapy. If you faint, stop the medication, call your doctor.

Do not take potassium or salt substitutes without informing your doctor.

Should not take medication if allergic to it or similar medications, such as Capoten and Vasotec.

Monitor vomiting, diarrhea, and heavy perspiration; dehydration can drop your blood pressure.

Before medical or dental surgery, tell your doctor or dentist you are taking this drug.

If a sore throat occurs, contact your doctor immediately.

Your kidney function should be monitored while taking this medication.

Accutane
∿∿∿∿∿∿∿∿∿∿∿∿∿∿∿∿∿∿∿∿∿∿∿∿∿∿∿∿∿∿∿∿∿∿∿

Generic name: Isotretinoin

Accutane is an anti-acne drug. It inhibits the production of sebum and the process of keratinization, which leads to severe acne. It is in the same chemical family as vitamin A.

℞ QUICK FACTS

Purpose

℞ Used to treat severe, disfiguring cystic acne which has not responded to antibiotics.

Dosage

 Take with food; follow the instructions carefully. After completing Accutane therapy, you should have a 2-month period of time off the medication. If your acne is still severe after this period, you may be prescribed a 2nd course of therapy. *Do not crush capsules.*

. . . .

 Usual adult dose: *initially*—0.5 to 1 milligram per 2.2 pounds of body weight per day, divided into 2 doses daily, for 15 to 20 weeks. Doctor may increase up to 2 milligrams per 2.2 pounds of body weight.

. . . .

 Usual child dose (adolescents only): *initially*—0.5 to 1 milligram per 2.2 pounds of body weight per day, divided into 2 doses daily, for 15 to 20 weeks. Doctor may increase up to 2 milligrams per 2.2 pounds of body weight.

. . . .

Missed dose: take as soon as possible, unless almost time for next dose. In that case, do not take missed dose; go back to regular schedule. *Do not double doses.*

Side Effects

Overdose symptoms: abdominal pain; dizziness; dry, cracked, inflamed lips; facial flushing; incoordination and clumsiness; headache; vomiting. If you suspect an overdose, immediately seek medical attention.

More common side effects: conjunctivitis (pinkeye); dry or fragile skin; dry, cracked, excessive scaling; inflamed lips; dry mouth; dry nose; itching, joint pains; nosebleed.

Less common side effects: bowel inflammation and pain, chest pain, decreased night vision, decreased tolerance to contact lenses, depression, fatigue, headache, nausea, peeling of palms or soles, rash, skin infections, stomach and intestinal discomfort, sunburn-sensitive skin, thinning hair, urinary discomfort, vision problems, vomiting.

Interactions

Inform your doctor before combining Accutane with vitamin supplements containing vitamin A.

No known food/other substance interactions.

Special Cautions

Do not use if pregnant; Accutane causes birth defects, including mental retardation and physical malformations. Women should have monthly pregnancy tests while taking Accutane; if you become pregnant, immediately stop taking Accutane and see your doctor. Women of childbearing age will receive verbal and written warnings

about avoiding pregnancy during Accutane therapy. You must sign an informed consent form before starting this medication. Women must test negative for pregnancy within 2 weeks prior to beginning therapy, and you must start Accutane on the 2nd or 3rd day of your menstrual period. May appear in breast milk; could affect a nursing infant.

 No special precautions apply to seniors.

 Follow doctor's instructions carefully for children.

 Stop taking Accutane if you experience: abdominal pain, bleeding from the rectum, or severe diarrhea.

Do not donate your blood while taking this medication, and for at least 1 month after finishing therapy.

Swelling of the optic nerve may occur; see a neurologist if you experience headache, nausea, or visual disturbances.

Use caution when driving at night; sudden decreases in night vision have been observed.

If you are sensitive to parabens, the preservative used in the capsules, you should not take Accutane.

Acebutolol Hydrochloride

see SECTRAL

Acetaminophen

see TYLENOL

Acetaminophen with Codeine

see TYLENOL WITH CODEINE

Acetaminophen with Oxycodone Hydrochloride

see PERCOCET

Acetazolamide

see DIAMOX

Achromycin V Capsules

Generic name: Tetracycline hydrochloride

Other brand names: Ala-Tet, Ala-V, Nor-Tet, Panmycin, Sumycin, Tetracyn, Tetralan-500

Achromycin V is a tetracycline antibiotic. It is used to prevent bacteria from multiplying and growing. It is an alternative drug for those who are allergic to penicillin.

℞ QUICK FACTS

Purpose

℞ Used to treat acne and a wide variety of bacterial infections.

Dosage

 Take exactly as prescribed. Finish the entire prescription. Shake liquid form well before using. *Do not use after expiration date; is highly toxic to the kidneys.* Take 1 hour before or 2 hours after a meal.

· ·

 Usual adult dose: *for most infections*—1 to 2 grams divided into 2 or 4 equal doses, depending on severity. *For brucellosis*—500 milligrams 4 times daily for 3 weeks, accompanied by streptomycin. *For syphilis*—a total of 30 to 40 grams taken in equally divided doses over a 10 to 15 day period. *For urethral, endocervical, or rectal infections in adults caused by* Chlamydia trachomatis—500 milligrams 4 times a day, for at least 7 days.

· ·

 Usual child dose: *for children 8 years and above*—10 to 20 milligrams per pound of body weight divided into 2 or 4 equal doses.

· ·

 Missed dose: *if taking 1 daily dose*—take as soon as possible, then take next dose 10 to 12 hours later. *If taking 2 daily doses*—take as soon as possible, then take next dose 5 to 6 hours later. *If taking 3 or more daily doses*—take as soon as possible, then take next dose 2 to 4 hours later. Then go back to regular schedule.

Side Effects

 Overdose symptom: may cause liver damage. If you suspect an overdose, immediately seek medical attention.

· ·

 More common side effects: anemia, blood disorders, blurred vision and headache (in adults), bulging soft spot on the head (in infants), diarrhea, difficult or painful swallowing, dizziness, extreme allergic reactions, genital or anal sores or rash, hives, inflammation of large bowel, inflammation of the tongue, inflammation of upper digestive tract, increased sensitivity to light, loss of appetite, nausea, rash, ringing in the ears, swelling due to fluid accumulation, vision disturbance, vomiting.

 Less common or rare side effects: inflamed skin, liver poisoning, muscle weakness, peeling, throat sores and inflammation.

Interactions

 Inform your doctor before combining Achromycin V with: antacids containing aluminum, calcium, or magnesium, such as Mylanta and Maalox; blood thinners such as Coumadin; oral contraceptives; Penicillin (Amoxil, Pen•Vee K, others).

 Foods, milk, and some dairy products interfere with the absorption of tetracyclines.

Special Cautions

 Not recommended for use during the last half of pregnancy. Can affect the development of the unborn child's bones and teeth. If pregnant or planning to become pregnant, inform your doctor immediately. Appears in breast milk; could affect a nursing infant.

 No special precautions apply to seniors.

 Not prescribed for children under 8 years.

 Do not take this medication if you have had an allergic reaction to this or other tetracycline medications.

Inform your doctor if you have kidney disease; a lower dose may be necessary.

Use caution in sunlight or ultraviolet light.

Sometimes antibiotics cause other infections; notify your doctor if you develop other infections.

If taking over a length of time, your blood, kidneys; and liver should be monitored.

Aclovate

∧∧∧∧∧∧∧∧∧∧∧∧∧∧∧∧∧∧∧∧∧∧∧∧∧∧∧∧∧∧∧∧∧∧∧∧∧∧∧

Generic name: Alclometasone dipropionate

Aclovate is a topical adrenocorticoid/anti-inflammatory. It interferes with the natural body mechanisms that produce rash, itching, or inflammation.

℞ QUICK FACTS

Purpose

℞   Used to relieve certain itchy rashes, including psoriasis.

Dosage

 Spread a thin film of cream or ointment over the rash; massage gently until medication disappears. For persistent rash, a thick layer of cream or ointment covered with a bandage may be required. For external use only; avoid getting into the eyes. *Do not bandage unless prescribed by your doctor.*

 Usual adult dose: apply thin film of cream or ointment to the affected skin areas; massage until medication disappears.

 Usual child dose: apply thin film of cream or ointment to the affected skin areas; massage gently until medication disappears.

Missed dose: apply as soon as possible, unless almost time for next dose. In that case, do not take missed dose; go back to regular schedule.

Side Effects

 Overdose symptoms: children—bulging soft spots on an infant's head, headache, nausea. If you suspect an overdose (child or adult), immediately seek medical attention.

 Side effects: abnormally excessive growth of hair, acne-like pimples, allergic rash, burning, dryness, infection, irritation, itching, maceration (sponginess) of the skin, pale (depigmented) spots, prickly heat, rash around the mouth, redness, skin inflammation, stretch marks on skin.

 No known less common or rare side effects.

Interactions

 Inform your doctor before using Aclovate with other, more potent steroids; may lead to large amounts of hormones in the bloodstream.

 No known food/other substance interactions.

Special Cautions

 If pregnant or planning to become pregnant, inform your doctor immediately. Medications absorbed from Aclovate may get into the fetal bloodstream or breast milk.

 No specific precautions apply to seniors.

 If used over extended periods, can affect a child's normal growth development. Children are more susceptible to Cushing's syndrome when Aclovate is used for extended periods over large areas of skin.

 Do not use if you have sensitivity or allergic reaction to: Alclometasone dipropionate or other corticosteroids, or any of the oils, waxes, alcohols, or other chemicals in the cream or ointment.

Use caution with Aclovate; some of the medication can be absorbed through the skin and into the bloodstream with prolonged use, leading to side effects elsewhere in the body.

Use for extended periods over large areas of skin may lead to Cushing's syndrome: moon-faced appearance, fattened neck and trunk, purplish streaks on the skin.

Actigall

Generic name: Ursodiol

Actigall is a gallstone dissolver. It reduces liver cholesterol production and blocks cholesterol absorption through the intestine.

℞ QUICK FACTS

Purpose

 Used to assist in dissolving gallstones. Is a good alternative to surgery.

Dosage

 Take exactly as prescribed, or the gallstones will dissolve slowly or not at all.

Usual adult dose: 8 to 10 milligrams per 2.2 pounds of body weight per day, divided into 2 or 3 doses.

 Usual child dose: not generally prescribed for children.

 Missed dose: take as soon as possible, or at the same time as the next dose.

Side Effects

 Most likely overdose symptom is diarrhea. If you suspect an overdose, immediately seek medical attention.

 Side effects: abdominal pain, anxiety, back pain, constipation, cough, depression, dry skin, fatigue, gas, hair thinning, headache, hives, indigestion, inflammation of the mouth or nose, itching, metallic taste, mild temporary diarrhea, muscle and joint pain, nausea, rash, severe pain in the upper right side of the abdomen, sleep disorders, sweating, vomiting.

 No known less common or rare side effects.

Interactions

 Inform your doctor before combining Actigall with: aluminum-based antacid medications (Alu-Cap, Alu-Tab, Rolaids, and others); certain cholesterol-lowering medications (Questran or Colestid); Estrogens such as Premarin; lipid-lowering medications (Lopid or Mevacor); oral contraceptives.

 No known food/other substance interactions.

Special Cautions

 If pregnant or planning to become pregnant, inform your doctor immediately. Actigall is not recommended during pregnancy. Not known if Actigall passes into breast milk.

 No special precautions apply to seniors.

 Not generally prescribed for children.

 Do not take if sensitivity to Actigall or other bile acid medications.

Your doctor must know if you have biliary tract (liver, gallbladder, bile duct) problems or certain liver and pancreas diseases before beginning Actigall therapy.

Most effective if gallstones are small or floatable (high cholesterol content).

Months of Actigall therapy required to dissolve gallstones. In some cases, they are not dissolved fully.

Actigall does not dissolve calcified cholesterol stones, radio-opaque stones, or radiolucent bile pigment stones.

Acyclovir
see ZOVIRAX

Adalat
see PROCARDIA

Adapin

see SINEQUAN

Advil

Generic name: Ibuprofen

Other brand names: Genpril, Medipren, Motrin, PediaProfen

Advil is a nonsteroidal anti-inflammatory drug (NSAID). It works by blocking the production of prostaglandins, which may trigger pain.

℞ QUICK FACTS

Purpose

℞ Used to treat the inflammation, swelling, stiffness, and joint pain with rheumatoid arthritis and osteoarthritis. Also used to relieve menstrual pain.

Dosage

 May take with food or antacid to prevent stomach irritation. Suspension form may be given with food if it causes stomach irritation in children.

 Usual adult dose: *for rheumatoid arthritis and osteoarthritis*—1,200 to 3,200 milligrams per day divided into 3 or 4 doses; not to exceed 3,200 milligrams per day. *For mild to moderate pain*—400 milligrams every 4 to 6 hours. *For menstrual pain*—400 milligrams every 4 hours. *Seniors*—doctors determine dose to the particular needs of the individual.

Usual child dose *(children 12 months to 12 years):* for fever reduction *(suspension only)*—5 milligrams per 2.2 pounds of body weight if temperature is less than 102.5° F, or 10 milligrams per 2.2 pounds of body weight if temperature is greater than 102.5° F. Do not exceed 40 milligrams per 2.2 pounds of body weight in one day.

Missed dose: take as soon as possible, unless almost time for next dose. In that case, do not take missed dose; go back to regular schedule. *Do not double doses.*

Side Effects

Overdose symptoms: abdominal pain, acute renal failure, blurred vision, disorientation, dizziness, drowsiness, gastric irritation, intense headache, lethargy, mental confusion, nausea, numbness, paresthesia, vomiting. If you suspect an overdose, immediately seek medical attention.

More common side effects: abdominal cramps or pain, abdominal discomfort, bloating and gas, constipation, diarrhea, dizziness, fluid retention and swelling, headache, heartburn, indigestion, itching, loss of appetite, nausea, nervousness, rash, ringing in ears, stomach pain, vomiting.

Less common or rare side effects: abdominal bleeding, anemia, black stool, blood in urine, blurred vision, changes in heartbeat, chills, confusion, congestive heart failure, depression, dry eyes and mouth, emotional volatility, fever, hair loss, hearing loss, hepatitis, high blood pressure, hives, inability to sleep, inflammation of nose, inflammation of the pancreas or stomach, kidney failure, severe allergic reactions, shortness of breath, skin eruptions, sleepiness, Stevens-Johnson syndrome (peeling skin), stomach or upper intestinal ulcer, ulcer of gums, vision loss, wheezing, yellow eyes and skin.

Interactions

 Do not take with Aspirin or other anti-inflammatory medications such as Naprosyn unless prescribed by your doctor. Inform your doctor before combining Advil with: blood pressure medications such as Vasotec and Aldomet; blood thinners such as Coumadin; diuretics such as Lasix and HydroDIURIL; Lithium (Lithonate); Methotrexate.

 Avoid using alcohol with this medication.

Special Cautions

 If pregnant or planning to become pregnant, inform your doctor immediately. May appear in breast milk, could affect a nursing infant.

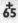 Doctor will vary dosage levels according to individual needs for seniors.

 Suspension form contains sucrose. Inform your doctor if your child monitors his or her sugar intake.

 Should not take Advil if you have sensitivity to Advil, Aspirin or similar drugs; asthma attacks caused by Aspirin or similar medications; or if you have angioedema (skin eruptions).

Peptic ulcers and bleeding may occur without warning.

Use with caution if you have kidney or liver disease.

Can cause water retention; use with caution if you have high blood pressure or poor heart function.

. . . .

If you have an infection, closely monitor it; Advil may mask the usual signs.

AeroBid

∧∧∧

Generic name: Flunisolide

Other brand names: AeroBid-M, Nasalide

AeroBid is a nasal adrenocorticosteroid hormone. It works by reducing inflammation of the mucosal lining of the nasal passages, making it easier to breathe.

℞ QUICK FACTS

Purpose

℞ Used to treat the symptoms of rhinitis (inflamed nasal passages). AeroBid therapy is for long-term, not occasional or short-term, relief.

Dosage

 Take exactly as prescribed; higher doses may affect the function of your adrenal glands. For maximum effectiveness, take at regularly spaced intervals. Going from tablet to inhaler therapy may cause allergic reactions that were controlled with tablet therapy.

. . . .

 Usual adult dose: *initially*—2 inhalations twice daily (morning and evening) for a total daily dose of 1 milligram. May be increased by doctor up to 4 inhalations twice a day, for a total daily dose of 2 milligrams.

 Usual child dose: *for children 6 to 15 years*— 2 inhalations twice daily, for a total daily dose of 1 milligram.

. . . .

Missed dose: take as soon as possible, unless almost time for next dose. In that case, do not take missed dose; go back to regular schedule. *Do not double doses.*

Side Effects

 No specific information is available regarding Aero-Bid overdose. If you suspect an overdose, immediately seek medical attention.

 More common side effects: cold symptoms, diarrhea, flu, headache, infection of upper respiratory tract, nasal congestion, nausea, sore throat, unpleasant taste, upset stomach, vomiting.

 Less common side effects: abdominal pain, chest congestion, chest pain, cough, decreased appetite, dizziness, ear infection, eczema (inflamed skin with sores and crusting), fever, heartburn, hoarseness, inflamed lining of the nose, irritability, itching, loss of smell or taste, menstrual disturbances, nervousness, phlegm, rapid or fluttering heartbeat, rash, runny nose, shakiness, sinus congestion, sinus drainage, sinus infection, sinus inflammation, sneezing, swelling due to fluid retention, wheezing, yeastlike fungal infection of the mouth and throat. Rare side effects: acne, anxiety, blurred vision, bronchitis, chest tightness, chills, constipation, depression, difficult or labored breathing, dry throat, earache, excessive restlessness, eye discomfort, eye infection, faintness, fatigue, gas, general feeling of illness, head stuffiness, high blood pressure, hives, inability to fall or stay asleep, increased appetite, indigestion, inflammation of the tongue, laryngitis, moodiness, mouth irritation, nasal irritation, nosebleed, numbness, pneumonia, rapid heart rate, sinus discomfort, sluggishness, sweating, swelling of the arms and legs, throat irritation, vertigo, weakness, weight gain.

Interactions

 No known drug interactions.

 No known food/other substance interactions.

Special Cautions

 If pregnant or planning to become pregnant, inform your doctor immediately. Is likely to pass into breast milk.

 No special precautions apply to seniors.

 Not generally prescribed for children under 6 years. Suppressed gland function and reduced bone growth in children can occur. Children using AeroBid are more susceptible to infection. *Keep from exposure to chicken pox and measles, which can be fatal.*

 Do not use if bronchodilators and other nonsteroid medications are effective.

Not for treatment of non-asthmatic bronchitis.

Inform your doctor if sensitive to AeroBid or other steroids.

Start AeroBid therapy when asthma is stable.

May cause yeastlike fungal infection of the mouth, throat, or voice box.

AeroBid-M

see AEROBID

Albuterol Sulfate

see PROVENTIL

Alclometasone Dipropionate

see ACLOVATE

Aldactazide

Generic name: Spironolactone with hydrochlorothiazide

Other brand names: Alazide, Spironazide, Spirozide

Aldactazide is a thiazide and potassium-sparing diuretic and a high blood pressure medication. It lowers blood pressure by helping the body produce and eliminate more urine.

℞ QUICK FACTS

Purpose

℞ Used to treat high blood pressure. Also reduces fluid accumulation caused by heart failure, cirrhosis of the liver, kidney disease, and the long-term use of some medications.

Dosage

 Take exactly as prescribed. Sudden discontinuance of this medication may worsen your condition.

Usual adult dose: *for congestive heart failure, cirrhosis, kidney disease*—100 milligrams each of spironolactone and hydrochlorothiazide daily, as a single dose or divided into 2 doses. *For high blood pressure*—50 milligrams to 100 milligrams each of spironolactone and hydrochlorothiazide daily, as a single dose, or divided into smaller doses.

 Usual child dose: 0.75 to 1.5 milligrams of spironolactone per pound of body weight.

 Missed dose: take as soon as possible, unless almost time for next dose. In that case, do not take missed dose; go back to regular schedule. *Do not double doses.*

Side Effects

 No specific information is available regarding Aldactazide overdose. If you suspect an overdose, immediately seek medical attention.

 Side effects: abdominal cramps, breast development in males, change in potassium levels, deepening of the voice, diarrhea, dizziness, dizziness on rising, drowsiness, excessive hairiness, fever, headache, hives, inflammation of blood or lymph vessels, inflammation of the pancreas, irregular menstruation, lack of coordination, loss of appetite, mental confusion, muscle spasms, nausea, postmenopausal bleeding, rash, red or purple spots on skin, restlessness, sensitivity to light, sexual dysfunction, sluggishness, stomach bleeding, stomach inflammation, stomach ulcers, tingling or pins and needles, vertigo, vomiting, weakness, yellow eyes and skin, yellow vision.

 No known less common or rare side effects.

Interactions

 Use extreme caution if taking Vasotec or other ACE-inhibitor medications. Inform your doctor before combining Aldactazide with: antigout medications such as Zyloprim; Digoxin (Lanoxin); diuretics such as Lasix and Midamor; Indomethacin (Indocin); Insulin or oral antidiabetic drugs such as Micronase; Lithium (Lithonate); Norepinephrine (Levophed); potassium supplements such as Slow-K; steroids such as Prednisone.

No known food/other substance interactions.

Special Cautions

 If pregnant or planning to become pregnant, inform your doctor immediately. Appears in breast milk; could affect a nursing infant.

 Doctor will vary dosage levels according to individual needs for seniors.

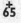 Follow doctor's instructions carefully for children.

 Do not take if sensitive to or had allergic reaction to: spironolactone, hydrochlorothiazide, or similar medications, or sulfa drugs.

Should not be used if you have: difficulty urinating, high potassium levels in the blood, inability to urinate, kidney disease, or liver failure.

If you have liver disease or lupus erythematosus, use cautiously.

Be careful not to lose too much water from the body; blood pressure lowers dramatically.

Before medical or dental surgery, tell your doctor or dentist you are taking this drug.

Aldactone

Generic name: Spironolactone

Aldactone is a thiazide and potassium-sparing diuretic and a high blood pressure medication. It lowers blood pressure by helping the body produce and eliminate more urine.

℞ QUICK FACTS

Purpose

℞ Used to treat high blood pressure. Also used to diagnose and treat hyperaldosteronism—excessive aldosterone secretion in the adrenal gland. Aldactone may also be used for: congestive heart failure, cirrhosis of the liver, kidney disease, and unusually low potassium levels.

Dosage

 Take exactly as prescribed. Sudden discontinuance of this medication may worsen your condition. Must be taken on a regular basis to be effective.

 Usual adult dose: *for high blood pressure*—50 to 100 milligrams per day in a single dose or divided into smaller doses. *For congestive heart failure, cirrhosis, or kidney disorder*—100 milligrams daily in a single dose or divided into smaller doses. Doctor may prescribe as low as 25 milligrams per day or as high as 200 milligrams daily. *For potassium loss*—25 to 100 milligrams per day. *To detect hyperaldosteronism*—400 milligrams per day for 3 to 4 weeks, known as the long test. *Short test to detect hyperaldosteronism—400 milligrams per day for 4 days.*

 Usual child dose: 1.5 milligrams per pound of body weight daily in a single dose or divided into smaller doses.

 Missed dose: take as soon as possible, unless almost time for next dose. In that case, do not take missed dose; go back to regular schedule. *Do not double doses.*

Side Effects

 No specific information is available regarding Aldactone overdose. If you suspect an overdose, immediately seek medical attention.

 Side effects: abdominal cramps, breast development in males, change in potassium levels, deepening of voice, diarrhea, drowsiness, excessive hairiness, fever, headache, hives, irregular menstruation, lack of coordination, lethargy, mental confusion, postmenopausal bleeding, sexual dysfunction, skin eruptions, stomach bleeding, stomach inflammation, ulcers, vomiting.

 No known less common or rare side effects.

Interactions

 Use extreme caution if taking Vasotec or other ACE-inhibitor medications. Inform your doctor before combining Aldactone with: Digoxin (Lanoxin), Indomethacin (Indocin), Norepinephrine (Levophed), other diuretics such as Lasix and HydroDIURIL, other high blood pressure medications such as Aldomet and Procardia XL.

No known food/other substance interactions.

Special Cautions

 If pregnant or planning to become pregnant, inform your doctor immediately. Appears in breast milk; could affect a nursing infant.

 No special precautions apply to seniors.

 Follow doctor's instructions carefully for children.

 Should not be used if you have: difficulty urinating, high potassium levels in the blood, inability to urinate, or kidney disease.

Avoid use of potassium supplements or other diuretics, such as Maxzide.

Be careful not to lose too much water from the body; blood pressure lowers dramatically.

Before medical or dental surgery, tell your doctor or dentist you are taking this drug.

Use with caution if you have liver disease.

Kidney function should be monitored with Aldactone use.

Aldomet

Generic name: Methyldopa

Aldomet is an antihypertensive. It is thought to act on the central nervous system to prevent the release of chemicals responsible for maintaining high blood pressure.

℞ QUICK FACTS

Purpose

 Used to treat high blood pressure.

Dosage

 Take exactly as prescribed. Aldomet must be taken on a regular basis to be effective; try not to miss any doses. It may take several weeks before any benefit is observed.

 Usual adult dose: 250 milligrams 2 or 3 times per day in the first 48 hours of treatment. Maintenance dose is 500 milligrams per day divided into 2 to 4 doses. Maximum dose is usually 3 grams.

 Usual child dose: 10 milligrams per 2.2 pounds of body weight daily, divided into 2 to 4 doses, adjusted until blood pressure is normal. Maximum daily dose is 65 milligrams per 2.2 pounds of body weight or 3 grams, whichever is less.

 Missed dose: take as soon as possible, unless almost time for next dose. In that case, do not take missed dose; go back to regular schedule. *Do not double doses.*

Side Effects

 Overdose symptoms: bloating, constipation, diarrhea, dizziness, extreme drowsiness, gas, light-headedness, nausea, severely low blood pressure, slow heartbeat, vomiting, weakness. If you suspect an overdose, immediately seek medical attention.

More common side effects: drowsiness at beginning of therapy, fluid retention or weight gain, headache, weakness.

 Less common or rare side effects: anemia, Bell's palsy (paralysis of the face), bloating, blood disorders, breast development in males, breast enlargement, changes in menstruation, chest pain, congestive heart failure, constipation, decreased mental ability, decreased sex drive, depression, diarrhea, dizziness when standing up, dry mouth, fever, gas, hepatitis, impotence, inflammation of the large intestine, inflammation of the pancreas, inflammation of the salivary glands, involuntary movements, joint pain, light-headedness, liver disorders, milk production, muscle pain, nasal stuffiness, nausea, nightmares, parkinsonism (tremors, shuffling walk, stooped posture, muscle weakness), rash, slow heartbeat, sore or "black" tongue, tingling or pins and needles, vomiting, yellow eyes and skin.

Interactions

 Inform your doctor before combining Aldomet with: Dextroamphetamine (Dexedrine), Imipramine (Tofranil), Lithium (Lithonate), other high blood pressure drugs, Phenylpropanolamine (decongestant used in Comprex, Entex LA, and others), Propranolol (Inderal), Tolbutamide (Orinase).

 No known food/other substance interactions.

Special Cautions

 If pregnant or planning to become pregnant, inform your doctor immediately. Using Aldomet during pregnancy is relatively safe. Appears in breast milk; could affect a nursing infant.

Doctor will vary dosage levels according to individual needs.

 Follow doctor's instructions carefully for children.

🛑 *Do not take if you have liver disease or cirrhosis, or developed liver disease from taking Aldomet.*

May cause drowsiness and impair your ability to drive a car or operate machinery. *Do not take part in any activity that requires alertness.*

Should not take if sensitive to or had allergic reaction to Aldomet, or if taking oral suspension Aldomet and had an allergic reaction to sulfites.

Before starting Aldomet therapy, your doctor should monitor your liver function.

May develop fever, jaundice within first 2 to 3 months of Aldomet therapy. If this occurs, stop taking immediately, contact your doctor.

Extended use may cause hemolytic anemia, a blood disorder that destroys red blood cells.

May experience elevated blood pressure after dialysis treatments.

Before medical or dental surgery, tell your doctor or dentist you are taking this drug.

Aleve

see ANAPROX

Allopurinol

see ZYLOPRIM

Alprazolam

see XANAX

Altace

^^

Generic name: Ramipril

Altace is an angiotensin-converting enzyme (ACE) inhibitor. It prevents angiotensin I, a blood chemical, from developing into angiotensin II, a stronger form that increases salt and water levels in the body.

℞ QUICK FACTS

Purpose

℞ Used to treat high blood pressure.

Dosage

 Take on an empty stomach, 1 hour before or 2 hours after a meal. Must be taken on a regular basis to be effective. It may take several weeks before any benefit is observed.

· ·

 Usual adult dose: *for patients not on diuretics*—2.5 milligrams, taken once daily to start. After blood pressure under control, dosage ranges from 2.5 to 20 milligrams per day in a single dose or divided into 2 equal doses.

· ·

Usual child dose: not generally prescribed for children.

 Missed dose: take as soon as possible, unless almost time for next dose. In that case, do not take missed dose; go back to regular schedule. *Do not double doses.*

Side Effects

 Primary sign of overdose: sudden drop in blood pressure. If you suspect an overdose, immediately seek medical attention.

 More common side effects: cough, headache.

 Less common or rare side effects: abdominal pain, angina (chest pain), anxiety, arthritis, bruises, change in taste, constipation, convulsions, depression, diarrhea, difficulty swallowing, dizziness, dry mouth, fainting, fatigue, feeling of general discomfort, fluid retention, hearing loss, heart attack, impotence, inability to sleep, increased salivation, indigestion, inflammation of the stomach and intestines, irregular heartbeat, itching, joint pain or inflammation, labored breathing, light-headedness, loss of appetite, low blood pressure, memory loss, muscle pain, nausea, nerve pain, nervousness, nosebleed, rash, ringing in ears, skin inflammation, skin sensitivity to light, sleepiness, sudden loss of strength, sweating, tingling or pins and needles, tremors, vertigo, very rapid heartbeat, vision changes, vomiting, weakness, weight gain.

Interactions

 Inform your doctor before combining Altace with: diuretics such as Hydrochlorothiazide and furosemide (Lasix), Lithium, potassium-sparing diuretics (found in Dyazide, Maxzide, Moduretic, and others),

Spironolactone (Aldactone), potassium supplements such as K-lyte and K-Tab, potassium-containing salt substitutes.

 Alcohol may increase sedative effects; *do not drink alcohol when taking this medication.*

Special Cautions

 Altace may cause birth defects, premature birth, and fetal and newborn death. If pregnant or planning to become pregnant, inform your doctor immediately. May appear in breast milk; could affect a nursing infant.

6̄5 Doctor will vary dosage levels according to individual needs.

 Not generally prescribed for children.

 In the event of chest pain, palpitations, or other heart effects, swelling of the face around the lips, tongue, or throat or difficulty swallowing, difficulty breathing, swelling of arms and legs or infection, sore throat, and fever, immediately contact your doctor.

Do not use salt substitutes with potassium without consulting with your doctor.

Kidney function assessment should be performed, with continual monitoring when taking Altace.

Use with caution if you have: connective tissue disease such as lupus erythematosus or scleroderma; diabetes; or liver disease.

Light-headedness may appear during the first days of therapy. If fainting occurs, stop taking Altace and immediately contact your doctor.

Dehydration, excessive sweating, severe diarrhea, vomiting could reduce body fluids, or taking high doses of diuretics can cause blood pressure to drop to dangerously low levels.

Alupent

Generic name: Metaproterenol sulfate

Other brand name: Metaprel

Alupent is a bronchodilator. It acts directly on the muscles of the bronchi (breathing tubes) to relieve bronchospasm, thereby allowing air to move to and from the lungs.

℞ QUICK FACTS

Purpose

℞ Used to prevent and relieve bronchial asthma and bronchial spasms (wheezing) associated with bronchitis and emphysema. Inhalation solution also used to treat acute asthma attacks in children 6 years and older.

Dosage

 Take exactly as prescribed. *Do not exceed doctor's recommended dose; fatalities have occurred with excessive use.*

 Usual adult dose: *Inhalation Aerosol*—2 to 3 inhalations, no more than every 3 to 4 hours, not to exceed 12 inhalations per day. *Inhalation Solution*—2 to 3 inhalations, no more than every 4 hours. *Inhalation Solution 0.5%*—10 inhalations; single dose of 5 to 15 inhalations can be prescribed. Usual single dose is 0.3 milliliter diluted in approximately 2.5

milliliters of saline solution. Dosage range is 0.2 to 0.3 milliliter. Administered by oral inhalation using intermittent positive pressure breathing (IPPB) apparatus or hand-bulb nebulizer. *Inhalation Solution 0.4% and 0.6% Unit Dose Vials*—1 vial per treatment. *Syrup*—2 teaspoonfuls 3 or 4 times a day. *Tablets*—20 milligrams taken 3 or 4 times per day.

 Usual child dose: *Inhalation Aerosol*—not recommended for children under 12 years. *Inhalation Solution*—not recommended for children under 12 years. *Syrup*—*For children 6 to 9 years or weighing under 60 pounds*—1 teaspoonful, 3 or 4 times a day. *For children over 9 years or weighing over 60 pounds*—2 teaspoonfuls, 3 or 4 times a day. *For children under 6 years*—1.3 to 2.6 milligrams per 2.2 pounds of body weight is usually tolerated well, although use in this age group is limited. *Tablets*—*For children 6 to 9 years or weighing under 60 pounds*—10 milligrams taken 3 or 4 times a day. *For children over 9 years or weighing over 60 pounds*—20 milligrams taken 3 or 4 times a day. *For children under 6 years, not recommended.*

 Missed dose: take as soon as possible. Take any remaining doses for the day at equal intervals thereafter. *Do not increase the total for the day; do not double doses.*

Side Effects

 Overdose symptoms: dizziness, dry mouth, fatigue, general feeling of bodily discomfort, headache, high or low blood pressure, inability to fall or stay asleep, irregular heartbeat, nausea, nervousness, rapid or strong heartbeat, severe or suffocating chest pain, tremors. If you suspect an overdose, immediately seek medical attention.

Side effects: cough, dizziness, exaggerated asthma symptoms, headache, high blood pressure, increased heart rate, nausea, nervousness, rapid or strong heartbeat, stomach upset, throat irritation, tremors, vomiting. Sometimes the container itself causes side effects; replacing container may solve problem.

 No known less common or rare side effects.

Interactions

 Do not use other inhaled medications with Alupent before checking with your doctor. Inform your doctor before combining Alupent with: MAO inhibitors (antidepressant drugs such as Nardil and Parnate), other beta-adrenergic aerosol bronchodilators such as Ventolin and Proventil, tricyclic antidepressants such as Elavil.

 No known food/other substance interactions.

Special Cautions

 If pregnant or planning to become pregnant, inform your doctor immediately. Not known if Alupent appears in breast milk.

 No special precautions apply to seniors.

 Follow doctor's instructions carefully for children.

 Do not take if you have an irregular, rapid heart rate.

If dose worsens or does not improve symptoms, immediately contact your doctor.

If sensitive to Alupent or other similar drugs, you should not use this medication.

. . . .

Check with your doctor if you have: diabetes mellitus, heart or convulsive disorder (epilepsy), high blood pressure or hyperthyroidism.

Alzapam

see ATIVAN

Ambien

Generic name: Zolpidem tartrate

Ambien is a sedative. It works to reduce the activity of certain chemicals in the brain. It is a relatively new drug, and is chemically different from Halcion and Dalmane.

℞ QUICK FACTS

Purpose

℞   Used to treat insomnia on a short-term basis.

Dosage

   Take before bed, exactly as prescribed by your doctor. If used every night for several weeks, medication loses its effectiveness. May cause dependency if used for a long time or in high doses.

. . . .

   Usual adult dose: 10 milligrams before bedtime, not to exceed 10 milligrams per day. Smaller doses may be prescribed if sensitive to medication. Seniors—5 milligrams before bedtime.

. . . .

Usual child dose: not generally prescribed for children.

 Missed dose: take only as needed. *Do not double doses.*

Side Effects

 Overdose symptoms: excessive sleepiness or even light coma. If you suspect an overdose, immediately seek medical attention. Symptoms more severe if taking other drugs that depress central nervous system; *multiple overdose has been fatal.*

 More common side effects: abdominal pain, abnormal vision, allergy, back pain, confusion, constipation, daytime drowsiness, depression, dizziness, double vision, drugged feeling, dry mouth, exaggerated feeling of well-being, flu-like symptoms, headache, indigestion, inflammation of the throat, insomnia, joint pain, lack of muscle coordination, lethargy, lightheadedness, nausea, rash, sinus inflammation, throbbing heartbeat, upper respiratory infection, urinary tract infection, vertigo.

 Less common side effects: abnormal dreams, agitation, amnesia, anxiety, arthritis, bronchitis, burning sensation, chest pain, constipation, coughing, daytime sleeping, decreased mental alertness, diarrhea, difficulty breathing, difficulty concentrating, difficulty swallowing, diminished sensitivity to touch, dizziness on standing, emotional instability, eye irritation, falling, fatigue, fever, gas, general discomfort, hallucination, hiccups, high blood pressure, high blood sugar, increased sweating, infection, lack of bladder control, loss of appetite, menstrual disorder, migraine, muscle pain, nasal inflammation, nervousness, numbness, paleness, prickling or tingling sensation, rapid heartbeat, ringing in the ears, sleep disorder, speech difficulties, swelling due to fluid retention, taste abnormalities, tremor, unconsciousness, vomiting, weakness. Rare side effects: abnormal tears or tearing, abscess, acne, aggravation of allergies, aggravation of high blood pressure, aggression, allergic reaction, altered production of saliva, anemia, belching, blisters, blood clot in lung, boils, breast pain, breast problems, breast tumors, bruising, chill with high temperature (followed by heat and perspiration), decreased sex drive, delusion, difficulties with blood circulation, difficulty urinating, excess hemoglobin in the blood, excessive urine production, eye pain, facial swelling due to fluid retention, fainting, false perceptions, feeling intoxicated, feeling strange, flushing, frequent urination, glaucoma, gout, heart attack, hemorrhoids, herpes infection, high cholesterol, hives, hot flashes, impotence, inability to urinate, increased appetite, increased tolerance to the drug, intestinal blockage, irregular heartbeat, joint degeneration, kidney failure, kidney pain, laryngitis, leg cramps, loss of reality, low blood pressure, mental deterioration, muscle spasms in arms and legs, muscle weakness, nosebleed, pain, painful urination, panic attacks, paralysis, pneumonia, rectal bleeding, rigidity, sciatica (lower back pain), sensation of seeing flashes of light or sparks, sensitivity to light, sleepwalking, speech difficulties, swelling of the eye, thinking abnormalities, thirst, tooth decay, uncontrolled leg movements, urge to go the bathroom, varicose veins, weight loss, yawning.

Interactions

Inform your doctor before combining Ambien with: the major tranquilizer Chlorpromazine (Thorazine); antidepressants such as Tofranil; other drugs that depress the central nervous system, including Valium, Percocet, and Benadryl.

Do not drink alcohol; can increase the side effects of this medication.

Special Cautions

 If pregnant or planning to become pregnant, inform your doctor immediately. Babies may have withdrawal symptoms after birth and may seem limp and flaccid. Not recommended for use by nursing mothers.

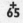 Seniors generally prescribed lower dosage levels.

 Not generally prescribed for children.

 Initially, may cause drowsiness and impair your ability to drive a car or operate machinery. *Do not take part in any activity that requires alertness.*

Immediately contact your doctor if you notice unusual changes in your thinking and/or behavior.

Can cause memory loss, avoid taking on overnight plane flights of less than 7 to 8 hours; "traveler's amnesia" may occur.

Use with caution if you have kidney disease.

Consult with your doctor before stopping if taking Ambien for more than 1 to 2 weeks. May cause withdrawal symptoms ranging from unpleasant feelings to vomiting and cramps.

Amcinonide

see CYCLOCORT

Amen
see PROVERA

Amiloride with Hydrochlorothiazide
see MODURETIC

Amitriptyline
see ELAVIL

Amitriptyline Hydrochloride with Perphenazine
see TRIAVIL

Amlodipine Besylate
see NORVASC

Amoxicillin
see AMOXIL

Amoxicillin with Clavulanate Potassium

see AUGMENTIN

Amoxil

Generic name: Amoxicillin

Other brand names: Amoxil Chewables, Biomox, Polymox, Trimox, Wymox

Amoxil is an antibiotic. It is used to prevent bacteria from multiplying and growing.

℞ QUICK FACTS

Purpose

℞ Used to treat infections, including: gonorrhea, middle ear, skin, upper and lower respiratory tract, genital and urinary tract.

Dosage

 To prevent stomach upset, may take with or without food. If using suspension, shake well before using. Take Amoxil for the entire amount of time your doctor has prescribed, especially with strep throat infections.

. . . .

 Usual adult dose: *for ear, nose, throat, skin, genital and urinary tract infections*—250 milligrams taken every 8 hours. *For infections of lower respiratory tract*—500 milligrams taken every 8 hours. *For gonorrhea*—3 grams in a single oral dose. *For gonococcal infections such as acute, uncomplicated anogenital and urethral infections*—3 grams as a single oral dose.

. . . .

Usual child dose: *for children weighing 44 pounds and over*—follow the recommended adult dose schedule. *For children weighing under 44 pounds*—dosage is determined by their weight. *Dosage of pediatric drops*—use dropper provided with medication to measure all doses. *For all infections except lower respiratory tract*—under 13 pounds: 0.75 milliliter every 8 hours; 13 to 15 pounds: 1 milliliter every 8 hours; 16 to 18 pounds: 1.25 milliliters every 8 hours. *For infections of the lower respiratory tract*—under 13 pounds: 1.25 milliliters every 8 hours; 13 to 15 pounds: 1.75 milliliters every 8 hours; 16 to 18 pounds: 2.25 milliliters every 8 hours. *Children weighing over 18 pounds*—should take oral liquid. Place suspension directly on tongue for swallowing. Can be added to formula, milk, fruit juice, water, ginger ale, or cold drinks. Take preparation immediately, and make sure entire preparation is taken.

 Missed dose: take as soon as possible. If almost time for next dose, and taking 2 doses a day, take missed dose, then next dose in 5 to 6 hours. If taking 3 or more doses a day, take missed dose, then next dose in 2 to 4 hours. Then go back to regular schedule. *Do not double doses.*

Side Effects

 Overdose symptoms: diarrhea, nausea, stomach cramps, vomiting. If you suspect an overdose, immediately seek medical attention.

 Side effects: agitation, anemia, anxiety, changes in behavior, confusion, diarrhea, dizziness, heartburn, hives, hyperactivity, insomnia, nausea, rash, vomiting.

 No known less common or rare side effects.

Interactions

 Inform your doctor before combining Amoxil with: Allopurinol (Lopurin), Chloramphenicol (Chloromycetin), Erythromycin (E.E.S., PCE, others), oral contraceptives, Probenecid (Benemid), Tetracycline (Achromycin V and others).

 No known food/other substance interactions.

Special Cautions

 If pregnant or planning to become pregnant, inform your doctor immediately. May appear in breast milk; could affect a nursing infant.

 Seniors should use with caution.

 Follow doctor's instructions carefully for children.

 Do not use if you are allergic to penicillin or cephalosporin antibiotics.

Stop using if you experience: bruising, fever, skin rash, itching, joint pain, swollen lymph nodes, or sores on the genitals, unless your doctor advises you to continue.

Consult with doctor if you have had: asthma, hives, hay fever, or other allergies, colitis, diabetes, kidney or liver disease.

If diabetic, may cause false positive urine glucose test results.

Ampicillin

see OMNIPEN

Anafranil

vvvvvvvvvvvvvvvvvvvvvvvvvvvvvvvvvvvvvvvvvvvvvvv

Generic name: Clomipramine hydrochloride

Anafranil is a tricyclic antidepressant. It blocks the movement of certain stimulant chemicals in and out of nerve endings.

℞ QUICK FACTS

Purpose

℞   Used to treat obsessive and compulsive disorders.

Dosage

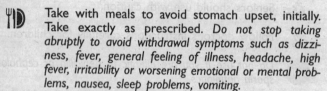 Take with meals to avoid stomach upset, initially. Take exactly as prescribed. *Do not stop taking abruptly to avoid withdrawal symptoms such as dizziness, fever, general feeling of illness, headache, high fever, irritability or worsening emotional or mental problems, nausea, sleep problems, vomiting.*

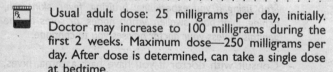 Usual adult dose: 25 milligrams per day, initially. Doctor may increase to 100 milligrams during the first 2 weeks. Maximum dose—250 milligrams per day. After dose is determined, can take a single dose at bedtime.

 Usual child dose: 25 milligrams per day, divided into smaller doses and taken with meals. Doctor may increase to maximum of 100 milligrams or 3 milligrams per 2.2 pounds of body weight per day, whichever is smaller. Maximum dose—200 milligrams or 3 milligrams per 2.2 pounds of body weight, whichever is smaller. Once dose is determined, can be taken in a single dose at bedtime.

Missed dose: if you take 1 dose at bedtime, consult your doctor. *Do not take missed dose in the morning.* If you take 2 or more doses per day, take missed dose as soon as possible, unless almost time for next dose. In that case, do not take missed dose; go back to regular schedule. *Do not double doses.*

Side Effects

Overdose symptoms: early signs—agitation, coma, convulsions, delirium, drowsiness, grimacing, exaggerated reflexes, loss of coordination, restlessness, rigid muscles, staggering gait, stupor, sweating, twitching, writhing. Other signs—bluish skin color, dilated pupils, excessive perspiration, fever, irregular heartbeat, little or no urine, low blood pressure, rapid heartbeat, shallow breathing, shock, vomiting. If you suspect an overdose, immediately seek medical attention. *Overdose can be fatal.*

More common side effects: abdominal pain, abnormal dreaming, abnormal milk secretion, abnormal tearing, agitation, allergy, anxiety, appetite loss, back pain, chest pain, confusion, constipation, coughing, depression, diarrhea, dizziness, dry mouth, extreme sleepiness, failure to ejaculate, fast heartbeat, fatigue, fever, flushing, fluttery heartbeat, frequent urination, gas, headache, hot flushes, impotence, inability to concentrate, increased appetite, increased sweating, indigestion, inflamed lining of the nose or sinuses, itching, joint pain, light-headedness upon standing up, memory problems, menstrual pain and disorders, middle ear infection (children), migraine, muscle pain or tension, nausea, nervousness, pain, rash, red or purple areas on the skin, ringing in the ears, sex-drive changes, sleeplessness, sleep disturbances, taste changes, tingling or pins and needles, tooth disorder, tremor, twitching, urinary problems, urinary tract infection, vision problems, vomiting, weight gain, weight loss (children), yawning.

 Less common side effects: abnormal skin odor (children), acne, aggression (children), eye allergy (children), anemia (children), bad breath (children), belching (children), breast enlargement, breast pain, chills, conjunctivitis (pinkeye), difficult or labored breathing (children), difficulty swallowing, difficulty or pain in urinating, dilated pupils, dry skin, emotional instability, eye twitching (children), fainting (children), hearing disorder (children), hives, irritability, lack of menstruation, loss of sense of identity, mouth inflammation (children), muscle weakness, nosebleed, panic, paralysis (children), skin inflammation, sore throat (children), stomach and intestinal problems, swelling due to fluid retention, thirst, unequal size of pupils of the eye (children), vaginal inflammation, weakness (children), wheezing, white or yellow vaginal discharge.

Interactions

Never take with antidepressant (MAO inhibitors) such as Nardil or Parnate; can cause serious, even fatal reactions. Inform your doctor before combining Anafranil with: antispasmodic drugs such as Donnatal, Cogentin, and Bentyl; barbiturates such as Phenobarbital; certain blood pressure drugs such as Ismelin and Catapres-TTS; Cimetidine (Tagamet); Digoxin (Lanoxin); Fluoxetine (Prozac); Haloperidol (Haldol); Methylphenidate (Ritalin); major tranquilizers such as Thorazine; Phenytoin (Dilantin); thyroid medications such as Synthroid; tranquilizers such as Xanax and Valium; Warfarin (Coumadin).

 Avoid alcohol while taking Anafranil.

Special Cautions

 If pregnant or planning to become pregnant, inform your doctor immediately. Should not be used during pregnancy unless absolutely necessary; babies born to women taking Anafranil sometimes experience withdrawal symptoms such as jitteriness, tremors, and seizure. Appears in breast milk; could affect a nursing infant.

 No special precautions apply to seniors.

 Follow doctor's instructions carefully for children.

 Can worsen narrow-angle glaucoma or urination difficulties.

Use with caution if you have: kidney function that is not normal; recently had a heart attack; tumor of the adrenal gland.

May cause skin sensitivity to sunlight.

Inform your doctor or dentist before surgery involving anesthesia.

May cause seizure; take special precautions operating machinery or driving a car. Risk of seizure increased by: history of alcoholism, brain damage, seizure, or if taking a medication that might cause seizures.

Anaprox

∿∿∿

Generic name: Naproxen sodium

Other brand names: Aleve, Anaprox DS, Naprosyn

Anaprox is a nonsteroidal anti-inflammatory drug (NSAID). It works by blocking the production of prostaglandins, which may trigger pain.

℞ QUICK FACTS

Purpose

Used to relieve mild to moderate pain and menstrual cramps. Also used to treat inflammation, swelling, stiffness, and joint pain associated with rheumatoid arthritis, osteoarthritis, juvenile arthritis, spinal arthritis, tendinitis, bursitis, and acute gout.

Dosage

May take with food to avoid stomach upset.

Usual adult dose: *for mild to moderate pain, menstrual cramps, acute tendinitis and bursitis*—550 milligrams every 6 to 8 hours, followed by 275 milligrams not to exceed 1,375 milligrams per day. *For rheumatoid arthritis, osteoarthritis, and spinal arthritis*—275 milligrams or 550 milligrams 2 times a day (morning and evening). *For acute gout*—825 milligrams, followed by 275 milligrams every 8 hours until symptoms subside. *For seniors*—your doctor may make adjustments to the usual adult dose based on your particular needs.

Usual child dose: *for juvenile arthritis*—a total of 10 milligrams per 2.2 pounds of body weight, divided into 2 doses, not to exceed 15 milligrams per 2.2 pounds per day.

 Missed dose: take as soon as possible, unless almost time for next dose. In that case, do not take missed dose; go back to regular schedule. *Do not double doses.*

Side Effects

 Overdose symptoms: agitation, change in pupil size, coma, disorientation, dizziness, double vision, drowsiness, headache, nausea, semiconsciousness, shallow breathing, stomach pain. If you suspect an overdose, immediately seek medical attention.

 More common side effects: abdominal pain, bruising, constipation, diarrhea, difficult or labored breathing, dizziness, drowsiness, headache, hearing changes, heartburn, indigestion, inflammation of the mouth, itching, light-headedness, nausea, rapid or fluttery heartbeat, red or purple spots on the skin, ringing in the ears, skin eruptions, sweating, swelling due to fluid retention, thirst, vertigo, vision changes.

 Less common or rare side effects: abdominal bleeding, black stools, blood in the urine, change in dream patterns, changes in hearing, chills and fever, colitis, congestive heart failure, depression, general feeling of illness, hair loss, inability to concentrate, inability to sleep, inflammation of the lungs, kidney disease or failure, menstrual problems, muscle weakness and/or pain, peptic ulcer, severe allergic reactions, skin inflammation due to sensitivity to light, skin rashes, vomiting, vomiting blood, yellow skin and eyes.

Interactions

Inform your doctor before combining Anaprox with: antiseizure drugs such as Dilantin; Aspirin; beta-blockers such as Inderal; blood thinners such as Coumadin; Lithium (Lithonate); loop diuretics such as Lasix; Methotrexate; Naproxen in other forms such as Naprosyn; oral diabetes drugs such as Micronase; Probenecid (Benemid).

Tell your doctor if you are on a low sodium diet; Anaprox contains sodium.

Special Cautions

If pregnant or planning to become pregnant, inform your doctor immediately. Appears in breast milk; could affect a nursing infant.

Doctor may make adjustments to dosage for seniors.

Follow doctor's instructions carefully for children.

May cause drowsiness and impair your ability to drive a car or operate machinery. *Do not take part in any activity that requires alertness.*

You should not take Anaprox if you have had any allergic reactions to: Anaprox, Aspirin, Motrin, or similar drugs, or if you have had asthma attacks caused by Aspirin or similar medications.

Ulcers or internal bleeding can occur without warning.

Use with caution if you have: heart disease, high blood pressure, or kidney or liver disease.

May cause vision problems or changes in vision; monitor closely, and report any changes to your doctor.

Ansaid

^^

Generic name: Flurbiprofen

Ansaid is a nonsteroidal anti-inflammatory drug (NSAID). It works by blocking the production of prostaglandins, which may trigger pain.

℞ QUICK FACTS

Purpose

℞ Used to treat the inflammation, swelling, stiffness and joint pain caused by rheumatoid arthritis and osteoarthritis.

Dosage

 Doctor may suggest taking with food or an antacid. Take exactly as prescribed.

 Usual adult dose: a total of 200 to 300 milligrams per day, divided into 2, 3, or 4 smaller doses, not to exceed 100 milligrams at any one time or 300 milligrams per day.

 Usual child dose: not generally prescribed for children.

 Missed dose: take as soon as possible, unless almost time for next dose. In that case, do not take missed dose; go back to regular schedule. *Do not double doses.*

Side Effects

 Overdose symptoms: agitation, change in pupil size, coma, disorientation, dizziness, double vision, drowsiness, headache, nausea, semiconsciousness, shallow breathing, stomach pain. If you suspect an overdose, immediately seek medical attention.

 More common side effects: abdominal bleeding, abdominal pain, anxiety, constipation, depression, diarrhea, dizziness, gas, general feeling of illness, headache, inflammation of the nose, indigestion, loss of memory, nausea, nervousness, rash, ringing in ears, sleepiness, swelling due to fluid retention, tremors, trouble sleeping, urinary tract infection, vision changes, vomiting, weakness, weight changes.

 Less common or rare side effects: altered sense of smell, anemia, asthma, blood in the urine, bloody diarrhea, bruising, chills and fever, confusion, conjunctivitis (pinkeye), heart failure, hepatitis, high blood pressure, hives, inflammation of the mouth and tongue, inflammation of the stomach, itching, kidney failure, lack of coordination, nosebleed, peptic ulcer, pins and needles, sensitivity of skin to light, severe allergic reaction, skin inflammation with or without sores and crusting, swelling of throat, twitching, vomiting blood, welts, yellow eyes and skin.

Interactions

 Inform your doctor before combining Ansaid with: Aspirin; beta-blockers such as Inderal and Tenormin; blood thinners such as Coumadin; Cimetidine (Tagamet); diuretics such as Lasix and Bumex; Methotrexate; oral diabetes drugs such as Micronase.

 No known food/other substance interactions.

Special Cautions

 If pregnant or planning to become pregnant, inform your doctor immediately. Appears in breast milk; could affect a nursing infant.

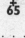 Seniors are most likely to develop kidney problems while taking this drug.

 Not generally prescribed for children.

 You should not take if you have had any allergic reactions to: Ansaid, Aspirin, Motrin, or similar drugs, or if you have had asthma attacks caused by Aspirin or similar medications.

Ulcers or internal bleeding can occur without warning.

Use with caution if you have heart disease, high blood pressure, kidney or liver disease, or if you are taking blood-thinning medication.

May cause vision problems; blurred and/or decreased vision has been observed when taking this medication.

Discuss the risks of using this drug for pain less serious than arthritis.

Antipyrine with Benzocaine and Glycerin
see AURALGAN

Antivert

~~~~~~

Generic name: Meclizine hydrochloride

Other brand names: Antrizine, Bonine, Dizmiss, Motion Cure, Ru-Vert-M, Wehvert

Antivert is an antihistamine/ anti-emetic. The antihistamine/ anti-emetic combination depresses middle-ear function.

℞ QUICK FACTS

Purpose

Used to treat nausea, vomiting, and dizziness from motion sickness. Also used to treat vertigo.

Dosage

Take exactly as prescribed.

Usual adult dose: *for motion sickness*—take 25 to 50 milligrams 1 hour prior to travel. May repeat dose every 24 hours for the duration of the travel. *For vertigo*—25 to 100 milligrams per day, divided into equal, smaller doses by your doctor.

Usual child dose: not generally prescribed for children under 12 years.

Missed dose: take as soon as possible, unless almost time for next dose. In that case, do not take missed dose, go back to regular schedule. *Do not double doses.*

Side Effects

No specific information is available regarding Antivert overdose. If you suspect an overdose, immediately seek medical attention.

More common side effects: drowsiness, dry mouth.

 Less common or rare side effect: blurred vision.

Interactions

 No known drug interactions.

 Do not combine alcohol with this medication; may intensify the effects of alcohol.

Special Cautions

 If pregnant or planning to become pregnant, inform your doctor. Not known if Antivert appears in breast milk.

 No special precautions apply to seniors.

 Not generally prescribed for children under 12 years.

 May cause drowsiness and impair your ability to drive a car or operate machinery. *Do not take part in any activity that requires alertness.*

Do not take Antivert if you have sensitivity to it or similar drugs. Inform your doctor of any reactions.

Check with your doctor before taking Antivert if you have asthma, glaucoma, or an enlarged prostate gland.

Antrizine

see ANTIVERT

Anusol-HC

∿∿∿∿∿∿∿∿∿∿∿∿∿∿∿∿∿∿∿∿∿∿∿∿∿∿∿∿∿∿∿∿∿∿∿

Generic name: Hydrocortisone

Other brand names: Alacort, Caldecort Light, Cortaid, Dermacort, Hytone, Lanacort, Penecort

Anusol-HC is a topical corticosteroid. It is unknown how it relieves inflammation.

℞ QUICK FACTS

Purpose

℞   Used to treat certain itchy rashes and other inflammatory skin conditions.

Dosage

    Use exactly as directed, and only for the condition for which it is prescribed. Use only on the skin, topically; keep away from eyes. Avoid using large amounts over extensive areas to prevent overabsorption.

    Usual adult dose: apply to affected area 2 to 4 times per day, depending on the severity. Doctor may advise using a bandage or covering over affected area for psoriasis or difficult conditions; remove bandage if infection occurs.

    Usual child dose: apply the least amount necessary, as directed by your doctor.

    Missed dose: apply as soon as possible, unless almost time for next dose. In that case, do not take missed dose; go back to regular schedule.

Side Effects

 Overdose symptoms: extensive or long-term use can cause Cushing's syndrome, glandular problems, higher than normal amounts of sugar in the blood, or high amounts of sugar in the urine. If you suspect an overdose, immediately seek medical attention.

 Side effects: acne-like skin eruptions, burning, dryness, growth of excessive hair, inflammation of the hair follicles, inflammation around the mouth, irritation, itching, peeling skin, prickly heat, secondary infection, skin inflammation, skin softening, stretch marks, unusual lack of skin color.

 No known less common or rare side effects.

Interactions

 No drug interactions reported.

 No known food/other substance interactions.

Special Cautions

 If pregnant or planning to become pregnant, inform your doctor. Not known if Anusol-HC appears in breast milk in sufficient amounts to harm nursing infant.

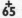 No special precautions apply to seniors.

 Children are particularly susceptible to overabsorption of hormone from Anusol-HC. Avoid covering treated area with waterproof diapers or plastic pants. Long-term use may interfere with growth and development.

Do not use if you have had an allergic reaction to Anusol-HC or any of its ingredients.

If irritation develops, stop using.

Anxanil

see ATARAX

Armour Thyroid

Generic name: Natural thyroid hormone

Other brand names: S-P-T, Thyrar, Thyroid Strong

Armour Thyroid is a thyroid hormone replacement. Hormones stimulate and regulate body functions.

℞ QUICK FACTS

Purpose

℞   Used to treat a thyroid gland incapable of producing enough hormone. Also used to treat or prevent goiter, and to diagnose an overactive thyroid in a suppression test.

Dosage

    Take exactly as prescribed, and at the same time each day. *Do not change brands without consulting your doctor.*

Usual adult dose: no usual dose, dose depends on how much thyroid hormone your body produces. *For an underactive thyroid gland*—may need to take medication indefinitely.

 Usual child dose: not generally prescribed for children.

 Missed dose: take as soon as possible, unless almost time for next dose. In that case, do not take missed dose; go back to regular schedule. *Do not double doses. Two or more missed doses in a row*—call your doctor. Dose may be adjusted if you have diabetes or underactive adrenal glands.

Side Effects

 Overdose symptoms: speeding up of all of the body's vital processes, causing physical and mental hyperactivity, increased appetite, excessive sweating, chest pain, increased pulse rate, palpitations, nervousness, intolerance to heat, tremors, rapid heartbeat. If you suspect an overdose, immediately seek medical attention.

 Side effects are rare when Armour Thyroid is taken exactly as prescribed. Taking too much or increasing dose too quickly may result in overstimulation of the thyroid gland. Symptoms of overstimulation: changes in appetite, diarrhea, fever, headache, increased heart rate, irritability, nausea, nervousness, sleeplessness, sweating, weight loss.

 No known less common or rare side effects.

Interactions

 Inform your doctor before combining Armour Thyroid with: asthma medications such as Theo-Dur; blood thinners such as Coumadin; Cholestyramine

(Questran); Colestipol (Colestid); Estrogen preparations, including birth control pills such as Ortho-Novum and Premarin; Insulin; oral diabetes medications such as Diabinese and Glucotrol.

No known food/other substance interactions.

Special Cautions

If pregnant or planning to become pregnant, inform your doctor. May use for thyroid deficiency during pregnancy with regular testing and medication adjustments by your doctor. May breastfeed while continuing treatment.

Seniors with angina (chest pain) should be prescribed a lower dose, and have regular checkups with your doctor.

Children may experience initial, temporary loss of hair when taking Armour Thyroid.

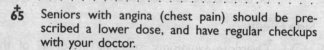

Not effective as a weight-loss medication and should not be used for that purpose. May cause severe side effects, especially if combined with appetite suppressants.

Should not take if you have or had: allergic reaction to this mediation, an overactive thyroid gland, or if your adrenal glands are not producing enough corticosteroid hormone.

Aggravates symptoms of diabetes.

Artane

Generic name: Trihexyphenidyl hydrochloride

Artane is an antiparkinsonism agent. It works by balancing certain chemicals in the brain.

℞ QUICK FACTS

Purpose

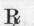

Used in conjunction with other drugs to treat certain symptoms of Parkinson's disease, a brain disorder that causes muscle tremor, stiffness, and weakness. Also used to control certain side effects induced by antipsychotic drugs such as Thorazine and Haldol.

Dosage

Take before or after meals, whichever is convenient. Take exactly as prescribe;, taking larger amounts can lead to overdose.

Usual adult dose: *for Parkinson's disease*—1 milligram on the first day, in tablet or liquid form. After first day, doctor may increase dose incrementally by 2 milligrams every 3 to 5 days, up to 6 to 10 milligrams per day. *For drug-induced parkinsonism*—ranges from 5 to 15 milligrams. *For use with Levodopa*—3 to 6 milligrams per day, divided into equal doses. *For tablets and liquid*—best if divided into 3 doses and taken at mealtimes. If taking high doses (more than 10 milligrams daily), doctor may divide into 4 parts. Once dosage level is stabilized, your doctor may switch you to sustained-release capsules, which are taken once or twice a day, swallowed whole.

Usual child dose: not generally prescribed for children.

 Missed dose: take as soon as possible, unless almost time for next dose. In that case, do not take missed dose; go back to regular schedule. *Do not double doses.*

Side Effects

 Overdose symptoms: clumsiness or unsteadiness, fast heartbeat, flushing of skin, seizures, severe drowsiness, shortness of breath or troubled breathing, trouble sleeping, unusual warmth. If you suspect an overdose, immediately seek medical attention.

 Common side effects: blurred vision, dry mouth, nausea, nervousness.

 Less common side effects: agitation, bowel obstruction, confusion, constipation, delusions, difficulty urinating, dilated pupils, disturbed behavior, drowsiness, hallucinations, headache, pressure in the eye, rapid heartbeat, rash, vomiting, weakness.

Interactions

 Inform your doctor before combining Artane with: Amantadine (Symmetral), Amitriptyline (Elavil), Chlorpromazine (Thorazine), Doxepine (Sinequan), Haloperidol (Haldol).

 No known food/other substance interactions.

Special Cautions

 If pregnant or planning to become pregnant, inform your doctor immediately. No information available about the effects of Artane during pregnancy or breastfeeding.

🕇 Seniors have high sensitivity to Artane; use with caution. If over 60, your doctor will individualize the dosage to your needs.

Not generally prescribed for children.

STOP Can impair the body's ability to perspire; avoid excessive sun or exercise that causes the body to overheat.

Tell your doctor if you have: enlarged prostate; glaucoma; heart, kidney, or liver disease; stomach/intestinal obstructive disease; or urinary tract obstructive disease.

Your doctor should check eyes frequently and watch for any allergic reactions while you take Artane.

Aspirin

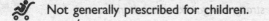

Generic name: Aspirin

Other brand names: A.S.A., Ascriptin, Bayer, Bufferin, Ecotrin, Empirin, Measurin, Norwich, Zorprin

Aspirin is an analgesic and anti-inflammatory agent. It reduces pain and inflammation.

℞ QUICK FACTS

Purpose

℞ Used to treat mild to moderate pain, fever, and inflammatory conditions such as rheumatoid arthritis. Has been shown to reduce the risk of small strokes and heart attacks in men with chest pain. Also temporarily relieves muscle aches, colds, flu, and menstrual discomfort.

Dosage

 Do not take more than the recommended dose. If it has a strong, vinegar-like odor, do not use.

 Usual adult dose: *for treatment of minor pain and fever*—1 or 2 tablets every 3 to 4 hours, up to 6 times per day. *For stroke prevention*—1 tablet 4 times per day or 2 tablets 2 times per day. *For heart attack prevention*—1 tablet daily. Your doctor may prescribe a higher dose.

 Usual child dose: consult your doctor before administering Aspirin to children.

 Missed dose: take as soon as possible, unless almost time for next dose. If so, skip missed dose; go back to regular schedule. *Do not double doses.*

Side Effects

 Overdose symptoms: nausea, neurologic abnormalities (coma, disorientation, seizures), vomiting. If you suspect an overdose, immediately seek medical attention.

 Side effects: bloody or tarry stools, dehydration, hyperactivity, hyperthermia, hyperventilation, heartburn, nausea and/or vomiting, possible involvement of stomach ulcers and bleeding, stomach pain, stomach upset.

 Less common side effects: loss of hearing or ringing in the ears, confusion, difficult or painful urination, difficulty in breathing, skin rash, unusual weakness.

Interactions

 Inform your doctor before combining Aspirin with: Acetazolamide (Diamox); ACE-inhibitor–type blood pressure medications such as Capoten; antigout medications such as Zyloprim; arthritis medications such as Motrin and Indocin; blood thinners such as Coumadin; certain diuretics such as Lasix; diabetes medications such as DiaBeta and Micronase; Diltiazem (Cardizem); Dipyridamole (Persantine); Insulin; seizure medications such as Depakene; steroids such as Prednisone.

 No known food/other substance interactions.

Special Cautions

 Do not use during last 3 months of pregnancy, unless specifically prescribed by a doctor. May cause problems in the fetus and complications during delivery. May appear in breast milk, could affect a nursing infant.

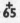 No special precautions apply to seniors.

 Consult your doctor before administering to children.

 Should not be given to children or teenagers for flu symptoms or chicken pox. Aspirin is associated with development of Reye's syndrome, a rare, life-threatening disorder.

Discontinue and call a doctor if you experience a continuous or high fever, severe or persistent sore throat, especially with a high fever, vomiting, and nausea.

Tell your doctor before taking Aspirin if you have or had: asthma, bleeding disorders, congestive heart failure, diabetes, glucose-6-phosphate dehydrogenase (G6PD) deficiency, gout, hemophilia, high blood pressure, kidney disease, liver disease, nasal polyps, peptic ulcers, or thyroid disease.

. . . .

Large doses may cause erroneous urine glucose test results.

Aspirin with Codeine

see EMPIRIN WITH CODEINE

Astemizole

see HISMANAL

Atarax

Generic name: Hydroxyzine hydrochloride

Other brand names: Anxanil, Vistaril

Atarax is an antihistamine. It works by blocking the effects of histamine, a body chemical that typically causes swelling and itching.

℞ QUICK FACTS

Purpose

℞ Used to treat common anxiety and tension, and in combination with other medications to treat anxiety resulting from physical illness. Also used to treat itching from allergic reactions, and as a sedative before and after general anesthesia.

. . . .

Dosage

 Take exactly as prescribed. Treatment that begins with injections can be continued in tablet form. Not intended for long-term use—no more than 4 months. If taking narcotics, non-narcotic analgesics, or barbiturates with Atarax, their dosage should be reduced.

 Usual adult dose: *for anxiety and tension*—50 to 100 milligrams 4 times per day. *For itching from allergies*— 25 milligrams, 3 or 4 times per day. *Before and after general anesthesia*—50 to 100 milligrams.

 Usual child dose—*For anxiety and tension under age 6*—50 milligrams per day total, divided into several smaller doses; *for anxiety and tension over age 6*— 50 to 100 milligrams per day, divided into smaller doses. *For itching from allergies under age 6*—50 milligrams per day total, divided into several smaller doses; *for itching from allergies over age 6*—50 to 100 milligrams per day, divided into several smaller doses. *Before and after general anesthesia*—0.6 milligrams per 2.2 pounds of body weight.

 Missed dose: take as soon as possible, unless almost time for next dose. If so, skip missed dose; go back to regular schedule. *Do not double doses.*

Side Effects

 Overdose symptoms: most common is oversedation; drop in blood pressure, although rare, is another symptom. If you suspect an overdose, immediately seek medical attention.

 Most common side effect: drowsiness.

Other side effects: convulsions, dry mouth, tremors, twitches.

Interactions

 Inform your doctor before combining Atarax with barbiturates such as Seconal and Phenobarbital, narcotics such as Demerol and Percocet, non-narcotic analgesics such as Motrin and Tylenol.

 Do not combine alcohol with this medication; may intensify the effects of alcohol.

Special Cautions

 If pregnant or planning to become pregnant, inform your doctor immediately. Should not be taken in early pregnancy. May appear in breast milk; could affect a nursing infant.

 No special precautions apply to seniors.

 Follow doctor's instructions carefully for children.

 May cause drowsiness and impair your ability to drive a car or operate machinery. *Do not take part in any activity that requires alertness.*

If allergic to Atarax, should not take.

Atenolol

see TENORMIN

Atenolol with Chlorthalidone

see TENORETIC

Ativan

Generic name: Lorazepam

Other brand name: Alzapam

Ativan is a benzodiazepine tranquilizer. It selectively reduces the activity of certain chemicals in the brain.

℞ QUICK FACTS

Purpose

 Used to treat anxiety disorders for short-term therapy (up to 4 months). Also prescribed for anxiety associated with depressive symptoms.

Dosage

 Take exactly as prescribed.

Usual adult dose: 2 to 6 milligrams per day total, divided into smaller doses, with largest dose taken at bedtime. *For anxiety*—2 to 3 milligrams per day divided into 2 or 3 smaller doses. *For insomnia due to anxiety*—2 to 4 milligrams in 1 single dose, usually at bedtime. *For seniors*—1 to 2 milligrams per day, divided into smaller doses.

 Usual child dose: not generally prescribed for children under 12 years.

Missed dose: if within an hour of the scheduled time, take missed dose. Otherwise, skip missed dose; go back to regular schedule. *Do not double doses.*

Side Effects

Overdose symptoms: coma, confusion, low blood pressure, sleepiness. If you suspect an overdose, immediately seek medical attention.

More common side effects: dizziness, sedation (excessive calm), unsteadiness, weakness.

Less common or rare side effects: agitation, change in appetite, depression, eye function disorders, headache, memory impairment, mental disorientation, nausea, skin problems, sleep disturbance, stomach and intestinal disorders. Side effects due to rapid decrease or abrupt withdrawal: abdominal and muscle cramps, convulsions, depressed mood, inability to fall or stay asleep, sweating, tremors, vomiting.

Interactions

Inform your doctor before combining Ativan with barbiturates (Phenobarbital, Seconal, or Amytal) or sedatives such as Valium and Halcion.

Do not combine alcohol with this medication; may intensify the effects of alcohol.

Special Cautions

Do not take Ativan if pregnant or planning to become pregnant. Increased risk of birth defects. Not known whether it appears in breast milk.

65 Doctor should monitor seniors for stomach and upper intestinal problems.

Not generally prescribed for children under 12 years.

STOP May cause drowsiness and impair your ability to drive a car or operate machinery. *Do not take part in any activity that requires alertness.*

Dependence and tolerance can develop with Ativan. Only doctor should discontinue dosage to avoid withdrawal symptoms.

Should not take if sensitive to Ativan or other similar medications such as Valium.

Everyday stress should not be treated with Ativan.

Should not take if you have narrow-angle glaucoma.

Tell your doctor if you have decreased kidney or liver function, or severe depression before taking this medication.

If using for a prolonged period of time, your doctor should monitor for stomach and upper intestinal problems.

Atretol

see TEGRETOL

Atrovent

Generic name: Ipratropium bromide

Atrovent is a bronchodilator. It works by opening airways in the lungs and relaxing smooth-muscle tissue (such as in the lungs) to improve breathing.

℞ QUICK FACTS

Purpose

 Used on a long-term basis to treat bronchial spasms (wheezing) associated with chronic obstructive pulmonary disease such as bronchitis and emphysema.

Dosage

 Take consistently to get the most benefit, as prescribed by your doctor.

 Usual adult dose: *aerosol*—2 inhalations 4 times per day, not to exceed 12 inhalations in 24 hours. *Solution*—1 unit dose vial taken 3 to 4 times per day via oral nebulizer.

 Usual child dose: not generally prescribed in children under 12 years.

 Missed dose: take as soon as possible, unless almost time for next dose. If so, skip missed dose; go back to regular schedule. *Do not double doses.*

Side Effects

 No specific information is available regarding Atrovent overdose. If you suspect an overdose, immediately seek medical attention.

 More common side effects: blurred vision, cough, dizziness, dry mouth, fluttering heartbeat, headache, irritation from aerosol, nausea, nervousness, rash, stomach and intestinal upset, worsening of symptoms.

 Less common or rare side effects: constipation, coordination difficulty, difficulty urinating, drowsiness, fatigue, flushing, hives, hoarseness, inability to fall or stay asleep, increased heart rate, itching, low blood pressure, loss of hair, mouth sores, sharp eye pain, tingling sensation, tremors.

Interactions

 No drug interactions reported.

 No known food/other substance interactions.

Special Cautions

 If pregnant or planning to become pregnant, inform your doctor immediately. Not known if Atrovent appears in breast milk.

 No special precautions apply to seniors.

 Not generally prescribed for children under 12 years.

 Unless directed otherwise by a doctor, do not take if you have: narrow-angle glaucoma, enlarged prostate, or obstruction of the neck of the bladder.

Not to be used for acute attacks of bronchial spasm.

Tell your doctor of any sensitivity or allergic reaction to this or similar medications.

Aerosol form accidentally sprayed in the eyes may temporarily blur vision.

A/T/S

see ERYTHROMYCIN, TOPICAL

Augmentin

∿∿∿∿∿∿∿∿∿∿∿∿∿∿∿∿∿∿∿∿∿∿∿∿∿∿∿∿∿∿∿∿∿∿∿

Generic name: Amoxicillin with clavulanate potassium

Other brand name: Augmentin Chewables

Augmentin is an antibiotic. It prevents bacteria from multiplying and growing. Clavulanate potassium prevents the breakdown of Amoxicillin in the body.

℞ QUICK FACTS

Purpose

℞ Used to treat lower respiratory, middle ear, sinus, skin, and urinary tract infections caused by certain bacteria.

Dosage

 To prevent stomach upset, may take with or without food. If taking suspension, shake well before using. Take exactly as prescribed.

. . . .

 Usual adult dose: one 250-milligram tablet every 8 hours. *For more severe infections and infections of the respiratory tract*—one 500-milligram tablet every 8 hours.

. . . .

 Usual child dose: total of 20 milligrams per 2.2 pounds of body weight per day, taken every 8 hours. *For middle ear infections, sinus infections, and lower respiratory infections*—40 milligrams per 2.2 pounds of weight, taken every 8 hours in divided doses. *For se-*

vere infections—higher than usual dose. For children weighing 88 pounds or more—take adult dose.

 Missed dose: take as soon as possible. If almost time for next dose, and taking 2 doses a day, take missed dose, then next dose in 5 to 6 hours. If taking 3 or more doses a day, take missed dose, then next dose 2 to 4 hours later. Then go back to regular schedule. *Do not double doses.*

Side Effects

 Augmentin is generally safe. Large amounts may cause overdose symptoms, including exaggerated side effects listed below. If you suspect an overdose, immediately seek medical attention.

 More common side effects: diarrhea/loose stools, itching or burning of the vagina, nausea or vomiting, skin rashes and hives.

 Less common side effects: abdominal discomfort, anemia, arthritis, black "hairy" tongue, blood disorders, fever, gas, headache, heartburn, indigestion, itching, joint pain, muscle pain, skin inflammation, skin peeling, sores and inflammation in the mouth and on the tongue and gums. Rare side effects: agitation, anxiety, behavioral changes, change in liver function, confusion, dizziness, hyperactivity, insomnia.

Interactions

 Inform your doctor before combining Augmentin with: Benemid, Probenecid, oral contraceptives, Zyloprim. *Do not take when using Antabuse (Disulfiram).*

 No known food/other substance interactions.

Special Cautions

 If pregnant or planning to become pregnant, inform your doctor immediately. Possible risk to the developing baby. May appear in breast milk; could affect a nursing infant.

 Seniors should use with caution.

 Follow doctor's instructions carefully for children.

 Allergic reactions can be serious and possibly fatal; inform your doctor of previous allergic reactions to penicillins or other medicines, food or other substances.

Consult with doctor if you have had: asthma, blood disorder, hives, hay fever, or other allergies, colitis, diabetes, kidney or liver disease, mononucleosis.

If diabetic, may cause false positive urine glucose test results.

Augmentin Chewables

see AUGMENTIN

Auralgan

Generic ingredients: Antipyrine with benzocaine and glycerin

Other brand names: Allergen Ear Drops, Auroto Otic, Otocalm Ear

Auralgan is an analgesic combination. The antipyrine works to relieve pain, benzocaine deadens nerves inside the ear that transmit painful impulses, and glycerin removes water present in the ear.

℞ QUICK FACTS

Purpose

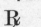 Used to reduce the inflammation and congestion and relieve the pain and discomfort of severe middle ear infections. Also used to remove excessive or impacted earwax.

Dosage

 Use exactly as prescribed. Discard dropper 6 months after first placed in solution. *Do not rinse dropper after use.*

 Usual adult dose: *for acute severe middle ear infection*—apply drops one at a time, enough to fill ear canal. Insert moist gauze into ear. Repeat every 1 to 2 hours until pain and congestion are relieved. *For removal of earwax*—apply drops 3 times per day for 2 to 3 days. Insert moist gauze into ear before and after removal of earwax.

 Usual child dose: same as adult dose.

 Missed dose: take as soon as possible, unless almost time for next dose. If so, skip missed dose; go back to regular schedule.

Side Effects

 No specific information is available regarding Auralgan overdose. If you suspect an overdose, immediately seek medical attention.

 No known more common side effects reported.

 No known less common side effects reported.

Interactions

 No drug interactions reported.

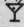 No known food/other substance interactions.

Special Cautions

 If pregnant or planning to become pregnant, inform your doctor immediately. Not known if Auralgan appears in breast milk.

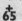 No specific precautions apply to seniors.

 Follow doctor's instructions carefully for children.

 Do not use if you have a punctured eardrum.

Tell your doctor of any sensitivity or allergies to the ingredients in Auralgan, or if any irritation or allergic reaction occurs.

Auranofin

see RIDAURA

Aventyl

see PAMELOR

Axid

^^^

Generic name: Nizatidine

Axid is an anti-ulcer agent. It relieves the symptoms and heals peptic ulcers.

℞ QUICK FACTS

Purpose

 Used to treat active duodenal ulcers. Used after ulcer has healed, as a long-term therapy at a reduced dose. Also used to treat heartburn and inflammation resulting from stomach acid flowing backward into esophagus.

Dosage

 Take exactly as prescribed.

 Usual adult dose: *for active duodenal ulcer*—300 milligrams once per day at bedtime, or 150 milligrams taken 2 times a day. *For maintenance of healed duodenal ulcer*—150 milligrams once per day at bedtime. *For seniors*—your doctor will prescribe dose based on your individual needs. Dose is reduced if kidney disease is present.

 Usual child dose: not generally prescribed for children.

 Missed dose: take as soon as possible, unless almost time for next dose. If so, skip missed dose; go back to regular schedule. *Do not double doses.*

Side Effects

 Overdose symptoms: no specific information is available regarding Axid overdose. If you suspect an overdose, immediately seek medical attention.

More common side effects: abdominal pain, diarrhea, dizziness, gas, headache, indigestion, inflammation of the nose, nausea, pain, sore throat, vomiting, weakness.

 Less common or rare side effects: abnormal dreams, anxiety, back pain, chest pain, constipation, dimmed vision, dry mouth, fever, inability to sleep, increased cough, infection, itching, loss of appetite, muscle pain, nervousness, rash, sleepiness, stomach/intestinal problems, tooth problems.

Interactions

 Inform your doctor before combining Axid with Aspirin in high doses.

 No known food/other substance interactions.

Special Cautions

 If pregnant or planning to become pregnant, inform your doctor immediately. Appears in breast milk; could affect a nursing infant.

 Appropriate dosage level is based on senior's individual needs.

 Not generally prescribed for children.

 Tell your doctor of any sensitivity to or allergic reaction to Axid or similar drugs, such as Zantac; if so, you should not take Axid.

Could mask stomach malignancy; if stomach problems continue, contact your doctor.

Azatadine Maleate with Pseudoephedrine Sulfate

see TRINALIN REPETABS

Azithromycin

see ZITHROMAX

Azmacort

^^

Generic name: Triamcinolone acetonide

Azmacort is a corticosteroid inhaler. It works to control inflammation of the mucosal lining of the bronchi, making it easier to breathe.

℞ QUICK FACTS

Purpose

℞ Used as a long-term therapy to treat bronchial asthma attacks.

Dosage

 Take exactly as prescribed, on a regular daily basis. For oral inhalation only. If using a bronchodilator inhalant, use before Azmacort inhalant, separated by several minutes.

 Usual adult dose: 2 inhalations (approximately 200 micrograms) taken 3 or 4 times per day, not to exceed 16 inhalations per day.

Usual child dose: *for children 6 to 12 years*—1 or 2 inhalations (approximately 100 to 200 micrograms) taken 3 or 4 times per day, not to exceed 12 inhalations per day. *For children under 6 years*—not generally prescribed.

 Missed dose: take as soon as possible, unless almost time for next dose. If so, skip missed dose; go back to regular schedule. *Do not double doses.*

Side Effects

 Overdose symptoms: most likely signaled by an increase in the side effects. If you suspect an overdose, immediately seek medical attention.

 More common side effects: dry mouth, dry throat, hoarseness, irritated throat.

 Less common side effects: facial swelling, increased wheezing and cough, mouth and throat infections.

Interactions

 Inform your doctor before combining Azmacort with alternate-day Prednisone treatment.

 No known food/other substance interactions.

Special Cautions

 If pregnant or planning to become pregnant, inform your doctor immediately. Not known whether Azmacort appears in breast milk.

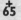 No specific precautions apply to seniors.

 Follow doctor's instructions carefully for children. Children are more susceptible to infection; try to avoid exposure to chicken pox and measles. Children's growth should be monitored by a doctor when using Azmacort.

 Do not use if occasional treatment for asthma is needed, if asthma can be controlled with nonsteroid medications, or if your bronchitis is not a result of asthma.

Notify your doctor before taking Azmacort if you have: extreme stress, herpes infections of the eye, recent surgery, tuberculosis, or untreated fungal, bacterial, or systemic viral infections.

Tell your doctor if you experience: depression, fungal infection in the mouth and throat, joint or muscular pain, light-headedness, weariness, or weight loss.

Azo-Standard
see PYRIDIUM

AZT
see RETROVIR

Azulfidine

Generic name: Sulfasalazine

Other brand names: Azaline, Azulfidine EN-tabs

Azulfidine is a sulfonamide and anti-inflammatory. Sulfa drugs work against infections in various parts of the body. An anti-inflammatory relieves inflammation.

℞ QUICK FACTS

Purpose

 Used to treat mild to moderate ulcerative colitis and severe ulcerative colitis. Also used to treat severe attacks of ulcerative colitis. Azulfidine EN-tabs are used when stomach and intestinal irritation (nausea and vomiting) is present.

Dosage

 Take in evenly spaced equal doses, preferably after meals or with food to avoid stomach upset, as directed by your doctor. Drink plenty of fluids to avoid kidney stones.

. . . .

 Usual adult dose: *initial therapy*—3 to 4 grams per day, divided into smaller doses; intervals (especially nighttime) should not exceed 8 hours. *For maintenance therapy*—2 grams per day.

. . . .

 Usual child dose: *for children 2 years and older*—40 to 60 milligrams per 2.2 pounds of body weight per a 24-hour period, divided into 4 to 6 doses. *For maintenance therapy*—30 milligrams per 2.2 pounds of body weight per a 24-hour period, divided into 4 doses, up to 2 grams per day.

. . . .

 Missed dose: take as soon as possible, unless almost time for next dose. If so, skip missed dose, go back to regular schedule. *Do not double doses.*

Side Effects

 Overdose symptoms: abdominal pain, convulsions, drowsiness, nausea, stomach upset, vomiting. If you suspect an overdose, immediately seek medical attention.

. . . .

More common side effects: headache, lack or loss of appetite, nausea, stomach distress, vomiting.

 Less common side effects: anemia, bluish discoloration of the skin, fever, hives, itching, skin rash. Rare side effects: abdominal pain, blood in the urine, bloody diarrhea, convulsions, diarrhea, drowsiness, hallucinations, hearing loss, hepatitis, inability to fall or stay asleep, inflammation of the mouth, itchy skin eruptions, joint pain, lack of muscle coordination, loss of hair, mental depression, red raised rash, ringing in the ears, sensitivity to light, severe allergic reaction, skin discoloration, skin disorders, swelling around the eye, urine discoloration, vertigo.

Interactions

 Inform your doctor before combining Azulfidine with: Digoxin (Lanoxin), or Folic acid (a B-complex vitamin).

 No known food/other substance reactions.

Special Cautions

 If pregnant or planning to become pregnant, inform your doctor immediately. Is secreted in breast milk; could affect a nursing infant.

 No specific precautions apply to seniors.

 Follow doctor's instructions carefully for children.

 Do not take if you have: intestinal or urinary obstruction or porphyria unless directed by your doctor.

Notify your doctor if you have allergic reactions, blood diseases, kidney or liver damage, changes in nerve and muscle impulses, or fibrosing alveolitis (inflammation of

the lungs); deaths have been reported when these conditions are present.

Inform your doctor before taking Azulfidine if you have kidney or liver damage or any blood disease.

Should not take if sensitivity or allergic reaction to Azulfidine, salicylates (Aspirin), or other sulfa drugs.

If EN-tabs are not disintegrated upon elimination, notify your doctor.

Men may temporarily experience infertility and low sperm count.

May experience yellow-orange cast to skin and urine.

Avoid over-exposure to the sun.

~~~~~~

Bacticort

see CORTISPORIN OPHTHALMIC SUSPENSION

Bactrim

see SEPTRA

Bactroban

~~~~~~

Generic name: Mupirocin

Bactroban is a topical antibiotic. It interferes with the production of certain biochemicals necessary for bacteria to sustain life.

℞ QUICK FACTS

Purpose

 Used to treat impetigo, eczema, inflammation of the hair follicles, and minor bacterial skin infections.

Dosage

 Use exactly as directed. Not for use in the eyes.

 Usual adult dose: apply ointment to affected area 3 times per day. Can cover treated area with gauze.

Usual child dose: same as adult dose.

 Missed dose: apply as soon as possible, unless almost time for next dose. In that case, do not take missed dose; go back to regular schedule.

Side Effects

 Overdose symptoms: no information available. If you suspect an overdose, immediately seek medical attention.

 More common side effects: burning, pain, stinging.

 Less common side effects: itching. Rare side effects: abnormal redness, dry skin, inflammation of the skin, nausea, oozing, skin rash, swelling, tenderness.

Interactions

 No known drug interactions.

 No known food/other substance interactions.

Special Cautions

 If pregnant or planning to become pregnant, inform your doctor immediately. May appear in breast milk; could affect a nursing infant.

 No special precautions apply to seniors.

 Follow doctor's instructions carefully for children.

 Contact your doctor if infection does not clear within 3 to 5 days, or if it gets worse.

If skin shows signs of an allergic reaction, stop using and call your doctor.

. . . .
Should not use if sensitive to Bactroban or similar drugs; inform your doctor of any allergic reactions.
. . . .
Prolonged use may result in bacteria that do not respond to Bactroban, causing a secondary infection.

Beclomethasone Dipropionate

see BECLOVENT INHALATION AEROSOL

Beclovent Inhalation Aerosol

Generic name: Beclomethasone dipropionate

Other brand names: Beconase AQ Nasal Spray, Beconase Inhalation Aerosol, Vancenase AQ Nasal Spray, Vancenase Nasal Inhaler, Vanceril Inhaler

Beclovent is a corticosteroid. It works to control inflammation of the mucosal lining of the bronchi, making it easier to breathe.

℞ QUICK FACTS

Purpose

 Used to treat respiratory problems, specifically bronchial asthma. Vanceril is also used to treat bronchial asthma. Beconase and Vancenase are used specifically to treat hay fever and to prevent recurrence of nasal polyps after surgical removal.

. . . .

Dosage

 Use exactly as prescribed. If combining with a bronchodilator, take it before using this medication. Leave several minutes between the medications. To avoid throat irritation, gargle or rinse mouth with water after each dose; *do not swallow the water.*

 Usual adult dose: *for oral inhalant*—2 inhalations 3 to 4 times per day or 4 inhalations 2 times per day, as prescribed. *For severe asthma*—12 to 16 inhalations per day, not to exceed 20 inhalations, as prescribed. *For nasal spray*—1 or 2 inhalations in each nostril 2 to 4 times per day.

 Usual child dose: *oral inhalant for children 6 to 12 years*—1 or 2 inhalations 3 or 4 times per day or 2 to 4 inhalations 2 times per day, as prescribed, not to exceed 10 inhalations per day. *Nasal spray for children 6 to 12 years*—1 inhalation in each nostril 3 times per day. *For children under 6 years*—generally not prescribed.

 Missed dose—take as soon as possible. Take remaining doses for the day at equal intervals. Skip missed dose if time for next dose. *Do not double doses.*

Side Effects

 Overdose symptoms: no specific overdose information. If you suspect an overdose, immediately seek medical attention.

 Side effects for inhalant: dry mouth, fluid retention, hives, hoarseness, skin rash, wheezing. Side effects for nasal spray: headache, light-headedness, nasal burning, nasal irritation, nausea, nose and throat infections, nosebleed, runny nose, sneezing, stuffy nose, tearing eyes.

No known less common or rare side effects.

Interactions

 No reported drug interactions.

 No known food/other substance interactions.

Special Cautions

 No information concerning pregnancy or breast-feeding.

 No special precautions apply to seniors.

 If on a high dose, avoid exposure to chicken pox or measles, which can be potentially fatal. Monitor children for reduced growth.

 Should not use if bronchodilators or other non-steroidal drugs are effective, or if quick relief is desired.

Not to be used for non-asthmatic bronchitis or occasional asthma treatment.

Inform your doctor of any sensitivity to or allergic reactions to this or similar medications.

Doctor should closely monitor if you are transferred from steroid tablets to inhalant or nasal spray; may experience "adrenal insufficiency."

If using oral inhalant, monitor for: facial swelling, increased bruising, mental disturbances, or weight gain.

Benadryl

~~~~~~

Generic name: Diphenhydramine hydrochloride

Other brand names: AllerMax, Banophen, Belix, Diphen Cough, Dormarex-2, Genahist, Hydramine, Nervine Nighttime, Nidryl, Nordryl, Nytol, Phendry, Sleep-Eze 3, Sominex, Twilite

Benadryl is an antihistamine. Antihistamines block the effects of histamine, a body chemical that causes swelling and itching.

℞ QUICK FACTS

Purpose

℞ Used to treat symptoms of allergy—red, inflamed eyes; itching, swelling and redness from hives and other rashes caused by allergies. Also used to relieve symptoms of seasonal allergies—sneezing, coughing, runny or stuffy nose. Is also used to treat allergic reactions to blood transfusions, to prevent and treat motion sickness, to prevent severe allergic reaction, and to treat Parkinson's disease.

Dosage

 Take exactly as prescribed.

 Usual adult dose: 25 to 50 milligrams 3 or 4 times per day. *As a sleep aid*—50 milligrams at bedtime. *For motion sickness*—first dose 30 minutes before motion, other doses before meals and at bedtime, as long as motion continues.

 Usual child dose (20 pounds and over): 12.5 to 25 milligrams 3 to 4 times per day, not to exceed 300

milligrams per day. *Do not use as a sleep aid for children under age 12.*

 Missed dose: take as soon as possible, unless almost time for next dose. In that case, do not take missed dose, go back to regular schedule. *Do not double doses.*

Side Effects

 Overdose symptoms: central nervous system depression or stimulation, especially in children; dry mouth; fixed, dilated pupils; flushing; stomach and intestinal symptoms. If you suspect an overdose, immediately seek medical attention.

 More common side effects: disturbed coordination, dizziness, excessive calm, increased chest congestion, sleepiness, stomach upset.

 Less common or rare side effects: anaphylactic shock (extreme allergic reaction), anemia, blurred vision, chills, confusion, constipation, convulsions, diarrhea, difficulty sleeping, double vision, dry mouth, dry nose, dry throat, early menstruation, excessive perspiration, excitation, fast or fluttery heartbeat, fatigue, frequent or difficult urination, headache, hives, inability to urinate, increased sensitivity to light, irregular heartbeat, irritability, loss of appetite, low blood pressure, nausea, nervousness, rapid heartbeat, rash, restlessness, ringing in the ears, stuffy nose, tightness of chest and wheezing, tingling or pins and needles, tremor, unreal or exaggerated sense of well-being, vertigo, vomiting.

Interactions

 Inform your doctor before combining Benadryl with: antidepressant drugs known as MAO inhibitors such as Parnate and Nardil; sedative/hypnotics such as

Halcion, Nembutal, and Seconal; tranquilizers such as Xanax and Valium.

· ·

 Alcohol may increase sedative effects; *do not drink alcohol when taking this medication.*

Special Cautions

 If pregnant or planning to become pregnant, inform your doctor immediately. Not advised for use when nursing an infant.

· ·

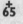 May cause dizziness, excessive calm, or low blood pressure.

· ·

 Follow doctor's instructions carefully for children, can cause excitability.

· ·

 Do not take if sensitivity to or allergic to this or other antihistamines.

· ·

May cause drowsiness and impair your ability to drive a car or operate machinery. *Do not take part in any activity that requires alertness.*

· ·

Use carefully if you have: difficulty urinating due to bladder obstruction, heart disease, high blood pressure, history of asthma or other chronic lung disease, intestinal blockage, narrow-angle glaucoma, narrowing of the stomach or intestine due to stomach problems, over-active thyroid, or symptoms of enlarged prostate.

Benazepril Hydrochloride

see LOTENSIN

Bentyl

~~~~~~

Generic name: Dicyclomine hydrochloride

Other brand names: Bemote, Byclomine, Di-Spaz

Bentyl is an antispasmodic. It slows bowel action and reduces stomach acid.

℞ QUICK FACTS

Purpose

 Used to treat irritable bowel syndrome.

Dosage

 Take exactly as prescribed.

 Usual adult dose: 160 milligrams per day divided into 4 equal doses. Doctor may start with 80 milligrams per day divided into 4 equal doses to decrease side effects. If not effective in 2 weeks, or lower than 80 milligrams is indicated, doctor may not continue therapy.

 Usual child dose: not generally prescribed for children.

 Missed dose: take as soon as possible, unless almost time for next dose. In that case, do not take missed dose; go back to regular schedule. *Do not double doses.*

Side Effects

 Overdose symptoms: blurred vision, central nervous system (brain and spinal cord) stimulation, difficulty in swallowing, dilated pupils, dizziness, dryness of the mouth, headache, hot or dry skin, nausea, nerve blockage causing weakness and possible paralysis, vomiting. If you suspect an overdose, immediately seek medical attention.

 Side effects: blurred vision, dizziness, drowsiness, dry mouth, light-headedness, nausea, nervousness, weakness.

 Side effects reported for similar drugs: abdominal pain, agitation, bloated feeling, coma, confusion or excitement, constipation, decreased anxiety, decreased sweating, difficulty in carrying out voluntary movements, difficulty urinating, disorientation, double vision, enlargement of the pupil of the eye, exaggerated feeling of well-being, eye paralysis, fainting, fast or fluttery heartbeat, fatigue, hallucinations, headache, hives, impotence, inability to fall or stay asleep, inability to urinate, itching, labored or difficult breathing, lack of coordination, lack or loss of appetite, nasal stuffiness or congestion, numbness, rapid heartbeat, rash, severe allergic reaction, short-term memory loss, sluggishness, sneezing, speech disturbance, suffocation, suppression of breast milk, taste loss, temporary cessation of breathing, throat congestion, tingling, vomiting.

Interactions

 Inform your doctor before combining Bentyl with: Amantadine (the Parkinson's disease drug Symmetrel); antacids such as Maalox; anti-arrhythmic drugs such as Quinidine (Quinidex); antiglaucoma drugs such as Pilocarpine; antihistamines such as Tavist; benzodiazepine tranquilizers such as Valium and Xanax; corticosteroids (Prednisone); Digoxin (Lanoxin); MAO inhibitors (antidepressants such as Nardil); Metoclopramide (gastrointestinal stimulant Reglan); narcotic analgesics (Demerol); nitrates and nitrites (heart medications such as Nitroglycerin); phenothiazines (antipsychotic drugs such as Proventil and Ventolin);

sympathomimetic airway-opening drugs such as Elavil and Tofranil.

 No known food/other substance interactions.

Special Cautions

 If pregnant or planning to become pregnant, inform your doctor immediately. Appears in breast milk; could affect a nursing infant.

 No special precautions apply to seniors.

 Not generally prescribed for children.

 Do not take if you have: blockage of urinary tract, stomach, or intestines; glaucoma; myasthenia gravis; reflux esophagitis; severe ulcerative colitis.

May cause drowsiness or blurred vision and impair your ability to drive a car or operate machinery. *Do not take part in any activity that requires alertness.*

Fever and heat stroke due to decreased sweating can occur when Bentyl is used in hot weather.

If diarrhea occurs, notify your doctor, especially if you have had bowel removals, an ileostomy or colostomy.

Notify your doctor if you have: autonomic neuropathy, congestive heart failure, coronary heart disease, hiatal hernia, high blood pressure, hyperthyroidism, known or suspected enlargement of the prostate, liver or kidney disease, rapid or irregular heartbeat.

Benzamycin

∿∿∿∿∿∿∿∿∿∿∿∿∿∿∿∿∿∿∿∿∿∿∿∿∿∿∿∿∿

Generic ingredients: Erythromycin with
benzoyl peroxide

Benzamycin is a combination antibiotic and antibacterial. It interferes with the production of certain biochemicals necessary for bacteria to sustain life.

℞ QUICK FACTS

Purpose

℞ Used to treat acne.

Dosage

  Apply to affected areas after thoroughly washing, rinsing with warm water, and drying gently.

  Usual adult dose: apply 2 times per day to affected areas, in the morning and evening.

  Usual child dose: not generally prescribed for children under age 12.

  Missed dose: apply as soon as possible, unless almost time for next dose. In that case, do not take missed dose; go back to regular schedule.

Side Effects

  Overdose symptoms: no information available. If you suspect an overdose, immediately seek medical attention.

  Side effects: abnormal redness of the skin, dryness, itching.

  No known less common or rare side effects.

Interactions

 Inform your doctor before combining Benzamycin with: any other prescription or over-the-counter acne remedy.

 No known food/other substance interactions.

Special Cautions

 If pregnant or planning to become pregnant, inform your doctor immediately. Not known if Benzamycin appears in breast milk.

 No special precautions apply to seniors.

 Not generally prescribed for children.

 Should not use if sensitive to ingredients of this drug; inform your doctor of any allergic reactions.

Use with caution, may bleach hair or colored fabric.

Monitor for any increased resistance of bacteria.

Benzonatate
see TESSALON

Benzoyl Peroxide
see DESQUAM-E

Benztropine Mesylate
see COGENTIN

Betagan
~~~~~~

Generic name: Levobunolol hydrochloride

Betagan is a beta-adrenergic blocking agent. It works to
reduce pressure in the eye.

℞ QUICK FACTS

Purpose

℞   Used to treat chronic open-angle glaucoma (increased pressure inside the eye) and ocular hypertension.

Dosage

    Use exactly as prescribed. Taper off use of medica-
tion slowly. In the case of overproduction of thyroid
hormone, abrupt withdrawal may provoke a rush of
the hormone.

    Usual adult dose: *starting dose*—1 drop of Betagan
0.5% in the affected eye(s) 1 time per day. *Maintenance dose*—1 or 2 drops of Betagan 0.25% 2 times
per day. *For more severe glaucoma*—doctor may prescribe Betagan 0.5% 2 times per day.

    Usual child dose: not generally prescribed for chil-
dren.

    Missed dose: *if taking 1 time per day*—take as soon
as possible, unless it is the next day. In that case, do

not take missed dose; go back to regular schedule. *Do not double doses. If taking 2 times per day*—take as soon as possible, unless almost time for next dose. In that case, do not take missed dose; go back to regular schedule. *Do not double doses.*

Side Effects

 Overdose symptoms: breathing difficulty, heart failure, low blood pressure, and/or slowed heartbeat. If you suspect an overdose, immediately seek medical attention.

 More common side effects: burning and stinging when applying eye drops, eye inflammation.

 Less common or rare side effects: chest pain, congestive heart failure, depression, diarrhea, difficult or labored breathing, dizziness, fainting, headache, heart palpitations, hives, low blood pressure, nasal congestion, nausea, pins and needles, rash, slow or irregular heartbeat, stroke, temporary heart stoppage, vision problems, weakness, wheezing.

Interactions

 Inform your doctor before combining Betagan with: calcium-blocking blood pressure medications such as Calan and Cardizem; Digitalis (heart medication Lanoxin); Epinephrine (EpiPen); oral beta-blockers such as Inderal and Tenormin; Reserpine (Serpasil).

 No known food/other substance interactions.

Special Cautions

 If pregnant or planning to become pregnant, inform your doctor immediately. Other beta-blocker medications do appear in breast milk, use with caution if breastfeeding.

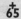 No special precautions apply to seniors.

 Not generally prescribed for children.

 Do not use more than 2 beta-blocker eye medications simultaneously.

Should not use Betagan if you have: asthma or other respiratory diseases, cardiogenic shock, certain heart irregularities, decreased heart function, diabetes, low blood sugar, severe chronic obstructive lung disease, slow heartbeat.

Betagan contains sulfites; monitor for allergic reactions.

Inform your doctor you are taking Betagan before surgery that requires anesthesia.

Medication may affect other parts of the body; use with caution.

Betamethasone Dipropionate

see DIPROLENE

Betaxolol Hydrochloride

see BETOPTIC

Betoptic

~~~~~~

Generic name: Betaxolol hydrochloride

Other brand names: Betoptic Ophthalmic Solution, Betoptic Ophthalmic Suspension, Kerlone

Betoptic is a beta-adrenergic blocking agent. It works to reduce pressure in the eye.

℞ QUICK FACTS

Purpose

 Used to treat open-angle glaucoma (Betoptic Ophthalmic Solution and Betoptic S Ophthalmic Suspension) and ocular hypertension.

Dosage

 Use exactly as prescribed. Shake suspension well before each dose.

. . . .

 Usual adult dose: *for Betoptic Solution*—1 to 2 drops in the affected eye(s) 2 times per day. *For Betoptic S Suspension*—1 to 2 drops in the affected eye(s) 2 times per day.

. . . .

 Usual child dose: not generally prescribed for children.

. . . .

 Missed dose: take as soon as possible, unless almost time for next dose. In that case, do not take missed dose; go back to regular schedule. *Do not double doses.*

Side Effects

☠ Overdose symptoms: *for oral beta-blockers*—heart failure, low blood pressure, slow heartbeat. If you

suspect an overdose, immediately seek medical attention.

 Most common side effect: temporary eye discomfort.

 Less common or rare side effects: allergic reactions, asthma, congestive heart failure, dead skin, decrease in corneal sensitivity, depression, difficulty breathing, difficulty sleeping or drowsiness, dizziness, hair loss, headache, hives, inflammation of the cornea, inflammation of the tongue, intolerance to light, itching, peeling skin, pupils of different sizes, red eyes and skin, slow heartbeat, sluggishness, tearing, thickening chest secretions, vertigo, wheezing.

Interactions

 Inform your doctor before combining Betoptic with: drugs that alter mood such as Nardil and Elavil; oral beta-blockers such as Inderal and Tenormin; Reserpine (Serpasil).

 No known food/other substance interactions.

Special Cautions

 If pregnant or planning to become pregnant, inform your doctor immediately. May appear in breast milk; could affect a nursing infant.

 No special precautions apply to seniors.

 Not generally prescribed for children.

 Do not use if sensitive to or allergic to this medication.

Inform your doctor before taking Betoptic if you have: asthma, diabetes, heart disease, thyroid disease.

May lose effectiveness for glaucoma if used over a long period of time.

If having surgery that requires general anesthesia, inform your doctor.

Biaxin

Generic name: Clarithromycin

Biaxin is a macrolide antibiotic. It works by killing bacteria directly or slowing the growth of bacteria so that the body's natural defenses can kill them.

℞ QUICK FACTS

Purpose

℞ Used to treat bacterial infections of the respiratory tract, including: pneumonia, sinusitis, skin infections, strep throat, and tonsillitis. Also prescribed for acute otitis media.

Dosage

 May take with or without food; take exactly as prescribed. Finish the entire treatment course.

 Usual adult dose: 250 to 500 milligrams every 12 hours for 7 to 14 days, depending on the type of infection and bacteria. Lower dosage may be required for kidney disease.

 Usual child dose: not generally prescribed for children under 12 years.

Missed dose: take as soon as possible, unless almost time for next dose. In that case, take the next dose 5 to 6 hours later, then go back to regular schedule.

Side Effects

 Overdose symptoms: no specific information regarding overdose. If you suspect an overdose, immediately seek medical attention.

 Side effects: abdominal pain and/or discomfort, altered sense of taste, diarrhea, headache, indigestion, nausea.

 No known less common or rare side effects.

Interactions

 Inform your doctor before combining Biaxin with: Carbamazepine (Tegretol) or Theophylline (Slo-Phyllin, Theo-Dur, others). Biaxin is in the same family of drugs as Erythromycin. Medications that interact with Erythromycin include: Astemizole (Hismanal); blood thinners such as Coumadin; Cyclosporine (Sandimmune); Digoxin (Lanoxin); Ergotamine (Caftergot); Hexobarbital; Phenytoin (Dilantin); Terfenadine (Seldane); Triazolam (Halcion).

 No known food/other substance interactions.

Special Cautions

 If pregnant or planning to become pregnant, inform your doctor immediately. May appear in breast milk; could affect a nursing infant. *May produce birth defects.*

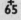 No special precautions apply to seniors.

 Not generally prescribed for children.

Do not use if sensitive to or allergic to this medication or similar antibiotics such as Tao or Zithromax. May cause pseudomembranous colitis, a potentially life-threatening diarrhea. Stop taking Biaxin and inform your doctor if you have prolonged or severe diarrhea.

Bleph-10

see SODIUM SULAMYD

Brethine

Generic name: Terbutaline sulfate

Other brand names: Brethaire, Bricanyl

Brethine is a bronchodilator. It works by opening airways in the lungs and relaxing smooth-muscle tissue (such as in the lungs) to improve breathing.

℞ QUICK FACTS

Purpose

℞ Used to prevent and relieve bronchial spasms in asthma, bronchitis, and emphysema.

Dosage

 Take exactly as prescribed, do not take more often than recommended.

 Usual adult dose: *for Brethine*—5 milligrams at approximately 6-hour intervals, 3 times per day during waking hours. May be reduced to 2.5 milligrams if experiencing many side effects. Do not exceed 15

milligrams in a 24-hour period. *For Brethaire—2 inhalations separated by 60-second interval, every 4
to 6 hours.*

 Usual child dose: *for children under 12 years—not
generally prescribed. For Brethine for children 12 to
15 years*—2.5 milligrams 3 times per day, not to exceed 7.5 milligrams in a 24-hour period. *For Brethaire
for children 12 years and older*—2 inhalations separated by 60-second interval, every 4 to 6 hours.

 Take as soon as possible, then take the remainder
of medication for that day in equally spaced doses.
Do not double doses.

Side Effects

 Overdose symptoms: same as the side effects. If you
suspect an overdose, immediately seek medical attention.

 More common side effects: chest discomfort, difficulty in breathing, dizziness, drowsiness, fast or fluttery heartbeat, flushed feeling, headache, increased
heart rate, nausea, nervousness, pain at injection
site, rapid heartbeat, sweating, tremors, vomiting,
weakness.

 Less common side effects: anxiety, dry mouth, muscle cramps. Rare side effects: dry throat, throat irritation, unusual taste.

Interactions

 Inform your doctor before combining Brethine with:
antidepressants known as MAO inhibitors (Nardil or
Parnate), beta-blockers (Inderal or Tenormin), other
bronchodilators (Proventil or Ventolin), tricyclic
antidepressants (Elavil or Tofranil).

No known food/other substance interactions.

Special Cautions

 If pregnant or planning to become pregnant, inform your doctor immediately. Not known if Brethine appears in breast milk.

 No special precautions apply to seniors.

 Not generally prescribed for children under 12 years.

 Should not use if sensitive to or had allergic reaction to this or similar medications such as Ventolin.

Inform your doctor before taking Brethine if you have: diabetes, heart disease, high blood pressure, irregular heart rate, an overactive thyroid gland, or seizures.

Bromocriptine Mesylate

see PARLODEL

Brompheniramine Maleate with Phenylpropanolamine Hydrochloride and Codeine Phosphate

see DIMETANE-DC

Bumetanide

see BUMEX

Bumex

∿∿∿∿∿∿∿∿∿∿∿∿∿∿∿∿∿∿∿∿∿∿∿∿∿∿∿∿∿∿∿∿∿∿∿

Generic name: Bumetanide

Bumex is a loop diuretic. It promotes water and salt loss in the body.

℞ QUICK FACTS

Purpose

℞ Used to treat fluid retention associated with congestive heart failure, and liver or kidney disease. Also occasionally prescribed to treat high blood pressure.

Dosage

 Take in the morning after breakfast with a single daily dose; with more than 1 dose per day, take last dose no later than 6:00 PM, as it may increase the frequency of urination, causing sleep loss if taken at night.

. . . .

 Usual adult dose: 0.5 to 2.0 milligrams per day, taken in a single daily dose. Doctor may increase if necessary, to 2 or 3 doses per day, not to exceed 10 milligrams. *For continuing control of fluid retention*—alternate days or for 3 to 4 days at a time with rest periods of 1 to 2 days in between. If prescribed dose is exceeded, can severely decrease water and mineral levels in the body, especially potassium.

. . . .

 Usual child dose: not generally prescribed for children.

. . . .

Missed dose: take as soon as possible, unless almost time for next dose. In that case, do not take missed dose; go back to regular schedule. *Do not double doses.*

Side Effects

Overdose symptoms: cramps, dizziness, lethargy, loss or lack of appetite, mental confusion, vomiting, weakness. Overdose may lead to: severe dehydration, reduction of blood volume, and severe problems with circulatory system. If you suspect an overdose, immediately seek medical attention.

More common side effects: dizziness, headache, low blood pressure, muscle cramps, nausea. Signs of too much potassium loss: dry mouth, irregular heartbeat, muscle cramps or pain, unusual tiredness or weakness.

Less common or rare side effects: abdominal pain, black stools, chest pain, dehydration, diarrhea, dry mouth, ear discomfort, fatigue, hearing loss, itching, joint pain, kidney failure, muscle and bone pain, nipple tenderness, premature ejaculation, rapid breathing, skin rash or hives, sweating, upset stomach, vertigo, vomiting, weakness.

Interactions

Inform your doctor before combining Bumex with: blood pressure medications such as Vasotec and Tenormin; Indomethacin (Indocin and other non-steroidal anti-inflammatory drugs), probenecid (Benemid). Combining with chemotherapy agent such as Cisplatin (Platinol) may cause hearing loss. Combining with Digitalis or Digoxin (Lanoxin) may cause changes in heartbeat. Combining with Lithium (Lithonate) may increase levels of lithium in the body to a poisonous level.

No known food/other substance interactions.

Special Cautions

 If pregnant or planning to become pregnant, inform your doctor immediately. Not known if Bumex appears in breast milk.

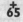 No special precautions apply to seniors.

 Not generally prescribed for children.

 Should not take if unable to urinate or are dehydrated.

Should not take if sensitive to or allergic to this or similar medications.

Inform your doctor of sensitivity to sulfur medications before taking Bumex.

Blood status should be regularly monitored when taking Bumex.

May require potassium supplement or doctor may recommend foods and fluids high in potassium.

If you experience light-headedness or if you faint when standing from a sitting or lying position, notify your doctor.

Bupropion Hydrochloride

see WELLBUTRIN

BuSpar

Generic name: Buspirone hydrochloride

BuSpar is an anti-anxiety drug. It reduces the activity of certain chemicals in the brain.

℞ QUICK FACTS

Purpose

 Used to treat anxiety disorders.

Dosage

 Take exactly as prescribed; full benefit may not be apparent for 1 to 2 weeks.

 Usual adult dose: 15 milligrams per day divided into 3 doses. Every 2 to 3 days doctor may increase 5 milligrams per day as needed, not to exceed 60 milligrams.

 Usual child dose: not generally prescribed for children.

 Missed dose: take as soon as possible, unless almost time for next dose. In that case, do not take missed dose; go back to regular schedule. *Do not double doses.*

Side Effects

 Overdose symptoms: dizziness, drowsiness, nausea or vomiting, severe stomach upset, unusually small pupils. If you suspect an overdose, immediately seek medical attention.

More common side effects: dizziness, dry mouth, fatigue, headache, light-headedness, nausea, nervousness, unusual excitement.

 Less common or rare side effects: anger/hostility, blurred vision, bone aches/pain, confusion, constipation, decreased concentration, depression, diarrhea, fast or fluttery heartbeat, incoordination, muscle pain/aches, numbness, pain or weakness in hands or feet, rapid heartbeat, rash, restlessness, stomach and abdominal upset, sweating/clamminess, tingling or pins and needles, tremor, urinary incontinence, vomiting, weakness.

Interactions

 Inform your doctor before combining with: Coumadin, Haloperidol (Haldol), MAO inhibitors (antidepressant drugs such as Nardil and Parnate), Trazodone (Desyrel).

 Avoid alcohol while taking BuSpar.

Special Cautions

 If pregnant or planning to become pregnant, inform your doctor immediately. Not known if BuSpar appears in breast milk.

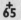 No special precautions apply to seniors.

 Not generally prescribed for children.

 Do not drive, operate machinery, or take part in any activity that requires alertness; effects of BuSpar on the central nervous system are unpredictable.

If sensitive to or had allergic reaction to this or similar medications, should not take.

Not for everyday stress-related anxiety or tension.

Should not use if you have severe kidney or liver damage.

Buspirone Hydrochloride
see BUSPAR

Butalbital with Acetaminophen and Caffeine
see FIORICET

Butalbital with Aspirin and Caffeine
see FIORINAL

Butalbital with Codeine Phosphate, Aspirin, and Caffeine
see FIORINAL WITH CODEINE

Butoconazole Nitrate

see FEMSTAT

Cafergot

Generic ingredients: Ergotamine tartrate
with Caffeine

Cafergot is an antimigraine vasoconstrictor. It acts by
constricting (narrowing) the blood vessels in the head,
thereby reducing blood flow, pressure, and pain.

℞ QUICK FACTS

Purpose

℞ Used to relieve or treat vascular headaches such as
migraines or cluster headaches.

Dosage

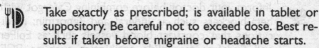 Take exactly as prescribed; is available in tablet or
suppository. Be careful not to exceed dose. Best re-
sults if taken before migraine or headache starts.

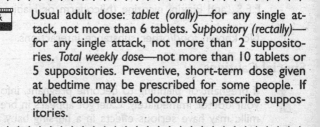 Usual adult dose: *tablet (orally)*—for any single at-
tack, not more than 6 tablets. *Suppository (rectally)*—
for any single attack, not more than 2 suppositories. *Total weekly dose*—not more than 10 tablets or
5 suppositories. Preventive, short-term dose given
at bedtime may be prescribed for some people. If
tablets cause nausea, doctor may prescribe suppositories.

Usual child dose: not generally prescribed for children.

Missed dose: take only when an attack threatens.

Side Effects

 Overdose symptoms: coma, convulsions, diminished or absent pulses, drowsiness, high or low blood pressure, numbness, shock, stupor, tingling, pain and bluish discoloration of the limbs, unresponsiveness, vomiting. If you suspect an overdose, immediately seek medical attention.

 Side effects: fluid retention, high blood pressure, itching, nausea, numbness, rapid heart rate, slow heartbeat, tingling or pins and needles, vertigo, vomiting, weakness. Complications caused by blood vessel constriction: bluish tinge to the skin, chest pain, cold arms and legs, gangrene, muscle pains.

 No known less common or rare side effects.

Interactions

 Inform your doctor before combining Cafergot with: beta-blockers such as Inderal and Tenormin; medications that constrict blood vessels such as EpiPen and Sudafed; macrolide antibiotics such as PCE, E.E.S., and Biaxin; nicotine (Nicoderm or Habitrol).

 No known food/other substance interactions.

Special Cautions

 If pregnant or planning to become pregnant, inform your doctor immediately. Cafergot appears in breast milk; may have serious effects in a nursing baby.

 No special precautions apply to seniors.

 Not generally prescribed for children.

Unless directed by your doctor, do not take if you have: coronary heart disease, circulatory problems, high blood pressure, impaired liver or kidney function, or if you are pregnant.

Excessive use can lead to ergot poisoning, which can lead to gangrene if not treated.

If sensitive to or had allergic reaction to ingredients in Cafergot, should not take this medication.

Can cause psychological dependence if used over a long period.

Discontinuance of Cafergot may cause sudden, severe headaches.

Take only for migraine and cluster headaches.

Calan

Generic name: Verapamil hydrochloride

Other brand names: Calan SR, Isoptin, Isoptin SR, Verelan

Calan is a calcium channel blocker. It increases the amount of oxygen that reaches the heart muscle.

℞ QUICK FACTS

Purpose

 Used to treat various types of chest pain (angina). Also used to treat irregular heartbeat and high blood pressure. Sustained release formula (SR) used for high blood pressure only. Has been prescribed to treat manic depression and panic attacks.

May be taken with or without food. Sustained release formulas should be taken with food, and must
be swallowed whole. Take exactly as prescribed,
even if you are feeling well. Take regularly; otherwise, condition may worsen.

 Usual adult dose: Calan and Isoptin: in general, no
more than 480 milligrams per day is ever prescribed.
For chest pain—80 to 120 milligrams 3 times per day.
*For chest pain in seniors or those with decreased liver
function*—40 milligrams 3 times per day. *For irregular
heartbeat*—people on Digitalis—240 to 320 milligrams per day, divided into 3 or 4 doses; people
not on Digitalis—240 to 480 milligrams per day, divided into 3 or 4 doses. *For high blood pressure only*—
80 milligrams 3 times per day, ranging from 360 to
480 milligrams total per day. *For high blood pressure
only in seniors and smaller individuals*—40 milligrams
3 times per day. Sustained Release and Verelan: *for
sustained release*—180 milligrams taken in the morning; smaller person may require 120 milligrams. *For
seniors*—120 milligrams taken in the morning.

 Usual child dose: not generally prescribed for children.

 Missed dose: take as soon as possible, unless almost
time for next dose. In that case, do not take missed
dose, go back to regular schedule. *Do not double
doses.*

Side Effects

 Overdose symptoms: no specific information available; however, if overdose is suspected, should be
under observation for 48 hours. If you suspect an
overdose, immediately seek medical attention.

More common side effects: congestive heart failure, constipation, dizziness, fatigue, fluid retention, headache, low blood pressure, nausea, rash, shortness of breath, slow heartbeat.

 Less common or rare side effects: angina, blurred vision, breast development in males, bruising, chest pain, confusion, diarrhea, difficulty sleeping, drowsiness, dry mouth, excessive milk secretion, fainting, fever and rash, flushing, hair loss, heart attack, hives, impotence, increased urination, joint pain, limping, loss of balance, muscle cramps, pounding heartbeat, rash, shakiness, skin peeling, sleepiness, spotty menstruation, sweating, tingling or pins and needles, upset stomach.

Interactions

 Inform your doctor before combining Calan with: Amiodarone (Cordarone); ACE inhibitor–type blood pressure medications such as Capoten and Vasotec; beta-blocker-type blood pressure medications such as Inderal, Lopressor, and Tenormin; Carbamazepine (Tegretol); Chloroquine (Aralen); Cimetidine (Tagamet); Cyclosporine (Sandimmune); Dantrolene (Dantrium); Digitalis (Lanoxin); Disopyramide (Norpace); diuretics such as Lasix and HydroDIURIL; Flecainide (Tambocor); Glipizide (Glucotrol); Imipramine (Tofranil); inhalation anesthetics; Lithium (Lithonate); nitrates such as Transderm Nitro and Isordil; Phenobarbital; Phenytoin (Dilantin); Quinidine (Quinidex); Rifampin (Rifadin); Theophylline (Theo-Dur); vasodilator-type blood pressure medications such as Loniten or other high blood pressure medications such as Minipress.

 No known food/other substance interactions.

Special Cautions

 If pregnant or planning to become pregnant, inform your doctor immediately. Appears in breast milk; could affect a nursing baby.

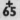 Lower dose is generally prescribed for seniors.

 Not generally prescribed for children.

 Do not take if sensitive to or had an allergic reaction to this or other brands, or other calcium channel blockers.

Should not take if you have: low blood pressure, certain types of heart disease, Duchenne's dystrophy, heartbeat irregularities, kidney disease, or liver disease.

Check with your doctor before major exertion or exercise.

Inform your doctor if you experience light-headedness.

Calcimar
ᴧᴧᴧᴧᴧᴧᴧᴧᴧᴧᴧᴧᴧᴧᴧᴧᴧᴧᴧᴧᴧᴧᴧᴧᴧᴧᴧᴧᴧᴧᴧᴧᴧᴧᴧ

Generic name: Calcitonin-salmon

Calcimar is a synthetic form of the thyroid hormone. It works to stimulate and regulate body functions.

℞ QUICK FACTS

Purpose

 Used to treat: Paget's disease (abnormal bone growth), hypercalcemia (abnormally high calcium blood levels), and postmenopausal osteoporosis.

Dosage

 Taken by injection, self or doctor administered. If self-administered, follow doctor's instructions carefully; must inject under the skin or into a muscle, *not into a vein.* To avoid nausea, vomiting, and skin flushing, take injection at bedtime. *Do not use Calcimar solution if it has a color change or particles floating in it.* If taking for postmenopausal osteoporosis, make sure your diet includes foods rich in calcium and vitamin D.

 Usual adult dose: prescribed according to individual's specific needs and condition being treated.

 Usual child dose: not generally prescribed for children.

 Missed dose: *if taking Calcimar 2 times per day*—take as soon as possible, unless within 2 hours of next dose. In that case, go back to regular schedule; if time for next dose, do not take missed dose; go back to regular schedule. *If taking Calcimar 1 time per day*—take as soon as possible, then go back to regular schedule; if you do not remember until the next day, skip the missed dose; go back to regular schedule. *If taking Calcimar every other day*—take as soon as possible, if it is the same day you are scheduled to take it; then go back to regular schedule. If you do not remember until the next day, skip a day, and start your schedule again. *If taking Calcimar 3 times a week*—take as soon as possible, or the next day, then set each injection back a day for the rest of the week. In the following week go back to your regular schedule. *Regardless of schedule, never double doses.*

Side Effects

 Overdose symptoms: nausea, vomiting. If you suspect an overdose, immediately seek medical attention.

. . . .

 More common side effects: inflamed skin at injection site, nausea, vomiting.

. . . .

 Less common side effects: flushed face, flushed hands, severe allergic reaction, skin rashes.

Interactions

 No known drug interactions.

. . . .

 No known food/other substance interactions.

Special Cautions

 If pregnant or planning to become pregnant, inform your doctor immediately. Not known whether Calcimar appears in breast milk; doctors usually advise women not to take while breastfeeding.

. . . .

 No special precautions apply to seniors.

. . . .

 Not generally prescribed for children.

. . . .

 Serious allergic reactions (shock, difficulty breathing, wheezing, and swelling of the throat or tongue) have been reported in some people.

. . . .

Should not use if sensitive or allergic to Calcimar; may want to have a skin test to determine whether sensitivity exists.

Monitor for: abnormally low blood level of calcium, resulting in cramps, spasms and twitches in the face, feet, and hands; and reduced effectiveness of medication.

If taking on a long-term basis, doctor should give periodic blood and urine tests.

Calcitonin-Salmon

see CALCIMAR

Calcitriol

see ROCALTROL

Capoten

Generic name: Captopril

Capoten is an antihypertensive and angiotensin-converting enzyme (ACE) inhibitor. It works to reduce blood pressure by preventing angiotensin I from converting into a more potent enzyme that increases salt and water retention.

℞ QUICK FACTS

Purpose

℞ Used to treat high blood pressure and congestive heart failure. Also used to improve survival in certain people who have had heart attacks, and to treat kidney disease in diabetics. Some doctors prescribe for crushing chest pain, Raynaud's phenomenon, and rheumatoid arthritis.

Dosage

Take 1 hour before meals. Must take regularly to be effective against high blood pressure. May take several weeks to see full benefit. If taking an antacid such as Maalox, take it 2 hours before taking Capoten. Follow instructions carefully, stopping medication abruptly can cause blood pressure to rise.

Usual adult dose: *for high blood pressure*—25 milligrams taken 2 or 3 times per day. (With kidney or major health problems, dose may be lower.) Doctor may increase to a total of 150 milligrams taken 2 or 3 times per day. *For heart failure*—25 milligrams taken 3 times per day, not to exceed 450 milligrams. *After heart attack*—6.25 milligrams taken once, followed by 12.5 milligrams taken 3 times per day. Doctor may increase to 25 milligrams taken 3 times per day, then to 50 milligrams taken 3 times per day over a span of several weeks. *For kidney disease in diabetes*—25 milligrams taken 3 times per day. *For seniors*—doctor will prescribe according to individual needs.

Usual child dose: not generally prescribed for children.

Missed dose: take as soon as possible, unless almost time for next dose. In that case, do not take missed dose, go back to regular schedule. *Do not double doses.*

Side Effects

Overdose symptoms: light-headedness and dizziness caused by sudden drop in blood pressure. If you suspect an overdose, immediately seek medical attention.

More common side effects: itching, loss of taste, low blood pressure, rash.

 Less common or rare side effects: abdominal pain, anemia, blisters, blurred vision, breast development in males, cardiac arrest, changes in heart rhythm, chest pain, confusion, constipation, cough, depression, diarrhea, difficulty swallowing, dizziness, dry mouth, fatigue, fever and chills, flushing, general feeling of ill health, hair loss, headache, heart attack, heart failure, impotence, inability to sleep, indigestion, inflammation of the nose, inflammation of the tongue, labored breathing, lack of coordination, loss of appetite, lung inflammation, muscle pain and/or weakness, nausea, nervousness, pallor, palpitations, peptic ulcer, rapid heartbeat, sensitivity to light, severe chest pain, skin inflammation, skin peeling, sleepiness, sore throat, stomach irritation, stroke, sudden fainting or loss of strength, swelling (of face, lips, tongue, throat, arms, or legs), tingling or pins and needles, vomiting, weakness, wheezing, yellow eyes and skin.

Interactions

 Inform your doctor before combining Capoten with: Allopurinol (Zyloprim), Aspirin, blood pressure beta-blockers such as Inderal and Tenormin, Cyclosporine (Sandimmune), Digoxin (Lanoxin), Nitroglycerin and similar heart medicines (Nitro-Dur or Transderm-Nitro), nonsteroidal anti-inflammatory drugs such as Indocin and Feldene, potassium preparations such as Micro-K and Slow-K, potassium-sparing diuretics such as Aldactone and Midamor. Do not use potassium-containing salt substitutes while taking Capoten.

 No known food/other substance interactions.

Special Cautions

 ACE inhibitor medicines such as Capoten have caused injury and death to the fetus when used by pregnant women during the 2nd and 3rd trimesters. If pregnant or planning to become pregnant, inform your doctor immediately. Appears in breast milk; could affect a nursing infant.

 Doctor will prescribe dosage according to individual needs.

 Not generally prescribed for children.

 Contact your doctor immediately if you develop: chest pain, difficulty swallowing, or swelling of the face around your lips, tongue, or throat. May be an emergency situation.

Should not take if sensitive or allergic to this or similar medications.

Before taking Capoten, doctor should assess kidney function, and continue to monitor during therapy.

If you experience yellowing of the skin or whites of the eyes, stop taking Capoten and call your doctor.

Check with your doctor before increasing physical activity if taking Capoten for heart problems.

Monitor for low blood pressure and light-headedness after first few doses. Taking a diuretic with Capoten, and dehydration (from excessive perspiration, vomiting, and /or diarrhea) may also cause low blood pressure.

Sore throat or fever may indicate a more serious illness; immediately inform your doctor if these symptoms appear.

Capozide

Generic ingredients: Captopril with Hydrochlorothiazide

Capozide is an antihypertensive/diuretic combination. Antihypertensives work to reduce blood pressure. Diuretics promote the loss of salt and water in the body and increase the diameter of the blood vessels, thereby lowering blood pressure.

℞ QUICK FACTS

Purpose

℞   Used to treat high blood pressure.

Dosage

    Must take regularly for it to be effective; continue taking Capozide even if feeling well.

    Usual adult dose: initial dose is one 25 milligram or 15 milligram tablet once a day. Doctor will adjust dose upward every 6 weeks if required. Daily dose should not exceed 150 milligrams Captopril and 50 milligrams Hydrochlorothiazide. *For seniors and people with decreased kidney function*—doctor will adjust dose according to specific needs.

    Usual child dose: not generally prescribed for children.

Missed dose: take as soon as possible, unless almost time for next dose. In that case, do not take missed dose, go back to regular schedule. *Do not double doses.*

Side Effects

Overdose symptoms: coma, hypermotility, lethargy, low blood pressure, sluggishness, stomach and intestinal irritation. If you suspect an overdose, immediately seek medical attention.

More common side effects: itching, loss of taste, low blood pressure, rash.

Less common or rare side effects: abdominal pain, blurred vision, breast development in males, bronchitis, bronchospasm, changes in heart rhythm, chest pain, confusion, constipation, cough, cramping, depression, diarrhea, dizziness, dizziness upon standing up, dry mouth, fainting, fatigue, fever, flushing, general feeling of ill health, hair loss, headache, heart attack, heart failure, hepatitis, hives, inability to sleep, indigestion, impotence, inflammation of nose, inflammation of tongue, labored breathing, lack of coordination, loss of appetite, low potassium levels leading to symptoms such as dry mouth, excessive thirst, weak or irregular heartbeat, muscle pain and/or weakness, muscle spasm, nausea, nervousness, pallor, peptic ulcer, rapid heartbeat, Raynaud's Syndrome (circulatory disorder), restlessness, sensitivity to light, severe allergic reactions, severe chest pain, skin inflammation and/or peeling, sleepiness, stomach irritation, stroke, swelling (of the arms, legs, face, lips, tongue, or throat), tingling or pins and needles, vomiting, vertigo, weakness, wheezing, yellow eyes and skin.

Interactions

 Inform your doctor before combining Capozide with: antigout drugs such as Zyloprim; barbiturates such as Phenobarbital and Seconal; calcium; cardiac glycosides such as Lanoxin; Cholestyramine (Questran); Colestipol (Colestid); corticosteroids such as Prednisone; diabetes medications; Diazoxide (Proglycem); Lithium (Lithonate); MAO inhibitors (Nardil or Parnate); Methenamine (Mandelamine); narcotics such as Percocet; Nitroglycerin or other nitrates such as Transderm-Nitro; nonsteroidal anti-inflammatory drugs such as Naprosyn; Norepinephrine (Levophed); oral blood thinners such as Coumadin; other blood pressure medications such as Vasotec and Procardia XL; potassium-sparing diuretics such as Moduretic; potassium supplements such as Slow-K; Probenecid (Benemid); salt substitutes containing potassium; Sulfinpyrazone (Anturane).

 Do not drink alcohol when taking Capozide.

Special Cautions

 ACE inhibitor medicines such as Capozide have caused injury and death to the fetus when used by pregnant women during the 2nd and 3rd trimesters. If pregnant or planning to become pregnant, inform your doctor immediately. Appears in breast milk; could affect a nursing infant.

 Doctor will prescribe dosage according to individual needs.

 Not generally prescribed for children.

 Contact your doctor immediately if you develop: chest pain, difficulty swallowing, or swelling of the face around your lips, tongue, or throat. May be an emergency situation.

Should not take if sensitive to or allergic to this or similar medications.

Should not take if unable to urinate.

Before taking Capoten, doctor should assess kidney function, and continue to monitor during therapy.

Sore throat or fever may indicate a more serious illness; immediately inform your doctor if these symptoms appear.

Use with caution if you have: congestive heart failure, impaired kidney function, liver disease or are on dialysis, or lupus erythematosus.

Excessive sweating, dehydration, severe diarrhea, or vomiting could deplete your fluids, thereby lowering blood pressure. Check with your doctor before increasing physical activity.

Captopril
see CAPOTEN

Captopril with Hydrochlorothiazide
see CAPOZIDE

Carafate

Generic name: Sucralfate

Carafate is an anti-ulcer medication. It works by forming a chemical barrier over an exposed ulcer, protecting it from stomach acid.

℞ QUICK FACTS

Purpose

℞ Used to treat active duodenal ulcers. Also used to treat ulcers in the mouth and esophagus caused by cancer therapy, digestive tract irritation caused by stomach ulcer drugs, and pain relief after tonsil removal.

Dosage

 Take on an empty stomach. Avoid taking antacids ½ hour before or after taking Carafate. Take exactly as prescribed.

 Usual adult dose: *for active duodenal ulcer*—1 gram (1 tablet or 2 teaspoonfuls of suspension) 4 times per day on an empty stomach. Should continue 4 to 8 weeks. *Maintenance therapy*—1 gram (1 tablet) 2 times per day.

 Usual child dose: not generally prescribed for children.

 Missed dose: take as soon as possible, unless almost time for next dose. In that case, do not take missed dose; go back to regular schedule. *Do not double doses.*

Side Effects

 Overdose symptoms: no specific information available. If you suspect an overdose, immediately seek medical attention.

 Most common side effect: constipation.

 Less common or rare side effects: back pain, diarrhea, dizziness, dry mouth, gas, headache, indigestion, insomnia, itching, nausea, possible allergic reactions including hives and breathing difficulty, rash, sleepiness, stomach upset, vertigo, vomiting.

Interactions

 Inform your doctor before combining Carafate with: antacids such as Maalox; blood-thinning drugs such as Coumadin; Cimetidine (Tagamet); Digoxin (Lanoxin); drugs for controlling spasms such as Bentyl; Ketoconazole (Nizoral); Phenytoin (Dilantin); Quinidine (Quinidex); Quinolone antibiotics such as Cipro and Floxin; Ranitidine (Zantac); Tetracycline (Achromycin V); Theophylline (Theo-Dur).

 No known food/other substance interactions.

Special Cautions

 If pregnant or planning to become pregnant, inform your doctor immediately. May appear in breast milk, could affect a nursing baby.

 No special precautions apply to seniors.

 Not generally prescribed for children.

 Use with caution if you have kidney failure or are on dialysis.

Carbamazepine

see TEGRETOL

Carbidopa with Levodopa

see SINEMET CR

Carbinoxamine Maleate with Pseudoephedrine Hydrochloride

see RONDEC

Carbodec

see RONDEC

Cardene

Generic name: Nicardipine hydrochloride
Other brand name: Cardene SR

Cardene is a calcium channel blocker. It increases the amount of oxygen that reaches the heart muscle.

℞ QUICK FACTS

Purpose

℞ Used to treat chronic stable chest pain (angina) and high blood pressure. Also used to prevent migraine headaches, and with other medications such as Amicar is used to manage neurological problems after a stroke. Using Cardene to treat congestive heart failure has been studied.

Dosage

 Take exactly as prescribed, even if symptoms disappear. Keep to your dosage schedule; if not taken regularly, condition may worsen. If taking Cardene SR, a long-acting form, must swallow whole.

· ·

 Usual adult dose: *for chest pain (immediate-release only)*—starting dose is 20 milligrams 3 times per day. Regular dose is 20 to 40 milligrams 3 times per day. *For high blood pressure*—starting dose is 20 milligrams 3 times per day. Regular dose is 20 to 40 milligrams 3 times per day. *For Cardene SR*—starting dose is 30 milligrams 2 times per day. Regular dose is 30 to 60 milligrams 2 times per day. *For seniors*— use with caution.

· ·

 Usual child dose: not generally prescribed for children.

· ·

 Missed dose: take as soon as possible, unless almost time for next dose. In that case, do not take missed dose; go back to regular schedule. *Do not double doses.*

Side Effects

 Overdose symptoms: confusion, drowsiness, severe low blood pressure, slow heartbeat, slurred speech.

If you suspect an overdose, immediately seek medical attention.

 More common side effects: dizziness, flushing, headache, increased chest pain, indigestion, nausea, pounding or rapid heartbeat, sleepiness, swelling of feet, weakness.

 Less common side effects: abnormal dreaming, constipation, difficulty sleeping, drowsiness, dry mouth, excessive nighttime urination, fainting, fluid retention, muscle pain, nervousness, rash, shortness of breath, tingling or pins and needles, tremors, vomiting, vague feeling of bodily discomfort. Rare side effects: allergic reactions, anxiety, blurred vision, confusion, dizziness when standing, depression, hot flashes, increased movements, infection, inflammation of the nose, inflammation of the sinuses, impotence, joint pain, low blood pressure, more frequent urination, ringing in ears, sore throat, unusual chest pain, vertigo, vision changes.

Interactions

 Inform your doctor before combining Cardene with: Amiodarone (Cordarone), Cimetidine (Tagamet), Cyclosporine (Sandimmune), Digoxin (Lanoxin), Phenytoin (Dilantin), Propranolol (Inderal).

 No known food/other substance interactions.

Special Cautions

 If pregnant or planning to become pregnant, inform your doctor immediately. May appear in breast milk; could affect a nursing baby.

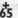 Seniors should use with caution.

Not generally prescribed for children.

 Should not take if you have advanced aortic steno-sis.

Use with caution if you have: congestive heart failure (especially if taking a beta-blocker), light-headedness or faint, liver disease or decreased liver function.

Should not take if sensitive to or allergic to this medication.

Check with your doctor before engaging in exercise or exertion.

Contact your doctor if you experience chest pain (increased) upon starting Cardene or when dosage is increased.

Cardizem

Generic name: Diltiazem hydrochloride

Other brand names: Cardizem CD, Cardizem SR, Dilacor XR

Cardizem is a calcium channel blocker. It increases the amount of oxygen that reaches the heart muscle.

℞ QUICK FACTS

Purpose

 Used to treat chest pain (angina) due to coronary artery spasm and chronic stable angina. Also used to treat high blood pressure, loss of circulation in the fingers and toes (Raynaud's Syndrome), involuntary movements (tardive dyskinesia), and to prevent second heart attack.

Dosage

 Take before meals and at bedtime; must swallow whole.

 Usual adult dose: 180 to 360 milligrams divided into 3 or 4 smaller doses. *For Cardizem SR (sustained release)—60 to 120 milligrams 2 times per day, up to 240 to 360 milligrams per day. For Cardizem CD (once-a-day form)—hypertension dose is 180 to 240 milligrams per day; angina dose is 120 to 180 milligrams per day.*

 Usual child dose: not generally prescribed for children.

 Missed dose: take as soon as possible, unless almost time for next dose. In that case, do not take missed dose; go back to regular schedule. *Do not double doses.*

Side Effects

 Overdose symptoms: fainting, dizziness, and irregular pulse due to heart block, heart failure, low blood pressure, very slow heartbeat. If you suspect an overdose, immediately seek medical attention.

 More common side effects: abnormally slow heartbeat (Cardizem SR and CD), dizziness, fluid retention, flushing (Cardizem SR and CD), headache, nausea, rash, weakness.

 Less common or rare side effects: abnormal dreams, amnesia, anemia, blood disorders, congestive heart failure, constipation, depression, diarrhea, difficulty sleeping, drowsiness, dry mouth, excessive urination at night, eye irritation, fainting, hair loss, hallucinations, heart attack, high blood sugar, hives, impotence, increased output of pale urine, indigestion, insomnia, irregular heartbeat, itching, joint pain, labored breathing, loss of appetite, low blood pressure, low blood sugar, muscle cramps, nasal congestion, nervousness, nosebleed, palpitations, personality change, rapid heartbeat, reddish or purplish spots on skin, ringing in ears, sexual difficulties, skin peeling, sensitivity to light, severe chest pain, sleepiness, taste alteration, thirst, tingling or pins and needles, tremor, unusual gait, vision changes, vomiting, weight increase, welts.

Interactions

Inform your doctor before combining Cardizem with: beta-blockers such as Tenormin and Inderal, Cimetidine (Tagamet), Cyclosporine (Sandimmune), Digoxin (Lanoxin), Ranitidine (Zantac).

No known food/other substance interactions.

Special Cautions

If pregnant or planning to become pregnant, inform your doctor immediately. Appears in breast milk; could affect a nursing baby.

No special precautions apply to seniors.

Not generally prescribed for children.

Do not take if you have low blood pressure or allergy to Cardizem.

Should not take Cardizem without a ventricular pacemaker if you have "sick sinus" syndrome or 2nd or 3rd degree heart block (irregular heartbeat).

Use with caution if you have: congestive heart failure, kidney or liver disease.

Monitor pulse rate, may cause heart rate to become too slow.

Cardura

Generic name: Doxazosin mesylate

Cardura is an antihypertensive agent. It works to reduce blood pressure.

℞ QUICK FACTS

Purpose

℞ Used to treat high blood pressure. Also used to treat benign prostatic hyperplasia (BPH), an abnormal enlargement of the prostate gland, and with other medications such as Digitalis and diuretics to treat congestive heart failure.

Dosage

 May be taken with or without food.

 Usual adult dose: 1 milligram taken once per day to start. May be increased to 2 milligrams per day, up to 16 milligrams per day. As dose increases, so does potential for side effects.

 Usual child dose: not generally prescribed for children.

 Missed dose: take as soon as possible, unless almost time for next dose. In that case, do not take missed

dose; go back to regular schedule. *Do not double doses.*

Side Effects

 Overdose symptom: low blood pressure is the most likely symptom. If you suspect an overdose, immediately seek medical attention.

 More common side effects: dizziness, drowsiness, fatigue, headache.

 Less common side effects: arthritis, constipation, depression, difficulty sleeping, eye pain, flushing, gas, inability to hold urine, indigestion, inflammation of conjunctiva (pink eye), itching joint pain, lack of muscle coordination, low blood pressure, motion disorders, muscle cramps, muscle pain, muscle weakness, nausea, nervousness, nosebleeds, rash, ringing in ears, shortness of breath, tingling or pins and needles, weakness. Rare side effects: abnormal thinking, abnormal vision, agitation, altered sense of smell, amnesia, back pain, breast pain, changeable emotions, changes in taste, chest pain, confusion, coughing, decreased sense of touch, diarrhea, dizziness when standing up, dry mouth, dry skin, earache, excessive urination, fainting, fecal incontinence, fever, fluid retention, flu-like symptoms, gout, hair loss, heart attack, hot flushes, inability to concentrate, inability to tolerate light, increased appetite, increased sweating, increased thirst, infection, inflammation of the nose, loss of appetite, loss of sense of personal identity, migraine headache, morbid dreams, nausea, nervousness, pain, pallor, rapid pounding heartbeat, sexual problems, sinus inflammation, slight or partial paralysis, sore throat, tremors, twitching, vertigo, weight gain, weight loss, wheezing.

Interactions

 No significant drug interactions reported with Cardura.

 No known food/other substance interactions.

 If pregnant or planning to become pregnant, inform your doctor immediately. May appear in breast milk; could affect a nursing baby.

 Seniors should use this medication with caution.

 Not generally prescribed for children.

 Avoid driving or any hazardous tasks within 24 hours of the first dose; may experience fainting, dizziness, or light-headedness. Additionally, may cause drowsiness; *do not take part in any activity that requires alertness.*

Should not take if sensitive to or allergic to this or medications such as Minipress or Hytrin.

Doctor should monitor closely if you have liver disease or are taking medications which affect liver function, and monitor blood counts.

Carisoprodol
see SOMA

Cataflam
see VOLTAREN

Catapres

~~~~~~

Generic name: Clonidine hydrochloride

Other brand name: Catapres-TTS

Catapres is an antihypertensive agent. It works to reduce blood pressure.

℞ QUICK FACTS

Purpose

℞ Used to treat high blood pressure. Also used to treat alcohol, nicotine, or tranquilizer withdrawal; migraine headaches; smoking cessation; Tourette's syndrome; premenstrual tension; and diabetic diarrhea.

Dosage

🍽 Take exactly as prescribed, even if you feel well. Follow schedule closely; if not taken consistently, condition may get worse.

💊 Usual adult dose: 0.1 milligram 2 times per day (morning and night) initially. Regular, ongoing dose ranges from 0.2 milligrams to 0.6 milligrams per day divided into smaller doses, not to exceed 2.4 milligrams per day. *Transdermal patch*—dose determined based on your blood pressure response.

🧸 Usual child dose: not generally prescribed for children under 12 years.

  Missed dose: take as soon as possible, then go back to regular schedule. If 2 or more doses in a row are missed, or if you forget to change the patch for days, contact your doctor.

Side Effects

 Overdose symptoms: changes in heart function, constriction of pupils in the eye, high blood pressure, irritability, low blood pressure, reduced rate of breathing, seizures, sleepiness, slow heartbeat, slowed reflexes, sluggishness, temporary failure to breath, vomiting, weakness. If you suspect an overdose, immediately seek medical attention.

 More common side effects: constipation, dizziness, drowsiness, dry mouth, sedation, skin reactions.

 Less common side effects: agitation, breast development in males, changes in heartbeat, changes in taste, decreased sexual activity, difficulty sleeping, difficulty urinating, dizziness on standing up, excessive nighttime urination, fatigue, fluid retention, hair loss, headache, hives, impotence, itching, joint pain, leg cramps, loss of appetite, loss of sexual drive, mental depression, muscle pain, nausea, nervousness, rash, retention of urine, sluggishness, vague bodily discomfort, vomiting, weakness, weight gain. Rare side effects: anxiety, behavior changes, blurred vision, burning eyes, congestive heart failure, delirium, dry eyes, dry nasal passages, fever, greater sensitivity to alcohol, hallucinations, hepatitis, pallor, restlessness, vivid dreams or nightmares.

Interactions

 Inform your doctor before combining Catapres with: barbiturates such as Nembutal and Seconal; sedatives such as Valium, Xanax, and Halcion; tricyclic antidepressants such as Elavil and Tofranil. If taking beta-blockers with Catapres, stop the beta-blockers *before* the gradual withdrawal of Catapres.

Do not drink alcohol while taking Catapres; may enhance the side effects of Catapres.

Special Cautions

 If pregnant or planning to become pregnant, inform your doctor immediately. Appears in breast milk; could affect a nursing baby.

 Initial dose for seniors may be lower.

 Not generally prescribed for children under 12 years.

 Do not take if sensitive to or allergic reaction to Catapres or any components of the transdermal patch.

Medication should not be abruptly discontinued; severe reactions such as disruption of brain function and death have been reported.

May cause drowsiness and impair your ability to drive a car or operate machinery. *Do not take part in any activity that requires alertness.*

If you have an allergic reaction to the patch, your doctor may switch you to tablets. May have similar allergic reaction to the tablet.

Take with caution if you have: disease of the blood vessels of the brain, severe heart disease, severe kidney disease, or if recovering from a heart attack.

Ceclor

Generic name: Cefaclor

Ceclor is a cephalosporin antibiotic. It interferes with the production of certain biochemicals necessary for bacteria to sustain life.

℞ QUICK FACTS

Purpose

 Used to treat ear, nose, throat, respiratory tract, urinary tract, and skin infections caused by bacteria, such as sore or strep throat, pneumonia, and tonsillitis.

Dosage

 Take exactly as prescribed; finish taking all medication. Works faster when taken on an empty stomach, but doctor may suggest taking with food to avoid stomach upset. Shake suspension well before taking; discard unused portion after 14 days.

 Usual adult dose: 250 milligrams every 8 hours.

 Usual child dose: 20 milligrams per 2.2 pounds of body weight per day divided into smaller doses, and taken every 8 hours. *For more severe infections—40 milligrams per 2.2 pounds of body weight per day divided into smaller doses, not to exceed 1 gram per day.*

 Missed dose: take as soon as possible, unless almost time for next dose. In that case, do not take missed dose; go back to regular schedule. *Do not double doses.*

Side Effects

Overdose symptoms: diarrhea, nausea, stomach upset, vomiting. If you suspect an overdose, immediately seek medical attention.

More common side effects: diarrhea, hives, itching.

 Less common or rare side effects: blood disorders, liver disorders, nausea, skin rashes accompanied by joint pain, vaginal inflammation, vomiting.

Interactions

 Inform your doctor before combining Ceclor with: certain antibiotics such as Amikin, certain diuretics such as Edecrin and Lasix, oral contraceptives, Probenecid (Benemid).

 No known food/other substance interactions.

Special Cautions

 If pregnant or planning to become pregnant, inform your doctor immediately. Appears in breast milk; could affect a nursing baby.

 No special precautions apply to seniors.

 Follow doctor's instructions carefully for children.

 Do not take if you have a history of gastrointestinal problems such as colitis.

If allergic to cephalosporins or penicillins, tell your doctor *before* taking Ceclor; could result in an extremely severe reaction.

May cause false positive reading with urine sugar tests for diabetics.

Before treating diarrhea, check with your doctor about which specific medications to take.

Cefaclor
see CECLOR

Cefadroxil Monohydrate
see DURICEF

Cefixime
see SUPRAX

Cefprozil
see CEFZIL

Ceftin

Generic name: Cefuroxime axetil

Ceftin is a cephalosporin antibiotic. It interferes with the production of certain biochemicals necessary for bacteria to sustain life.

℞ QUICK FACTS

Purpose

℞ Used to treat mild to moderate bacterial infections of the throat, lungs, ears, skin, and urinary tract, and to treat gonorrhea.

Dosage

 Take exactly as prescribed; finish taking all medication. May be taken with or without food; works faster when taken after meals. Treatment for children is in tablet form only. Since tablets have a strong, bitter taste, they may be crushed and mixed with food.

 Usual adult dose (and children 12 years and older): 250 milligrams taken 2 times per day. *For more severe infections*—up to 500 milligrams taken 2 times per day. *For urinary tract infections*—125 milligrams taken 2 times per day, up to 250 milligrams taken 2 times per day for a severe infection. *For gonorrhea*— a single dose of 1 gram.

 Usual child dose: children up to 12 years—125 milligrams taken 2 times per day. *For middle ear infections*: children under 2 years—125 milligrams taken 2 times per day; children over 2 years—250 milligrams 2 times per day.

 Missed dose: *for 1 dose per day*—take as soon as possible, unless almost time for next dose. In that case, take missed dose, and the next dose 10 to 12 hours later, then go back to regular schedule. *For 2 doses per day*—take as soon as possible, unless almost time for next dose. In that case, take missed dose, and the next dose 5 to 6 hours later, then go back to regular schedule. *Do not double doses.*

Side Effects

 Overdose symptoms: overdose can cause brain irritation leading to convulsions. If you suspect an overdose, immediately seek medical attention.

More common side effects: colitis; diarrhea; nausea; skin rashes, redness, or itching; vomiting.

 Less common or rare side effects: dizziness, headache, seizures, vaginal inflammation, yeast infection.

Interactions

 Inform your doctor before combining Ceftin with: Probenecid, a gout medication; and antidiarrheal medications such as Lomotil, which may cause diarrhea side effect to worsen.

 No known food/other substance interactions.

Special Cautions

 If pregnant or planning to become pregnant, inform your doctor immediately. Appears in breast milk; could affect a nursing baby.

 No special precautions apply to seniors.

 Follow doctor's instructions carefully for children.

 If allergic to cephalosporins or penicillins, tell your doctor *before* taking Ceftin; could result in an extremely severe reaction.

May cause false positive reading with urine sugar tests for diabetics.

If you develop diarrhea, contact your doctor immediately; colitis has been associated with using Ceftin.

Cefuroxime Axetil

see CEFTIN

Cefzil

∿∿

Generic name: Cefprozil

Cefzil is a cephalosporin antibiotic. It interferes with the production of certain biochemicals necessary for bacteria to sustain life.

℞ QUICK FACTS

Purpose

℞ Used to treat mild to moderately severe bacterial infections of the throat, ear, respiratory tract, and skin, such as strep throat, tonsillitis, bronchitis, and pneumonia.

Dosage

 Take exactly as prescribed; finish taking all medication. Works faster when taken on an empty stomach, but doctor may suggest taking with food to avoid stomach upset. Shake suspension well before taking; discard unused portion after 14 days.

. . . .

 Usual adult dose: *for throat and respiratory tract infections*—500 milligrams taken once per day for 10 days. *For skin infections*—250 milligrams taken 2 times per day, or 500 milligrams taken 1 or 2 times per day for 10 days.

. . . .

 Usual child dose: *for children 2 to 12 years*—7.5 milligrams for each 2.2 pounds of body weight, taken 2 times per day for 10 days (for throat infections and tonsillitis). *For infants and children 6 months to 12 years*—15 milligrams for each 2.2 pounds of body weight, taken 2 times per day for 10 days (for ear infections). *For infants under 6 months*—not generally prescribed.

. . . .

Missed dose: take as soon as possible, unless almost time for next dose. In that case, do not take missed dose; go back to regular schedule. *Do not double doses.*

Side Effects

 Overdose symptoms: no specific information available. If you suspect an overdose, immediately seek medical attention.

 Most common side effect: nausea.

 Less common or rare side effects: abdominal pain, confusion, diaper rash, diarrhea, difficulty sleeping, dizziness, genital itching, headache, hives, hyperactivity, nervousness, rash, sleepiness, superinfection (additional infection), vaginal inflammation, vomiting, yellow eyes and skin.

Interactions

 Inform your doctor before combining Cefzil with: other antibiotics such as Amikin, diuretics such as Edecrin and Lasix, oral contraceptives, Probenecid (Benemid), Propantheline (Pro-Banthine).

 No known food/other substance interactions.

Special Cautions

 If pregnant or planning to become pregnant, inform your doctor immediately. May appear in breast milk; could affect a nursing baby.

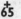 No special precautions apply to seniors.

 Follow doctor's instructions carefully for children.

If allergic to cephalosporins or penicillins, tell your doctor *before* taking Cefzil; could result in an extremely severe reaction.

If you develop diarrhea, contact your doctor immediately, colitis has been associated with using Cefzil.

Doctor should check kidney function before treatment, and monitor while on treatment.

Use with caution if: taking a strong diuretic, or if you have had stomach and intestinal disease such as colitis.

May need to be treated with another antibiotic if you get a new infection.

Can alter urine sugar test results (for diabetes).

Cephalexin Hydrochloride
see KEFLEX

Chlordiazepoxide
see LIBRIUM

Chlordiazepoxide Hydrochloride with Clidinium Bromide
see LIBRAX

Chlorhexidine Gluconate
see PERIDEX

Chlorothiazide
see DIURIL

Chlorpheniramine Maleate with d-Pseudoephedrine Hydrochloride
see DECONAMINE

Chlorpromazine
see THORAZINE

Chlorpropamide
see DIABINESE

Chlorthalidone
see HYGROTON

Chlorzoxazone
see PARAFON FORTE DSC

Cholestyramine
see QUESTRAN

Choline Magnesium Trisalicylate
see TRILISATE

Chronulac Syrup

Generic name: Lactulose

Other brand names: Cephulac, Cholac, Constilac, Duphalac, Enulose

Chronulac Syrup is a laxative. It works by increasing the stool's fluid content, promoting bowel evacuation.

℞ QUICK FACTS

Purpose

℞ Used to treat constipation. For chronic constipation, increases the number and frequency of bowel movements.

Dosage

 Take exactly as prescribed. May take with water, fruit juice, or milk. *Do not take if you are on a low-galactose diet.*

 Usual adult dose: 1 to 2 tablespoonfuls (15 to 30 milliliters) per day, up to 60 milliliters per day.

 Usual child dose: *for portal-systemic encephalopathy only*—30 to 45 milliliters 3 or 4 times per day.

 Missed dose: take as soon as possible, *do not double doses.*

Side Effects

 Overdose symptoms: abdominal cramps, diarrhea. If you suspect an overdose, immediately seek medical attention.

 Side effects: diarrhea, gas, intestinal cramps, nausea, potassium and fluid loss, vomiting.

 No known less common or rare side effects.

Interactions

 Inform your doctor before taking Chronulac syrup with non-absorbable antacids such as Maalox and Mylanta.

 No known food/other substance interactions.

Special Cautions

 If pregnant or planning to become pregnant, inform your doctor immediately. May appear in breast milk; could affect a nursing baby.

No special precautions apply to seniors.

 Not generally prescribed for children except in the case of portal-systemic encephalopathy.

 May take 24 to 48 hours to have a normal bowel movement.

Use with caution if you are diabetic.

Notify your doctor of unusual diarrhea.

Ciclopirox Olamine
see LOPROX

Cimetidine
see TAGAMET

Cipro
~~~~~~

Generic name: Ciprofloxacin hydrochloride

Other brand name: Ciloxan Eyedrops

Cipro is an antibiotic and antibacterial. It interferes with the production of certain biochemicals necessary for bacteria to sustain life.

℞ QUICK FACTS

Purpose

 Used to treat lower respiratory tract, skin, bone and joint, and urinary tract infections. Also used to treat infectious diarrhea, serious ear infections, tuberculosis, infections common in AIDS patients, and ocular infections.

Dosage

 May be taken with or without food, best tolerated when taken 2 hours after a meal. Drink plenty of fluids while taking Cipro. Take medication exactly as prescribed—consistently, at evenly spaced intervals.

 Usual adult dose: 250 milligrams taken every 12 hours. *For more serious infections*—500 milligrams taken every 12 hours. *For lower respiratory tract, skin, bone and joint infections*—500 milligrams taken every 12 hours; more serious infections may require 750 milligrams taken every 12 hours. *For infectious diarrhea*—500 milligrams every 12 hours. *Eyedrops*—1 or 2 drops in affected eye several times per day, as prescribed by your doctor.

 Usual child dose: not generally prescribed for children.

 Missed dose: take as soon as possible, unless almost time for next dose. In that case, do not take missed dose; go back to regular schedule. *Do not double doses.*

Side Effects

 Overdose symptoms: no specific information. If you suspect an overdose, immediately seek medical attention.

More common side effects: abdominal pain, diarrhea, headache, nausea, rash, restlessness, vomiting.

 Less common side effects: abnormal dread or fear, achiness, bleeding in the stomach and/or intestines, blood clots in the lungs, blurred vision, change in visual perception of colors, chills, confusion, constipation, convulsions, coughing up blood, decreased vision, depression, difficulty swallowing, dizziness, double vision, drowsiness, eye pain, fainting, fever, flushing, gas, gout flare-up, hallucinations, hearing loss, heart attack, hiccups, high blood pressure, hives, inability to fall or stay asleep, inability to urinate, indigestion, intestinal inflammation, involuntary eye movement, irregular heartbeat, irritability, itching, joint or back pain, joint stiffness, kidney failure, labored breathing, lack of muscle coordination, lack or loss of appetite, large volumes of urine, light-headedness, loss of sense of identity, loss of sense of smell, mouth sores, neck pain, nightmares, nosebleed, pounding heartbeat, ringing in the ears, seizures, sensitivity to light, severe allergic reaction, skin peeling, redness, sluggishness, speech difficulties, swelling (of the face, neck, lips, eyes, hands, or throat), tender red bumps on the skin, tingling sensation, tremors, unpleasant taste, unusual darkening of the skin, vaginal inflammation, vague feeling of illness, weakness, yellowed eyes and skin.

Interactions

 Inform your doctor before combining Cipro with: Cyclophosphamide (Cytoxan), Cyclosporine (Sandimmune), Metoprolol (Lopressor), Phenytoin (Dilantin), Probenecid (Benemid), Sucralfate (Carafate), Theophylline (Theo-Dur), Warfarin (Coumadin). *Taking Cipro with Theophylline (Theo-Dur) has caused serious and fatal reactions, including cardiac arrest, seizures,*

continuous attacks of epilepsy with no periods of consciousness, and respiratory failure.

 Cipro may increase the effects of caffeine. Products with iron, multivitamins containing zinc, and antacids containing magnesium, aluminum, or calcium may interfere with absorption of Cipro.

Special Cautions

 If pregnant or planning to become pregnant, inform your doctor immediately. Appears in breast milk; could affect a nursing baby.

 No special precautions apply to seniors.

 Not generally prescribed for children.

 Notify your doctor immediately if a skin rash or other allergic reaction occurs. Although rare, serious and occasionally fatal allergic reactions—some following the first dose—have been reported. If sensitive to or had an allergic reaction to this or similar drugs, you should not take this medication.

May cause dizziness or light-headedness and impair your ability to drive a car or operate machinery. *Do not take part in any activity that requires alertness.*

Convulsions have been reported; if you experience a seizure or convulsions, notify your doctor immediately.

Prolonged use may result in a secondary infection not treatable by Cipro; doctor should monitor your condition on a regular basis.

Tell your doctor before taking Cipro if you have a known or suspected central nervous system disor-

der such as epilepsy, or hardening of the arteries in
the brain.

May become sensitive to light while taking Cipro.

Doctor should monitor your urine, kidney and liver
function, and blood if taking Cipro for an extended
period.

Ciprofloxacin Hydrochloride

see CIPRO

Cisapride

see PROPULSID

Clarithromycin

see BIAXIN

Claritin

Generic name: Loratadine

Claritin is an antihistamine. Antihistamines block the effects of histamine, a body chemical that causes swelling
and itching.

℞ QUICK FACTS

Purpose

 Used to treat the symptoms of hay fever—itching, runny nose, sneezing, stuffiness, and teary eyes.

Dosage

 Take on an empty stomach, and exactly as prescribed.

 Usual adult dose: one 10-milligram tablet taken one time per day. *For people with liver disease—one 10-milligram tablet taken every other day.*

 Usual child dose: *for children 12 years and older only—*same as adult dose.

 Missed dose: take as soon as possible, unless almost time for next dose. In that case, do not take missed dose; go back to regular schedule. *Do not double doses.*

Side Effects

 Overdose symptoms: headache, rapid heartbeat, sleepiness. If you suspect an overdose, immediately seek medical attention.

 More common side effects: dry mouth, fatigue, headache, sleepiness.

Less common or rare side effects: abdominal discomfort or pain, abnormal dreams, aggravated allergy, agitation, anxiety, back pain, blurred vision, breast enlargement, breast pain, bronchitis, change in salivation, change in taste, chest pain, chills and fever, confusion, conjunctivitis (pink eye), constipation, coughing up blood, decreased sensitivity to touch, decreased sex drive, depression, diarrhea, difficult or labored breathing, difficulty concentrating, difficulty speaking, discoloration of urine, dizziness, dry hair, dry skin, earache, eye pain, fainting, fever, flushing, gas, general feeling of illness, hair loss, hepatitis, high blood pressure, hives, hyperactivity, impotence, inability to fall or stay asleep, increased appetite, increased or decreased eye tearing, increased sweating, indigestion, inflammation of the mouth, itching, joint pain, laryngitis, leg cramps, loss of appetite, low blood pressure, memory loss, menstrual changes, migraine, muscle pain, nasal congestion, nasal dryness and inflammation, nausea, nervousness, nosebleeds, palpitations, rapid heartbeat, rash, red or purple spots on the skin, ringing in ears, seizures, sensitivity to light, sinus inflammation, skin eruptions, skin inflammation, sneezing, sore throat, stomach inflammation, swelling caused by allergic reaction, swelling of extremities, thirst, tingling or pins and needles, toothache, tremor, twitching of the eye, upper respiratory infection, urinary changes, vaginal inflammation, vertigo, vomiting, weakness, weight gain, wheezing, yellow eyes and skin.

Interactions

 Inform your doctor before combining Claritin with: certain antibiotics, Cimetidine (Tagamet), Ketoconazole (Nizoral), Ranitidine (Zantac), Theophylline (Theo-Dur).

 No known food/other substance interactions.

Special Cautions

 If pregnant or planning to become pregnant, inform your doctor immediately. Appears in breast milk; could affect a nursing baby.

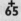 Can cause excessive sleepiness in seniors.

Not generally prescribed for children under 12 years.

 Do not take if sensitive or had allergic reaction to Claritin or any of its ingredients.

If you have liver disease, doctor should prescribe a lower starting dose.

May cause excessive sleepiness in people with kidney or liver disease.

Clemastine Fumarate

see TAVIST

Cleocin T

Generic name: Clindamycin phosphate

Cleocin T is an antibiotic. It slows the growth of bacteria that form acne pustules.

℞ QUICK FACTS

Purpose

 Used to treat acne.

Dosage

 Use exactly as prescribed, overuse may dry or irritate skin.

 Usual adult dose: apply thin film of gel, solution, or lotion to affected area 2 times per day. If using lotion, shake well before using. Apply carefully to avoid eyes, nose, mouth or skin abrasions.

 Usual child dose: not generally prescribed for children under 12 years.

 Missed dose: apply as soon as possible, unless almost time for next dose. In that case, do not apply missed dose, go back to regular schedule.

Side Effects

 Overdose symptoms: no specific information available. If you suspect an overdose, immediately seek medical attention.

 Most common side effect: dry skin.

 Less common or rare side effects: abdominal pain, bloody diarrhea, burning or abdominal redness of skin, colitis, diarrhea, oily skin, peeling skin, skin inflammation and irritation, stomach and intestinal disturbances.

Interactions

 Inform your doctor before combining Cleocin T with: antidiarrheal medications, especially Lomotil.

 Should not use products containing paregoric.

Special Cautions

 If pregnant or planning to become pregnant, inform your doctor immediately. May appear in breast milk; could affect a nursing baby.

65 No special precautions apply to seniors.

Not generally prescribed for children under 12 years.

 There have been severe and even fatal cases of colitis when taken internally. Do not take if you have had an intestinal inflammation, ulcerative colitis, or antibiotic-associated colitis.

Medication can be absorbed into the bloodstream.

If sensitive to or have had an allergic reaction to this or similar medications, you should not use.

Use with caution if you have asthma, eczema, or hay fever.

Clindamycin Phosphate

see CLEOCIN T

Clinoril

Generic name: Sulindac

Clinoril is a nonsteroidal anti-inflammatory drug (NSAID). It works by blocking the production of prostaglandins, which may trigger pain.

℞ QUICK FACTS

Purpose

 Used to treat the swelling, stiffness and joint pain associated with rheumatoid arthritis, osteoarthritis, and ankylosing spondylitis* (stiffness and progressive spine arthritis). Also used to treat bursitis, tendinitis, acute gouty arthritis, and other types of pain.

Dosage

 Take exactly as prescribed. If taking for arthritis, take on a regular basis.

 Usual adult dose: *for osteoarthritis, rheumatoid arthritis, or ankylosing spondylitis*—150 milligrams taken 2 times per day, not to exceed 400 milligrams per day. Take with food. *For acute gouty arthritis or arthritic shoulder and joint condition*—400 milligrams taken in doses of 200 milligrams 2 times per day. Length of therapy is usually 7 to 14 days for painful shoulder, and 7 days for acute gouty arthritis.

 Usual child dose: not generally prescribed for children.

 Missed dose: take as soon as possible, unless almost time for next dose. In that case, do not take missed dose; go back to regular schedule. *Do not double doses.*

Side Effects

 Overdose symptoms: coma, low blood pressure, reduced output of urine, stupor. If you suspect an overdose, immediately seek medical attention.

 More common side effects: abdominal pain, constipation, diarrhea, dizziness, gas, headache, indigestion, itching, loss of appetite, nausea, nervousness, rash, ringing in the ears, stomach cramps, swelling due to fluid retention, vomiting.

 Less common or rare side effects: abdominal bleeding, abdominal inflammation, anemia, appetite change, bloody diarrhea, blurred vision, change in color of urine, chest pain, colitis, congestive heart failure, depression, fever, hair loss, hearing loss, hepatitis, high blood pressure, inability to sleep, inflammation of lips and tongue, kidney failure, liver failure, loss of sense of taste, low blood pressure, muscle and joint pain, nosebleed, painful urination, pancreatitis, peptic ulcer, sensitivity to light, shortness of breath, skin eruptions, sleepiness, Stevens-Johnson syndrome (blisters in mouth and eyes), vaginal bleeding, weakness, yellow eyes and skin.

Interactions

 Inform your doctor before combining Clinoril with: antigout medication such as Benemid; Aspirin; blood thinners such as Coumadin; Cyclosporine (Sandimmune); Diflunisal (Dolobid); Dimethyl sulfoxide (DMSO); Lithium; loop diuretics such as Lasix; Methotrexate; oral diabetes medications (Glucotrol).

 No known food/other substance interactions.

Special Cautions

 If pregnant or planning to become pregnant, inform your doctor immediately. *Drugs of this class are known to cause birth defects.* May appear in breast milk; could affect a nursing baby.

 No special precautions apply to seniors.

 Not generally prescribed for children.

 Immediately stop using Clinoril if you develop pancreatitis; do not restart.

May cause drowsiness and impair your ability to drive a car or operate machinery. *Do not take part in any activity that requires alertness.*

Safety and effectiveness for people with rheumatoid arthritis who are incapacitated, bedridden, in wheelchairs, or unable to care for themselves are not known.

Doctor should monitor your condition frequently; ulcers or internal bleeding can occur with no warning.

If sensitive to or had an allergic reaction to this medication, aspirin or similar drugs, or asthma attacks caused by aspirin or similar drugs, should not take Clinoril.

Use with caution if you have: heart disease or high blood pressure, kidney or liver disease.

Can hide the symptoms of infection; inform your doctor of any infection you may have.

May cause changes in vision; contact your doctor if vision changes.

Clobetasol Propionate

see TEMOVATE

Clomid

Generic name: Clomiphene citrate

Other brand names: Milophene, Serophene

Clomid is a fertility drug. It stimulates release of the hormones that result in ovulation.

℞ QUICK FACTS

Purpose

 Used to treat ovulatory failure in women who are trying to become pregnant.

Dosage

 Take exactly as prescribed.

 Usual adult dose: 50 milligrams (1 tablet daily) for the first course of treatment—5 days. If ovulation does not occur, doctor may prescribe up to 2 more courses of treatment.

 Usual child dose: not prescribed for children.

Missed dose: take as soon as possible. If time for next dose, take the 2 doses together, then go back to your regular schedule. If more than one dose is missed, contact your doctor.

Side Effects

 Overdose symptoms: no information available. If you suspect an overdose, immediately seek medical attention.

 More common side effects: abdominal discomfort, enlargement of the ovaries, hot flushes.

 Less common side effects: abnormal uterine bleeding, breast tenderness, depression, dizziness, fatigue, hair loss, headache, hives, inability to fall or stay asleep, increased urination, inflammation of the skin, light-headedness, nausea, nervousness, ovarian cysts, visual disturbances, vomiting, weight gain.

Interactions

 No known drug interactions.

 No known food/other substance interactions.

Special Cautions

 If you become pregnant, immediately inform your doctor. You should not be pregnant and taking Clomid.

 No special precautions apply to seniors.

 Not prescribed for children.

 Do not use if you have: abnormal uterine bleeding of undetermined origin, an abnormality of the brain such as a pituitary gland tumor, an uncontrolled thyroid or adrenal gland, liver disease or history of liver problems, ovarian cysts or enlargement of the ovaries not caused by polycystic ovarian syndrome, unless directed by your doctor.

Ovarian hyperstimulation syndrome (OSS, enlargement of the ovaries) could occur. Can progress and rapidly become serious. Early warning signs include: nausea, severe pelvic pain, vomiting, and weight gain. Contact your doctor immediately if you experience any of these signs.

Likelihood of getting pregnant decreases with each course of therapy.

Should have a pelvic exam before and after each course of treatment.

Before treatment, doctor should evaluate your liver function and estrogen levels.

Clomid increases the possibility of multiple births and birth defects.

Drive a car or operate machinery with caution; blurring and other visual symptoms can occur. Notify your doctor of any visual disturbances.

Clomiphene Citrate
see CLOMID

Clomipramine Hydrochloride
see ANAFRANIL

Clonazepam
see KLONOPIN

Clonidine Hydrochloride
see CATAPRES

Clopra
see REGLAN

Clorazepate Dipotassium
see TRANXENE

Clotrimazole
see GYNE-LOTRIMIN

Clotrimazole with Betamethasone Dipropionate
see LOTRISONE

Clozapine
see CLOZARIL

Clozaril

Generic name: Clozapine

Clozaril is an antipsychotic. It works by calming certain areas of the brain while enabling the rest of the brain to function properly, screening the transmission of some nerve impulses but restricting others.

℞ QUICK FACTS

Purpose

 Used to treat severe schizophrenia in cases where standard treatments have failed.

Dosage

 Take exactly as directed. Clozaril is distributed *only* via the Clozaril Patient Management Systems, ensuring weekly testing prior to the delivery of the pill supply.

Usual adult dose: ½ of a 25-milligram tablet (12.5 milligrams) 1 or 2 times per day. Doctor may increase in increments of 25 to 50 milligrams a day, up to 300 to 450 milligrams per day total, by the end of 2 weeks. Dosage may increase up to 900 milligrams per day, at weekly increments of 100 milligrams.

 Usual child dose: not prescribed for children under 16 years.

 Missed dose: take as soon as possible, unless almost time for next dose. In that case, do not take missed dose; go back to regular schedule. *Do not double doses.*

Side Effects

 Overdose symptoms: coma, delirium, drowsiness, excess salivation, faintness, low blood pressure, rapid heartbeat, seizures, shallow breathing. If you suspect an overdose, immediately seek medical attention.

 More common side effects: abdominal discomfort, agitated state, constipation, disturbed sleep, dizziness, drowsiness, dry mouth, fainting, fever, headache, heartburn, high blood pressure, loss of muscle movement, low blood pressure, nausea, nightmares, rapid heartbeat and other heart conditions, restlessness, salivation, sedation, sweating, tremors, vertigo, vision problems, weight gain.

 Less common side effects: abdominal distension, abnormal stools, anemia, anxiety, appetite increase, back pain, belching, bitter taste, blood clots, bloodshot eyes, bluish tinge to the skin, breast pain or discomfort, bronchitis, chills, confusion, constant involuntary eye movement, coughing, depression, diarrhea, difficult or labored breathing, dilated pupils, disorientation, dry throat, ear disorders, ejaculation problems, excessive movement, eyelid disorder, fast or fluttery heartbeat, fatigue, fluid retention, frequent urination, hallucinations, hives, hot flashes, impotence, inability to sit down, inability to urinate, increase or decrease in sex drive, inflamed stomach and intestines, involuntary movement, irritability, itching, jerky movements, joint pain, lack of coordination, leg pain, lethargy, light-headedness, loss of appetite, loss of speech, low body temperature, memory loss, muscle pain or ache, muscle spasm, muscle weakness, neck pain, nervous stomach, nosebleed, numbness, painful menstruation, pallor, paranoia, pneumonia-like symptoms, poor coordination, rapid breathing, rash, rectal bleeding, rigidity, runny nose, seizures, severe chest pain, shakiness, shortness of breath, skin inflammation, redness, scaling, sleeplessness, slow heartbeat, slurred speech, sneezing, sore throat, sore or numb tongue, stomach pain, stomach ulcer, stuffy nose, stupor, stuttering, thirst, throat discomfort, twitching, urination problems, vaginal infection, vaginal itch, vague feeling of sickness, vomiting, vomiting blood, weakness, wheezing.

Interactions

 Inform your doctor before combining Clozaril with: blood pressure medications such as Aldomet; Cimetidine (Tagamet); Digoxin (Lanoxin); drugs that affect the central nervous system such as Valium, Xanax, and Seconal; drugs that contain atropine such as Donnatal and Levsin; epilepsy drugs such as Tegretol and Dilantin; Epinephrine; other antipsychotic and mood-altering medications; Warfarin (Coumadin).

 No known food/other substance interactions.

Special Cautions

 If pregnant or planning to become pregnant, inform your doctor immediately. Clozaril should be discontinued during pregnancy unless absolutely necessary. May appear in breast milk; could affect a nursing baby.

 No special precautions apply to seniors.

 Not prescribed for children under 16 years.

 May cause granulocytosis, a potentially fatal white blood cell disorder; approximately 1% develop this disorder and must stop taking Clozaril. As a result, the medication is carefully controlled through weekly blood tests. Before receiving the following week's supply of medication, the blood cell counts must be normal. Early warning signs include: fever, general feeling of illness, flu-like feeling, lethargy, sore throat, ulcer of the lips, ulcer of the mouth or mucous membranes, or weakness.

May cause drowsiness or seizures and impair your ability to drive a car or operate machinery, swim or climb. *Do not take part in any activity that requires alertness.*

Seizures occur in approximately 5% of people who take Clozaril. The higher the dosage, the higher the risk of seizure.

Because of the risks of taking Clozaril, should only be prescribed when other antipsychotic medications such as Haldol or Mellaril have not worked.

Should not take Clozaril if you have: abnormal white blood cell count, bone marrow disease or disorder, or if you are taking drugs that could decrease your white blood cell count such as Tegretol.

Doctor should monitor if you have: enlarged prostate; history of seizures; kidney, liver, lung, or heart disease; or narrow-angle glaucoma.

Clozaril may cause Neuroleptic Malignant Syndrome; symptoms include: changes in heart rhythm, excessive perspiration, high fever, irregular pulse or blood pressure, muscle rigidity, or rapid heartbeat.

Cogentin

Generic name: Benztropine mesylate

Cogentin is an anticholinergic and antiparkinsonism agent. It works by slowing the action of the bowel and reducing the amount of stomach acid.

℞ QUICK FACTS

Purpose

℞ Used to treat the symptoms of parkinsonism: muscle rigidity, tremors, difficulty with posture and balance.

Dosage

 Take exactly as prescribed. Is suitable for bedtime.

 Usual adult dose: orally—1 to 2 milligrams per day. Can range from 0.5 to 6 milligrams per day. May take 2 to 3 days to notice the effects of Cogentin. Doctor may lower dosage in hot weather.

 Usual child dose: not generally prescribed for children under 3 years. Follow doctor's instructions for dosage.

 Missed dose: take as soon as possible, unless within 2 hours of next dose. In that case, do not take missed dose, go back to regular schedule. *Do not double doses.*

Side Effects

 Overdose symptoms: may include side effects listed, plus coma, convulsions, delirium, difficulty swallowing or breathing, dizziness, flushed and/or dry skin, glaucoma, headache, high blood pressure, high body temperature, inability to sweat, muscle weakness, palpitations, shock, uncoordinated movements. If you suspect an overdose, immediately seek medical attention.

 Side effects: blurred vision, bowel blockage, confusion, constipation, depression, dilated pupils, disorientation, dry mouth, fever, hallucinations, heat stroke, impaired memory, inability to urinate, listlessness, nausea, nervousness, numbness in fingers, painful urination, rapid heartbeat, rash, vomiting.

 No known less common or rare side effects.

Interactions

 Inform your doctor before combining Cogentin with: Amantadine (Symmetral), Doxepine (Sinequan), antihistamines such as Benadryl and Tavist, other anticholinergic agents such as Bentyl. *Has caused bowel blockage or heat stroke that is dangerous or fatal when taking Cogentin with: antipsychotic medications (Thorazine, Stelazine, Haldol) or tricyclic antidepressants (Elavil, Norpramine, Tofranil).* Antacids (Tums, Maalox, Mylanta) may decrease effects of Cogentin; *do not take within 1 hour of taking Cogentin.*

 No known food/other substance interactions.

Special Cautions

 If pregnant or planning to become pregnant, inform your doctor immediately. Not known if Cogentin appears in breast milk.

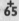 No special precautions apply to seniors.

 Not prescribed for children under 3 years.

 Do not take if sensitive or allergic to this or similar medications, or you have angle-closure glaucoma.

May impair your ability to drive a car or operate machinery. *Do not take part in any activity that requires alertness.*

If taking another medication similar to Cogentin, gradually discontinue use when you start taking Cogentin; do not abruptly stop the other medication.

Tell your doctor if you experience any noticeable muscle weakness.

Should not be given to treat tardive dyskinesia; may worsen condition.

. . . .

Inform your doctor if you have: enlarged prostate or excessively rapid heartbeats.

. . . .

As Cogentin has a drying effect, use with caution if taking with other medications that have a drying effect. May be at risk for anhidrosis (inability to sweat), heat stroke, or death from high fever. This risk may be increased by: chronic illness, alcoholism, central nervous system disease, or heavy manual labor in a hot environment.

Cognex

Generic name: Tacrine hydrochloride

Cognex is a cholinesterase inhibitor. It works by balancing certain chemicals in the brain.

℞ QUICK FACTS

Purpose

℞ Used to treat mild to moderate Alzheimer's disease.

Dosage

 Take exactly as prescribed; *do not change the dose unless instructed by your doctor.* Abruptly stopping the treatment can cause the condition to worsen; increasing dose also causes serious problems. More effective if taken at regular intervals, between meals. If irritating to the stomach, doctor may prescribe taking Cognex with meals.

Usual adult dose: 10 milligrams taken 4 times per day, for at least 6 weeks. Doctor may increase up to 20 milligrams 4 times per day. *Restarting Cognex therapy*—10 milligrams taken 4 times per day for 6 weeks.

 Usual child dose: not prescribed for children.

 Missed dose: take as soon as possible, unless within 2 hours of next dose. In that case, do not take missed dose; go back to regular schedule. *Do not double doses.*

Side Effects

 Overdose symptoms: collapse, convulsions, *extreme muscle weakness (possibly ending in death if breathing muscles affected),* low blood pressure, nausea, salivation, slowed heart rate, sweating, vomiting. If you suspect an overdose, immediately seek medical attention.

 More common side effects: abdominal pain, abnormal thinking, agitation, anxiety, chest pain, clumsiness or unsteadiness, confusion, constipation, coughing, depression, diarrhea, dizziness, fatigue, flushing, frequent urination, gas, headache, inflamed nasal passages, insomnia, indigestion, liver function disorders, loss of appetite, muscle pain, nausea, rash, sleepiness, upper respiratory infection, urinary tract infection, vomiting, weight loss.

 Less common side effects: back pain, hallucinations, hostile attitude, purple or red spots on the skin, skin discoloration, tremor, weakness.

Interactions

 Inform your doctor before combining Cognex with: antispasmodic drugs such as Bentyl and Cogentin;

Bethanechol chloride (Urecholine); Cimetidine (Tagamet); Theophylline (Theo-Dur).

 No known food/other substance interactions.

Special Cautions

 If pregnant or planning to become pregnant, inform your doctor immediately. Not known if Cognex appears in breast milk.

 No special precautions apply to seniors.

 Not prescribed for children.

 Do not take if there is sensitivity to or allergic reaction to Cognex.

Discuss any medical problems of the person you are caring for with the doctor before starting Cognex therapy, especially any history of asthma, heart disorders, liver disease, or stomach ulcers.

Monitor for nausea, vomiting, loose stools, or diarrhea at the start of therapy. Later, monitor for rash, yellowing of the eyes and skin, or changes in the color of the stool.

Notify doctor before any surgery, including dental, that the person is being treated with Cognex.

Can cause seizures and difficulty urinating.

Doctor will schedule weekly blood tests to monitor liver function for the first 18 weeks of therapy, then every 3 months thereafter. If dose increased, weekly monitoring will resume.

Colace

~~~~~~

Generic name: Docusate sodium

Colace is an emollient laxative. It works by increasing the stool's fluid content, promoting bowel evacuation.

℞ QUICK FACTS

Purpose

℞ Used to soften stools, helpful for people who have had rectal surgery, those with heart problems or high blood pressure, hernias, and women who have just had babies.

Dosage

🍽 Take in a half glass of milk or fruit juice. Can also be added to infant formula. May use with a retention or flushing enema. For short-term use only.

. . . .

💊 Usual adult dose: 50 to 200 milligrams per day. *In enemas*—add 50 to 100 milligrams of Colace or 5 to 10 milliliters of Colace liquid to a retention or flushing enema, as prescribed.

. . . .

🧸 Usual child dose: *for children 12 year and older*— same as adult dose. *For children 6 to 12 years*—40 to 120 milligrams per day. *For children 3 to 6 years*— 20 to 60 milligrams per day. *For children under 3 years*—10 to 40 milligrams.

. . . .

◢ Missed dose: take medication on an as-needed basis only.

Side Effects

☠ Overdose symptoms: none reported with normal use of Colace. If you suspect an overdose, immediately seek medical attention.

. . . .

More common side effects: bitter taste, throat irritation, nausea.

 Less common side effect: rash.

Interactions

 No drug interactions reported.

 No known food/other substance interactions.

Special Cautions

 If pregnant or planning to become pregnant, inform your doctor before using this medication. Not known if Colace appears in breast milk.

 No special precautions apply to seniors.

 Follow doctor's instructions carefully.

 Usually takes 2 to 3 days to achieve laxative effect, in some cases 4 to 5 days.

Colestid

^^

Generic name: Colestipol hydrochloride

Colestid is an antihyperlipidemic (blood fat reducer). It works by binding bile salts in the gastrointestinal tract to prevent cholesterol production.

℞ QUICK FACTS

Purpose

℞ Used to treat high levels of cholesterol.

Dosage

 Mix with liquids such as: carbonated beverages, flavored drinks, milk, orange juice, pineapple juice, pulpy fruit (crushed peaches, pears, or pineapple), soup with a high liquid content, tomato juice, water.

 Usual adult dose: 5 to 10 grams per day, up to 30 grams per day divided into smaller, equal doses or one single dose per day.

 Usual child dose: doctor will determine dosage for children.

 Missed dose: take as soon as possible, unless almost time for the next dose. In that case, do not take missed dose; go back to regular schedule. *Do not double doses.*

Side Effects

 Overdose symptoms: none specifically reported. Most likely sign of overdose would be obstruction of the stomach and/or intestines. If you suspect an overdose, immediately seek medical attention.

 Most common side effects: constipation, worsening of hemorrhoids.

 Less common side effects: abdominal discomfort, abdominal pain, anxiety, arthritis, belching, diarrhea, distended abdomen, dizziness, drowsiness, fatigue, gas, headache, hives, loss of appetite, muscle and joint pain, nausea, shortness of breath, skin inflammation, vertigo, vomiting, weakness.

Interactions

 Inform your doctor before combining Colestid with: Chlorothizide (Diuril); Digitalis (Lanoxin); Furosemide (Lasix); Gemfibrozil (Lopid); Penicillin G, including brands such as Pentids; phosphate supplements; Propranolol (Inderal); Tetracycline drugs such as Sumycin; vitamins such as A, D, and K. Take other drugs at least 1 hour before or 4 hours after taking Colestid, may delay absorption of other medications.

 May prevent absorption of vitamins A, D, and K.

Special Cautions

 If pregnant or planning to become pregnant, inform your doctor before using this medication. Not known if Colestid appears in breast milk.

 No special precautions apply to seniors.

 Dose is individualized by your doctor for children.

 Take caution not to accidentally inhale Colestid—NEVER take in dry form. Should always be mixed with water or other liquids BEFORE taking.

Should not use if allergic to any of the ingredients of Colestid.

Prior to taking Colestid: doctor should test (and treat) you for any diseases that may contribute to increased cholesterol—hypothyroidism, diabetes, nephrotic syndrome, dysproteinemia, and obstructive liver disease; and you should be on a low-cholesterol diet, and a weight loss diet if necessary.

Cholesterol and triglyceride levels should be monitored on a regular basis while taking Colestid.

May cause or worsen constipation, people with coronary heart disease should be careful. Constipation may worsen hemorrhoids.

Colestipol Hydrochloride

see COLESTID

Compazine

Generic name: Prochlorperazine

Other brand names: Compazine Spansules, Compazine Suppositories, Compazine Syrup

Compazine is an antinauseant. It works to reduce the urge to vomit.

℞ QUICK FACTS

Purpose

℞ Used to treat severe nausea and vomiting. Also used to treat schizophrenia, and occasionally anxiety.

Dosage

 Take exactly as prescribed, otherwise serious side effects may occur. Should not be stopped suddenly; can cause change in appetite, dizziness, nausea, vomiting, and tremors.

 Usual adult dose: *for severe nausea and vomiting*—one 5-milligram or 10-milligram tablet 3 or 4 times a day; Spansule capsules—one 15-milligram capsule on getting out of bed or one 10-milligram capsule every 12 hours; Rectal suppository—25 milligrams taken 2 times per day. *For nonpsychotic anxiety*—Tablets—5 milligrams taken 3 or 4 times per day; Spansule capsules—one 15-milligram capsule on getting up or one 10-milligram capsule every 12 hours. Treatment is up to 12 weeks, not exceeding 20 milligrams per day. *For mild psychotic disorders*—5 or 10 milligrams taken 3 or 4 times daily. *For moderate to severe psychotic disorders*—10 milligrams taken 3 or 4 times per day; doctor may increase up to 50 to 70 milligrams per day. *For more severe psychotic disorders*—100 to 150 milligrams per day. Seniors—prescribed lower doses.

 Usual child dose: *for severe nausea and vomiting*—one day of oral or rectal dose, as follows: *children 20 to 29 pounds*—2.5 milligrams 1 or 2 times per day, not to exceed 7.5 milligrams. *Children 30 to 39 pounds*—2.5 milligrams 2 or 3 times per day, not to exceed 10 milligrams. *Children 40 to 85 pounds*—2.5 milligrams 3 times per day or 5 milligrams 2 times per day. Total daily amount not to exceed 15 milligrams. *For psychotic disorders*—*children 2 to 5 years*—oral or rectal, 2.5 milligrams 2 or 3 times per day, not to exceed 10 milligrams on 1st day, and 20 milligrams thereafter. *Children 6 to 12 years*—oral or rectal, 2.5 milligrams 2 or 3 times per day, not to exceed 10 milligrams on the 1st day and 25 milligrams thereafter.

 Missed dose: take as soon as possible, unless almost time for the next dose. In that case, do not take missed dose; go back to regular schedule. *Do not double doses.*

Side Effects

 Overdose symptoms: agitation, coma, convulsions, dry mouth, extreme sleepiness, fever, intestinal blockage, irregular heart rate, restlessness. If you suspect an overdose, immediately seek medical attention.

 Side effects: abnormal muscle rigidity; abnormal secretion of milk; abnormal sugar in urine; abnormalities of posture and movement; agitation; anemia; appetite changes; asthma; blurred vision; breast development in males; chewing movements; constipation; convulsions; difficulty swallowing; discolored skin tone; dizziness; drooling; drowsiness; dry mouth; ejaculation difficulties; exaggerated reflexes; fever; fluid retention; head arched backward; headache; heart attack; heels bent back on legs; high or low blood sugar; hives; impotence; inability to urinate; increase in psychotic symptoms; increase in weight; infection; insomnia; intestinal obstruction; involuntary movements of arms, hands, legs, and feet; involuntary movements of face, tongue, and jaw; irregular movements; jerky movements; jitteriness; light sensitivity; low blood pressure; mask-like face; menstrual irregularities; narrowed or dilated pupils; nasal congestion; nausea; pain in the shoulder and neck area; painful muscle spasm; parkinsonism-like symptoms; persistent and/or painful erections; pill-rolling motion; protruding tongue; puckering of the mouth; puffing of the cheeks; rigid arms, feet, head, and muscles; rotation of eyeballs or state of fixed gaze; shock; shuffling gait; skin peeling; rash and inflammation; sore throat, mouth, and gums; spasms in back, feet and ankles, jaw, and neck; swelling and itching skin; swelling in throat; tremors; yellowed eyes and skin.

 No known less common or rare side effects.

Interactions

 Inform your doctor before combining Compazine with: anticonvulsants such as Dilantin and Tegretol; anticoagulants such as Coumadin; Guanethidine (Ismelin); narcotic painkillers such as Demerol and Tylenol with Codeine; other central nervous system depressants such as Xanax, Valium, Seconal, and Halcion; Propranolol (Inderal); Thiazide diuretics such as Dyazide.

Large amounts of alcohol may cause serious problems.

Special Cautions

 If pregnant or planning to become pregnant, inform your doctor before using this medication. May cause false-positive pregnancy tests. Not generally prescribed for pregnant women, unless potential benefits outweigh risks if used for severe nausea and vomiting. May appear in breast milk; could affect a nursing infant.

 Seniors are usually prescribed lower doses. Risk of developing low blood pressure is present when taking Compazine. Senior women are susceptible to tardive dyskinesia, causing involuntary muscle spasms and twitches in the face and body.

 Follow doctor's instructions closely for children.

 Do not take if sensitive to or allergic to Prochlorperazine or other phenothiazine medications such as Thorazine, Prolixin, Triavil, Mellaril, or Stelazine.

May impair your ability to drive a car or operate machinery. *Do not take part in any activity that requires alertness.*

May cause tardive dyskinesia, involuntary muscle spasms and twitches in the face and body. Can be a permanent condition. Senior women have higher risk.

Inform your doctor if you are being treated for: brain tumor, intestinal blockage, heart disease, glaucoma, or abnormal blood condition such as leukemia, or are exposed to extreme heat or pesticides.

Avoid sunlight; skin and eyes may develop sensitivity.

Use caution in hot weather; ability to sweat can be compromised by Compazine usage.

Conjugated Estrogens

see PREMARIN

Corgard

Generic name: Nadolol

Corgard is a beta-blocker. It slows the heart rate and reduces high blood pressure.

℞ QUICK FACTS

Purpose

Used to treat angina (chest pain) and to reduce high blood pressure.

Dosage

May take with or without food. Take as prescribed, even if symptoms disappear. Must take regularly for it to be effective with high blood pressure; may take a few weeks before you observe full effect of medication. Medication should not be stopped abruptly, may increase chest pain or cause a heart attack.

Usual adult dose: *for angina*—initially, 40 milligrams once per day. Long-term dose is 40 to 80 milligrams, once per day, up to 160 to 240 milligrams once per day. *For high blood pressure*—initially, 40 milligrams once per day. Long-term dose is 40 to 80 milligrams once per day, up to 240 to 320 milligrams once per day. *Seniors*—dose will reflect individual needs.

Usual child dose: not generally prescribed for children.

Missed dose: take as soon as possible, unless within 8 hours of the next dose. In that case, do not take missed dose; go back to regular schedule. *Do not double doses.*

Side Effects

Overdose symptoms: difficulty in breathing, heart failure, low blood pressure, slow heartbeat. If you suspect an overdose, immediately seek medical attention.

More common side effects: behavior change, change in heartbeat, dizziness or light-headedness, mild drowsiness, slow heartbeat, weakness or tiredness.

Less common or rare side effects: abdominal discomfort, asthma-like symptoms, bloating, confusion, constipation, cough, decreased sex drive, diarrhea, dry eyes, dry mouth, dry skin, facial swelling, gas, headache, heart failure, impotence, indigestion, itching, loss of appetite, low blood pressure, nasal stuffiness, nausea, rash, ringing in ears, slurred speech, vision changes, vomiting, weight gain.

Interactions

Inform your doctor before combining Corgard with: antidiabetic medications including Insulin and oral medications such as Micronase; certain blood pressure medications such as Diupres and Ser-Ap-Es; Epinephrine (EpiPen).

No known food/other substance interactions.

Special Cautions

 If pregnant or planning to become pregnant, inform your doctor immediately. Appears in breast milk; could affect a nursing baby.

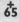 Dose will reflect individual needs in seniors.

 Not generally prescribed for children.

 May impair your ability to drive a car or operate machinery. *Do not take part in any activity that requires alertness.*

Should not take if you have: slow heartbeat, heartbeat irregularity, cardiogenic shock, or active heart failure.

Use with caution if you have: asthma, chronic bronchitis, emphysema, seasonal allergies or other bronchial conditions, kidney disease, or liver disease.

Monitor pulse rate, may have slowed rate while taking Corgard.

If diabetic, be aware that Corgard can mask the symptoms of low blood sugar, or alter blood sugar levels.

Notify your doctor or dentist that you are taking Corgard before surgery or in an emergency situation.

Cortaid
see ANUSOL-HC

Cortisporin Ophthalmic Suspension

Generic ingredients: Polymyxin B sulfate with neomycin sulfate and hydrocortisone

Other brand name: Bacticort

Cortisporin Ophthalmic Suspension is a combination drug/antibiotic. It is used to prevent bacteria from multiplying and growing, and to relieve inflammatory conditions.

℞ QUICK FACTS

Purpose

℞   Used to treat irritation, swelling, redness, and general eye discomfort, and bacterial eye infections.

Dosage

 Use the entire prescription, even if symptoms have disappeared.

 Usual adult dose: 1 or 2 drops in the affected eye every 3 or 4 hours. May mask the existence of an infection or worsen an existing one if using this medication for more than 10 days.

 Usual child dose: not generally prescribed for children.

 Missed dose: apply as soon as possible, unless almost time for the next dose. In that case, do not apply missed dose; go back to regular schedule.

Side Effects

 Overdose symptoms: no specific information available. If you suspect an overdose, immediately seek medical attention.

 Side effects: cataract formation, delayed wound healing, increased eye pressure with possible development of glaucoma or optic nerve damage, irritation when drops applied, local allergic reactions (itching, swelling, redness), other infections such as fungal infections of the cornea and bacterial eye infection.

 No known less common or rare side effects.

Interactions

 No drug interactions reported.

 No known food/other substance interactions.

Special Cautions

 If pregnant or planning to become pregnant, inform your doctor immediately. Appears in breast milk; could affect a nursing baby.

 No special precautions apply to seniors.

 Not generally prescribed for children.

 Use with extreme caution if you have herpes simplex.

Long-term use (more than 10 days) may result in glaucoma or suppress immune system, leading to secondary eye infections. Doctor may periodically measure your eye pressure.

Should not use if you have: viral or fungal eye disease, or if sensitive to or allergic to any ingredients of this medication. Allergic reaction subsides once medication is stopped.

Corzide

Generic ingredients: Nadolol with bendroflumethiazide

Corzide is a thiazide diuretic and beta-blocker combination. It works to reduce blood pressure.

℞ QUICK FACTS

Purpose

 Used to treat high blood pressure.

Dosage

 Must take regularly for Corzide to be effective. May take several weeks before the full effect of the medication is observed. Can take with or without food.

 Usual adult dose: one Corzide 40/5 milligram tablet per day, or one 80/5 milligram tablet per day.

 Usual child dose: not generally prescribed for children.

 Missed dose: take as soon as possible, unless within 8 hours of the next dose. In that case, do not take missed dose; go back to regular schedule. *Do not double doses.*

Side Effects

 Overdose symptoms: abdominal irritation, central nervous system depression, coma, extremely slow heartbeat, heart failure, lethargy, low blood pressure, wheezing. If you suspect an overdose, immediately seek medical attention.

 More common side effects: asthma-like symptoms, changes in heart rhythm, cold hands and feet, dizziness, fatigue, low blood pressure, low potassium levels, slow heartbeat.

 Less common or rare side effects: abdominal discomfort, anemia, bloating, blurred vision, certain types of irregular heartbeat, change in behavior, constipation, cough, diarrhea, dry eyes, dry mouth, dry skin, facial swelling, gas, headache, heart failure, hepatitis, impotence, indigestion, inflammation of the pancreas, itching, loss of appetite, lowered sex drive, muscle spasm, nasal stuffiness, nausea, rash, ringing in ears, sedation, sensitivity to light, slurred speech, sweating, tingling or pins and needles, vertigo, vomiting, weakness, weight gain, wheezing, yellowed eyes and skin.

Interactions

 Inform your doctor before combining Corzide with: Amphotericin B; antidepressant drugs such as Nardil and Parnate; antidiabetic drugs such as Micronase; antigout drugs such as Benemid; barbiturates such as Phenobarbital; blood thinners such as Coumadin; blood pressure drugs such as Diupres and Ser-Ap-Es; calcium salt; Cholestyramine (Questran); Colestipol (Colestid); Diazoxide (Proglycem); digitalis medications such as Lanoxin; Lithium (Lithonate); Methenamine (Mandelamine); narcotics such as Percocet; nonsteroidal anti-inflammatory drugs such as Motrin, Naprosyn, and Nuprin; other antihypertensives such as Vasotec; steroid medications such as Prednisone; Sulfinpyrazone (Anturane).

 Do not drink alcohol with this medication; it may intensify the effects of alcohol.

Special Cautions

 If pregnant or planning to become pregnant, inform your doctor immediately. Appears in breast milk; could affect a nursing baby.

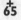 Doctor will prescribe amount based on seniors' particular needs.

 Not generally prescribed for children.

 May impair your ability to drive a car or operate machinery. *Do not take part in any activity that requires alertness.*

Should not take if you have: active congestive heart failure, bronchial asthma, certain heartbeat, emphysema, inability to urinate, inadequate blood supply to the circulatory system, kidney or liver disease, slow heartbeat, or sensitivity or allergic reaction to Corzide.

Monitor pulse rate. Corzide can cause heartbeat to slow.

May mask symptoms of low blood sugar or altered blood sugar levels.

Notify your doctor or dentist that you are taking Corzide before surgery or in an emergency situation.

Coumadin

^^

Generic name: Warfarin sodium

Other brand name: Sofarin

Coumadin is an anticoagulant/blood thinner. It works by decreasing the production of blood-clotting substances by the liver.

℞ QUICK FACTS

Purpose

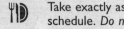 Used to treat and/or prevent blood clots: within a blood vessel; from reaching the lungs; or to prevent heart attack or stroke.

Dosage

 Take exactly as prescribed, adhere strictly to dosage schedule. *Do not change drug brand without consulting your doctor.*

. . . .

 Usual adult dose: 2 to 5 milligrams per day to start. Maintenance dose ranges from 2 to 10 milligrams per day. Dose is highly variable; doctor will individualize carefully for your specific needs.

. . . .

 Usual child dose: not prescribed for children under 18 years.

. . . .

 Missed dose: take as soon as possible, then go back to regular schedule. *Do not double doses.*

Side Effects

Overdose symptoms: blood in stools or urine, excessive menstrual bleeding, black stools, reddish or purplish spots on skin, excessive bruising, persistent bleeding from superficial injuries. If you suspect an overdose, immediately seek medical attention.

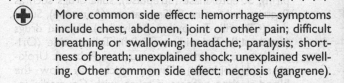

More common side effect: hemorrhage—symptoms include chest, abdomen, joint or other pain; difficult breathing or swallowing; headache; paralysis; shortness of breath; unexplained shock; unexplained swelling. Other common side effect: necrosis (gangrene).

Less common side effects: abdominal and other cramping, allergic reactions, diarrhea, fever, hives, liver damage, loss of hair, nausea, purple toes, severe or long-lasting inflammation of the skin.

Interactions

Inform your doctor before combining Coumadin with: Acetaminophen (Tylenol), Allopurinol (Zyloprim), Aminosalicylic acid, Amiodarone hydrochloride (Cordarone), anabolic steroids such as Anadrol-50, antibiotics such as Cipro, Anistreplase (Eminase), Bromelains (Bromase), Chenodiol, Chloral hydrate (Noctec), Chlorpropamide (Diabinese), Chymotrypsin, Cimetidine (Tagamet), Clofibrate (Atromid-S), Dextrothyroxine (Choloxin), Diazoxide (Proglycem), Diflunisal (Dolobid), Disulfiram (Antabuse), diuretics such as Hydromox, Ethacrynic acid (Edecrin), Fenoprofen (Nalfon), Glucagon, hepatotoxic drugs, Ibuprofen (Motrin), Indomethacin (Indocin), influenza virus vaccine (Flu-Immune), Lovastatin (Mevacor), Mefenamic acid (Ponstel), Methyldopa (Aldomet), Methylphenidate (Ritalin), Metronidazole (Flagyl), Moconazole (Monistat), MAO inhibitors (antidepressants such as Nardil or Parnate), Moricizine hydrochloride (Ethmozine), Nalidixic acid (NegGram), Naproxen (Naprosyn), narcotics taken for long periods such as Demerol and Percocet, Pentoxifylline (Trental), Phenobarbital in drugs such as Donnatal, Phenylbutazone (Butazolidin), Phenytoin (Dilantin),

Propafenone (Rythmol), Quinidine (Quinidex), Quinine (Quinamm), Ranitidine (Zantac), salicylates (Aspirin), Streptokinase (Streptase), sulfa drugs such as Bactrim and Septra, Sulfinpyrazone (Anturane), Sulindac (Clinoril), Tamoxifen (Nolvadex), thyroid drugs (Synthroid), Ticlopidine (Ticlid), Tolbutamide (Orinase), topical pain relievers such as Anbesol, Urokinase (Abbokinase). Drugs which may slow the blood-clotting process if taken with Coumadin include: adrenocortical steroids such as Prednisone, Aminoglutethimide (Cytadren), antacids such as Maalox, antihistamines such as Benadryl, barbiturates such as Phenobarbital, Carbamazepine (Tegretol), Chloral hydrate (Noctec), Chlordiazepoxide (Librium), Cholestyramine (Questran), diuretics such as Hydromox, Ethchlorvynol (Placidyl), Glutethimide (Doriden), Griseofulvin (Gris-PEG), Haloperidol (Haldol), Meprobamate (Miltown), Moricizine hydrochloride (Ethmozine), Nafcillin (Unipen), oral contraceptives, Paraldehyde, Primidone (Mysoline), Ranitidine (Zantac), Rifampin (Rifadin), Sucralfate (Carafate), Trazodone (Desyrel), vitamin C.

Do not eat large amounts of leafy green vegetables; they contain vitamin K, and may counteract the effects of Coumadin. Avoid alcohol, as well as any drastic change in diet.

Special Cautions

Coumadin passes through the placental barrier, possibly causing fatal hemorrhage in the fetus. Reports of malformed babies born to mothers taking Coumadin, as well as spontaneous abortions and stillbirths. If pregnant or planning to become pregnant, inform your doctor immediately. May appear in breast milk, could affect a nursing baby.

65 No special precautions apply to seniors.

Not generally prescribed for children.

 Do not take if you are being treated for: a tendency to hemorrhage, abnormal blood condition, aneurysms, bleeding tendencies (associated with ulceration of the stomach, intestines, respiratory tract, or genital or urinary system), eclampsia, excessive bleeding of brain blood vessels, inflammation due to bacterial infection of the membrane lining the heart, malignant hypertension, preeclampsia, pregnancy, recent or contemplated traumatic surgery, recent or future central nervous system or eye surgery, threatened abortion.

Blood clot risk increased if you have: an infectious disease or intestinal disorder, family history of blood clots, dental procedures, inflammation of a blood vessel, moderate to severe high blood pressure, moderate to severe kidney or liver dysfunction, polycythemia vera, severe allergic disorders, severe diabetes, trauma resulting in internal bleeding.

Doctor should monitor the time it takes for your blood to clot on a continuous basis.

Notify your doctor if you experience: diarrhea; infection or fever; pain, swelling or discomfort; prolonged bleeding from cuts; increased menstrual flow; vaginal bleeding; nosebleeds; bleeding of gums from brushing; unusual bleeding or bruising; red or dark brown urine; or red or tarry black stool.

Monitor for purple toes syndrome, which may occur 3 to 10 weeks after taking Coumadin.

If you have congestive heart failure, you should be monitored by your doctor for sensitivity to Coumadin.

. . . .

Serious risk of hemorrhage and gangrene associated with Coumadin, resulting in death or permanent disability.

. . . .

Should carry identification card indicating you are taking Coumadin.

Cromolyn Sodium

see INTAL

Cyclobenzaprine Hydrochloride

see FLEXERIL

Cyclocort

Generic name: Amcinonide

Cyclocort is a topical adrenocorticoid/anti-inflammatory. It interferes with the natural body mechanisms that produce rash, itching or inflammation.

℞ QUICK FACTS

Purpose

℞   Used to treat inflammatory and itchy symptoms of skin disorders.

Dosage

 Use exactly as prescribed. For external use only; keep out of and away from eyes. Apply sparingly; rub gently into skin. Avoid using large amounts of Cyclocort over large areas, thus reducing risk of absorption into bloodstream. Use only for the disorder for which it is prescribed.

 Usual adult dose: apply thin film 2 or 3 times per day. *Cyclocort lotion*—may be applied 2 times per day, used particularly for hairy areas.

 Usual child dose: use in a small, limited amount.

 Missed dose: apply as soon as possible. Use remaining doses for the day at equally spaced intervals. *Do not double doses.*

Side Effects

 Overdose symptoms: severe overdose unlikely. Long-term use may cause unwanted side effects. If you suspect an overdose, immediately seek medical attention.

 More common side effects: burning, itching, soreness, stinging.

 Less common side effects: dryness, excessive growth of hair, infection, inflammation of skin around the mouth, irritation, prickly heat, skin eruptions resembling acne, softening of the skin, stretch marks.

Interactions

 No drug interactions reported.

No known food/other substance interactions.

Special Cautions

 If pregnant or planning to become pregnant, inform your doctor immediately. Not known if Cyclocort appears in breast milk.

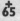 No special precautions apply to seniors.

 Long-term use may result in growth and development problems in children.

 Unless specifically instructed by doctor, do not cover Cyclocort with bandages or airtight dressings. Use special caution with infants being treated in the diaper area.

If sensitive to or had allergic reaction to this or other steroid medications, you should not use.

Cyclophosphamide
see CYTOXAN

Cyclosporine
see SANDIMMUNE

Cylert

Generic name: Pemoline

Other brand name: Cylert Chewables

Cylert is known as an analeptic. It calms the central nervous system in children, and acts as a stimulant in adults.

℞ QUICK FACTS

Purpose

 Used to treat children with attention deficit disorder, adults with narcolepsy, and as a mild stimulant for seniors.

Dosage

 Take once per day, in the morning.

 Usual adult dose: 50 to 200 milligrams per day, in equally divided doses after breakfast and lunch. *As a stimulant*—20 to 50 milligrams per day, in equally divided doses after breakfast and lunch.

 Usual child dose: *initial dose*—37.5 milligrams per day, then between 56.25 to 75 milligrams per day, not to exceed 112.5 milligrams per day.

 Missed dose: take as soon as possible, unless it is the next day. In that case, do not take missed dose; go back to regular schedule. *Do not double doses.*

Side Effects

 Overdose symptoms: agitation, coma, confusion, convulsions, delirium, dilated pupils, exaggerated feeling of well-being, extremely high temperature, flushing, hallucinations, headache, high blood pressure, increased heart rate, increased reflex reactions, muscle twitches, sweating, tremors, vomiting. If you suspect an overdose, immediately seek medical attention.

More common side effect: insomnia.

Less common side effects: dizziness, drowsiness, hallucinations, headache, hepatitis and other liver problems, increased irritability, involuntary fragmented movements (of the face, eyes, lips, tongue, arms, and legs), loss of appetite, mild depression, nausea, seizures, skin rash, stomachache, suppressed growth (in children), uncontrolled vocal outbursts (such as grunts, shouts and obscene language), weight loss, yellowing of skin or eyes. Rare side effects: rare form of anemia with symptoms including bleeding gums, bruising, chest pain, fatigue, headache, nosebleeds, and abnormal paleness.

Interactions

 Inform your doctor before combining Cylert with: anti-epileptic medications such as Tegretol; other drugs that affect the central nervous system, such as Ritalin.

 No known food/other substance interactions.

Special Cautions

 If pregnant or planning to become pregnant, inform your doctor immediately. Not known if Cylert appears in breast milk.

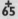 No special precautions apply to seniors.

 May affect a child's growth; doctor should carefully monitor your child if taking Cylert on a long-term basis. Children with psychotic disorders may experience more disordered thoughts and behavioral disturbances when taking Cylert.

 Should not use if sensitive to or allergic to Cylert, or if kidney or liver problems are present.

May cause dizziness; alert your child to be careful when participating in activities requiring mental alertness.

If you have a history of drug or alcohol abuse, use Cylert with caution, can be potentially addictive.

Cyproheptadine Hydrochloride

see PERIACTIN

Cytotec

Generic name: Misoprostol

Cytotec is a synthetic prostaglandin/anti-ulcer agent. It works to relieve and promote the healing of ulcers.

℞ QUICK FACTS

Purpose

℞ Used to treat and prevent stomach ulcers in people who take Aspirin and other nonsteroidal anti-inflammatory medications.

Dosage

 Take with meals, exactly as prescribed.

 Usual adult dose: 200 micrograms 4 times per day with food. Take last dose at bedtime. Doctor may adjust down to 100 micrograms if you cannot tolerate higher level.

Usual child dose: not generally prescribed for children.

 Missed dose: take as soon as possible, unless almost time for the next dose. In that case, do not take missed dose; go back to regular schedule. *Do not double doses.*

Side Effects

 Overdose symptoms: abdominal pain, breathing difficulty, convulsions, diarrhea, fever, heart palpitations, low blood pressure, sedation (extreme drowsiness), slowed heartbeat, stomach or intestinal discomfort, tremors. If you suspect an overdose, immediately seek medical attention.

 More common side effects: abdominal cramps, diarrhea, nausea. Other side effects: constipation, gas, indigestion, headache, heavy menstrual bleeding, menstrual disorder, menstrual pain or cramps, paleness, spotting (between periods), stomach or intestinal bleeding, uterine bleeding, vomiting.

 No known less common or rare side effects.

Interactions

 No reported drug interactions.

 No known food/other substance interactions.

Special Cautions

 If pregnant or planning to become pregnant, inform your doctor immediately. *Cytotec can cause miscarriage. Women of childbearing age must take a pregnancy test 2 weeks prior to Cytotec treatment.* Not known if Cytotec appears in breast milk.

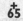 No special precautions apply to seniors.

 Not generally prescribed for children.

 Do not take if sensitive to or allergic to Cytotec or other prostaglandin medications.

May cause uterine bleeding, even in women who have gone through menopause. If you notice any bleeding, notify your doctor.

May cause diarrhea. Use with caution if you have inflammatory bowel disease or any other condition in which the loss of fluid would be dangerous. Take Cytotec with food to help prevent diarrhea. Avoid taking magnesium-containing antacids such as Maalox, Digel, and Mylanta. Have ongoing checkups.

Cytoxan

Generic name: Cyclophosphamide

Cytoxan is an alkylating agent. It works to prevent the multiplication and growth of cancer cells.

℞ QUICK FACTS

Purpose

 Used to treat the following cancers: breast, leukemias, malignant lymphomas, multiple myeloma, advanced mycosis fungoides, neuroblastoma, ovarian, retinoblastoma. Also used to treat "minimal change" nephrotic syndrome (kidney damage) in children who don't respond to steroid medications.

Dosage

Take exactly as prescribed, preferably on an empty stomach, unless you experience severe stomach upset. May be prescribed in oral solution if unable to swallow tablet form. Drink 3 or 4 liters of fluid per day to help prevent bladder problems.

Usual adult dose: *for malignant diseases*—1 to 5 milligrams per 2.2 pounds of body weight per day.

Usual child dose: *for malignant diseases*—1 to 5 milligrams per 2.2 pounds of body weight per day. *For kidney damage*—2.5 to 3 milligrams per 2.2 pounds of body weight for 60 to 90 days.

Missed dose: *do not take missed dose.* Go back to regular schedule; contact your doctor. *Do not double doses.*

Side Effects

Overdose symptoms: no specific information available. If you suspect an overdose, immediately seek medical attention.

More common side effects: loss of appetite, nausea and vomiting, temporary hair loss.

Less common or rare side effects: abdominal pain, anemia, bleeding, inflamed colon, darkening of skin and changes in fingernails, decreased sperm count, diarrhea, impaired wound healing, mouth sores, new tumor growth, prolonged impairment of fertility or temporary sterility in men, rash, severe allergic reaction, temporary failure to menstruate, yellowing of eyes and skin.

Interactions

 Inform your doctor before combining Cytoxan with: adrenal steroid hormones, Adriamycin (anticancer drug), Allopurinol (Zyloprim), Anectine (used in anesthesia), Digoxin (Lanoxin), Phenobarbital.

 No known food/other substance interactions.

Special Cautions

 Can cause defects in an unborn baby. If pregnant or planning to become pregnant, inform your doctor immediately. Appears in breast milk; could affect a nursing baby.

 No special precautions apply to seniors.

 Follow doctor's instructions carefully for children.

 Do not take if sensitive to or allergic to Cytoxan.

Inform your doctor of allergic reactions to other cancer drugs such as Alkeran, CeeNU, Emcyt, Leukeran, Myleran, or Zanosar.

At increased risk for toxic side effects if you have: blood disorder, bone marrow tumors, kidney disorder, liver disorder, past anticancer therapy, past x-ray therapy.

Adults should not take for any kidney disease.

Possible side effect is secondary cancer, typically of the bladder, lymph nodes, or bone marrow.

Immune system activity may be lowered, causing infection.

May cause bladder damage, including bladder infection with bleeding and fibrosis of the bladder.

Doctor will monitor your white blood cell count through frequent blood tests. Should not take if you are unable to produce normal blood cells.

Dalmane

Generic name: Flurazepam hydrochloride

Dalmane is a benzodiazepine/sedative-hypnotic. It works by selectively reducing the activity of certain chemicals in the brain.

℞ QUICK FACTS

Purpose

 Used to treat insomnia.

Dosage

 Take exactly as prescribed. Changes in the dosage or discontinuance of this medication should be regulated by your doctor to avoid serious side effects.

 Usual adult dose: 30 milligrams at bedtime; 15 milligrams may be adequate. *Seniors*—usual starting dose is 15 milligrams.

 Usual child dose: not prescribed for children under 15 years.

 Missed dose: take as soon as possible, unless within one hour of next dose. In that case, do not take missed dose; go back to regular schedule. *Do not double doses.*

Side Effects

Overdose symptoms: coma, confusion, low blood pressure, sleepiness. If you suspect an overdose, immediately seek medical attention.

More common side effects: dizziness, drowsiness, falling, lack of muscular coordination, light-headedness, staggering.

Less common or rare side effects: apprehension, bitter taste, blurred vision, body and joint pain, burning eyes, chest pains, confusion, constipation, depression, diarrhea, difficulty focusing, dry mouth, exaggerated feeling of well-being, excessive salivation, excitement, faintness, flushes, genital and urinary tract disorders, hallucinations, headache, heartburn, hyperactivity, irritability, itching, loss of appetite, low blood pressure, nausea, nervousness, rapid or fluttery heartbeat, restlessness, shortness of breath, skin rash, slurred speech, stimulation, stomach and intestinal pain, stomach upset, sweating, talkativeness, vomiting, weakness. Side effects due to abrupt withdrawal from Dalmane: abdominal and muscle cramps, convulsions, depressed mood, inability to fall or stay asleep, sweating, tremors, vomiting.

Interactions

Inform your doctor before combining Dalmane with: antidepressants such as Elavil and Tofranil, antihistamines such as Benadryl and Tavist, barbiturates such as Seconal and phenobarbital, major tranquilizers such as Mellaril and Thorazine, narcotic painkillers such as Demerol and Tylenol with Codeine, sedatives such as Xanax and Halcion, tranquilizers such as Librium and Valium.

Do not drink alcohol while taking this medication; alcohol intensifies the effects of Dalmane.

Special Cautions

 Do not take Dalmane if pregnant or planning to become pregnant; increases risks of birth defects. May appear in breast milk; could affect a nursing infant.

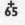 Seniors are prescribed a lower dosage to avoid oversedation, dizziness, confusion, or lack of muscle coordination.

 Not generally prescribed for children under 15 years.

 May cause drowsiness and impair your ability to drive a car or operate machinery. *Do not take part in any activity that requires alertness.*

If sensitive to or have allergic reaction to this or similar medications, should not take.

Consult with your doctor before taking Dalmane if you have: chronic respiratory or lung disease, decreased kidney or liver function, or severe depression.

D-AMP

see OMNIPEN

Darvocet-N

Generic ingredients: Propoxyphene napsylate with acetaminophen

Other brand names: Darvon-N (propoxyphene napsylate), Darvon (propoxyphene hydrochloride), Darvon Compound-65 (propoxyphene hydrochloride, aspirin, caffeine)

Darvocet-N is a narcotic analgesic. It works by altering the response to mild to moderate painful stimuli.

℞ QUICK FACTS

Purpose

 Used to treat mild to moderate pain, with or without fever—Darvocet-N and Darvon Compound-65. Darvon-N and Darvon used to treat mild to moderate pain.

Dosage

 Take exactly as prescribed to avoid dependence.

 Usual adult dose: take every 4 hours as needed for pain. *Darvocet-N 50*—2 tablets; *Darvocet-N 100*—1 tablet; *Darvon*—1 capsule; *Darvon Compound-65*—1 capsule. Doctor may lower dosage for individuals with kidney or liver problems. Should not exceed more than 6 capsules per day of Darvon or Darvon Compound-65. *Seniors*—doctor may lengthen time between doses.

 Usual child dose: not generally prescribed for children.

 Missed dose: take as soon as possible, unless almost time for next dose. In that case, do not take missed dose; go back to regular schedule. *Do not double doses.*

Side Effects

Extreme overdose may lead to unconsciousness and death. Overdose symptoms: *for propoxyphene*—bluish tinge to the skin, coma, convulsions, decreased or difficult breathing to the point of temporary stoppage, decreased heart function, extreme sleepiness, irregular heartbeat, low blood pressure, pinpoint pupils becoming dilated later, stupor. *Additional symptoms with Darvocet-N*—abdominal pain, excessive sweating, general feeling of illness, kidney failure, liver problems, loss of appetite, nausea, vomiting. *Additional symptoms with Darvon Compound-65*—confusion, deafness, excessive perspiration, headache, mental dullness, nausea, rapid breathing, rapid pulse, ringing in the ears, vertigo, vomiting. If you suspect an overdose, immediately seek medical attention.

More common side effects: drowsiness, dizziness, nausea, sedation, vomiting.

Less common side effects: abdominal pain, constipation, feelings of elation or depression, hallucinations, headache, kidney problems, light-headedness, liver problems, minor visual disturbances, skin rashes, weakness, yellowed eyes and skin.

Interactions

Inform your doctor before combining Darvocet-N with: anticonvulsant medications such as Tegretol (severe neurologic disorders have occurred when taken with Darvocet-N), antidepressant drugs such as Elavil, antihistamines such as Benadryl, muscle relaxants such as Flexeril, narcotic pain relievers such as Demerol, sleep aids such as Halcion, tranquilizers such as Xanax and Valium, warfarin-like drugs such as Coumadin.

Avoid alcohol while taking Darvocet-N; heavy use may cause overdose symptoms.

Special Cautions

 Do not take Darvocet-N if pregnant or planning to become pregnant, or in the last 3 months of pregnancy unless directed by a doctor; may cause temporary drug dependence in newborns. Does appear in breast milk; no adverse effects have been found in nursing infants.

 Seniors may be directed by their doctor to lengthen time between doses.

 Not generally prescribed for children.

 May cause drowsiness and impair your ability to drive a car or operate machinery. *Do not take part in any activity that requires alertness.*

If sensitive to or allergic to Darvocet-N or similar drugs, you should not take.

Consult with your doctor before taking Darvocet-N if you have: kidney or liver disease, blood clotting problem, ulcer.

Due to association between aspirin and Reye's syndrome, children and teenagers with chicken pox or flu should not take Darvon Compound-65 unless directed by a doctor.

If you have experienced asthma attacks from aspirin, contact your doctor before taking Darvon Compound-65.

Darvon
see DARVOCET-N

Daypro

Generic name: Oxaprozin

Daypro is a nonsteroidal anti-inflammatory drug (NSAID). It works by blocking the production of prostaglandins, which may trigger pain.

℞ QUICK FACTS

Purpose

 Used to treat the inflammation, swelling, stiffness, and joint pain associated with rheumatoid arthritis and osteoarthritis.

Dosage

 Take with a full glass of water. Although pain relief may be delayed, can take with food, milk, or an antacid if Daypro upsets your stomach. Avoid lying down for 20 minutes after taking Daypro to prevent upper digestive tract irritation.

Usual adult dose: *for rheumatoid arthritis*—1,200 milligrams (two 600-milligram caplets) once a day. *For osteoarthritis*—1,200 milligrams (two 600-milligram caplets) once a day. Daily dosage should not exceed 1,800 milligrams divided into smaller doses, or 26 milligrams per 2.2 pounds of body weight, whichever is lower.

 Usual child dose: not generally prescribed for children.

Missed dose: try to take at the same time each day. If you miss a dose and remember later that day, take the missed dose. Otherwise, *do not double the dose the next day; return to your regular schedule as soon as possible.*

Side Effects

 Overdose symptoms: coma, drowsiness, fatigue, nausea, pain in the stomach, stomach and intestinal bleeding, vomiting. Rarely: acute kidney failure, high blood pressure, slowdown in breathing. If you suspect an overdose, immediately seek medical attention.

 More common side effects: constipation, diarrhea, indigestion, nausea, rash.

 Less common side effects: abdominal pain, confusion, depression, frequent or painful urination, gas, loss of appetite, ringing in the ears, sleep disturbances, sleepiness, vomiting. Rare side effects: anemia, blood in the urine, blood pressure changes, blurred vision, bruising, changes in kidney and liver function, decreased menstrual flow, fluid retention, general feeling of illness, hemorrhoid or rectal bleeding, hepatitis, hives, inflammation of the mouth, irritated eyes, itching, peptic ulcerations, respiratory infection, sensitivity to light, severe allergic reaction, stomach and intestinal bleeding, weakness, weight gain or loss.

Interactions

 Inform your doctor before combining Daypro with: aspirin, beta-blocking blood pressure medications such as Inderal and Tenormin, blood thinners such as Coumadin, diuretics such as Lasix and Midamor, lithium (Lithonate).

Should not use alcohol while taking Daypro.

Special Cautions

 If pregnant or planning to become pregnant, inform your doctor immediately. Not known if Daypro appears in breast milk.

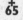 No special precautions apply to seniors.

 Not generally prescribed for children.

 Do not use if you are planning to have surgery in the immediate future.

Ulcers and internal bleeding may occur without warning; doctor should give regular checkups.

If sensitive to or had allergic reaction to Daypro, should not take. Inform your doctor if you have: asthma, nasal tumors, or other allergic reactions to aspirin or other NSAIDs.

Use with caution if you have: heart disease, high blood pressure, kidney or liver disease.

Doctor should monitor for anemia if you are taking Daypro for a prolonged period of time.

Since Daypro may cause sensitivity, avoid excessive sunlight.

DDAVP

Generic name: Desmopressin acetate

Other brand name: Stimate

DDAVP is a posterior pituitary hormone. Hormones stimulate and regulate body functions.

℞ QUICK FACTS

Purpose

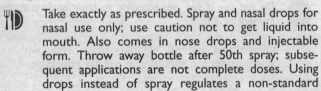

Used to treat frequent urination and water loss associated with diabetes insipidus. Also used to treat frequent urination and increased thirst in individuals with brain injuries, individuals undergoing pituitary surgery, and childhood bedwetting.

Dosage

Take exactly as prescribed. Spray and nasal drops for nasal use only; use caution not to get liquid into mouth. Also comes in nose drops and injectable form. Throw away bottle after 50th spray; subsequent applications are not complete doses. Using drops instead of spray regulates a non-standard dosage.

Usual adult dose: 0.1 to 0.4 milliliter per day, as a single dose or divided into 2 or 3 doses. Dosage level is increased or decreased based on length of sleep without urination and amount of urine your kidneys produce.

Usual child dose: *for children 3 months to 12 years*— 0.05 to 0.3 milliliter per day, as a single dose or divided into 2 doses.

Missed dose: take as soon as possible. *For 1 daily dose*—if you remember the next day, skip missed dose; go back to regular schedule. *For more than 1 dose per day*—if almost time for next dose, skip missed dose; go back to regular schedule. *Do not double doses.*

Side Effects

 Overdose symptoms: abdominal cramps, flushing, headache, nausea, stuffy or irritated nose. If you suspect an overdose, immediately seek medical attention.

 More common side effects: *from too high a dosage*—flushing, headache, irritation of the nose, mild abdominal cramps, nausea, stuffy nose. *Post DDAVP therapy*—cold or other upper respiratory infections, cough, nosebleed, sore throat.

 Other side effects: abdominal pain, chills, disruption in output of tears, dizziness, eye swelling, inflamed eyelids, nostril pain, stomach or intestinal upset, weakness.

Interactions

 Inform your doctor before combining DDAVP with: any drug used to increase blood pressure, clofibrate (Atromid-S), glyburide (Micronase), epinephrine (EpiPen).

 No known food/other substance interactions.

Special Cautions

 If pregnant or planning to become pregnant, inform your doctor immediately. Not known if DDAVP appears in breast milk.

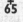 Seniors should limit fluid intake; there is a limited risk of water intoxication.

 Follow doctor's instructions carefully for children. Children with diabetes should limit fluid intake; there is a limited risk of water intoxication.

· ·

 Do not use if sensitive to or had an allergic reaction to DDAVP.

· ·

Use caution before swimming; unabsorbed DDAVP washes out of the nose.

· ·

If you experience nasal swelling, your doctor may prescribe injectable form.

· ·

Use cautiously if you have: coronary artery disease, cystic fibrosis, electrolyte imbalance, or high blood pressure.

Decadron Tablets

Generic name: Dexamethasone

Other brand names: Dexameth, Dexone, Hexadrol

Decadron is an anti-inflammatory/corticosteroid. It works by stimulating the synthesis of enzymes needed to decrease the inflammatory response.

℞ QUICK FACTS

Purpose

℞ Used to treat inflammation and symptoms of several disorders including: rheumatoid arthritis, severe asthma, and a lack of sufficient adrenal hormone. Also used to treat: allergic conditions (severe), blood disorders, certain cancers, connective tissue diseases, digestive tract disease, high serum levels of calcium associated with cancer, fluid retention due to kidney damage, eye diseases, lung diseases, skin diseases.

· ·

Dosage

 Take exactly as prescribed. Doctor may suggest taking with meals to prevent peptic ulcers. Consult with your doctor before abruptly stopping medication.

 Usual adult dose: 0.75 to 9 milligrams per day. After the achieved response occurs, dosage will be lowered by your doctor.

 Usual child dose: not generally prescribed for children.

 Missed dose: take as soon as possible, unless almost time for next dose. In that case, do not take missed dose; go back to regular schedule. *Do not double doses.*

Side Effects

 Overdose symptoms: no specific symptoms have been reported. If you suspect an overdose, immediately seek medical attention.

 Side effects: abdominal distension, allergic reactions, blood clots, bone fractures and degeneration, bruises, cataracts, congestive heart failure, convulsions, "cushingoid" symptoms (moon face, weight gain, high blood pressure, emotional disturbances, growth of facial hair in women), emotional disturbances, excessive hairiness, fluid and salt retention, general feeling of illness, glaucoma, headache, hiccups, high blood pressure, hives, increased appetite, increased eye pressure, increased sweating, increases in amounts of Insulin or hypoglycemic medications needed in diabetes, inflammation of esophagus, inflammation of pancreas, irregular menstruation, loss of muscle mass, low potassium levels in blood, muscle weakness, nausea, osteoporosis, peptic ulcer, perforated small and large bowel, poor healing of wounds, protruding eyeballs, ruptured tendons, suppression of growth in children, thin skin, tiny red or purplish spots on the skin, vertigo, weight gain.

 No known less common or rare side effects.

Interactions

 Inform your doctor before combining Decadron Tablets with: aspirin; blood thinners such as Coumadin and Panwarfin; ephedrine; indomethacin (Indocin); phenobarbital; phenytoin (Dilantin); potassium-depleting diuretics such as HydroDIURIL; rifampin (Rifadin or Rimactane).

 No known food/other substance interactions.

Special Cautions

 If pregnant or planning to become pregnant, inform your doctor immediately. Adrenal problems may occur in infants whose mothers take corticosteroids during pregnancy. Corticosteroids appear in breast milk and can suppress growth in infants.

 No special precautions apply to seniors.

 Not generally prescribed for children.

 Do not use if you have a fungal infection, or are sensitive to or allergic to the ingredients in Decadron.

Do not get a smallpox vaccination while you are taking Decadron.

Inform your doctor before taking Decadron if you have: allergies to cortisone-like drugs, cirrhosis, diabetes, diverticulitis, eye infection (herpes simplex), glaucoma, high blood pressure, impaired thyroid function, kidney disease, myasthenia gravis, osteoporosis, peptic ulcer, recent heart attack, tuberculosis, ulcerative colitis.

. . . .

May experience lowered resistance to infections, or may mask the signs of infection. Immediately inform your doctor if exposed to measles or chicken pox; can be serious or fatal in adults.

. . . .

May alter your body's reaction to unusual stress; higher dosage may be prescribed by your doctor.

. . . .

Dormant tuberculosis may be activated by Decadron. Your doctor should prescribe anti-tuberculosis medication if taking Decadron for a prolonged period.

. . . .

After Decadron therapy ends, may experience withdrawal symptoms such as fever, muscle or joint pain, and a feeling of illness.

. . . .

Can alter male fertility.

. . . .

May cause or aggravate existing emotional problems; notify your doctor if you experience mood changes.

. . . .

Inform your doctor of recent trips to the tropics as well as any diarrhea.

Decadron Turbinaire and Respihaler

$\wedge$

Generic name: Dexamethasone sodium phosphate

Other brand name: Dexacort

Decadron Turbinaire and Respihaler is an adrenocorti-costeroid/anti-asthmatic/anti-inflammatory. It works by stimulating the synthesis of enzymes needed to decrease the inflammatory response.

℞ QUICK FACTS

Purpose

 Used to treat hay fever and other nasal allergies, and to treat nasal polyps. Respihaler is used to treat bronchial asthma.

Dosage

 Take exactly as prescribed, carefully follow directions for use. Dosage is gradually reduced once symptoms start to disappear, and stopped as soon as possible. Oral steroid medications should be reduced or stopped before Respihaler dosage is reduced.

 Usual adult dose: Turbinaire—2 sprays in each nostril 2 or 3 times per day, not to exceed 12 sprays per day. Respihaler—3 inhalations 3 or 4 times per day, not to exceed 3 inhalations per dose, 12 inhalations per day.

 Usual child dose (6 to 12 years): Turbinaire—1 or 2 sprays in each nostril 2 times per day, not to exceed 8 sprays per day. Respihaler—2 inhalations 3 or 4 times per day, not to exceed 8 inhalations per day.

Missed dose: take as soon as possible, unless time for next dose. In that case, take remaining doses for the day at equally spaced intervals. Do not double doses.

Side Effects

 Overdose symptoms: *in rare cases poisoning and death occur following steroid overdose.* If you suspect an overdose, immediately seek medical attention.

 More common side effects: *Turbinaire*—nasal dryness, nasal irritation. *Respihaler*—coughing, fungal infections in the throat, hoarseness, throat irritation.

 Less common side effects: *Turbinaire*—bronchial asthma, headache, hives, light-headedness, loss of smell, nausea, nosebleeds, perforated nasal septum, rebound nasal congestion, throat discomfort. Side effects when Decadron is absorbed into the bloodstream: abdominal distension, abnormal skin redness, allergic skin reactions, blood clots, cataracts, congestive heart failure, convulsions, development of Cushing's syndrome (moon face, weight gain, high blood pressure, emotional disturbances, growth of facial hair in women), diabetes, dizziness, emotional disturbances, excessive hairiness, fractures of the vertebrae, fragile skin, glaucoma, headache, hiccups, high blood pressure, hives, increased appetite, increased eye pressure, increased pressure in the head, increased sweating, loss of muscle mass, menstrual irregularities, muscle diseases resulting from steroid use, muscle weakness, nausea, osteoporosis, perforated small or large bowel, poor wound healing, potassium loss, protruding eyeballs, reddish or purplish spots on the skin, ruptured tendons, salt and fluid retention, stomach ulcer, vague feeling of weakness, weight gain.

Interactions

 Do not get a smallpox vaccination while taking Decadron. Inform your doctor before combining Decadron with: aspirin; blood thinners such as Coumadin; ephedrine; phenobarbital; phenytoin (Dilantin); potassium-depleting diuretics such as Diazide and Esidrix; rifampin (Rifadin or Rimactane).

 No known food/other substance interactions.

Special Cautions

 If pregnant or planning to become pregnant, inform your doctor immediately. Adrenal problems may occur in infants whose mothers take corticosteroids during pregnancy. Corticosteroids appear in breast milk and can suppress growth in infants.

 No special precautions apply to seniors.

 Follow doctor's instructions carefully for children. Not recommended for children under 6 years. Can affect growth and development of children.

 Do not use if you have a fungal infection, or are sensitive to or allergic to the ingredients in Decadron.

Stop if you develop an infection of the voice box; immediately notify your doctor.

Inform your doctor before taking Decadron if you have: cirrhosis, diverticulitis, high blood pressure, kidney disease, myasthenia gravis, osteoporosis, peptic ulcer, recent heart attack, tuberculosis, ulcerative colitis, underactive thyroid.

Should be used for asthma when bronchodilators or other medications are not effective. Not for rapid relief.

May experience lowered resistance to infections, or may mask the signs of infection. Immediately inform your doctor if exposed to measles or chicken pox, can be serious or fatal in adults.

May alter your body's reaction to unusual stress; higher dosage may be prescribed by your doctor.

Dormant tuberculosis may be activated by Decadron. Your doctor should prescribe anti-tuberculosis medication if taking Decadron for a prolonged period.

After Decadron therapy ends, may experience withdrawal symptoms such as fever, muscle or joint pain, and a feeling of illness.

Can alter male fertility.

May cause or aggravate existing emotional problems; notify your doctor if you experience mood changes.

Inform your doctor of recent trips to the tropics as well as any diarrhea.

If used for prolonged period, may cause cataracts, glaucoma, and eye infections.

Monitor for: increase in salt and water retention, increase in potassium loss, raised blood pressure.

Deconamine

Generic ingredients: Chlorpheniramine maleate with d-pseudoephedrine hydrochloride

Other brand names: Allerest, Anamine, Brexin, Chlorafed, Chlor-Trimeton, Dorcol, Duralex, Isoclor, Kronofed, Naspril, Rhinosyn, Sudafed Plus

Deconamine is an antihistamine/decongestant. It works by blocking the effects of histamine (a body chemical that narrows air passages), reducing swelling and itching, and drying secretions.

℞ QUICK FACTS

Purpose

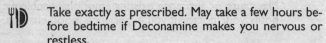

℞ Used on a temporary basis to treat persistent runny nose, sneezing, and nasal congestion caused by the common cold, sinus inflammation, or hay fever. Also used to clear nasal passages and drain sinuses, and relieve sinus pressure.

Dosage

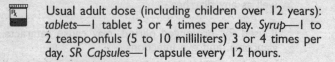

Take exactly as prescribed. May take a few hours before bedtime if Deconamine makes you nervous or restless.

. . . .

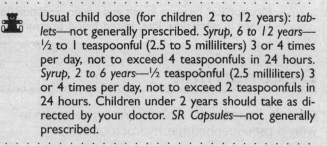

Usual adult dose (including children over 12 years): *tablets*—1 tablet 3 or 4 times per day. *Syrup*—1 to 2 teaspoonfuls (5 to 10 milliliters) 3 or 4 times per day. *SR Capsules*—1 capsule every 12 hours.

. . . .

Usual child dose (for children 2 to 12 years): *tablets*—not generally prescribed. *Syrup, 6 to 12 years*— ½ to 1 teaspoonful (2.5 to 5 milliliters) 3 or 4 times per day, not to exceed 4 teaspoonfuls in 24 hours. *Syrup, 2 to 6 years*—½ teaspoonful (2.5 milliliters) 3 or 4 times per day, not to exceed 2 teaspoonfuls in 24 hours. Children under 2 years should take as directed by your doctor. *SR Capsules*—not generally prescribed.

. . . .

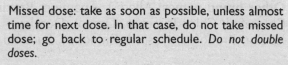

Missed dose: take as soon as possible, unless almost time for next dose. In that case, do not take missed dose; go back to regular schedule. *Do not double doses.*

. . . .

Side Effects

Overdose symptoms: clumsiness or unsteadiness; convulsions; flushing; hallucinations; ongoing headaches; severe drowsiness; severe dryness of mouth, nose, and throat; shortness of breath and/or difficulty breathing; sleep problems; slow or rapid heartbeat. If you suspect an overdose, immediately seek medical attention.

Most common side effect: mild to moderate drowsiness.

Less common or rare side effects: anxiety, blurred vision, breathing difficulty, chills, confusion, constipation, diarrhea, difficulty sleeping, disturbed coordination, dizziness, double vision, dry mouth, dry nose, dry throat, early menstruation, exaggerated sense of well-being, excessive perspiration, excitation, extreme allergic reaction, extreme calm, fatigue, fear, fever, frequent or difficult urination, hallucinations, headache, hives, hysteria, increased chest congestion, irregular heartbeat, irritability, light-headedness, loss of appetite, low blood pressure, mood changes, nausea, nervousness, nightmares, painful urination, pallor, pounding heartbeat, rapid heartbeat, restlessness, ringing in ears, sensitivity to light, skin rash, sore throat, stomach upset or pain, stuffy nose, thickening of bronchial secretions, tightness of chest, tingling in arms and legs, tremor, unusual bleeding or bruising, unusual tiredness, urinary retention, vertigo, vomiting, weakness, wheezing.

Interactions

Inform your doctor before combining Deconamine with: antidepressants such as Nardil, Parnate, Tofranil, and Elavil; asthma medications such as Ventolin and Proventil; blood pressure medications such as Inderal and Tenormin; bromocriptine (Parlodel);

methyldopa (Aldomet); narcotic painkillers such as Demerol and Percocet; phenytoin (Dilantin); sleep aids such as Halcion and Seconal; tranquilizers such as Valium and Xanax.

 Avoid alcohol while taking Deconamine; increases sedative effect of the medication.

Special Cautions

 If pregnant or planning to become pregnant, inform your doctor immediately. Deconamine appears in breast milk; could affect a nursing infant.

 No special precautions apply to seniors.

 Follow doctor's instructions carefully for children. Monitor child for excitability.

 May cause drowsiness or dizziness and impair your ability to drive a car or operate machinery. *Do not take part in any activity that requires alertness.*

Do not use if you have: sensitivity or allergic reaction to antihistamines, severe heart disease, severe high blood pressure, or if taking a MAO inhibitor such as Nardil or Parnate.

Can cause nervousness or sleeplessness.

Use with extreme caution if you have: difficulty urinating, glaucoma, peptic ulcer or certain gastric obstructions, or symptoms of enlarged prostate.

Use cautiously if you have: bronchial asthma, diabetes, or an overactive thyroid.

May produce central nervous system stimulation resulting in convulsions or cardiovascular collapse with low blood pressure.

Decotan Tablets

see RYNATAN

Deltasone

Generic name: Prednisone

Other brand names: Liquipred, Meticorten, Orasone, Panasol-S, Prednicen-M, Sterapred

Deltasone is an adrenocorticosteroid/anti-inflammatory. It works by stimulating the synthesis of enzymes needed to decrease the inflammatory response.

℞ QUICK FACTS

Purpose

℞ Used to treat inflammation and symptoms of several disorders, including rheumatoid arthritis, severe asthma, and a lack of sufficient adrenal hormone. Also used to treat: allergic conditions (severe), blood disorders, certain cancers, connective tissue diseases, eye diseases, flare-ups of multiple sclerosis, fluid retention due to kidney damage, lung diseases, prevention of organ rejection, severe flare-ups of ulcerative colitis or inflammation of the intestines, skin diseases, trichinosis (with complications).

Dosage

 Take exactly as prescribed. Doctor may suggest taking with meals to prevent peptic ulcers. Consult with doctor before abruptly stopping medication. For long-term therapy, doctor may prescribe alternate-day therapy. If on alternate-day therapy, take Deltasone in the morning, with breakfast.

 Usual adult dose: 5 to 60 milligrams per day, depending on what you are being treated for, and your tolerance to the medication. *For multiple sclerosis—* 200 milligrams per day for one week. Lower dose may be prescribed if you have: cirrhosis of the liver or underactive thyroid.

 Usual child dose: not generally prescribed for children.

 Missed dose: *for 1 daily dose*—take as soon as possible, unless you remember the next day. In that case, do not take missed dose; go back to regular schedule. *For several doses per day*—take as soon as possible, then go back to regular schedule. If you remember when it is time to take the next dose, take 2 doses. *For every-other-day dose*—take as soon as possible (if in the morning), then go back to regular schedule. If you remember in the afternoon, skip the next morning; go back to regular schedule.

Side Effects

 Overdose symptoms: long-term use may cause Cushing's syndrome (moon face, weight gain, high blood pressure, emotional disturbances, growth of facial hair in women). If you suspect an overdose, immediately seek medical attention.

 Side effects: Cushing's syndrome, euphoria, eye problems, fluid retention, high blood pressure, insomnia, mood changes, personality changes, psychotic behavior, severe depression.

 Other potential side effects: bone fractures, bulging eyes, convulsions, distended abdomen, face redness, glaucoma, headache, hives and other allergic-type reactions, increased pressure inside eyes or skull, inflamed esophagus or pancreas, irregular menstrual periods, muscle weakness or disease, osteoporosis, peptic ulcer, poor healing of wounds, stunted growth (in children), sweating, thin or fragile skin, vertigo.

Interactions

 Do not get a smallpox vaccination while taking Deltasone. Inform your doctor before combining Deltasone with: amphotericin B (Fungizone); aspirin; carbamazepine (Tegretol); cyclosporine (Sandimmune); estrogen drugs such as Premarin; ketoconazole (Nizoral); oral contraceptives; oral medications for diabetes such as Insulin; phenytoin (Dilantin); potent diuretics such as Lasix; rifampin (Rifadin).

 No known food/other substance interactions.

Special Cautions

 If pregnant or planning to become pregnant, inform your doctor immediately. Not known if Deltasone appears in breast milk.

 No special precautions apply to seniors.

 Not generally prescribed for children. If prescribed, be aware that Deltasone may stunt growth if taken for a prolonged period.

 Do not take if sensitive to or had an allergic reaction to Deltasone.

. . . .

Use with extreme caution if you have an eye infection caused by herpes simplex.

. . . .

May experience lowered resistance to infections, or may mask the signs of infection. Immediately inform your doctor if exposed to measles or chicken pox; can be serious or fatal in adults.

. . . .

Should not take if you have a fungus infection throughout your body, such as candidiasis or cryptococcosis.

. . . .

Dormant tuberculosis may be activated by Deltasone. Doctor should prescribe anti-tuberculosis medication if taking Deltasone for a prolonged period.

. . . .

Use with caution if you have: diverticulitis, high blood pressure, kidney disorder, myasthenia gravis, osteoporosis, peptic ulcer, ulcerative colitis.

Demerol

Generic name: Meperidine hydrochloride

Other brand names: Pethadol, Pheperidine Hydrochloride

Demerol is a narcotic analgesic. It works by altering the response to painful stimuli.

℞ QUICK FACTS

Purpose

℞ Used to treat moderate to severe pain.

. . . .

Dosage

 Take exactly as prescribed. If using syrup form, take with a half glass of water.

 Usual adult dose: 50 to 150 milligrams every 3 or 4 hours. *Seniors:* doctor may reduce dosage.

 Usual child dose: 0.5 to 0.8 milligram per pound of body weight, every 3 or 4 hours.

 Missed dose: take as soon as possible, unless almost time for next dose. In that case, do not take missed dose; go back to regular schedule. *Do not double doses.*

Side Effects

 Overdose symptoms: bluish discoloration of the skin, cold and clammy skin, coma or extreme sleepiness, limp and/or weak muscles, low blood pressure, slow heartbeat, troubled or slowed breathing. *Severe overdose may result in breathing stoppage, heart attack, or death.* If you suspect an overdose, immediately seek medical attention.

 More common side effects: dizziness, light-headedness, nausea, sedation, sweating, vomiting.

 Less common or rare side effects: agitation, constipation, difficulty urinating, disorientation, dry mouth, fainting, fast heartbeat, feeling of elation or depression, flushing of the face, hallucinations, headache, hives, impairment of physical performance, itching, low blood pressure, mental sluggishness or clouding, palpitations, rashes, restlessness, severe convulsions, slow heartbeat, tremors, troubled and slowed breathing, uncoordinated muscle movements, visual disturbances, weakness.

Interactions

 Do not take with MAO inhibitors such as Nardil or Parnate. Inform your doctor before combining Demerol with: antidepressants such as Elavil and Tofranil; antihistamines such as Benadryl; cimetidine (Tagamet); major tranquilizers such as Mellaril and Thorazine; other narcotic painkillers such as Percocet and Tylenol with Codeine; phenytoin (Dilantin); sedatives such as Halcion and Restoril; tranquilizers such as Xanax and Valium.

 Do not drink alcohol while taking Demerol; slows brain activity and intensifies the effects of alcohol.

Special Cautions

 If pregnant or planning to become pregnant, inform your doctor immediately. Demerol appears in breast milk; could affect a nursing infant.

 Doctor may reduce dosage for seniors.

 Follow doctor's instructions carefully for children.

 May impair your ability to drive a car or operate machinery. May also cause dizziness or light-headedness. *Do not take part in any activity that requires alertness.*

Should not take if sensitive to, or had an allergic reaction to Demerol or other narcotic painkillers.

Monitor for mental and physical tolerance if you take Demerol on an ongoing basis, or if you have had a drug abuse problem.

Use with extreme caution if you have a severe asthma attack, if you have recurring lung disease, if unable to inhale or exhale extra air when needed.

Use with caution if you have: Addison's disease, an enlarged prostate, convulsions, head injury, irregular heartbeat, severe abdominal condition, severe liver or kidney disorder, underactive thyroid gland, or urethral stricture.

Notify your doctor that you are taking Demerol before having surgery.

Depakene

~~~~~~

Generic name: Valproic acid

Depakene is an anticonvulsant. It reduces excessive stimulation in the brain.

℞ QUICK FACTS

Purpose

℞ Used to treat seizures and convulsions.

Dosage

 May take with food to avoid digestive system irritation. Swallow capsules whole to prevent mouth and throat irritation. Depakene should be stopped gradually, as directed by your doctor.

 Usual adult dose: 15 milligrams per 2.2 pounds of body weight per day, up to 60 milligrams per 2.2 pounds per day.

 Usual child dose: follow doctor's instructions carefully for children.

 Missed dose: *for 1 dose per day*—take as soon as possible, unless it is the next day. In that case, do not take missed dose; go back to regular schedule. *For multiple doses*—take as soon as possible, if within 6 hours of scheduled time. Take the rest of the doses for the day at equally spaced intervals. *Do not double doses.*

Side Effects

Overdose symptoms: coma, extreme drowsiness, heart problems. If you suspect an overdose, immediately seek medical attention.

More common side effects: indigestion, nausea, vomiting.

Less common or rare side effects: abdominal cramps, aggression, anemia, bleeding, blood disorders, breast enlargement, breast milk not associated with pregnancy or nursing, bruising, changes in behavior, coma, constipation, depression, diarrhea, difficulty in speaking, dizziness, double vision, drowsiness, emotional upset, fever, hair loss (temporary), hallucinations, headache, involuntary eye movements, involuntary jerking or tremors, irregular menstrual periods, itching, lack of coordination, liver disease, loss of bladder control, loss of or increased appetite, overactivity, rash, sedation, sensitivity to light, skin eruptions or peeling, spots before the eyes, swelling of the arms and legs due to fluid retention, swollen glands, weakness, weight loss or gain.

Interactions

Inform your doctor before combining Depakene with: aspirin; barbiturates such as phenobarbital and Seconal; blood thinners such as Coumadin; carbamazepine (Tegretol); clonazepam (Klonopin); cyclosporine (Sandimmune); Dicumarol; ethosuximide (Zarontin); felbamate (Felbatol); isoniazid (Nydrazid); oral contraceptives; phenytoin (Dilantin); primidone

(Mysoline). Watch for extreme drowsiness if you take Halcion, Restoril, or Xanax with Depakene.

 Alcohol causes extreme drowsiness if used while taking Depakene.

Special Cautions

 Depakene may cause harm to a fetus and should not be taken unless it is essential for seizure control. If pregnant or planning to become pregnant, inform your doctor immediately. Depakene appears in breast milk; could affect a nursing infant.

 No special precautions apply to seniors.

 Follow doctor's instructions carefully for children. Children under 2 years are especially at risk, more so if they are taking other anticonvulsant medicines, or are mentally retarded.

 May cause drowsiness and impair your ability to drive a car or operate machinery. *Do not take part in any activity that requires alertness.*

Can cause serious liver damage, often within the first 6 months of therapy. Risk of liver damage decreases with age. Should not take if you have liver disease.

If you have had an allergic reaction to Depakene, you should not take.

Your doctor will test your blood regularly due to the potential for side effects such as bruising, hemorrhaging, or clotting.

Inform your doctor or dentist that you are taking Depakene before surgical or dental procedures.

Depakote

∿∿∿∿∿∿∿∿∿∿∿∿∿∿∿∿∿∿∿∿∿∿∿∿∿∿∿∿∿∿∿∿∿∿∿

Generic name: Divalproex sodium (valporic acid)

Depakote is an anticonvulsant. It reduces excessive stimulation in the brain.

℞ QUICK FACTS

Purpose

℞   Used to treat seizures and convulsions.

Dosage

   May take with food to avoid stomach upset, swallowing tablet whole. Sprinkle capsule—can swallow whole or open it and mix the contents with soft food, swallowing without chewing.

. . . .

   Usual adult dose: 15 milligrams per 2.2 pounds of body weight per day, up to 60 milligrams. For total daily doses over 250 milligrams, your doctor may advise you to take smaller, separate doses.

. . . .

   Usual child dose: 15 milligrams per 2.2 pounds of body weight per day, up to 60 milligrams per 2.2 pounds of body weight per day. For daily doses over 250 milligrams, your doctor may advise you to take smaller, separate doses.

. . . .

   Missed dose: *for 1 dose per day*—take as soon as possible, unless it is the next day. In that case, do not take missed dose; go back to regular schedule. *For multiple doses*—take as soon as possible, if within 6 hours of scheduled time. Take the rest of the doses for the day at equally spaced intervals. *Do not double doses.*

. . . .

Side Effects

 Overdose symptoms: coma, extreme sleepiness, heart problems. If you suspect an overdose, immediately seek medical attention.

 More common side effects: indigestion, nausea, vomiting.

 Less common or rare side effects: abdominal cramping, abnormal milk secretion, aggression, anemia, behavior problems, bleeding, blood disorders, breast enlargement, bruising, coma, constipation, depression, diarrhea, dizziness, double vision, drowsiness, emotional upset, fever, hallucinations, headache, increased appetite, involuntary rapid movement of eyeball, irregular menstruation, itching, jerky movements, lack of muscular coordination, liver problems, loss of appetite, loss of bladder control, overactivity, sedation, seeing spots before your eyes, sensitivity to light, skin eruptions or peeling, skin rash, speech difficulties, swelling of arms due to fluid retention, swollen glands, temporary hair loss, tremor, weakness, weight loss or gain.

Interactions

 Inform your doctor before combining Depakote with: aspirin; barbiturates such as phenobarbital and Seconal; blood thinners such as Coumadin; cyclosporine (Sandimmune); felbamate (Felbatol); isoniazid (Nydrazid); oral contraceptives; other seizure medications including carbamazepine (Tegretol), clonazepam (Klonopin), ethosuximide (Zarontin), and phenytoin (Dilantin); primidone (Mysoline); sleep aids such as Halcion; tranquilizers such as Valium and Xanax.

 Do not drink alcohol during Depakote therapy; its effects are increased.

Special Cautions

 Depakote may cause harm to a fetus and should not be taken unless it is essential for seizure control. If pregnant or planning to become pregnant, inform your doctor immediately. Depakote appears in breast milk; could affect a nursing infant.

 No special precautions apply to seniors.

 Follow doctor's instructions carefully for children. Children under 2 years are especially at risk, more so if taking other anticonvulsant medicines, or are mentally retarded.

 May cause drowsiness and impair your ability to drive a car or operate machinery. *Do not take part in any activity that requires alertness.*

Can cause serious liver damage, often within the first 6 months of therapy. Risk of liver damage decreases with age. Should not take if you have liver disease.

If you have had an allergic reaction to Depakote or other epilepsy drugs, you should not take.

Monitor bleeding; Depakote prolongs the time it takes blood to clot.

Inform your doctor or dentist that you are taking Depakote before surgical or dental procedures.

Depo-Provera
see PROVERA

Desipramine Hydrochloride
see NORPRAMIN

Desmopressin Acetate
see DDAVP

Desonide
see TRIDESILON

DesOwen
see TRIDESILON

Desoximetasone
see TOPICORT

Desquam-E
∧∧∧

Generic name: Benzoyl peroxide

Other brand names: Benzac W, Benzagel,
BenzaShave, PanOxyl, Persa-Gel, Theroxide

Desquam-E is a topical gel. It treats skin disorders with
minimal effects throughout the body.

℞ QUICK FACTS

Purpose

 ℞ Used to treat acne.

Dosage

 Clean treatment area, gently rub in Desquam-E. For external use only; avoid eyes, nose, or throat.

 Usual adult dose: rub gel into affected areas 1 or 2 times per day.

 Usual child dose: *for children over 12 years*—rub gel into affected areas 1 or 2 times per day.

 Missed dose: apply as soon as you remember, then go back to regular schedule.

Side Effects

 Overdose symptoms: excessive scaling of the skin, reddening skin, or swelling due to fluid retention. If you suspect an overdose, immediately seek medical attention.

 Side effects: allergic reaction (itching, rash), excessive drying.

 No known less common or rare side effects.

Interactions

 No known drug interactions.

 May cause temporary skin discoloration if used with sunscreens containing PABA.

Special Cautions

 If pregnant or planning to become pregnant, inform your doctor immediately. May appear in breast milk; could affect a nursing infant.

 No special precautions apply to seniors.

 Follow doctor's instructions carefully for children.

 Do not use if sensitive to or allergic to benzoyl peroxide.

If sensitive to benzoic acid or cinnamon, you may have sensitivity to this medication.

Use with caution; may bleach hair or colored fabric.

Desyrel

Generic name: Trazodone hydrochloride

Other brand name: Desyrel Dividose

Desyrel is an antidepressant. It increases the concentration of chemicals involved in nerve transmission in the brain.

℞ QUICK FACTS

Purpose

℞ Used to treat depression.

Dosage

 Take exactly as prescribed. May take after a meal or light snack to avoid dizziness or light-headedness. Most patients notice improvement after 2 weeks, although it may take up to 4 weeks.

Usual adult dose: 150 milligrams per day, divided into 2 or more doses, up to 400 milligrams per day total, divided into smaller doses.

 Usual child dose: not generally prescribed for children.

 Missed dose: take as soon as possible, unless within 4 hours of the next dose. In that case, do not take missed dose, go back to regular schedule. *Do not double doses.*

Side Effects

 Desyrel overdose combined with other drugs can be fatal. Overdose symptoms: breathing failure, drowsiness, irregular heartbeat, prolonged and/or painful erection, seizures, vomiting. If you suspect an overdose, immediately seek medical attention.

 More common side effects: abdominal or stomach disorder, aches or pains in muscles and bones, allergic skin reaction, anger or hostility, blurred vision, brief loss of consciousness, confusion, constipation, decreased appetite, diarrhea, dizziness or lightheadedness, drowsiness, dry mouth, excitement, fast or fluttery heartbeat, fatigue, fluid retention and swelling, headache, impaired memory, inability to fall or stay asleep, low blood pressure, nasal or sinus congestion, nausea, nervousness, nightmares or vivid dreams, rapid heartbeat, sudden loss of strength or fainting, tremors, uncoordinated movements, vomiting, weight gain or loss.

 Less common side effects: allergic reactions, anemia, bad taste in mouth, blood in urine, chest pain, delayed urine flow, decrease in concentration, decrease in sex drive, disorientation, early menstruation, ejaculation problems, excess salivation, fullness or heaviness in the head, gas, general feeling of illness, hallucinations or delusions, high blood pressure, impaired memory, impaired speech, impotence, increased appetite, increased sex drive, itchy eyes, missed menstrual periods, more frequent urination, muscle twitches, numbness, prolonged erections, red eyes, restlessness, ringing in the ears, shortness of breath, sweating or clammy skin, tingling or pins and needles, tired eyes.

Interactions

 Inform your doctor before combining Desyrel with: antidepressants known as MAO inhibitors, including Parnate and Nardil; barbiturates such as Seconal; central nervous system depressants such as Demerol and Halcion; chlorpromazine (Thorazine); digoxin (Lanoxin); high blood pressure drugs such as Catapres and Wytensin; other antidepressants such as Prozac and Norpramin; phenytoin (Dilantin).

 Do not drink alcohol during Desyrel therapy; its effects are increased.

Special Cautions

 If pregnant or planning to become pregnant, inform your doctor immediately. May appear in breast milk; could affect a nursing infant.

 No special precautions apply to seniors.

 Not generally prescribed for children.

 May cause drowsiness and impair your ability to drive a car or operate machinery. *Do not take part in any activity that requires alertness.*

If sensitive to or allergic to Desyrel, should not take.

Inform your doctor or dentist that you are taking Desyrel before surgical or dental procedures.

Use with caution if you have heart disease.

Dexacort
see DECADRON TURBINAIRE AND RESPIHALER

Dexamethasone
see DECADRON TABLETS

Dexamethasone Sodium Phosphate
see DECADRON TURBINAIRE AND RESPIHALER

Dexamethasone Sodium Phosphate with Neomycin Sulfate
see NEODECADRON OPHTHALMIC OINTMENT AND SOLUTION

Dexchlor
see POLARAMINE

Dexchlorpheniramine Maleate

see POLARAMINE

Dexedrine
∿∿

Generic name: Dextroamphetamine sulfate

Other brand names: DextroStat, Ferndex, Oxydess II, Spancap No. 1

Dexedrine is a stimulant. It calms the central nervous system in children, and acts as a stimulant in adults.

℞ QUICK FACTS

Purpose

℞ Used on a short-term basis to treat: narcolepsy, attention deficit disorder (ADD) with hyperactivity, obesity. *Do not use this medication to improve mental alertness or to stay awake.*

Dosage

 Take exactly as prescribed. Swallow sustained-release Spansule whole. Use with caution; can become dependent on this medication. Your doctor may periodically stop Dexedrine therapy to evaluate whether you still require the medication. *Do not increase dosage unless directed by your doctor.*

 Usual adult dose: *for narcolepsy*—5 to 60 milligrams per day, divided into equal doses. *For obesity*—one 10-milligram or 15-milligram Spansule taken in the morning, or up to 30 milligrams daily, divided into smaller doses, taken 30 to 60 minutes before meals.

Usual child dose: *for narcolepsy—children 6 to 12 years*—5 milligrams per day; *children 12 years and older*—10 milligrams per day, doctor may prescribe up to 60 milligrams per day. May be reduced if insomnia or anorexia appears. *For ADD—children 3 to 5 years*—2.5 milligrams daily; *children 6 years and older*—5 milligrams 1 or 2 times per day. Children should take the first dose upon waking up, then the remaining at intervals determined by your doctor. *For obesity*—not prescribed for children under 12 years for this use.

Missed dose: *for 1 daily dose*—take as soon as possible, unless within 6 hours of bedtime. If you remember the next day, do not take missed dose; return to regular schedule. *For 2 or 3 doses per day*—take as soon as possible unless within 1 hour of next dose. In that case, do not take missed dose; return to regular schedule. *Do not double doses.*

Side Effects

Dexedrine overdose can be fatal. Overdose symptoms: abdominal cramps, assaultiveness, coma, confusion, convulsions, depression, diarrhea, fatigue, hallucinations, high fever, heightened reflexes, high or low blood pressure, irregular heartbeat, nausea, panic, rapid breathing, restlessness, tremor, vomiting. If you suspect an overdose, immediately seek medical attention.

More common side effects: excessive restlessness, overstimulation.

Other side effects: changes in sex drive, constipation, diarrhea, dizziness, dry mouth, exaggerated feeling of well-being or depression, headache, heart palpitations, high blood pressure, hives, impotence, rapid heartbeat, sleeplessness, stomach and intestinal disturbances, tremors, uncontrollable twitching or jerking, unpleasant taste in the mouth. Effects of chronic heavy abuse of Dexedrine: hyperactivity, irritability, personality changes, schizophrenia-like thoughts and behavior, severe insomnia, severe skin disease.

Interactions

 Inform your doctor before combining Dexedrine with: ammonium chloride; chlorpromazine (Thorazine); glutamic acid hydrochloride; guanethidine (Ismelin); haloperidol (Haldol); lithium carbonate (Lithonate); methenamine (Urised); reserpine (Diupres); sodium acid phosphate. *Substances that boost the effects of Dexedrine*—acetazolamide (Diamox); baking soda; Diuril; MAO-inhibitor antidepressants such as Nardil and Parnate; propoxyphene (Darvon). *Substances that decrease their effectiveness with Dexedrine*—antihistamines such as Benedryl; blood pressure medications such as Catapres, Hytrin, and Minipress; ethosuximide (Zarontin); veratrum alkaloids (found in certain blood pressure medications). *Substances that increase their effectiveness with Dexedrine*—antidepressants such as Norpramin and Vivactil; meperidine (Demerol); Norepinephrine (Levophed); phenobarbital; phenytoin (Dilantin). *Do not take for at least 14 days after MAO-inhibitor antidepressant therapy; may cause life-threatening rise in blood pressure.*

 Fruit juices and vitamin C dampen the effects of Dexedrine.

Special Cautions

 Dexedrine can cause premature births or babies with low birth weight. If pregnant or planning to become pregnant, inform your doctor immediately.

Appears in breast milk; nursing mothers should not use.

 No special precautions apply to seniors.

 Follow doctor's instructions carefully for children. Monitor children on Dexedrine therapy; may stunt growth.

 May cause drowsiness and impair your ability to drive a car or operate machinery. *Do not take part in any activity that requires alertness.*

Do not take if sensitive to or allergic to Dexedrine.

Your doctor will not start you on Dexedrine therapy if you have: agitation, cardiovascular disease, glaucoma, hardening of the arteries, high blood pressure, overactive thyroid gland, substance abuse.

Dexedrine contains tartrazine—yellow food coloring—which can cause severe allergic reaction.

Dextroamphetamine Sulfate
see DEXEDRINE

DiaBeta
see MICRONASE

Diabinese

~~~~~~

Generic name: Chlorpropamide

Diabinese is an oral antidiabetic. It induces the pancreas to secrete more Insulin.

℞ QUICK FACTS

Purpose

 Used to treat Type II (non-insulin-dependent) diabetes.

Dosage

 Usually taken once a day with breakfast. To avoid stomach upset, your doctor may suggest dividing the dose into smaller doses taken throughout the day. Follow the exercise and diet suggested by your doctor closely.

. . . .

 Usual adult dose: 250 milligrams, up to 750 milligrams, depending on the severity of the diabetes. *Seniors*—100 to 125 milligrams.

. . . .

 Usual child dose: not generally prescribed for children.

. . . .

 Missed dose: take as soon as possible, unless almost time for next dose. In that case, do not take missed dose, go back to regular schedule. *Do not double doses.*

Side Effects

 Overdose symptom: low blood sugar. If you suspect an overdose, immediately seek medical attention.

. . . .

 More common side effects: diarrhea, hunger, itching, loss of appetite, nausea, stomach upset, vomiting.

Less common or rare side effects: anemia and other blood disorders, hives, inflammation of the rectum and colon, sensitivity to light, yellowing of the skin and eyes. May cause hypoglycemia; symptoms of mild hypoglycemia: cold sweat, drowsiness, fast heartbeat, headache, nausea, nervousness. Symptoms of severe hypoglycemia: coma, pale skin, seizures, shallow breathing.

Interactions

 Inform your doctor before combining Diabinese with: anabolic steroids; aspirin in large doses; barbiturates such as Seconal; beta-blockers such as Inderal and Tenormin; calcium-blockers such as Cardizem and Procardia; chloramphenicol (Chloromycetin); Coumarin (Coumadin); diuretics such as Diuril and HydroDIURIL; epinephrine (EpiPen); estrogen medications such as Premarin; isoniazid (Nydrazid); major tranquilizers such as Mellaril and Thorazine; MAO inhibitors such as Nardil and Parnate; nicotinic acid (Nicobid or Nicolar); nonsteroidal anti-inflammatory agents such as Advil, Motrin, Naprosyn, and Nuprin; oral contraceptives; phenothiazines; phenylbutazone (Butazolidin); phenytoin (Dilantin); probenecid (Benemid or ColBENEMID); steroids such as prednisone; sulfa drugs such as Bactrim and Septra; thyroid medications such as Synthroid.

 Excessive alcohol usage while taking Diabinese can cause low blood sugar, breathlessness, and facial flushing.

Special Cautions

 If pregnant or planning to become pregnant, inform your doctor immediately. Appears in breast milk; nursing mothers should not use. Your doctor may prescribe Insulin injections during pregnancy to maintain normal blood sugar levels. To lower risk of low blood sugar in newborns, Diabinese, if prescribed, should be discontinued at least 1 month prior to delivery.

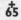 Seniors are prescribed lower doses of Diabinese.

 Not generally prescribed for children.

 Do not take if you have diabetic ketoacidosis—a life-threatening medical emergency brought on by insufficient insulin and evidenced by excessive thirst, nausea, fatigue, pain below the breastbone, and fruity breath odor.

If you suffer from impaired liver or kidneys, or are malnourished, a lower dosage of Diabinese will be prescribed.

Diabinese is not an oral form of insulin, and cannot substitute for insulin.

Should not take if you have an allergic reaction to Diabinese.

Inform your doctor before taking Diabinese if you have a heart problem.

Doctor should monitor your blood and urine periodically for abnormal sugar levels.

Effectiveness may decrease over time due to a reduced responsiveness or a worsening of the diabetes.

Diamox

Generic name: Acetazolamide

Other brand names: Ak-Zol, Dazamide, Diamox Sequels

Diamox is a carbonic anhydrase inhibitor. It has the effect of a weak diuretic.

℞ QUICK FACTS

Purpose

℞ Used to treat glaucoma, epilepsy, and fluid retention due to congestive heart failure or drugs. Also used to treat acute mountain sickness.

Dosage

 Take exactly as prescribed.

. . . .

 Usual adult dose: *for glaucoma*—250 milligrams to 1 gram per 24 hours, in 2 or more smaller doses. *For secondary glaucoma*—250 milligrams every 4 hours. Diamox Sequels—1 capsule (500 milligrams) twice a day, in the morning and evening. *For epilepsy*—8 to 30 milligrams per 2.2 pounds of body weight in 2 or more doses. Typical dosage is 375 to 1,000 milligrams per day. *For congestive heart failure*—250 milligrams to 375 milligrams per day or 5 milligrams per 2.2 pounds of body weight, taken in the morning. Works best when taken every other day. *For edema due to medication*—250 milligrams to 375 milligrams daily for 1 or 2 days, followed by a day of rest. *For acute mountain sickness*—500 milligrams to 1,000 milligrams a day in 2 or more doses. Therapy should start 1 or 2 days prior to reaching high altitudes.

. . . .

 Usual child dose: *for epilepsy*—8 milligrams to 30 milligrams per 2.2 pounds of body weight.

. . . .

 Missed dose: take as soon as possible, unless almost time for next dose. In that case, do not take missed

dose; go back to regular schedule. *Do not double doses.*

Side Effects

 Overdose symptoms: no specific information available. If you suspect an overdose, immediately seek medical attention.

 More common side effects: change in taste or metallic taste, diarrhea, increase in the amount or frequency of urination, loss of appetite, nausea, ringing in the ears, tingling or pins and needles in hands or feet, vomiting.

 Less common or rare side effects: anemia, black or bloody stools, blood in urine, confusion, convulsions, drowsiness, fever, hives, liver dysfunction, nearsightedness, paralysis, rash, sensitivity to light, severe allergic reaction, skin peeling.

Interactions

 Inform your doctor before combining Diamox with: amitriptyline (Elavil); amphetamines such as Dexedrine; aspirin; cyclosporine (Sandimmune); lithium (Lithonate); methenamine (Urex); oral diabetes drugs such as Micronase; quinidine (Quinidex).

 No known food/other substance interactions.

Special Cautions

 If pregnant or plan to become pregnant, inform your doctor immediately. May appear in breast milk, could affect a nursing infant.

 Seniors should use with caution.

Follow doctor's instructions carefully for children.

 Do not take Diamox if you have serious liver, kidney, or Addison's disease; low blood sodium; low potassium.

Development of: rash, sore throat, bruises, or fever may signal allergic reaction. Immediately contact your doctor if you experience any of these.

If you are taking large doses of aspirin, use caution when combining with Diamox.

If you have emphysema or other breathing disorders, use this medication with caution.

Long-term use for chronic noncongestive angle-closure glaucoma should be avoided.

If you take Diamox to help in rapid ascent of a mountain, must come down promptly if signs of severe mountain sickness appear.

Diazepam
see VALIUM

Diclofenac Sodium
see VOLTAREN

Dicloxacillin Sodium
see PATHOCIL

Dicyclomine Hydrochloride

see BENTYL

Diethylpropion Hydrochloride

see TENUATE

Diflorasone Diacetate

see PSORCON

Diflucan

Generic name: Fluconazole

Diflucan is an antifungal agent. It destroys and prevents the growth of fungi.

℞ QUICK FACTS

Purpose

℞   Used to treat fungal infections known as candidiasis (thrush or yeast infections). Also used to treat throat infections and fungal infections throughout the body including urinary tract, abdomen, kidney, liver, spinal cord or brain (meningitis), and in patients with AIDS.

Dosage

 Take exactly as prescribed. May take with or without food. Even if you feel better, continue taking medication for the amount of time your doctor has prescribed.

 Usual adult dose: *for throat infections*—200 milligrams on the first day, then 100 milligrams once a day, for 2 to 3 weeks. For esophagus infection, treatment should continue for at least 2 weeks after symptoms have stopped. *For bodywide infections*—400 milligrams on the first day, followed by 200 milligrams once a day, for a minimum of 4 weeks. *For cryptococcal meningitis*—400 milligrams on the first day, then 200 milligrams once a day for 10 to 12 weeks. *For AIDS patients*—200 milligrams once a day. Dosages may be reduced if you have kidney disease.

 Usual child dose: not generally prescribed for children, although a small number have been treated safely with Diflucan. Dosage is prescribed according the child's specific needs.

 Missed dose: take as soon as possible, unless almost time for next dose. In that case, do not take missed dose; go back to regular schedule. *Do not double doses.*

Side Effects

 Overdose symptoms: hallucinations, paranoia. If you suspect an overdose, immediately seek medical attention.

 Most common side effect: nausea.

 Less common side effects: abdominal pain, diarrhea, headache, skin rash, vomiting.

Interactions

 Inform your doctor before combining Diflucan with: antidiabetic drugs (Orinase, DiaBeta, or Glucotrol); antihistamines such as Hismanal; blood thinners (Coumadin); cyclosporine (Sandimmune); hydro-chlorothiazide (HydroDIURIL); phenytoin (Dilantin); rifampin (Rifadin); ulcer medications such as Tagamet.

 No known food/other substance interactions.

Special Cautions

 If pregnant or plan to become pregnant, inform your doctor immediately. Appears in breast milk; could affect a nursing infant.

 No special precautions apply to seniors.

 Follow doctor's instructions carefully for children.

 Do not take if sensitive to any ingredients in Diflucan, or similar medications such as Nizoral.

Although rare, strong allergic reactions have been reported. Symptoms—hives, itching, swelling, sudden drop in blood pressure, difficulty breathing or swallowing, diarrhea, abdominal pain.

Doctor should monitor your kidney function while taking Diflucan.

If you have low immunity and develop a rash, inform your doctor; this condition should be monitored.

Diflunisal
see DOLOBID

Digoxin
see LANOXIN

Dihydrocodeine Bitartrate with Aspirin and Caffeine
see SYNALGOS-DC

Dilantin

Generic name: Phenytoin sodium

Other brand names: Diphenylan Sodium, Phenytoin Sodium Extended

Dilantin is an anticonvulsant. It reduces excessive stimulation in the brain.

℞ QUICK FACTS

Purpose

℞ Used to treat grand mal seizures and temporal lobe seizures. Also used to prevent and treat seizures during and after neurosurgery.

Dosage

 Strictly follow therapy regimen. If using Suspension form, shake well before using; swallow Kapseals whole. Infatabs can be chewed thoroughly and swallowed, or swallowed whole. Infatabs are not for once-a-day dosing. *Do not switch brands without advice from your doctor.*

Usual adult dose: *standard daily dose*—one 100-milligram capsule 3 times per day. On an ongoing basis, one capsule 3 to 4 times per day is standard. *For 1 dose a day*—one 300-milligram capsule per day, if your seizures are controlled by three 100-milligram capsules.

 Usual child dose: 5 milligrams per 2.2 pounds of body weight per day, divided into 2 or 3 equal doses, up to 300 milligrams per day to start. Ongoing dose—4 to 8 milligrams per 2.2 pounds of body weight.

 Missed dose: *1 dose per day*—take as soon as possible, unless you remember the next day. In that case, do not take missed dose; go back to regular schedule. *More than 1 dose per day*—take as soon as possible, unless within 4 hours of the next dose. In that case, do not take missed dose; go back to regular schedule. If you forget to take this medication for more than 2 days in a row, call your doctor. *Do not double doses.*

Side Effects

 Overdose symptoms: coma, difficulty pronouncing words correctly, involuntary eye movement, lack of muscle coordination, low blood pressure, nausea, sluggishness, slurred speech, tremors, vomiting. If you suspect an overdose, immediately seek medical attention.

 More common side effects: decreased coordination, involuntary eye movement, mental confusion, slurred speech.

 Other side effects: abnormal hair growth, abnormal muscle tone, blood disorders, coarsening of facial features, constipation, dizziness, enlargement of lips, fever, headache, inability to fall asleep or stay asleep, joint pain, nausea, nervousness, overgrowth of gum tissue, Peyronie's disease, rapid and spastic involuntary movement, skin peeling or scaling, skin rash, tremors, twitching, vomiting, yellowing of skin and eyes.

Interactions

Inform your doctor before combining Dilantin with: amiodarone anti-arrhythmics such as Cordarone; antacids containing calcium; blood thinners such as Coumadin; carbamazepine (Tegretol); chloramphenicol (Chloromycetin); chlordiazepoxide (Librium); diazepam (Valium); Dicumarol; digitoxin (Crystodigin); disulfiram (Antabuse); doxycycline (Vibramycin); estrogens such as Premarin; ethosuximide (Zarontin); felbamate (Felbatol); furosemide (Lasix); isoniazid (Nydrazid); major tranquilizers such as Mellaril and Thorazine; methylphenidate (Ritalin); molindone hydrochloride (Moban); oral contraceptives; phenobarbital; phenylbutazone (Butazolidin); quinidine (Quinidex); reserpine (Diupres); rifampin (Rifadin); salicylates such as aspirin; steroid drugs such as prednisone; succinimides (anticonvulsant medications); sucralfate (Carafate); sulfonamides; theophylline (Theo-Dur); tolbutamide (Orinase); trazodone (Desyrel); ulcer medications such as Tagamet and Zantac; valproic acid (Depakene). Tricyclic antidepressants (Elavil or Norpramin) may cause seizures.

Avoid alcohol while taking Dilantin.

Special Cautions

Anti-epileptic medications such as Dilantin can cause birth defects. If pregnant or plan to become pregnant, inform your doctor immediately. Appears in breast milk; could affect a nursing infant.

Seniors should use cautiously, may show signs of drug poisoning.

 Follow doctor's instructions carefully for children.

 Do not stop Dilantin therapy abruptly, may cause status epilepticus, a possibly fatal condition.

If allergic to or sensitive to phenytoin or similar epilepsy medications, do not take Dilantin.

Monitor for hyperglycemia (high blood sugar).

Should not be used for seizures due to hypoglycemia (low blood sugar) or petit mal seizures.

Notify doctor if a skin rash appears (measles-like or scale-like).

May be a link between Dilantin therapy and the development of certain lymph system diseases, including Hodgkin's disease.

Use cautiously if you have porphyria (skin disorder).

Maintain good dental hygiene during Dilantin therapy.

May cause abnormal bone softening due to interference with vitamin D metabolism.

Dilaudid

Generic name: Hydromorphone hydrochloride

Other brand name: HydroStat

Dilaudid is a narcotic analgesic. It works by altering the response to painful stimuli.

℞ QUICK FACTS

Purpose

 Used to treat moderate to severe pain caused by: bilary colic (obstruction of the gallbladder or bile duct), burns, cancer, heart attack injury, renal colic (sharp lower back and groin pain from passing a stone), surgery. Is prescribed with caution after surgery or for patients with lung disease, as Dilaudid suppresses the cough reflex.

Dosage

 Take exactly as prescribed; consult with your doctor to increase the amount.

 Usual adult dose: *tablets*—2 to 4 milligrams every 4 to 6 hours. *Liquid*—½ to 2 teaspoonfuls every 3 to 6 hours. *Suppositories*—1 suppository inserted rectally every 6 to 8 hours. *Seniors*—dosage will be prescribed according to individual needs. Mental and physical dependence may result from high doses taken repeatedly.

 Usual child dose: not generally prescribed for children.

 Missed dose: take as soon as possible, unless almost time for next dose. In that case, do not take missed dose, go back to regular schedule. *Do not double doses.*

Side Effects

Overdose symptoms: bluish tinge to the skin, cold and clammy skin, constricted pupils, coma, extreme sleepiness progressing to unresponsiveness, labored or slow breathing, limp, weak muscles, low blood pressure, slow heart rate. If you suspect an overdose, immediately seek medical attention.

More common side effects: anxiety, constipation, dizziness, drowsiness, fear, impairment of mental and physical performance, inability to urinate, mental clouding, mood changes, nausea, restlessness, sedation, sluggishness, troubled and slowed breathing, vomiting.

Less common side effects: agitation, blurred vision, chills, cramps, diarrhea, difficulty urinating, disorientation, double vision, dry mouth, exaggerated feelings of depression or well-being, failure of breathing or heartbeat, faintness/fainting, flushing, hallucinations, headache, increased pressure in the head, insomnia, involuntary eye movements, itching, lightheadedness, loss of appetite, low or high blood pressure, muscle rigidity or tremor, muscle spasms of the throat or air passages, palpitations, rashes, shock, slow or rapid heartbeat, small pupils, sudden dizziness on standing, sweating, taste changes, tingling and/or numbness, tremor, uncoordinated muscle movements, visual disturbances, weakness.

Interactions

Inform your doctor before combining Dilaudid with: anti-emetics such as Compazine and Phenergan; anti-histamines such as Benadryl; general anesthetics; other central nervous system depressants such as Nembutal and Restoril; other narcotic analgesics such as Demerol and Percocet; phenothiazines such as Thorazine; sedative/hypnotics such as Valium and Halcion; tranquilizers such as Xanax; tricyclic antidepressants such as Elavil and Tofranil.

Do not drink alcohol during Dilaudid therapy; its effects are increased.

Special Cautions

 Newborns may experience drug dependence if the mother has taken narcotics on a regular basis during pregnancy. If pregnant or plan to become pregnant, inform your doctor immediately. May appear in breast milk; could affect a nursing infant.

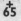 Dosage will be prescribed according to individual needs for seniors.

 Not generally prescribed for children.

 May cause drowsiness and impair your ability to drive a car or operate machinery. *Do not take part in any activity that requires alertness.*

If sensitive to or allergic to Dilaudid or other narcotics, should not take.

Use with caution if you have: Addison's disease (adrenal gland failure), enlarged prostate, head injury, low blood pressure, severe liver or kidney disease, underactive thyroid gland, urethral stricture.

Use with extreme caution if you have breathing difficulties.

Monitor for sudden or severe abdominal conditions; narcotics may mask symptoms.

May aggravate existing condition of convulsions.

Diltiazem Hydrochloride

see CARDIZEM

Dimetane-DC

^^

Generic ingredients: Brompheniramine maleate with phenylpropanolamine hydrochloride and codeine phosphate

Other brand names: Bromaline, Bromarest, Bromatapp, Bromfed-DM, Bromphen, Diamine, Dimaphen, Dimetapp, Genatapp, Myphetapp, Partapp, Veltane

Dimetane-DC is an antihistamine/decongestant combination. It works by blocking the effects of histamine, a body chemical that narrows air passages, reducing swelling and itching, drying secretions, and suppressing coughing.

℞ QUICK FACTS

Purpose

 Used to treat coughs and nasal condition caused by allergies and the common cold.

Dosage

 Take exactly as prescribed.

 Usual adult dose (for adults and children 12 years and older): 2 teaspoonfuls every 4 hours; *do not exceed more than 6 doses in 24 hours.*

Usual child dose: *for children 6 to 11 years*—1 teaspoonful every 4 hours. *For children 2 to 5 years*—½ teaspoonful every 4 hours. *For children 6 months to under 2 years*—doctor will determine appropriate dosage; *do not take more than 6 doses in 24 hours.*

 Missed dose: take as soon as possible, unless almost time for next dose. In that case, do not take missed

dose; go back to regular schedule. *Do not double doses.*

Side Effects

 Overdose symptoms: anxiety, breathing difficulty, convulsions, dilated pupils, excessive excitement or stimulation, extreme sleepiness leading to unconsciousness, hallucinations, heart attack, high blood pressure, irregular heartbeat, rapid heartbeat, restlessness, tremors. *Antihistamine overdose may cause death, especially in infants.* If you suspect an overdose, immediately seek medical attention.

 More common side effects: dizziness or light-headedness, drowsiness, dry mouth, dry nose, dry throat, sedation, thickening of phlegm.

 Less common or rare side effects: anemia, constipation, convulsions, diarrhea, difficulty sleeping, difficulty urinating, disturbed coordination, exaggerated sense of well-being or depression, frequent urination, headache, high blood pressure, hives, increased sensitivity to light, irregular heartbeat, irritability, itching, loss of appetite, low blood pressure, nausea, nervousness, rash, shortness of breath, stomach upset, tightness in chest, tremor, vision changes, vomiting, weakness, wheezing.

Interactions

 Inform your doctor before combining Dimetane-DC with: MAO inhibitors such as Nardil and Parnate; high blood pressure drugs such as Aldomet; sedatives/ hypnotics such as Phenobarbital, Halcion, and Seconal; tranquilizers such as Xanax, BuSpar, Librium, and Valium.

Do not drink alcohol during Dimetane-DC therapy; its effects are increased.

Special Cautions

 If pregnant or plan to become pregnant, inform your doctor immediately. Should not take if you are breastfeeding.

 No special precautions apply to seniors.

 Follow doctor's instructions carefully for children. May cause excitedness in young children. Newborns should not be given this medication.

 Do not take if you have: severe high blood pressure or heart disease.

May cause drowsiness and impair your ability to drive a car or operate machinery. *Do not take part in any activity that requires alertness.*

Dimetane-DC should not be prescribed to treat asthma or other breathing disorders.

Should not take if sensitive to or allergic to any of the ingredients of this medication.

Use with caution if you have: bronchial asthma; heart disease; high blood pressure; narrow-angle glaucoma; stomach, intestinal or bladder obstruction; thyroid disease.

Monitor dependence of this medication with ongoing use.

Dipentum

Generic name: Olsalazine sodium

Dipentum is a bowel anti-inflammatory. It works by blocking the production of prostaglandins, which may trigger pain.

℞ QUICK FACTS

Purpose

℞ Used to treat the symptoms of ulcerative colitis—chronic inflammation and ulceration of the large intestine and rectum.

Dosage

 Take as prescribed by your doctor, even once you start to feel better. Should take with food.

 Usual adult dose: 1 gram per day divided into 2 equal doses.

 Usual child dose: not generally prescribed for children.

 Missed dose: take as soon as possible, unless almost time for next dose. In that case, do not take missed dose; go back to regular schedule. *Do not double doses.*

Side Effects

 Overdose symptoms: no reports of Dipentum overdose. However, if you suspect an overdose, immediately seek medical attention.

 More common side effects: diarrhea, loose stools.

Other side effects: abdominal pain/cramping, bloating, depression, dizziness, drowsiness, fatigue, feeling of tiredness, headache, heartburn, increased blood in stool, indigestion, inflamed mucous lining in mouth, insomnia, joint pain, light-headedness, loss of appetite, nausea, rectal bleeding, skin itching, skin rash, sluggishness, upper respiratory infection, vertigo, vomiting. Rare side effect: hepatitis.

Interactions

 Inform your doctor before combining Dipentum with warfarin (Coumadin).

 No known food/other substance interactions.

Special Cautions

 If pregnant or plan to become pregnant, inform your doctor immediately. Not known if Dipentum appears in breast milk.

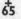 No special precautions apply to seniors.

 Not generally prescribed for children.

 Monitor kidney function if you have kidney disease; Dipentum may cause more damage.

Do not take if allergic to salicylates such as aspirin.

Contact your doctor if you experience diarrhea.

Diphenhydramine Hydrochloride

see BENADRYL

Diphenoxylate Hydrochloride with Atropine Sulfate

see LOMOTIL

Dipivefrin Hydrochloride

see PROPINE

Diprolene

Generic name: Betamethasone dipropionate

Other brand names: Alphatrex, Betatrex, Beta-Val, Diprosone, Lotrisone, Maxivate, Teladar, Valisone

Diprolene is a topical corticosteroid. It interferes with the natural body mechanisms that produce rash, itching or inflammation.

℞ QUICK FACTS

Purpose

 Used to treat itchy rashes and other inflammatory skin conditions.

Dosage

 Apply a thin film, as prescribed. For use on the skin only; keep out of eyes. Use only for the skin condition for which this medication is prescribed. To prevent unwanted side effects, avoid using large amounts

over large areas; *do not use airtight bandages. Do not use for longer than prescribed.*

 Usual adult dose: *cream or ointment*—apply thin film 1 or 2 times per day, up to 45 grams per week. *Lotion*—apply a few drops 1 or 2 times per day, up to 50 milliliters per week, and 14 days. *Gel*—apply thin layer 1 or 2 times per day, up to 50 grams per week, and 14 days.

 Usual child dose: not generally prescribed for children under 12 years.

 Missed dose: apply as soon as possible, unless almost time for next dose. In that case, do not apply missed dose, go back to regular schedule.

Side Effects

 Overdose symptoms: Cushing's syndrome, high blood sugar (moon face, weight gain, high blood pressure, emotional disturbances, growth of facial hair in women), sugar in the urine. Cushing's syndrome may lead to diabetes mellitus and could become serious. If you suspect an overdose, immediately seek medical attention.

 Most common side effect: stinging or burning where medication is applied to the skin.

 Other side effects: acne-like eruptions, atrophy, broken capillaries, cracking or tightening, dryness, infected hair follicles, irritation, itching, prickly heat, rash, redness, sensitivity.

Interactions

 No drug interactions reported with this medication.

 No known food/other substance interactions.

Special Cautions

 If pregnant or planning to become pregnant, inform your doctor immediately. Not known if Diprolene appears in breast milk.

 No special precautions apply to seniors.

 Not generally prescribed for children under 12 years.

 Do not use if sensitive to or allergic to Diprolene.

Dipyridamole
see PERSANTINE

Disopyramide Phosphate
see NORPACE

Ditropan

Generic name: Oxybutynin chloride

Ditropan is an antispasmodic/anticholinergic. It slows the action of the bowel and reduces the amount of stomach acid.

℞ QUICK FACTS

Purpose

 Used to relax the bladder muscle and reduce spasms. Treats the symptoms associated with inability to control the bladder.

Dosage

 Take exactly as prescribed.

 Usual adult dose: *tablets*—one 5-milligram tablet taken 2 to 3 times per day, up to 4 tablets per day. *Syrup*—one teaspoonful 2 to 3 times per day, up to 4 times per day. *Seniors*—not usually prescribed for older seniors.

 Usual child dose (children over 5 years): *tablets*—one 5-milligram tablet taken 2 times per day, up to 3 tablets per day. *Syrup*—one teaspoonful 2 times per day, up to 3 times per day. Not generally prescribed for children under 5 years.

 Missed dose: take as soon as possible, unless almost time for next dose. In that case, do not take missed dose; go back to regular schedule. *Do not double doses.*

Side Effects

 Overdose symptoms: coma, convulsions, delirium, difficulty breathing, fever, flushing, hallucinations, irritability, low or high blood pressure, nausea, paralysis, rapid heartbeat, restlessness, tremor, vomiting. If you suspect an overdose, immediately seek medical attention.

⊕ Side effects: constipation, decreased production of tears, decreased sweating, difficulty falling or staying asleep, dilation of the pupils, dim vision, dizziness, drowsiness, dry mouth, eye paralysis, hallucinations, impotence, inability to urinate, nausea, palpitations, rapid heartbeat, rash, restlessness, suppression of milk production, weakness.

 No known less common or rare side effects.

Interactions

 Inform your doctor before combining Ditropan with sedatives such as Halcion or Restoril.

 Alcohol may cause increased drowsiness.

Special Cautions

 If pregnant or planning to become pregnant, inform your doctor immediately. May appear in breast milk, could affect a nursing infant.

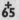 Not usually prescribed for older seniors.

 Not generally prescribed for children under 5 years.

 Do not take if sensitive to or allergic to this medication.

May cause drowsiness and impair your ability to drive a car or operate machinery. *Do not take part in any activity that requires alertness.*

May cause heat prostration; use with caution if you are exposed to high temperatures.

Should not take if you have: abnormal muscle weakness, certain types of untreated glaucoma, partial or complete gastrointestinal tract blockage, obstructed bowel, severe colitis, or urinary tract obstruction.

Immediately contact your doctor if you have an ileostomy or colostomy and develop diarrhea.

Use with caution if you have: kidney or liver disease, or nervous system disorder.

May experience aggravation if you suffer from the following: congestive heart failure, enlarged prostate, heart disease, irregular or rapid heartbeat, or overactive thyroid.

Diuril

Generic name: Chlorothiazide

Other brand names: Diurigen, Diupres

Diuril is a diuretic. Diuretics promote the loss of salt and water in the body and increase the diameter of the blood vessels, thereby lowering blood pressure.

℞ QUICK FACTS

Purpose

℞ Used to treat high blood pressure and other conditions requiring elimination of excess fluid from the body, including congestive heart failure, cirrhosis, corticosteroid and estrogen therapy, and kidney disease.

Dosage

 Take exactly as prescribed. If stopped suddenly, condition may worsen. Must take regularly for it to be effective against high blood pressure. May take several weeks before you notice the full benefit of the medication; continue taking even if you feel well.

Doctor may recommend potassium-rich foods while taking Diuril, as it can lower your normal levels.

 Usual adult dose: *for swelling due to excess water*— 0.5 gram to 1 gram, 1 or 2 times per day. *For high blood pressure*—0.5 gram to 1 gram per day, taken as one dose or 2 or more doses. *Seniors*—dosage is determined according to individual needs.

 Usual child dose: generally 10 milligrams per pound of body weight daily in 2 doses. *Under 6 months*— up to 15 milligrams per pound of body weight daily in 2 doses. *Under 2 years*—125 milligrams to 375 milligrams per day in 2 doses. Liquid—½ to 1½ teaspoonfuls per day. *2 to 12 years*—375 milligrams to 1 gram daily in 2 doses. Liquid—1½ to 4 teaspoonfuls per day.

 Missed dose: take as soon as possible, unless almost time for next dose. In that case, do not take missed dose; go back to regular schedule. *Do not double doses.*

Side Effects

 Overdose symptoms: dehydration, symptoms of low potassium (dry mouth, excessive thirst, weak or irregular heartbeat, muscle pain or cramps). If you suspect an overdose, immediately seek medical attention.

 Side effects: abdominal cramps, anemia, changes in blood sugar, constipation, diarrhea, difficulty breathing, dizziness, dizziness on standing up, fever, fluid in lungs, hair loss, headache, high levels of sugar in urine, hives, hypersensitivity reactions, impotence, inflammation of the pancreas, inflammation of the salivary glands, light-headedness, loss of appetite, low blood pressure, low potassium, lung inflammation, muscle spasms, nausea, rash, reddish or purplish spots on skin, restlessness, sensitivity to light, Stevens-Johnson syndrome, stomach irritation, stomach upset, tingling or pins and needles, vertigo, vision changes, vomiting, weakness, yellow eyes and skin.

 No known less common or rare side effects.

Interactions

 Inform your doctor before combining Diuril with: barbiturates such as phenobarbital and Seconal; cholesterol-lowering drugs such as Questran and Colestid; drugs to treat diabetes such as insulin and Micronase; lithium (Lithonate); nonsteroidal anti-inflammatory drugs such as Naprosyn and Motrin; norepinephrine (Levophed); other drugs for high blood pressure such as Capoten and Procardia XL; steroids such as prednisone.

Do not drink alcohol during Diuril therapy; its effects are increased.

Special Cautions

 If pregnant or planning to become pregnant, inform your doctor immediately. Appears in breast milk; could affect a nursing infant.

 Dosage for seniors is determined according to individual needs.

 Follow doctor's instructions carefully for children.

 Should not take if you cannot urinate.

 If sensitive to or allergic to this or similar medications, or sulfa drugs, should avoid taking. May be at higher risk if you have bronchial asthma or a history of allergies.

Your doctor should monitor your kidney function during Diuril therapy.

Use with caution if you have: diabetes, gout, liver disease, lupus erythematosus, or severe kidney disease.

Monitor your body's depletion of body fluids; too much depletion can lower your blood pressure.

Inform your doctor or dentist that you are taking Diuril before surgery, or in an emergency.

Divalproex Sodium

see DEPAKOTE

Docusate Sodium

see COLACE

Dolobid

Generic name: Diflunisal

Dolobid is a nonsteroidal anti-inflammatory (NSAID). It works by blocking the production of prostaglandins, which may trigger pain.

℞ QUICK FACTS

Purpose

 Used to treat mild to moderate pain and relieve the symptoms of rheumatoid arthritis and osteoarthritis.

Dosage

 Should take with food or food and an antacid, with a full glass of water or milk. Not to be taken on an empty stomach. Swallow tablets whole.

 Usual adult dose: *for mild to moderate pain*—1,000 milligrams, followed by 500 milligrams every 8 to 12 hours. *For osteoarthritis and rheumatoid arthritis*—500 to 1,000 milligrams per day in 2 doses of 250 milligrams or 500 milligrams. Dosage should not exceed 1,500 milligrams per day.

 Usual child dose: not generally prescribed for children under 12 years.

 Missed dose: take as soon as possible, unless almost time for next dose. In that case, do not take missed dose, go back to regular schedule. *Do not double doses.*

Side Effects

 Overdose symptoms: abnormally rapid heartbeat, coma, diarrhea, disorientation, drowsiness, hyperventilation, nausea, ringing in the ears, stupor, sweating, vomiting. If you suspect an overdose, immediately seek medical attention.

 More common side effects: abdominal pain, constipation, diarrhea, dizziness, fatigue, gas, headache, inability to sleep, indigestion, nausea, rash, ringing in ears, sleepiness, vomiting.

Less common or rare side effects: abdominal bleeding, anemia, blurred vision, confusion, depression, disorientation, dry mouth and nose, fluid retention, flushing, hepatitis, hives, inflammation of lips and tongue, itching, kidney failure, light-headedness, loss of appetite, nervousness, painful urination, peptic ulcer, pins and needles, protein or blood in urine, rash, sensitivity to light, skin eruptions, Stevens-Johnson syndrome, vertigo, weakness, yellow eyes and skin.

Interactions

 Inform your doctor before combining Dolobid with: acetaminophen (Tylenol); antacids taken regularly; aspirin; cyclosporine (Sandimmune); hydrochlorothiazide; methotrexate (Rheumatrex); naproxen (Naprosyn); oral anticoagulants (blood thinners); sulindac (Clinoril).

 No known food/other substance interactions.

Special Cautions

 If pregnant or planning to become pregnant, inform your doctor immediately. Appears in breast milk, could affect a nursing infant.

 No special precautions apply to seniors.

 Not generally prescribed for children under 12 years.

 May cause drowsiness and impair your ability to drive a car or operate machinery. *Do not take part in any activity that requires alertness.*

Internal bleeding or ulcers may occur without warning; should have ongoing check-ups with your doctor if taking medication on a regular basis.

. . . .

Should not take if sensitive to or allergic to Dolobid, Aspirin or similar drugs, or if you have experienced asthma attacks from aspirin or similar drugs.

. . . .

Use with caution if you have: heart disease, high blood pressure, kidney disease, liver disease, or are taking a blood-thinning medication.

. . . .

Infections may be masked while taking this medication; tell your doctor of any infections you have.

. . . .

If your vision changes, inform your doctor.

Donnatal

Generic ingredients: Phenobarbital with hyoscyamine sulfate, atropine sulfate, and scopolamine hydrobromide

Other brand names: Barophen, Donnamor, Donnapine, Donna-Sed, Hyosophen, Malatal, Myphentol, Relaxadon, Spaslin, Spasmophen, Susano

Donnatal is an anticholinergic/antispasmodic. It slows the action of the bowel and reduces the amount of stomach acid.

℞ QUICK FACTS

Purpose

 Used to treat cramps and stomach, intestinal, and bowel pain.

Dosage

 Take ½ hour to 1 hour before meals, as prescribed.

 Usual adult dose: *tablets or capsules*—1 or 2 tablets or capsules 3 or 4 times per day. *Liquid*—1 or 2 teaspoonfuls 3 or 4 times per day. *Donnatal Extentabs*—1 tablet every 8 or 12 hours as prescribed by your doctor.

 Usual child dose: elixir is determined by body weight. Usual dosage is given every 4 to 6 hours.

 Missed dose: take as soon as possible, unless almost time for next dose. In that case, do not take missed dose; go back to regular schedule. *Do not double doses.*

Side Effects

 Overdose symptoms: blurred vision, central nervous system stimulation, difficulty swallowing, dilated pupils, dizziness, dry mouth, headache, hot and dry skin, nausea, vomiting. If you suspect an overdose, immediately seek medical attention.

 Side effects: agitation, allergic reaction, bloated feeling, blurred vision, constipation, decreased sweating, difficulty sleeping, difficulty urinating, dilation of the pupil of the eye, dizziness, drowsiness, dry mouth, excitement, fast or fluttery heartbeat, headache, hives, impotence, lessened sense of taste, muscular and bone pain, nausea, nervousness, rapid heartbeat, skin rash or hives, suppression of lactation, vomiting, weakness.

 No known less common or rare side effects.

Interactions

 Inform your doctor before combining Donnatal with: antidepressants such as Elavil and Tofranil; antihistamines such as Benadryl; antispasmodics such as Bentyl and Cogentin; barbiturates such as Seconal; blood thinners such as Coumadin; diarrhea medications that contain either kaolin or attapulgite; digitalis (Lanoxin); MAO inhibitors such as Nardil and Parnate; narcotics such as Percocet; potassium supplements (Slow-K or K-Dur); steroids such as Medrol and Deltasone; tranquilizers such as Valium. Take antacids at least 1 hour before taking Donnatal.

 Donnatal can intensify the effects of alcohol; check with your doctor before using alcohol.

Special Cautions

 If pregnant or planning to become pregnant, inform your doctor immediately. Not known if Donnatal appears in breast milk.

 No special precautions apply to seniors.

 Follow doctor's instructions carefully for children.

 Do not take if you have been drug dependent; Donnatal contains phenobarbital, which can be habit-forming.

Do not take if you have: glaucoma, diseases that block the urinary or gastrointestinal tract, or myasthenia gravis.

May cause drowsiness and impair your ability to drive a car or operate machinery. *Do not take part in any activity that requires alertness.*

Avoid use if you have: acute intermittent porphyria, hiatal hernia, intestinal atony, severe ulcerative colitis, or unstable cardiovascular status, or if phenobarbital makes you excited instead of calm.

Should not take if sensitive or allergic to this or similar medications.

Use with caution if you have: gastric ulcer, heart disease, high blood pressure, irregular or rapid heartbeat, kidney or liver disease, or overactive thyroid.

Monitor for heat prostration when in high temperatures, Donnatal can decrease sweating.

If you experience diarrhea, contact your doctor immediately, especially if you have an ileostomy or colostomy.

Doral

Generic name: Quazepam

Doral is a benzodiazepine sedative. It selectively reduces the activity of certain brain chemicals.

℞ QUICK FACTS

Purpose

℞ Used to treat insomnia on a short-term basis.

Dosage

 Take exactly as prescribed—one dose per day at bedtime. If you respond well, doctor may cut your dosage in half after a few nights. Follow doctor's instruction for gradually stopping this medication, otherwise you may experience withdrawal symptoms. Is potentially addictive, and your body may get used to this medication; important to use only as prescribed.

 Usual adult dose: 15 milligrams per day; may be reduced to 7.5 milligrams per day. Seniors or people with lower health status may be prescribed early dosage reduction.

 Usual child dose: not generally prescribed for children.

 Missed dose: take medication only as needed.

Side Effects

 Overdose symptoms: coma, confusion, extreme sleepiness. If you suspect an overdose, immediately seek medical attention.

 More common side effects: drowsiness during the day, headache.

 Less common side effects: changes in sex drive, dizziness, dry mouth, fatigue, inability to urinate, incontinence, indigestion, irregular menstrual periods, irritability, muscle spasms, slurred or otherwise abnormal speech, yellowed eyes and skin. Rare side effects: agitation, hallucinations, sleep disturbances, or stimulation—the *opposite* of desired effect; immediately contact your doctor if you experience these.

Interactions

Inform your doctor before combining Doral with: antihistamines such as Benadryl, antiseizure medications such as Dilantin and Tegretol, mood-altering medications such as Thorazine and Clozaril, other central nervous system depressants such as Xanax and Valium.

Do not drink alcohol, may increase the effect of Doral.

Special Cautions

Doral may harm a fetus and should not be taken during pregnancy. Babies born to mothers taking Doral may be flaccid, instead of having normal muscle tone. If pregnant or planning to become pregnant, inform your doctor immediately. Not known if Donnatal appears in breast milk.

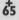

Seniors may have sensitivity; dosage can be reduced after 1 or 2 nights.

Not generally prescribed for children.

May decrease your daytime alertness and impair your ability to drive a car or operate machinery. *Do not take part in any activity that requires alertness.*

Do not take if sensitive to or allergic to this or other Valium-type medications.

Should not take if you have sleep apnea or if you are pregnant.

Use with special caution if you have a history of alcohol or drug abuse, or if you suffer from depression.

. . . .

Inform your doctor immediately if the medication does not seem to work any longer.

Doryx

∧∧

Generic name: Doxycycline hyclate

Other brand names: Doxy-Caps, Doxychel Hyclate, Vibramycin, Vibra-Tabs

Doryx is a tetracycline antibiotic. It interferes with the production of certain biochemicals necessary for bacteria to sustain life.

℞ QUICK FACTS

Purpose

℞ Used to treat a range of bacterial infections, including: Rocky Mountain spotted fever and other fevers caused by ticks, fleas, and lice; amoebic dysentery; some gonococcal infections in adults; severe acne; trachoma; and urinary tract infections. Also used to prevent malaria on trips of 4 months or less.

Dosage

Take with a full glass of water or other liquid to avoid throat or stomach irritation. May be taken with or without food. Tablets should be swallowed whole. If taking oral suspension, shake well before using; *do not use expired medication.*

Usual adult dose: 200 milligrams on the first day of treatment, followed by a maintenance dose of 100 milligrams per day. Maintenance dose may be as a single dose or 50 milligrams every 12 hours. *For chronic urinary tract infections*—100 milligrams every 12 hours. *For uncomplicated gonorrhea (except anorec-*

tal infections in men)—100 milligrams orally, 2 times per day for 7 days, *or* 300 milligrams in a single dose followed by 300 milligrams 1 hour later. *For primary and secondary syphilis*—200 milligrams a day, divided into equal doses for 14 days. *For prevention of malaria*—100 milligrams a day, starting 1 to 2 days before travel to destination where malaria is found, then daily during travel, and 4 weeks after leaving.

Usual child dose (for children over 8 years): *if weighing 100 pounds or less*—2 milligrams per pound of body weight, divided into 2 doses on day one, then 1 milligram per pound of body weight as a single dose or 2 doses on the following days. *For severe infections*—up to 2 milligrams per pound of body weight. *For prevention of malaria*—2 milligrams per 2.2 pounds of body weight up to 100 milligrams.

Missed dose: take as soon as possible. *If taking 1 dose per day*—take next dose 10 to 12 hours after missed dose, then return to regular schedule. *If taking 2 doses per day*—take next dose 5 to 6 hours after missed dose, then return to regular schedule. *If taking 3 doses per day*—take next dose 2 to 4 hours after missed dose, then return to regular schedule.

Side Effects

Overdose symptoms: no specific information available on overdose. If you suspect an overdose, immediately seek medical attention.

More common side effects: angioedema (chest pain; swelling of face, lips, tongue, throat, arms and legs; difficulty swallowing), bulging foreheads in infants, diarrhea, difficulty swallowing, discolored teeth in infants and children, inflammation of the tongue, loss of appetite, nausea, rash, rectal or genital itching, severe allergic reaction (hives, itching, swelling), skin sensitivity to light, vomiting.

 Less common or rare side effects: aggravation of lupus erythematosus, skin inflammation and peeling, throat inflammation and ulcerations.

Interactions

 Inform your doctor before combining Doryx with: antacids containing aluminum, calcium, magnesium, or iron-containing preparations such as Maalox and Mylanta; barbiturates such as phenobarbital; bismuth subsalicylate (Pepto-Bismol); blood thinners such as Coumadin; carbamazepine (Tegretol); oral contraceptives; penicillin (V-Cillin K or Pen•Vee K); phenytoin (Dilantin); sodium bicarbonate. May decrease effectiveness of oral contraceptives containing estrogen.

 No known food/other substance interactions.

Special Cautions

 Should not use if pregnant; can damage developing teeth during the last half of pregnancy. If pregnant or planning to become pregnant, inform your doctor immediately. Tetracyclines appear in breast milk; can affect a nursing infant.

 No special precautions apply to seniors.

 Follow doctor's instructions carefully for children.

 May permanently discolor developing teeth; should not be taken by pregnant women or children under 8 years.

. . . .

Should not take if sensitive to or allergic to this or similar medications. If you have asthma, use very cautiously.

Monitor for secondary infection.

. . . .

May cause sensitivity to sunlight; immediately notify your doctor if you develop a skin rash.

Doxazosin Mesylate

see CARDURA

Doxepin Hydrochloride

see SINEQUAN

Doxycycline Hyclate

see DORYX

Duphalac

see CHRONULAC SYRUP

Duricef

Generic name: Cefadroxil monohydrate

Other brand name: Ultracef

Duricef is a cephalosporin antibiotic. It interferes with the production of certain biochemicals necessary for bacteria to sustain life.

℞ QUICK FACTS

Purpose

 Used to treat nose, throat, urinary tract, and skin infections caused by bacteria such as staph, strep, and *E. coli.*

Dosage

 Take exactly as prescribed, finishing the entire prescription.

 Usual adult dose: *for uncomplicated urinary tract infections*—1 to 2 grams per day as a single dose or 2 smaller doses. For other urinary tract infections, 2 grams per day taken in 2 doses. *For skin and skin structure infections*—1 gram per day as a single dose or 2 smaller doses. *For throat infections*—*strep throat and tonsillitis*—1 gram per day as a single dose or 2 smaller doses for 10 days. *Seniors*—may be prescribed reduced dose.

 Usual child dose: *for urinary tract and skin infections*—30 milligrams per 2.2 pounds of body weight per day, divided into 2 doses taken every 12 hours. *For throat infections*—30 milligrams per 2.2 pounds of body weight as a single dose or 2 smaller doses. Take up to 10 days for strep throat.

Missed dose: take as soon as possible. *If taking 1 dose per day*—take next dose 10 to 12 hours after missed dose, then return to regular schedule. *If taking 2 doses per day*—take next dose 5 to 6 hours after missed dose, then return to regular schedule. *If taking 3 doses per day*—take next dose 2 to 4

hours after missed dose, then return to regular
schedule.

Side Effects

 Overdose symptoms: generally safe; however, large
amounts may cause seizures or side effects. If you
suspect an overdose, immediately seek medical attention.

 Most common side effect: diarrhea.

 Less common or rare side effects: inflammation of
the bowel (colitis), nausea, redness and swelling of
skin, skin rash and itching, vaginal inflammation,
vomiting.

Interactions

 No significant drug interactions reported.

 No known food/other substance interactions.

Special Cautions

 If pregnant or planning to become pregnant, inform
your doctor immediately. May appear in breast milk;
could affect a nursing infant.

 Seniors may be prescribed reduced dose.

 Follow doctor's instructions carefully for children.

 Inform your doctor *before* taking Duricef if allergic
to penicillin or cephalosporin antibiotics; reaction
may be very severe.

If you experience allergies to drugs or often have diarrhea when taking other antibiotics, tell your doctor *before* taking Duricef.

Use with caution if you have a history of colitis or other gastrointestinal disease.

Monitor for development of secondary infection.

Dyazide

Generic ingredients: Hydrochlorothiazide with triamterene

Dyazide is a diuretic. Diuretics promote the loss of salt and water in the body and increase the diameter of the blood vessels, thereby lowering blood pressure.

℞ QUICK FACTS

Purpose

℞ Used to treat high blood pressure and other conditions requiring elimination of excess fluid.

Dosage

 Take early in the day. May take with food to avoid stomach irritation. Must take regularly to be effective against high blood pressure, and can take several weeks before full effects are observed. Continue to take even if feeling well.

 Usual adult dose: 1 or 2 capsules one time per day. Potassium levels should be monitored by your doctor.

Usual child dose: not generally prescribed for children.

 Missed dose: take as soon as possible, unless almost time for next dose. In that case, do not take missed dose; go back to regular schedule. *Do not double doses.*

Side Effects

 Overdose symptoms: fever, flushed face, nausea, production of large amounts of pale urine, vomiting, weakness, weariness. If you suspect an overdose, immediately seek medical attention.

 Side effects: abdominal pain, anemia, blurred vision, breathing difficulty, change in potassium level, constipation, diabetes, diarrhea, dizziness, dizziness when standing up, dry mouth, fatigue, fluid in the lungs, headache, hives, impotence, irregular heartbeat, kidney failure, kidney stones, muscle cramps, nausea, rash, sensitivity to light, strong allergic reaction, tingling or pins and needles, vertigo, vision changes, vomiting, weakness, worsening of lupus, yellow eyes and skin.

 No known less common or rare side effects.

Interactions

 Inform your doctor before combining Dyazide with: ACE inhibitors such as Capoten and Vasotec; adrenocorticotropic hormone (ACTH); amphotericin B (Fungizone); blood thinners such as Coumadin; corticosteroids such as Deltasone; diabetes medications such as Micronase; gout medications such as Zyloprim; laxatives; lithium (Lithonate); low-salt milk; Methenamine (Urised); nonsteroidal anti-inflammatory drugs such as Voltaren and Dolobid;

norepinephrine (Levophed); other drugs that minimize potassium loss or contain potassium; other high blood pressure medications such as Minipress and Vasotec; salt substitutes containing potassium; sodium polystyrene sulfonate (Kayexalate).

 No known food/other substance interactions.

Special Cautions

 If pregnant or planning to become pregnant, inform your doctor immediately. Appears in breast milk, could affect a nursing infant.

 No special precautions apply to seniors.

 Not generally prescribed for children.

 Do not use potassium-containing salt substitutes. Only take potassium supplements under the direction of your doctor. Doctor should monitor potassium level on an ongoing basis.

If you are: unable to urinate, have serious kidney disease, high potassium levels in the blood, or if you are taking other medications to prevent potassium loss, you should not take Dyazide.

If sensitive to or allergic to ingredients in this medication or similar medications, or sulfa drugs, should not take.

Use with caution if you have: liver disease, diabetes, cirrhosis of the liver, heart failure, or kidney stones.

Kidney function should be monitored regularly if you have kidney disease.

Monitor for dehydration when exercising or in hot weather if you have a salt deficiency.

Not recommended to be in sunlight for prolonged periods.

Dynacin

see MINOCIN

DynaCirc

Generic name: Isradipine

DynaCirc is a calcium channel blocker. It increases the amount of oxygen that reaches the heart muscle.

℞ QUICK FACTS

Purpose

℞ Used to treat high blood pressure.

Dosage

 Take exactly as prescribed. Try not to miss doses; condition may worsen if you miss doses. Must take regularly to be effective against high blood pressure, and can take several weeks before full effects are observed. Continue to take even if feeling well.

 Usual adult dose: 2.5 milligrams 2 times per day. Then may be increased by 5 milligrams per day at 2 to 4 weeks, in intervals up to 20 milligrams per day. *If you have kidney or liver disease*—2.5 milligrams

2 times per day. *Seniors*—effects of drug may be stronger, same dose is prescribed.

Usual child dose: not generally prescribed for children.

Missed dose: take as soon as possible, unless almost time for next dose. In that case, do not take missed dose; go back to regular schedule. *Do not double doses.*

Side Effects

Overdose symptoms: no specific information available about DynaCirc; however, overdose symptoms associated with calcium channel blockers are drowsiness, severe low blood pressure, slow heartbeat. If you suspect an overdose, immediately seek medical attention.

More common side effects: chest pain, dizziness, fatigue, fluid retention, flushing, headache, pounding heartbeat.

Less common side effects: diarrhea, nausea, rapid heartbeat, rash, shortness of breath, stomach upset, unusually frequent urination, vomiting, weakness. Rare side effects: changes in heartbeat, constipation, cough, decreased sex drive, depression, difficulty sleeping, drowsiness, dry mouth, excessive nighttime urination, excessive sweating, fainting, heart attack, heart failure, hives, impotence, itching, leg and foot cramps, low blood pressure, nervousness, numbness, severe dizziness, sluggishness, stroke, throat discomfort, tingling or pins and needles, vision changes.

Interactions

 Inform your doctor before combining DynaCirc with: beta-blockers such as Inderal, Lopressor, and Tenormin; carbamazepine (Tegretol); phenytoin (Dilantin).

 No known food/other substance interactions.

Special Cautions

 If pregnant or planning to become pregnant, inform your doctor immediately. May appear in breast milk; could affect a nursing infant.

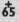 Seniors may experience stronger effects of drug; however, dose is not lowered.

 Not generally prescribed for children.

 If sensitive to or allergic reaction to this or other calcium channel blockers, should not take.

Monitor for light-headedness or feeling faint; can cause low blood pressure.

Use with caution if you have congestive heart failure and are taking beta-blockers.

Notify doctor or dentist that you are taking DynaCirc before surgery.

Dynapen
see PATHOCIL

~~~~~~

Echothiopate Iodide

see PHOSPHOLINE IODINE

Econazole Nitrate

see SPECTAZOLE CREAM

E.E.S.

see ERYTHROMYCIN, ORAL

Effexor

~~~~~~

Generic name: Venlafaxine hydrochloride

Effexor is an antidepressant. It blocks the movement of certain stimulant chemicals in and out of nerve endings.

℞ QUICK FACTS

Purpose

℞   Used to treat major depression.

Dosage

 Take with food, exactly as prescribed. *Do not abruptly discontinue taking this medication without supervision from your doctor; may cause withdrawal symptoms.*

 Usual adult dose: 75 milligrams per day divided into 2 or 3 smaller doses, taken with food. Doctor may increase dose to 150 to 225 milligrams per day. *With kidney or liver disease*—dose will be adjusted.

 Usual child dose: not generally prescribed for children.

 Missed dose: not necessary to make up missed dose. You do not need to take missed dose, continue with next scheduled dose. *Do not double doses.*

Side Effects

 Overdose symptoms: convulsions, rapid heartbeat, sleepiness. If you suspect an overdose, immediately seek medical attention.

 More common side effects: abnormal dreams, abnormal ejaculation/orgasm, anxiety, blurred vision, chills, constipation, diarrhea, dizziness, dry mouth, extreme muscle tension, flushing, frequent urination, gas, headache, impotence, inability to sleep, indigestion, loss of appetite, nausea, nervousness, prickling or burning sensation, rash, sleepiness, sweating, tremor, vomiting, weakness, yawning.

 Less common side effects: abnormal thinking, abnormal vision, accidental injury, agitation, belching, blood in the urine, bronchitis, bruising, changeable emotions, chest pain, confusion, decreased sex drive, depression, difficult or painful urination, difficulty in breathing, difficulty swallowing, dilated pupils, ear pain, high or low blood pressure, inflammation of the vagina, injury, itching, lack of orgasm, light-headedness on standing up, lockjaw, loss of touch with reality, menstrual problems, migraine headache, neck pain, orgasm disturbance, rapid heartbeat, ringing in the ears, taste changes, twitching, uterine bleeding between menstrual periods, vague feeling of illness, vertigo, weight loss or gain. Rare side effects: abnormal movements, abnormal sensitivity to sound, abnormal speech, abnormally slow movements, abortion, abuse of alcohol, acne, alcohol intolerance, allergic reaction, anemia, apathy, appendicitis, arthritis, asthma, bad breath, black stools, bleeding gums, blocked intestine, blood clots, blood clots in the lungs, blood disorders, bluish color to the skin, body odor, bone disease and/or pain, including osteoporosis, breast enlargement or swelling, breast pain, brittle nails, bulging eyes, cancerous growth, cataracts, changed sense of smell, chest congestion, cold hands and feet, colitis, confusion, conjunctivitis, coughing up blood, crushing chest pain, deafness, delusions, depression, diabetes, double vision, drug withdrawal symptoms, dry eyes, dry skin, ear infection, eczema, enlarged abdomen, enlarged thyroid gland, exaggerated feeling of well-being, excessive hair growth, excessive menstrual flow, eye disorders, eye pain, fainting, fungus infection, gallstones, glaucoma, gout, hair discoloration, hair loss, hallucinations, hangover effect, heart disorders, hemorrhoids, hepatitis, herpes infections, high cholesterol, hives, hostility, hyperventilation, inability to communicate, increased mucus, increased physical activity, increased salivation, increased sensitivity to touch, increased sex drive, inflammation (of the stomach, intestines, anus and rectum, gums, tongue, eyelid, or inner ear), intolerance to light, involuntary eye movements, irregular or slow heartbeat, kidney disorders, lack of menstruation, large amounts of urine, laryngitis, loss of consciousness, loss of muscle movement, low or high blood sugar, menstrual problems, middle ear infection, mouth fungus, mouth sores, muscle spasms, muscle weakness, nosebleeds, over- and underactive thyroid gland, overdose, paranoia, pelvic pain, pinpoint pupils, pins and needles around the mouth, pneumonia, prolonged erection, psoriasis, rectal hemorrhage, reduced menstrual flow, restlessness, secretion of milk, sensitivity to light, skin disorders, skin eruptions or hemorrhage, skin inflammation, sleep disturbance, soft stools, stiff neck, stomach or peptic ulcer, stroke, stupor, sugar in the urine, swelling due to fluid retention, swollen or discolored tongue, taste loss, temporary failure to breathe, thirst, twisted neck, ulcer, unconsciousness, uncoordinated movements, urgent need to urinate, urination at night, uterine and vaginal hemorrhage, varicose veins, voice changes, vomiting blood, yellowed eyes and skin.

Interactions

 Inform your doctor before combining Effexor with: MAO inhibitors such as Nardil and Parnate—may cause a fatal reaction; central nervous system medications, including narcotic painkillers, sleep aids, tranquilizers, and other antidepressants; Tagamet.

 Avoid alcohol while taking this medication.

Special Cautions

 If pregnant or planning to become pregnant, inform your doctor immediately. May appear in breast milk, could affect a nursing infant.

 Seniors should inform their doctors if they are taking Tagamet.

 Not generally prescribed for children.

May cause drowsiness and impair your ability to drive a car or operate machinery. *Do not take part in any activity that requires alertness.*

Use with caution if you have: high blood pressure; heart, liver or kidney disease; history of seizures; mania.

Inform your doctor of any drug addition before starting Effexor.

If you develop a skin rash or hives, contact your doctor.

Efudex

Generic name: Fluorouracil

Other brand name: Fluoroplex Topical Solution

Efudex is an antineoplastic. It prevents the growth of rapidly dividing cells, such as cancer cells.

℞ QUICK FACTS

Purpose

 Used to treat actinic or solar keratoses (growths caused by overexposure to ultraviolet radiation or the sun)—which may develop into skin cancer. Also used to treat superficial basal cell carcinomas, or slow-growing malignant face tumors.

Dosage

 Use carefully around the eyes, nose, and mouth. Wash hands thoroughly after application. Comes in cream or solution. If your doctor suggests covering affected area with a bandage after applying medication, use a porous gauze to avoid inflammation.

 Usual adult dose: *for actinic or solar keratosis*—apply cream or solution 2 times per day, covering affected area. Continue to use until the skin wears away, a sore forms and the skin cells die. Treatment is usually 2 to 4 weeks. *For superficial basal cell carcinomas*—only use 5% solution, applying 2 times per day, covering the affected area. Treatment is usually 3 to 6 weeks.

 Usual child dose: not generally prescribed for children.

 Missed dose: apply as soon as possible, unless more than a few hours have passed. In that case, do not take missed dose; go back to regular schedule. If more than 1 dose is missed, call your doctor.

Side Effects

 Overdose symptoms: no specific information available. If you suspect an overdose, immediately seek medical attention.

 More common side effects: burning, discoloration of the skin, itching, pain.

 Less common side effects: allergic skin inflammation, pus, scaling, scarring, soreness, swelling, tenderness.

Interactions

 No known drug interactions.

 No known food/other substance interactions.

Special Cautions

 If pregnant or planning to become pregnant, inform your doctor immediately. Not known if Efudex appears in breast milk.

 No special precautions apply to seniors.

 Not generally prescribed for children.

 Should not use if sensitive to or allergic to this or similar medications.

May experience unsightly skin during and for weeks after treatment.

Avoid repeated exposure to ultraviolet rays.

Doctor may order a biopsy if the condition does not clear up with Efudex therapy.

If treated for superficial basal cell carcinoma, your doctor will order follow-up biopsies.

Elavil

Generic name: Amitriptyline

Other brand names: Amitril, Endep, Enovil

Elavil is a tricyclic antidepressant. It increases the concentration of the chemicals necessary for nerve transmission in the brain, thereby relieving depression.

℞ QUICK FACTS

Purpose

 Used to relieve the symptoms of mental depression; also used to treat bulimia, chronic pain, prevention of migraines, and pathological laughing and weeping associated with multiple sclerosis.

Dosage

 Take exactly as prescribed. Take with water or food to lessen stomach irritation, unless otherwise prescribed by doctor. May take 2 to 3 weeks before effects of medication are observed.

. . . .

 Usual adult dose: 75 milligrams per day divided into 2 or more doses, up to 150 milligrams per day, not to exceed 200 milligrams per day. *Alternate therapy*— 50 milligrams to 100 milligrams at bedtime, increasing dose by 25 or 50 milligrams, up to 150 milligrams per day. *Long-term use*—40 to 100 milligrams taken one time per day, usually at bedtime. *Seniors*—10 milligrams taken 3 times per day, with 20 milligrams taken at bedtime.

. . . .

 Usual child dose (for children 12 years and older): 10 milligrams taken 3 times per day, with 20 milligrams taken at bedtime.

. . . .

 Missed dose: take as soon as possible, unless almost time for next dose. In that case, do not take missed dose; go back to regular schedule. *Do not double doses. If prescribed one daily dose at bedtime, do not take missed dose in the morning; may cause side effects during the day.*

Side Effects

 Elavil overdose can be fatal. Overdose symptoms: abnormally low blood pressure, congestive heart failure, convulsions, dilated pupils, drowsiness, rapid or irregular heartbeat, reduced body temperature, stupor, unresponsiveness or coma. Symptoms contrary to the effect of this medication: agitation, extremely high body temperature, rigid muscles, vomiting. If you suspect an overdose, immediately seek medical attention.

Side effects: abnormal movements, anxiety, black tongue, blurred vision, breast development in males, breast enlargement, coma, confusion, constipation, delusions, diarrhea, difficult or frequent urination, difficulty in speech, dilation of pupils, disorientation, disturbed concentration, dizziness on getting up, dizziness or light-headedness, drowsiness, dry mouth, excessive or spontaneous flow of milk, excitement, fast or fluttery heartbeat, fatigue, fluid retention, hair loss, hallucinations, headache, heart attack, high or low blood sugar, hives, impotence, inability to sleep, increased or decreased sex drive, increased perspiration, increased pressure within the eye, inflammation of the mouth, intestinal obstruction, irregular heartbeat, lack or loss of coordination, loss of appetite, low blood pressure, nausea, nightmares, numbness, rapid heartbeat, rash, red or purple spots on skin, restlessness, ringing in the ears, seizures, sensitivity to light, stomach upset, strange taste, stroke, swelling due to fluid retention in the face and tongue, swelling of testicles, swollen glands, tingling and pins and needles in the arms and legs, tremors, vomiting, weakness, weight gain or loss, yellowed eyes and skin. Side effects due to rapid decrease or abrupt withdrawal from Elavil: headache, nausea, vague feeling of bodily discomfort. Side effects due to gradual dosage reduction: dream and sleep disturbances, irritability, restlessness.

No known less common or rare side effects.

Interactions

 Inform your doctor before combining Elavil with: parkinsonism drugs such as Cogentin; quinidine (Quinidex); seizure medications such as Tegretol and Dilantin; sleep medications such as Halcion and Dalmane; thyroid hormones (Synthroid); tranquilizers such as Librium and Xanax; vitamin C in large doses; warfarin (Coumadin).

. . . .

 Alcohol may increase sedative effects; *do not drink alcohol when taking this medication.*

Special Cautions

 If pregnant or planning to become pregnant, inform your doctor immediately. Appears in breast milk; could affect a nursing infant.

. . . .

 Seniors are prescribed lower doses.

. . . .

 Not prescribed for children under 12 years.

. . . .

 If you have or have had: asthma, diabetes, electroshock therapy, enlarged prostate gland, epilepsy, glaucoma or other chronic eye conditions, heart or circulatory system disorder, liver or kidney problems, mental illness, seizures, stomach or intestinal problems, thyroid disease, or urinary retention, notify your doctor before taking Elavil.

. . . .

You may feel dizzy or light-headed or faint when standing up from a lying or sitting position. If standing slowly is not helpful, notify your doctor.

. . . .

Urine may turn blue-green; this effect is harmless.

. . . .

May experience increased sensitivity to sunlight; avoid the sun as much as possible.

. . . .

Before medical or dental surgery, tell your doctor or dentist you are taking this drug.

Eldepryl

Generic name: Selegiline hydrochloride

Eldepryl is an antiparkinsonism agent/monoamine oxidase (MAO inhibitor). It works by balancing certain chemicals in the brain.

℞ QUICK FACTS

Purpose

Used to treat Parkinson's disease. Is used with Sinemet when it loses its effectiveness. Eldepryl is effective only when used with levodopa or Sinemet.

Dosage

Take exactly as prescribed.

Usual adult dose: 10 milligrams per day divided into 2 smaller doses, taken at breakfast and lunch.

Usual child dose: not generally prescribed for children.

Missed dose: take as soon as possible, unless almost time for next dose. In that case, do not take missed dose, go back to regular schedule. *Do not double doses.*

Side Effects

Overdose symptoms: no specific information available; however, Eldepryl is a MAO inhibitor, which has the following overdose symptoms: agitation, chest pain, clammy skin, coma, convulsions, dizziness, drowsiness, extremely high fever, faintness, fast and irregular pulse, hallucinations, headache (severe), high blood pressure, hyperactivity, inability to breathe, irritability, lockjaw, low blood pressure (severe), shallow breathing, spasms of the entire body, sweating. *After large overdose, symptoms may take 12 to 24 hours to manifest. An overdose can be fatal.* If you suspect an overdose, immediately seek medical attention.

Side effects: abdominal pain, abnormal movements, abnormally fast walking, aches, agitation, anxiety, apathy, asthma, back pain, behavior or mood changes, bleeding from the rectum, blurred vision, body ache, burning lips and mouth or throat, chills, confusion, constipation, crushing chest pain, delusions, depression, diarrhea, difficulty swallowing, disorientation, dizziness, double vision, drowsiness, dry mouth, excessive urination at night, eyelid spasm, facial grimace, facial hair, fainting, falling down, freezing, frequent urination, general feeling of illness, hair loss, hallucinations, headache, heartburn, heart palpitations, heart rhythm abnormalities, "heavy leg," high blood pressure, hollow feeling, inability to carry out purposeful movements, inability to urinate, increased sweating, increased tremor, insomnia, involuntary movements, irritability, lack of appetite, leg pain, lethargy, light-headedness upon standing up, loss of balance, low blood pressure, lower back pain, migraine, muscle cramps, nausea, nervousness, numbness in toes/fingers, overstimulation, pain over the eyes, personality change, poor appetite, rapid heartbeat, rash, restlessness, ringing in the ear, sensitivity to light, sexual problems, shortness of breath, sleep disturbance, slow heartbeat, slow urination, slowed body movements, speech problems, stiff neck, stomach and intestinal bleeding, swelling of the ankles or arms and legs, taste disturbance, tension, tiredness, twitching, urinary problems, vertigo, vivid dreams or nightmares, vomiting, weakness, weight loss.

 No known less common or rare side effects.

Interactions

 Inform your doctor before combining Eldepryl with: amphetamines such as Dexedrine; antidepressants such as Elavil and Tofranil; diabetes medications such as insulin and Micronase; fluoxetine (Prozac); narcotic painkillers such as Demerol, Percocet, and Tylenol with Codeine. Should wait 5 weeks after Prozac therapy to begin taking Eldepryl. Should wait 14 days after Eldepryl therapy to begin taking Prozac.

 As a MAO inhibitor, may interact with: aged cheeses and meats, pickled herring, beer, and wine, causing a potentially fatal surge in blood pressure. Monitor your diet, and never take more than the prescribed dose.

Special Cautions

 If pregnant or planning to become pregnant, inform your doctor immediately. Not known if Eldepryl appears in breast milk or causes birth defects.

 No special precautions apply to seniors.

 Not generally prescribed for children.

 Do not take if sensitive to or allergic to this medication.

Immediately call your doctor at the onset of a severe headache.

Elocon

Generic name: Mometasone furoate

Elocon is a topical corticosteroid. It interferes with the natural body mechanisms that produce rash, itching or inflammation.

℞ QUICK FACTS

Purpose

 Used to treat itchy rashes and other inflammatory skin conditions.

Dosage

 Apply thin film of cream or ointment, or a few drops of lotion to affected area. Keep out of eyes. *Do not cover with a bandage, tight diaper, plastic pants, or any other airtight dressing; and do not use longer than doctor prescribes to avoid absorption through the skin into the bloodstream. Do not use for conditions Elocon is not specifically prescribed for.*

 Usual adult dose: apply one time per day.

Usual child dose: limit use—steroid use over a prolonged period may interfere with growth and development in children.

 Missed dose: apply as soon as possible, unless almost time for next dose. In that case, do not take missed dose, go back to regular schedule.

Side Effects

 Overdose symptoms: long-term use may cause Cushing's syndrome (moon face, weight gain, high blood pressure, emotional disturbances, growth of facial hair in women). May be serious if left untreated. Cushing's syndrome may also lead to diabetes mellitus. If you suspect an overdose, immediately seek medical attention.

 Side effects: acne-like pimples, allergic skin rash, boils, burning, damaged skin, dryness, excessive hairiness, infected hair follicles, infection of the skin, irritation, itching, light-colored patches on skin, prickly heat, rash around the mouth, skin atrophy and wasting, softening of the skin, stretch marks, tingling or stinging.

 No known less common or rare side effects.

Interactions

 No known drug interactions.

 No known food/other substance interactions.

Special Cautions

 If pregnant or planning to become pregnant, inform your doctor immediately. Should not be used during pregnancy. May appear in breast milk; could affect a nursing infant.

 No special precautions apply to seniors.

 Prescribed for children on a limited basis, follow doctor's instructions carefully.

 Do not use if sensitive to or allergic to this or similar steroid medications.

Empirin
see ASPIRIN

Empirin with Codeine

Generic name: Aspirin with Codeine

Other brand names: Anexsia with Codeine, Emcodeine

Empirin with Codeine is an analgesic and anti-inflammatory agent. It reduces pain and inflammation, is a narcotic pain reliever, and has both pain-relieving and cough-suppressing properties.

℞ QUICK FACTS

Purpose

℞ Used to treat mild, moderate, and moderate to severe pain and tension headaches.

Dosage

  May take with food or a full glass of milk to avoid stomach upset. More effective if taken at onset of pain than when pain intense. Can be habit-forming if taken over a long period of time or in high doses; take exactly as prescribed.

  Usual adult dose: *for Empirin with Codeine No. 3*—1 or 2 tablets every 4 hours as needed. For *Empirin with Codeine No. 4*—1 tablet every 4 hours as needed.

  Usual child dose: not generally prescribed for children.

  Missed dose: take as soon as possible, unless almost time for next dose. If so, skip missed dose; go back to regular schedule. *Do not double doses.*

Side Effects

 Overdose symptoms: *adults*—bluish skin color due to lack of oxygen, circulatory collapse, clammy skin, coma, constricted pupils, delirium, delusions, difficult or labored breathing, double vision, excitability, flabby muscles, garbled speech, hallucinations, restlessness, skin eruptions, slow and shallow breathing, stupor, vertigo. *Children*—confusion, convulsions, dehydration, difficulty hearing, dim vision, dizziness, drowsiness, extremely high body temperature, headache, nausea, rapid breathing, ringing in ears, sweating, thirst, vomiting. If you suspect an overdose, immediately seek medical attention.

 More common side effects: constipation, dizziness, drowsiness, flushing, light-headedness, loss of appetite, nausea, shallow breathing, sweating, vomiting.

 Less common side effects: abdominal pain, aggravation of peptic ulcer, anaphylactic shock (severe allergic reaction), asthma, bruising or bleeding, confusion, dizziness, drowsiness, exaggerated sense of well-being or depression, excessive bleeding following injury or surgery, fatigue, headache, hearing problems, heartburn, hives, indigestion, itching, nausea, rapid heartbeat, ringing in ears, runny nose, skin rashes, sweating, thirst, vision problems, vomiting, weakness.

Interactions

 Inform your doctor before taking Empirin with Codeine with blood thinners such as Coumadin; furosemide (Lasix); insulin; MAO inhibitors such as Nardil; mercaptopurine; methotrexate (Rheumatrex); nonsteroidal anti-inflammatory drugs such as Advil, Motrin, and Indocin; oral diabetes medications such as Diabinese and Tolinase; other narcotic analgesics such as Percodan and Tylox; para-amino salicylic acid; penicillin; probenecid (Benemid); sedatives such as phenobarbital and Nembutal; steroids such as Medrol and prednisone; sulfa drugs such as Azo Gantrisin and Septra; sulfinpyrazone (Anturane); tranquilizers such as Xanax and Valium; vitamin C.

 Alcohol may increase sedative effects; do not drink alcohol when taking this medication.

Special Cautions

 If pregnant or planning to become pregnant, inform your doctor immediately. Appears in breast milk, could affect a nursing infant.

 Seniors in a weakened condition should use with caution.

 Consult your doctor before administering to children.

 May cause drowsiness and impair your ability to drive a car or operate machinery. *Do not take part in any activity that requires alertness.*

Codeine may hide symptoms of serious abdominal conditions.

Can cause severe allergic reactions including difficulty breathing, bluish skin color caused by lack of oxygen, fever, rash or hives, irregular pulse, convulsions, or collapse.

With a peptic ulcer, open sores in the stomach or intestines, may cause bleeding. May also prolong bleeding after an injury or surgery.

. . . .
Use with caution after head or brain injury; can slow breathing, cause drowsiness, increase pressure in your head.
. . . .
Use with caution if you have: Addison's disease, breathing disorder, enlarged prostate or narrowing of the urethra, gallstones or gallbladder disease, inflamed stomach or intestines, irregular heartbeat, severe kidney or liver disease, underactive thyroid gland.

Sensitivity reactions are relatively common in people with asthma or nasal polyps. Use caution if you have allergies.

Enalapril Maleate

see VASOTEC

Enalapril Maleate with Hydrochlorothiazide

see VASERETIC

Enoxacin

see PENETREX

Entex LA

Generic ingredients: Guaifenesin with phenylpropanolamine hydrochloride

Other brand names: Exgest LA, Gentab LA, Nolex LA, Vanex LA

Entex LA is a decongestant-expectorant combination. Decongestants constrict blood vessels in the nose and sinuses to open air passages. Expectorants change a nonproductive cough into a productive cough (producing phlegm).

℞ QUICK FACTS

Purpose

 Used to treat bronchitis, the common cold, sinus inflammation, nasal congestion, and sore throat.

Dosage

 May break tablets in half for easier swallowing; must swallow whole, not crushed or chewed.

 Usual adult dose: 1 tablet every 12 hours.

 Usual child dose (for children 6 to 12 years): ½ tablet every 12 hours.

 Missed dose: take as soon as possible, unless almost time for next dose. If so, skip missed dose; go back to regular schedule. *Do not double doses.*

Side Effects

 Overdose symptoms: coma, convulsions, high blood pressure. If you suspect an overdose, immediately seek medical attention.

Side effects: difficulty urinating (for men with enlarged prostate), headache, inability to sleep or difficulty sleeping, irritated stomach, nausea, nervousness, restlessness.

 No known less common or rare side effects.

Interactions

 Do not take concurrently with MAO inhibitors such as Nardil and Parnate. Avoid Proventil, Ventolin, and many decongestants. Inform your doctor before combining Entex LA with: bromocriptine (Parlodel), methyldopa (Aldomet).

 No known food/other substance interactions.

Special Cautions

 If pregnant or planning to become pregnant, inform your doctor immediately. Not known if Entex LA appears in breast milk.

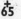 No special precautions apply to seniors.

 Follow doctor's instructions carefully for children 6 to 12 years.

 Inform your doctor *before* taking Entex LA if you have: diabetes, heart disease, or high blood pressure.

Should not use if sensitive to other stimulants such as Dristan Decongestant.

Use with caution if you have: glaucoma, hyperthyroidism, or prostate enlargement.

Epitol
see TEGRETOL

Equanil
see MILTOWN

Ergoloid Mesylates
see HYDERGINE

Ergotamine Tartrate with Caffeine
see CAFERGOT

EryPed
see PEDIAZOLE

Erythromycin Ethylsuccinate with Sulfisoxazole Acetyl
see PEDIAZOLE

Erythromycin, Oral

Brand names: E.E.S. 200 Liquid, E.E.S. 400 Filmtab, Eramycin, Eryc, EryPed, Erythrocin, E-Mycin, Ery-Tab, Ilosone, PCE, Robimycin Robitabs

Erythromycin is a macrolide antibiotic. It is used to treat a variety of bacterial infections.

℞ QUICK FACTS

Purpose

℞ Used to treat several infections including: chlamydia, diphtheria, ear infections, gonorrhea, intestinal infections, Legionnaires' disease, rheumatic fever, skin infections, syphilis, upper and lower respiratory tract infections, urinary tract infections, whooping cough. Also used to prevent heart infections.

Dosage

 Take exactly as prescribed. Can take with or without food; however, food may decrease the effectiveness. In those cases your doctor will suggest taking this medication 30 minutes to 2 hours before or after meals. For maximum effectiveness there should be a constant amount of Erythromycin in the blood—strictly adhere to dose schedule.

 Usual adult dose: *for streptococcal infections*—250 milligrams every 6 hours, 333 milligrams every 8 hours, or 500 milligrams every 12 hours. May be increased up to 4 grams per day. *For streptococcal infections of the upper respiratory tract*—take for 10 days. *To prevent recurrence of rheumatic fever*—250 milligrams 2 times per day. *For gonorrhea*—3 grams in a single oral dose. *To prevent bacterial endocarditis*—1 gram taken 30 minutes to 2 hours before dental surgery or surgical procedures of the upper respiratory tract, followed by 500 milligrams every 6 hours, for 8 doses. *For urinary tract infections due to chlamydia during pregnancy*—500 milligrams orally 4 times per day, or 666 milligrams every 8 hours on an empty stomach for 7 days. Decreased dose—500 milligrams every 8 hours, or 250 milligrams 4 times per day for 14 days. *For uncomplicated urinary tract or rectal infections caused by chlamydia when tetracycline is not tolerated*—500 milligrams 4 times per day, or 333 milligrams every 8 hours for at least 7 days. *For nongonococcal urethral infections when tetracycline is not tolerated*—500 milligrams 4 times per day, or 666 milligrams every 8 hours for at least 7 days. *For syphilis*—30 to 40 grams divided into smaller doses over 10 to 15 days. *For intestinal infections*—500 milligrams every 12 hours, 333 milligrams every 8 hours, or 250 milligrams every 6 hours for 10 to 14 days. *For Legionnaires' disease*—1 to 4 grams daily, divided into smaller doses for 21 days.

. . . .

Usual child dose: 30 to 50 milligrams per day for each 2.2 pounds of body weight, divided into equal doses. *For more severe infections*—double dose, not to exceed 4 grams per day. *For children over 44 pounds*—follow adult dose schedule. *For conjunctivitis in newborn caused by chlamydia*—50 milligrams for each 2.2 pounds of body weight per day, divided into 4 doses for at least 2 weeks. *For pneumonia in infants caused by chlamydia*—50 milligrams for each 2.2 pounds of body weight per day, divided into 4 doses for at least 3 weeks. *For whooping cough*—40 to 50 milligrams for each 2.2 pounds of body weight per day, divided into smaller doses for 5 to 14 days.

. . . .

Missed dose: take as soon as possible, unless almost time for next dose. If so, skip missed dose; go back to regular schedule. *Do not double doses.*

. . . .

Side Effects

 Overdose symptoms: diarrhea, nausea, stomach cramps, vomiting. If you suspect an overdose, immediately seek medical attention.

 More common side effects: abdominal pain, diarrhea, loss of appetite, nausea, vomiting.

 Less common side effects: hives, rash, skin eruptions, yellow eyes and skin. Rare side effects: chest pain, confusion, dizziness, hallucinations, hearing loss (temporary), inflammation of large intestine, palpitations, rapid heartbeat, seizures, severe allergic reaction, vertigo.

Interactions

 Inform your doctor before combining erythromycin with: alfentanil (Alfenta), astemizole (Hisminal), blood thinners such as Coumadin, bromocriptine (Parlodel), carbamazepine (Tegretol), cyclosporine (Sandimmune), digoxin (Lanoxin), disopyramide (Norpace), ergotamine (Cafergot), felodipine (Plendil), hexobarbital, lovastatin (Mevacor), Midazolam (Ver-sed), other antibiotics, penicillin (Amoxil or Omnipen), phenytoin (Dilantin), terfenadine (Seldane), theophylline (Theo-Dur), triazolam (Halcion).

No known food/other substance interactions.

Special Cautions

 If pregnant or planning to become pregnant, inform your doctor immediately. Appears in breast milk; could affect a nursing infant.

 Seniors should use with caution.

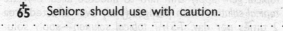

Follow doctor's instructions carefully for children.

 Inform your doctor *before* taking erythromycin if you have or had liver disease.

Should not use if sensitive to or allergic to this medication.

May cause new infections that need to be treated with a different antibiotic.

Erythromycin, Topical

Brand names: Akne-Mycin, A/T/S, Erycette, Erygel, T-STAT

Erythromycin topical is a macrolide antibiotic. It is used to treat a variety of bacterial infections.

℞ QUICK FACTS

Purpose

℞ Used to treat acne.

Dosage

 Use exactly as prescribed. Wash affected area with soap and water before applying medication, and wash hands after application.

 Usual adult dose: *A/T/S topical solution*—apply 2 times per day to affected area, morning and night. *A/T/S topical gel*—apply thin film to affected area. *Erycette topical solution*—rub pledget (pad) over affected area 2 times per day. *T-STAT topical solution*—apply solution or pads over affected areas 2 times per day.

Usual child dose: not generally prescribed for children.

 Missed dose: apply as soon as possible, unless almost time for next dose. If so, skip missed dose; go back to regular schedule.

Side Effects

 Overdose symptoms: is unlikely; however, not recommended to use in excess. If you suspect an overdose, immediately seek medical attention.

 Side effects: burning sensation, dryness, hives, irritation of eyes, itching, oiliness, peeling, scaling, tenderness, unusual redness of the skin.

 No known less common or rare side effects.

Interactions

 Inform your doctor before combining Erythromycin Topical with other topical acne medications.

 No known food/other substance interactions.

Special Cautions

 If pregnant or planning to become pregnant, inform your doctor immediately. May appear in breast milk; could affect a nursing infant.

 No special precautions apply to seniors.

 Not generally prescribed for children.

 Should not use if sensitive to or allergic to this medication.

May cause new infections that need to be treated with a different antibiotic.

. . . .

If you use other topical acne medications, may experience irritation.

Erythromycin with Benzoyl Peroxide

see BENZAMYCIN

Estazolam

see PROSOM

Estrace

see ESTRADERM

Estracon

see PREMARIN

Estraderm

Generic name: Estradiol

Other brand names: Estrace Cream, Estrace Tablet

Estraderm is a form of estrogen. It replaces estrogen in the body.

℞ QUICK FACTS

Purpose

Used to treat and/or reduce menopause symptoms—warmth in face, neck, and chest; and hot flashes. Also used to treat other conditions caused by lack of estrogen—dry, itchy external genitals; vaginal irritation; osteoporosis; low levels of estrogen; and relief in breast or prostate cancer.

Dosage

Apply patch directly to skin, to a clean, dry area on the trunk of your body. *Do not apply to breasts or waist.* Firmly press patch for 10 seconds after applying to skin. Rotate application side on at least a weekly basis. Also comes in tablet and vaginal cream forms.

Usual adult dose: *for menopause, Estraderm*—0.05 milligram applied to skin 2 times per week; dosage is decreased at 3-to-6-month intervals. *For menopause, Estrace*—1 or 2 milligrams per day, 3 weeks on and 1 week off. *For osteoporosis, Estraderm*—0.05 milligram per day. *For osteoporosis, Estrace*—0.5 milligram per day for 3 weeks, 1 week off. *For low estrogen levels*—1 or 2 milligrams per day. *For breast cancer*—10 milligrams 3 times per day for at least 3 months. *For prostate cancer*—1 to 2 milligrams 3 times per day. *For vaginal itching and dryness*—2 to 4 grams inserted vaginally one time per day, for 1 to 2 weeks.

Usual child dose: not generally prescribed for children.

Missed dose: *tablets*—take as soon as possible, unless almost time for next dose. If so, skip missed dose; go back to regular schedule. *Do not double doses. Patch*—apply as soon as possible, unless almost time to change patch. If so, skip missed dose; go back to regular schedule. *Do not use more than 1 patch at a time.*

Side Effects

Overdose symptoms: nausea, vomiting, withdrawal bleeding. If you suspect an overdose, immediately seek medical attention.

Most common side effects: skin redness and irritation at patch site.

Less common or rare side effects: abdominal cramps, bloating, breakthrough bleeding, breast enlargement, breast tenderness, change in cervical secretions, change in menstrual flow, change in sex drive, change in weight, darkening of skin, dizziness, fluid retention, growth of benign fibroid tumors in the uterus, headache, intolerance to contact lenses, migraine, nausea, rash, severe allergic reaction, spotting, vomiting, yellowing of eyes and skin. Other side effects with Estraderm: abnormal withdrawal bleeding, certain cancers, cardiovascular disease, depression, excessive growth of hair, gallbladder disease, hair loss, high blood pressure, reddened skin, skin discoloration, skin eruptions, twitching, vaginal yeast infections.

Interactions

Inform your doctor before combining Estraderm with: barbiturates such as phenobarbital; blood thinners such as Coumadin; epilepsy drugs such as Tegretol and Dilantin; rifampin (Rifadin); tricyclic antidepressants such as Elavil and Tofranil.

No known food/other substance interactions.

Special Cautions

 Should not use during pregnancy. If pregnant or planning to become pregnant, inform your doctor immediately. May appear in breast milk, could affect a nursing infant.

 No special precautions apply to seniors.

 Not generally prescribed for children.

 Doctor should take complete medical history *before* you start taking Estraderm, with physical exams on at least a yearly basis thereafter.

Should have regular checkups while taking Estraderm, increased risk of endometrial cancer; immediately contact your doctor if you have unusual vaginal bleeding.

Should not use if sensitive to or allergic to Estraderm.

Avoid use if you have blood clots or blood clotting disorder, with or without estrogen use. Increased risk for blood clots, potentially leading to stroke, heart attack, or other serious disorders.

If using Estraderm post-menopause, may develop gallbladder disease.

Immediately contact your doctor if you experience: abdominal pain, tenderness, or swelling; abnormal vaginal bleeding; breast lumps; coughing up blood; pain in chest or calves; severe headache; dizziness or faintness; sudden shortness of breath; vision changes; yellowing of skin.

Use with caution if you have: asthma, epilepsy, migraine, or heart or kidney disease.

Estradiol
see ESTRADERM

Estrogen and Progestin
see ORAL CONTRACEPTIVES

Estropipate
see OGEN

Etodolac
see LODINE

Eulexin

Generic name: Flutamide

Eulexin is an antineoplastic agent. It prevents the growth of rapidly dividing cells, such as cancer cells.

℞ QUICK FACTS

Purpose

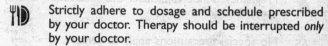

℞ Used to treat prostate cancer. Is prescribed with medications such as Lupron.

Dosage

Strictly adhere to dosage and schedule prescribed by your doctor. Therapy should be interrupted *only* by your doctor.

Usual adult dose: 2 capsules 3 times per day at 8-hour intervals, up to 750 milligrams per day.

Usual child dose: not generally prescribed for children.

Missed dose: take as soon as possible, unless almost time for next dose. If so, skip missed dose; go back to regular schedule. *Do not double doses.*

Side Effects

Overdose symptoms: breast development or tenderness. If you suspect an overdose, immediately seek medical attention.

More common side effects: breast tissue swelling and tenderness, diarrhea, hot flashes, impotence, loss of sex drive, nausea, vomiting.

Less common side effects: confusion, decreased sexual ability, jaundice and liver damage, rash, sun sensitivity, urine discoloration.

Interactions

Inform your doctor before combining Eulexin with blood thinners such as Coumadin. Doctor should monitor you closely; may lower your dosage of the other medications.

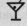 No known food/other substance interactions.

Special Cautions

 Pregnancy is not applicable; this medication is only prescribed for men.

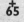 No special precautions apply to seniors.

 Not generally prescribed for children.

 Do not take if sensitive to or allergic to this medication, or any of the ingredients of this medication.

Doctor should check your liver function *before* Eulexin therapy; may cause liver damage.

F

Famotidine

see PEPCID

Fastin

Generic name: Phentermine hydrochloride

Other brand names: Adipex-P, Dapex, Fastin, Ionamin, Obenix, Obephen, Obermine, Obestin-30, Parmine, Phentrol, Profast-SR, Tora, Unifast Unicelles, Wilpowr, Zantryl

Fastin is a nonamphetamine appetite suppressant. It relieves hunger by altering nerve impulses to the appetite control center of the brain.

℞ QUICK FACTS

Purpose

℞ Used for weight reduction on a short-term basis.

Dosage

  Take after breakfast, not in the evening. Ionamin capsules should be swallowed whole. Fastin should be used in conjunction with a behavior modification program. Avoid suddenly stopping Fastin after prolonged use; may cause depression or trouble sleeping.

Usual adult dose: *Fastin*—1 capsule 2 hours after breakfast. *Ionamin*—1 capsule per day, taken before breakfast or 10 to 14 hours before bedtime.

 Usual child dose: not generally prescribed for children under 12 years.

 Missed dose: skip missed dose completely; return to schedule.

Side Effects

 Overdose symptoms: abdominal cramps, aggressiveness, confusion, diarrhea, exaggerated reflexes, hallucinations, high or low blood pressure, irregular heartbeat, nausea, panic states, rapid breathing, restlessness, tremors, vomiting. If you suspect an overdose, immediately seek medical attention. Fatigue and depression may appear after stimulant effects of Fastin. *With fatal poisoning, convulsions and coma usually precede death.*

 Side effects: changes in sex drive, constipation, diarrhea, dizziness, dry mouth, exaggerated feelings of depression or elation, headache, high blood pressure, hives, impotence, inability to fall or stay asleep, increased heart rate, overstimulation, restlessness, stomach or intestinal problems, throbbing heartbeat, tremors, unpleasant taste.

 No known less common or rare side effects.

Interactions

 Inform your doctor before combining Fastin with: MAO inhibitors such as Nardil and Parnate, diabetes medications such as Insulin and Micronase, or high blood pressure medications such as Ismelin.

May intensify effects of alcohol; avoid use when taking Fastin.

Special Cautions

 If pregnant or planning to become pregnant, inform your doctor immediately. Not known if Fastin appears in breast milk.

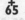 No special precautions apply to seniors.

 Not generally prescribed for children under 12 years.

 Do not take if you have: hardening of the arteries, heart or blood vessel disease, overactive thyroid, glaucoma, or moderate to severe high blood pressure.

Should not take if you: are agitated, have abused drugs, or have taken MAO inhibitors within the last 14 days.

If sensitive to or allergic to this or medications that stimulate the nervous system, should not take.

May impair your ability to operate machinery or perform potentially hazardous activities; use with extreme caution.

Monitor for psychological dependence; contact your doctor if you become dependent.

Overuse can cause: inability to fall or stay asleep, irritability, hyperactivity, personality changes, or severe skin disorders.

Use with caution if you have mildly high blood pressure.

Felbamate

see FELBATOL

Felbatol

Generic name: Felbamate

Felbatol is an anticonvulsant. It selectively reduces excessive brain stimulation.

℞ QUICK FACTS

Purpose

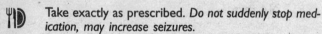 Used to treat epilepsy and certain types of seizures. Also used to treat Lennox-Gastaut syndrome.

Dosage

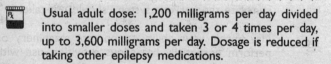 Take exactly as prescribed. *Do not suddenly stop medication, may increase seizures.*

Usual adult dose: 1,200 milligrams per day divided into smaller doses and taken 3 or 4 times per day, up to 3,600 milligrams per day. Dosage is reduced if taking other epilepsy medications.

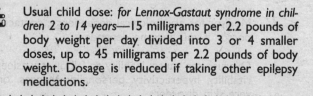 Usual child dose: *for Lennox-Gastaut syndrome in children 2 to 14 years*—15 milligrams per 2.2 pounds of body weight per day divided into 3 or 4 smaller doses, up to 45 milligrams per 2.2 pounds of body weight. Dosage is reduced if taking other epilepsy medications.

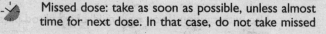 Missed dose: take as soon as possible, unless almost time for next dose. In that case, do not take missed

dose; go back to regular schedule. *Do not double doses.*

Side Effects

 Overdose symptoms: mild stomach upset, unusually fast heartbeat. If you suspect an overdose, immediately seek medical attention.

 Side effects with Felbatol taken *alone*: acne, anxiety, constipation, diarrhea, double vision, ear infection, facial swelling, fatigue, headache, inability to fall or stay asleep, indigestion, loss of appetite, menstrual irregularities, nausea, nasal inflammation, rash, upper respiratory infection, urinary tract infection, vomiting, weight decrease. Side effects with Felbatol when taken *with other medications*: abdominal pain, abnormal stride, abnormal sense of taste, abnormal vision, anxiety, chest pain, constipation, depression, diarrhea, dizziness, double vision, dry mouth, fatigue, fever, headache, inability to fall or stay asleep, indigestion, lack of muscle coordination, loss of appetite, muscle pain, nausea, nervousness, pins and needles, rash, sinus inflammation, sleepiness, sore throat, stupor, tremor, upper respiratory infection, vomiting. Side effects with Felbatol *in children who take other medications*: abnormal stride, abnormal thinking, abnormally small pupils, constipation, coughing, diarrhea, ear infection, fatigue, fever, headache, hiccups, inability to control urination, inability to fall or stay asleep, indigestion, lack of muscle coordination, loss of appetite, mood changes, nausea, nervousness, pain, rash, red or purple spots on skin, sleepiness, sore throat, taste changes, unstable emotions, upper respiratory infection, upset stomach, vomiting, weight decrease.

No known less common or rare side effects.

Interactions

 Inform your doctor before combining Felbatol with other epilepsy drugs such as Dilantin, Depakene, and Tegretol.

· ·

 No known food/other substance interactions.

Special Cautions

 If pregnant or planning to become pregnant, inform your doctor immediately. Appears in breast milk; could affect a nursing infant.

· ·

 No special precautions apply to seniors.

· ·

 Follow doctor's instructions carefully for children.

· ·

 Doctor should closely monitor your reaction when beginning Felbatol therapy.

Feldene

Generic name: Piroxicam

Feldene is a nonsteroidal anti-inflammatory (NSAID). It works by blocking the production of prostaglandins, which may trigger pain.

℞ QUICK FACTS

Purpose

℞ Used to treat the swelling, stiffness, and joint pain from rheumatoid arthritis and osteoarthritis.

· ·

Dosage

 Always take with food or antacid and a full glass of water to avoid digestive problems.

 Usual adult dose: *for rheumatoid arthritis and osteo-arthritis*—20 milligrams per day in a single dose. Doctor may divide dose into smaller ones. Can take 7 to 12 days to observe the medicine's full effects. *Seniors*—dosage determined by individual needs.

 Usual child dose: not generally prescribed for children.

 Missed dose: take as soon as possible, unless almost time for next dose. In that case, do not take missed dose, go back to regular schedule. *Do not double doses.*

Side Effects

 Overdose symptoms: no specific information available. If you suspect an overdose, immediately seek medical attention.

 More common side effects: abdominal pain or discomfort, anemia, constipation, diarrhea, dizziness, fluid retention, gas, general feeling of ill health, headache, heartburn, indigestion, inflammation inside mouth, itching, loss of appetite, nausea, rash, ringing in the ears, sleepiness, stomach upset, vertigo.

 Less common or rare side effects: abdominal bleeding, allergic reaction (severe), angioedema (swelling of lips, face, tongue, and throat), black stools, blood in urine, blurred vision, bruising, colicky pain, congestive heart failure worsening, depression, dry mouth, eye irritations, fatigue, fever, flu-like symptoms, hepatitis, high blood pressure, hives, inability to sleep, joint pain, labored breathing, low or high blood sugar, nervousness, nosebleed, serum sickness (fever, painful joints, enlarged lymph nodes, skin rash), skin allergy to sunlight, Stevens-Johnson syndrome, sweating, swollen eyes, vomiting blood, weight loss or gain, wheezing, worsening of angina, yellow eyes and skin.

Interactions

 Inform your doctor before combining Feldene with aspirin, blood thinners such as Coumadin, or lithium. Avoid aspirin during Feldene therapy.

 Avoid using alcohol during Feldene therapy.

Special Cautions

 If pregnant or planning to become pregnant, inform your doctor immediately. Should not take if you are pregnant or nursing.

 Dosage for seniors determined by individual needs.

 Not generally prescribed for children.

 With long-term use, may cause stomach ulcers or bleeding. Immediately contact your doctor if you experience abdominal or stomach cramps, pain or burning in the stomach, and black tarry stools.

If sensitive to or had allergic reaction to this or similar medications, or aspirin, should not take.

Use with caution if you have: heart disease, high blood pressure, other conditions causing fluid retention, or kidney or liver disease.

Inform your doctor if you experience visual problems.

Felodipine
see PLENDIL

Femstat

Generic name: Butoconazole nitrate

Femstat is an antifungal. It destroys and prevents the growth of fungi.

℞ QUICK FACTS

Purpose

℞ Used to treat fungal infections of the vulva and vagina.

Dosage

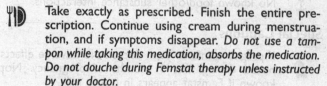

Take exactly as prescribed. Finish the entire prescription. Continue using cream during menstruation, and if symptoms disappear. *Do not use a tampon while taking this medication, absorbs the medication. Do not douche during Femstat therapy unless instructed by your doctor.*

Usual adult dose: *for nonpregnant women*—1 applicator filled with cream inserted vaginally at bedtime for 3 days. Doctor may extend 3 more days if necessary. *For pregnant women*—1 applicator filled with cream inserted vaginally at bedtime for 6 days.

Usual child dose: not generally prescribed for children.

Missed dose: apply as soon as possible, unless almost time for next dose. In that case, do not apply missed dose; go back to regular schedule.

Side Effects

 Overdose symptoms: no overdoses reported. However, if you suspect an overdose, immediately seek medical attention.

 Side effects: itching of the fingers, soreness, swelling, vaginal discharge, vulvar itching, vulvar or vaginal bleeding.

 No known less common or rare side effects.

Interactions

 No drug interactions reported.

 No known food/other substance interactions.

Special Cautions

 If pregnant, inform your doctor. No adverse effects noted during first 3 months of pregnancy. Not known if Femstat appears in breast milk.

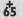 No special precautions apply to seniors.

 Not generally prescribed for children.

 If sensitive to or allergic to any ingredients of Femstat, should not use.

Notify your doctor if symptoms remain, or if you experience allergic reaction or irritation.

Finasteride

see PROSCAR

Fioricet

~~~~~~

Generic ingredients: Butalbital with acetaminophen and caffeine

Other brand names: Amaphen, Anoquan, Bancap, Butace, Endolor, Esgic, Esgic Plus, Femcet, G-1, Medigesic, Phrenilin, Phrenilin Forte, Repan, Sedapap-10, Triaprin, Two-Dyne

Fioricet is a non-narcotic analgesic combination. It reduces the activity of certain brain chemicals and relieves pain.

℞ QUICK FACTS

Purpose

℞   Used to treat tension headaches and migraines.

Dosage

   Take exactly as prescribed. May experience mental and physical dependence if medication taken in higher than prescribed doses over a prolonged period. *Do not increase dosage without consulting your doctor.*

   Usual adult dose: *Fioricet*—1 or 2 tablets every 4 hours as needed, not to exceed 6 tablets per day. *Esgic Plus*—1 tablet every 4 hours as needed, not to

exceed 6 tablets per day. *Seniors*—dosage determined based on individual needs.

 Usual child dose: not generally prescribed for children under 12 years.

 Missed dose: take as soon as possible, unless almost time for next dose. In that case, do not take missed dose; go back to regular schedule. *Do not double doses.*

Side Effects

 Overdose symptoms: *due to barbiturate component of medication*—coma, confusion, drowsiness, low blood pressure, shock, slow or troubled breathing. *Due to acetaminophen component of medication*—kidney or liver damage induced by low blood sugar, or liver failure. Liver damage symptoms: excess perspiration, feeling of bodily discomfort, nausea, vomiting. If you suspect an overdose, immediately seek medical attention.

 More common side effects: dizziness, drowsiness.

 Less common or rare side effects: depression, gas, light-headedness, mental confusion, nausea, rash, skin peeling, vomiting.

Interactions

 Inform your doctor before combining Fioricet with: antihistamines such as Benadryl; antidepressants such as Elavil; antipsychotics such as Haldol and Thorazine; muscle relaxants such as Flexeril; narcotic pain relievers such as Darvon; sleep aids such as Halcion; tranquilizers such as Xanax and Valium. May decrease the effects of blood thinners.

Fioricet intensifies the effects of alcohol; avoid alcohol use while taking this medication.

Special Cautions

 If pregnant or planning to become pregnant, inform your doctor immediately. Appears in breast milk; could affect a nursing infant.

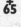 May cause excitement, depression, and confusion in seniors; dosage is determined based on individual needs.

 Not generally prescribed for children under 12 years.

 Do not take if you have porphyria unless specifically instructed by your doctor.

May cause drowsiness and impair your ability to drive a car or operate machinery. *Do not take part in any activity that requires alertness.*

Inform your doctor *before* taking Fioricet if you are being treated for severe depression or have a history of severe depression or drug abuse.

Should not take if sensitive to or allergic to barbiturates, acetaminophen, caffeine, or medications similar to Fioricet.

Fiorinal

Generic ingredients: Butalbital with aspirin and caffeine

Other brand names: Axotal, B-A-C, Butalbital Compound, Fiorgen PF, Isollyl Improved, Lanorinal, Marnal

Fiorinal is a non-narcotic analgesic combination. It reduces the activity of certain brain chemicals and relieves pain.

℞ QUICK FACTS

Purpose

℞ Used to treat tension headaches and migraines.

Dosage

 Take as soon as a headache begins. To avoid stomach irritation, take with a full glass of water or food. *Do not take if medication has a strong vinegar odor. Do not increase dosage without consulting your doctor.*

 Usual adult dose: 1 or 2 tablets or capsules every 4 hours, not to exceed 6 tablets or capsules per day.

 Usual child dose: not generally prescribed for children under 12 years.

 Missed dose: if taking on a regular schedule, take as soon as possible, unless almost time for next dose. In that case, do not take missed dose; go back to regular schedule. *Do not double doses.*

Side Effects

 Overdose symptoms: *due to barbiturate component of medication*—coma, confusion, drowsiness, low blood pressure, shock, slow or troubled breathing. *Due to aspirin and caffeine components of medication*—abdominal pain, deep and/or rapid breathing, delirium, high fever, inability to fall or stay asleep, rapid or irregular heartbeat, restlessness, ringing in the ears, seizures, tremor, vomiting. If you suspect an overdose, immediately seek medical attention.

 More common side effects: dizziness, drowsiness.

 Less common or rare side effects: gas, light-headedness, nausea, rash, skin problems, vomiting.

Interactions

 Inform your doctor before combining Fiorinal with: acetazolamide (Diamox); antidepressants such as Elavil, Norpramin, Nardil, and Parnate; beta-blockers such as Inderal and Tenormin; blood thinners such as Coumadin; narcotic pain relievers such as Darvon and Percocet; oral contraceptives; oral diabetes medications such as Micronase; sleep aids such as Halcion, Nembutal, and phenobarbital; steroid medications such as prednisone; theophylline (Theo-Dur); tranquilizers such as Librium, Valium, and Xanax; valproic acid (Depakene or Depakote).

 Fiorinal intensifies the effects of alcohol; avoid alcohol use while taking this medication.

Special Cautions

 If pregnant or planning to become pregnant, inform your doctor immediately. Butalbital and aspirin appear in breast milk; could affect a nursing infant.

 No special precautions apply to seniors.

 Not generally prescribed for children under 12 years.

 Do not take if you have porphyria unless specifically instructed by your doctor.

. . . .

May cause drowsiness and impair your ability to drive a car or operate machinery. *Do not take part in any activity that requires alertness.*

. . . .

Do not administer to children or teenagers suffering from flu or chicken pox; may cause Reye's syndrome.

. . . .

Tell your doctor if you have an ulcer or a disorder affecting the blood clotting process *before* taking Fiorinal.

. . . .

May experience dependence if taken for prolonged periods of time.

. . . .

Should not take if sensitive to or allergic to similar medications to butalbital, barbiturates, aspirin, or other sedatives or pain relievers.

. . . .

Consult with your doctor if chronic tension headaches continue after taking this medication.

Fiorinal with Codeine

Generic ingredients: Butalbital with codeine phosphate, aspirin, and caffeine

Fiorinal with Codeine is a narcotic-analgesic combination. It reduces the activity of certain brain chemicals and relieves pain.

℞ QUICK FACTS

Purpose

℞   Used to treat tension headaches and migraines.

. . . .

Dosage

Take exactly as prescribed. To avoid stomach irritation, take with a full glass of water or food. *Do not take if medication has a strong vinegar odor. Do not increase dosage without consulting your doctor.*

Usual adult dose: 1 or 2 capsules every 4 hours as needed, not to exceed 6 capsules per day.

Usual child dose: not generally prescribed for children under 12 years.

Missed dose: if taking on a regular schedule, take as soon as possible, unless almost time for next dose. In that case, do not take missed dose; go back to regular schedule. *Do not double doses.*

Side Effects

Overdose symptoms: *due to barbiturate component of medication*—coma, confusion, dizziness, drowsiness, low blood pressure, shock, slow or troubled breathing. *Due to codeine component of medication*—convulsions, loss of consciousness, pinpoint pupils, troubled and slowed breathing. *Due to aspirin component of medication*—abdominal pain, deep and/or rapid breathing, delirium, high fever, restlessness, ringing in the ears, seizures, vomiting. *Due to caffeine poisoning*—delirium, insomnia, irregular heartbeat, rapid heartbeat, restlessness, tremor. If you suspect an overdose, immediately seek medical attention.

More common side effects: abdominal pain, dizziness, drowsiness, nausea. Additional side effects caused by components of this medication: anemia, blocked air passages, hepatitis, high blood sugar, internal bleeding, intoxicated feeling, irritability, kidney damage, lack of clotting, light-headedness, peptic ulcer, stomach upset, tremors.

No known less common or rare side effects.

Interactions

 Inform your doctor before combining Fiorinal with Codeine with: acetazolamide (Diamox); antidepressants such as Elavil, Norpramin, Nardil, and Parnate; antigout medications such as Zyloprim; antihistamines such as Benadryl; beta-blockers such as Inderal and Tenormin; blood thinners such as Coumadin; 6-mercaptopurine; methotrexate (Rheumatrex); narcotic pain relievers such as Darvon and Vicodin; nonsteroidal anti-inflammatory medications such as Motrin and Indocin; oral contraceptives; oral diabetes medications such as Micronase; sleep aids such as Nembutal and phenobarbital; steroid medications such as prednisone; theophylline (Theo-Dur); tranquilizers such as Librium, Valium, and Xanax; valproic acid (Depakene or Depakote).

 Intensifies the effects of alcohol; avoid alcohol use while taking this medication, may cause overdose symptoms.

Special Cautions

 If pregnant or planning to become pregnant, inform your doctor immediately. Butalbital, aspirin, codeine, and caffeine appear in breast milk; could affect a nursing infant.

 No special precautions apply to seniors.

 Not generally prescribed for children under 12 years.

 Do not take if you have: asthma due to aspirin or other anti-inflammatory medications, nasal polyps, peptic ulcer, porphyria, tendency to bleed excessively, severe liver

damage, severe vitamin K deficiency, or swelling from fluid retention, unless specifically instructed by your doctor.

. . . .

May cause drowsiness and impair your ability to drive a car or operate machinery. *Do not take part in any activity that requires alertness.*

. . . .

Do not administer to children or teenagers suffering from flu or chicken pox; may cause Reye's syndrome.

. . . .

If you have: drug dependence (or a history of), kidney, liver, or blood clotting disorder, inform your doctor *before* starting this medication.

. . . .

Use with extreme caution if you are older or have a weakened condition.

. . . .

Codeine use may result in: difficulty in monitoring head-injury patients, increased pressure as a result of fluid surrounding the brain and spinal cord in the case of a head injury, or unusually slow or troubled breathing.

. . . .

Should not take if sensitive to or allergic to similar medications to butalbital, codeine, aspirin, caffeine, or other pain relievers.

. . . .

Consult with your doctor if chronic tension headaches continue after taking this medication.

. . . .

Monitor for internal bleeding in the case of an ulcer or bleeding disorder.

. . . .

Codeine may mask signs of severe abdominal problems.

Flagyl

∿∿∿∿∿∿∿∿∿∿∿∿∿∿∿∿∿∿∿∿∿∿∿∿∿∿∿∿∿∿∿∿∿∿

Generic name: Metronidazole

Other brand names: Femazole, Metizol, MetroGel, Metryl, Protostat, Satric

Flagyl is an amoebicide/antibiotic. It acts by killing bacteria or parasites.

℞ QUICK FACTS

Purpose

℞ Used to treat vaginal and urinary tract infections in men and women; amoebic dysentery and liver abscesses; infections of the abdomen, skin, bones, joints, brain, lungs, and heart caused by bacteria.

Dosage

 Take medication consistently and on schedule. Works best when the body maintains a constant level of the medication. If treated for trichomoniasis (sexually transmitted infection), your doctor may also treat your partner, even if there are no symptoms. Avoid sexual intercourse during treatment until cured, or use a condom. Can take with or without food.

 Usual adult dose: *for trichomoniasis*—*I day treatment*—2 grams in a single dose or divided into 2 doses; *7 day treatment*—250 milligrams taken 3 times per day for 7 consecutive days. *For acute amoebic dysentery*—750 milligrams taken orally 3 times per day for 5 to 10 days. *For amoebic liver abscess*—500 milligrams or 750 milligrams taken orally 3 times per day for 5 to 10 days. *For anaerobic bacterial infections*—7.5 milligrams per 2.2 pounds of body weight taken orally every 6 hours. *Seniors*—doctor may adjust dosage.

 Usual child dose: 35 to 50 milligrams per 2.2 pounds of body weight per day, divided into 3 doses, taken for 10 days.

 Missed dose: take as soon as possible, unless almost time for next dose. In that case, do not take missed dose; go back to regular schedule. *Do not double doses.*

Side Effects

 Overdose symptoms: lack of muscle coordination, nausea, vomiting. If you suspect an overdose, immediately seek medical attention.

 More common side effects: abdominal cramps, constipation, diarrhea, headache, loss of appetite, nausea, upset stomach, vomiting.

 Less common side effects: blood disorders, confusion, dark urine, decreased sex drive, depression, difficulty sleeping, dizziness, dry mouth, dry vagina or vulva, fever, flushing, furry tongue, hives, inability to hold urine, increased production of pale urine, inflamed mouth or tongue, inflammation of the rectum, irritability, lack of muscle coordination, metallic taste, occasional joint pain, pain during sexual intercourse, painful or difficult urination, pelvic pressure, rash, stuffy nose, vaginal yeast infection, vertigo, weakness. *If you experience seizures and numbness or tingling in the arms, legs, hands, and feet, stop taking the medication and immediately contact your doctor.*

Interactions

 Inform your doctor before combining Flagyl with: blood thinners such as Coumadin; cholestyramine

(Questran); cimetidine (Tagamet); disulfiram (Antabuse); lithium (Lithonate); phenobarbital; phenytoin (Dilantin).

 Do not drink alcohol during Flagyl therapy and for 24 hours after final dose. Also avoid medications containing alcohol such as cough and cold syrups.

Special Cautions

 If pregnant or planning to become pregnant, inform your doctor immediately. Appears in breast milk; could affect a nursing infant. Should not use during first trimester of pregnancy.

 Doctor may adjust dosage for seniors.

 Follow doctor's instructions carefully for children.

 Do not take if sensitive to or allergic to Flagyl or similar medications.

Inform your doctor if you have liver disease.

Yeast infections may appear or worsen during Flagyl therapy.

Flavoxate Hydrochloride
see URISPAS

Flecainide Acetate
see TAMBOCOR

Flexeril

∿∿∿∿∿∿∿∿∿∿∿∿∿∿∿∿∿∿∿∿∿∿∿∿∿∿∿∿∿∿∿∿∿∿∿∿∿

Generic name: Cyclobenzaprine hydrochloride

Flexeril is a muscle relaxant. It is thought to work by blocking the reflexes involved in producing and maintaining muscle spasms.

℞ QUICK FACTS

Purpose

 Used to relieve muscle spasms. Also provides relief of muscular stiffness and pain.

Dosage

 Can take with or without food. Is for short-term use (3 weeks or less) only.

. . . .

 Usual adult dose: 10 milligrams taken 3 times per day, not to exceed 60 milligrams per day.

. . . .

 Usual child dose: not generally prescribed for children under 15 years.

. . . .

 Missed dose: take as soon as possible, unless almost within an hour of next dose. In that case, do not take missed dose; go back to regular schedule. *Do not double doses.*

Side Effects

Overdose symptoms: agitation, coma, confusion, congestive heart failure, convulsions, dilated pupils, disturbed concentration, drowsiness, hallucinations, high or low temperature, increased heartbeats, irregular heart rhythms, muscle stiffness, overactive reflexes, severe low blood pressure, stupor, vomiting. High doses may also cause side effects listed below. If you suspect an overdose, immediately seek medical attention.

 More common side effects: dizziness, drowsiness, dry mouth.

 Less common or rare side effects: abnormal heartbeats, abnormal sensations, abnormal thoughts or dreams, agitation, anxiety, bloated feeling, blurred vision, confusion, constipation, convulsions, decreased appetite, depressed mood, diarrhea, difficulty falling or staying asleep, difficulty speaking, disorientation, double vision, excitement, fainting, fatigue, fluid retention, gas, hallucinations, headache, heartburn, hepatitis, hives, increased heart rate, indigestion, inflammation of the stomach, itching, lack of coordination, liver diseases, loss of sense of taste, low blood pressure, muscle twitching, nausea, nervousness, palpitations, rash, ringing in the ears, severe allergic reaction, stomach and intestinal pain, sweating, swelling of the tongue or face, thirst, tingling in hands or feet, tremors, unpleasant taste in the mouth, urinating less than usual, vague feeling of bodily discomfort, vertigo, vomiting, weakness, yellow eyes and skin.

Interactions

 Inform your doctor before combining Flexeril with: antispasmodic medications such as Donnatal and Bentyl; barbiturates such as phenobarbital; guanethidine (Esimil or Ismelin) and other blood pressure medications; other medications that slow central nervous system such as Halcion and Xanax. *Should not take if currently taking* MAO *inhibitors (Nardil or Parnate) or have taken them within the last 14 days; may cause fatal reaction.*

 Should not drink alcohol while taking this medication.

Special Cautions

 If pregnant, inform your doctor. Not known if Flexeril appears in breast milk; however, medications related to the ingredients in Flexeril do appear in breast milk.

 No special precautions apply to seniors.

 Not generally prescribed for children under 15 years.

 May cause drowsiness and impair your ability to drive a car or operate machinery. *Do not take part in any activity that requires alertness.*

If sensitive to or allergic to this medication, should not take.

Use with caution if you have glaucoma or the inability to urinate.

If you have: an overactive thyroid, congestive heart failure, irregular heartbeat, or recent heart attack, should not take Flexeril.

Flexeril does not relieve other types of pain.

This medication is not a substitute for physical therapy, rest, or exercise needed for proper healing of spasms.

Florone

see PSORCON

Floxin

Generic name: Ofloxacin

Floxin is a fluoraquinolone antibiotic. It inhibits the growth of bacteria by chemically interfering with their ability to survive.

℞ QUICK FACTS

Purpose

 Used to treat lower respiratory tract infections, sexually transmitted diseases, and infections of the urinary tract, prostate gland, and skin. Not effective in treating syphilis, and may hide or delay symptoms.

Dosage

 Take exactly as prescribed, finishing the entire prescription. Drinks lots of fluids during Floxin therapy.

Usual adult dose: *for lower respiratory tract infections—Worsening of chronic bronchitis*—400 milligrams every 12 hours for 10 days, up to 800 milligrams per day. *Pneumonia*—400 milligrams every 12 hours for 10 days, up to 800 milligrams per day. *For sexually transmitted diseases—Gonorrhea*—400 milligrams taken once. *Infections of the cervix or urethra*—300 milligrams every 12 hours for 7 days, up to 600 milligrams per day. *For mild to moderate skin infections*—400 milligrams every 12 hours for 10 days, up to 800 milligrams per day. *For urinary tract infections—Bladder infections*—200 milligrams every 12 hours, totaling 400 milligrams per day. Taken 3 days for *E. coli* or *K. pneumonia;* taken 7 days for other microbes. *Complicated urinary tract infections*—200 milligrams every 12 hours for 10 days, totaling 400 milligrams per day. *Prostatitis*—300 milligrams every 12 hours for 6 weeks, totaling 600 milligrams per day.

 Usual child dose: not generally prescribed for children.

 Missed dose: take as soon as possible, unless almost time for next dose. In that case, do not take missed dose, go back to regular schedule. *Do not double doses.*

Side Effects

 Overdose symptoms: no specific information available. If you suspect an overdose, immediately seek medical attention.

 More common side effects: diarrhea, difficulty sleeping, dizziness, headache, itching of genital area in women, nausea, vaginal inflammation, vomiting.

 Less common or rare side effects: abdominal pain and cramps, aggressiveness or hostility, agitation, anemia, anxiety, asthma, blood in urine, blurred vision, body pain, bruising, burning or rash of the female genitals, burning sensation in the upper chest, changeable emotions, changes in thinking and perception, chest pain, confusion, conjunctivitis (pink eye), continual runny nose, constipation, cough, decreased appetite, depression, difficult or labored breathing, disorientation, disturbed dreams, disturbed sense of smell, double vision, dry mouth, exaggerated sense of well-being, excessive perspiration, fainting, fatigue, fear, fever, fluid retention, frequent urination, gas, hallucinations, hearing disturbance or loss, hepatitis, hiccups, high or low blood pressure, high or low blood sugar, hives, inability to urinate, increased urination, indigestion, inflammation of the colon, inflammation or rupture of tendons, intolerance to light, involuntary eye movement, itching, joint pain, kidney problems, lack of coordination, light-headedness, liver problems, menstrual changes, muscle pain, nervousness, nightmares, nosebleed, pain, pain in arms and legs, painful or difficult urination, purple or red spots on the skin, rapid heartbeat, rash, reddened skin, restlessness, ringing in the ears, seizures, sensitivity to light, severe allergic reaction, skin inflammation and flaking or eruptions, sleepiness, sleep problems, sore mouth or throat, Stevens-Johnson syndrome, stomach and intestinal upset or bleeding, taste distortion, thirst, throbbing or fluttering heartbeat, tingling or pins and needles, tremor, unexplained bleeding from the uterus, vaginal discharge, vaginal yeast infection, vague feeling of illness, vertigo, visual disturbances, weakness, weight loss, yellowing of eyes and skin.

Interactions

Inform your doctor before combining Floxin with: antacids containing aluminum, magnesium, or calcium; blood thinners such as Coumadin; calcium supplements such as Caltrate; cyclosporine (Sandimmune); insulin; iron supplements such as Feosol; multivitamins with zinc; nonsteroidal anti-inflammatory medications such as Motrin and Naprosyn; oral diabetes medications such as Diabinese and Micronase; sucralfate (Carafate); theophylline (Theo-Dur).

Do not take with food. Do not take mineral supplements, vitamins with iron or minerals, or antacids with calcium, aluminum, or magnesium within 2 hours of taking this medication.

Special Cautions

Should not use during pregnancy. If pregnant or planning to become pregnant, inform your doctor immediately. Appears in breast milk; could affect a nursing infant.

 No special precautions apply to seniors.

 Not generally prescribed for children.

 Do not take if sensitive to or allergic to this or other quinolone antibiotics such as Cipro and Noroxin.

May cause drowsiness and impair your ability to drive a car or operate machinery. *Do not take part in any activity that requires alertness.*

Immediately stop taking Floxin and contact your doctor if you develop a skin rash or other allergic reaction. *In rare cases, serious and fatal allergic reactions occur after the first dose. Signs of allergic reaction: swelling of the face and throat, shortness of breath, difficulty swallowing, rapid heartbeat, tingling, itching, and hives.*

Stop taking Floxin if you experience: convulsions, increased pressure in the head, psychosis, tremors, restlessness, light-headedness, nervousness, confusion, depression, nightmares, insomnia, or hallucinations.

Inform your doctor and use with caution if you have: brain disorder, epilepsy, or seizures due to kidney disease.

To prevent sun poisoning, avoid long exposure to the sun.

Fluconazole
see DIFLUCAN

Flunisolide

see AEROBID

Fluocinonide

see LIDEX

Fluorometholone

see FML

Fluoroplex Topical Solution

see EFUDEX

Fluorouracil

see EFUDEX

Fluoxetine Hydrochloride

see PROZAC

Flurazepam Hydrochloride

see DALMANE

Flurbiprofen
see ANSAID

Flutamide
see EULEXIN

Fluvastatin Sodium
see LESCOL

FML

Generic name: Fluorometholone

Other brand names: Flarex, Fluor-Op, FML Forte, FML Liquifilm, FML Ointment

FML is an ophthalmic anti-inflammatory corticosteroid. It inhibits the growth of bacteria in the eyes by chemically interfering with their ability to survive.

℞ QUICK FACTS

Purpose

℞ Used to treat inflammation of the eye and eyelid.

Dosage

 Use exactly as prescribed. Doctor may suggest that you not wear contacts while using FML; may increase the chance of infection from contact lenses.

Do not discontinue medication without doctor authorization. To avoid spreading infection, do not share this prescription. Do not continue using beyond what your doctor specifically prescribes; may risk eye damage. If you have recurring eye problems, do not use leftover prescription unless specifically advised by your doctor to do so.

 Usual adult dose: *ointment*—apply ½ ribbon between lower eyelid and eyeball 1 to 3 times per day. In first 2 days of therapy, doctor may prescribe 1 dose every 4 hours. *Liquifilm*—place 1 drop between the lower eyelid and eyeball 2 to 4 times per day. In first 2 days of therapy, doctor may prescribe 1 dose every 4 hours.

 Usual child dose: not generally prescribed for children under 2 years.

 Missed dose: apply as soon as possible, unless almost time for next dose. In that case, do not apply missed dose; go back to regular schedule. *Do not double doses.*

Side Effects

 Overdose symptoms: FML does not usually cause severe problems. If accidentally swallowed, drink plenty of fluids to dilute medication. However, if you suspect an overdose, immediately seek medical attention.

 Side effects: cataract formation, corneal ulcers, dilation of the pupil, drooping eyelids, eye inflammation and infection including conjunctivitis, glaucoma, increased eye pressure, slow wound healing.

 No known less common or rare side effects.

Interactions

 No specific drug interactions reported.

 No known food/other substance interactions.

Special Cautions

 If pregnant or planning to become pregnant, inform your doctor immediately. May appear in breast milk; could affect a nursing infant.

 No special precautions apply to seniors.

 Not generally prescribed for children under 2 years.

 Do not use if sensitive to or allergic to this or similar medications such as Decadron.

Not prescribed for certain viral, fungal, and bacterial eye infections.

Ongoing use may cause glaucoma, cataract formation, or development or worsening of eye infection.

FML and similar steroids may cause punctures when used with diseases that thin the cornea or the sclera.

Doctor should monitor internal eye pressure during FML therapy.

Use with caution if you have cataract surgery.

If condition worsens after 48 hours, stop taking medication and contact your doctor.

Fosinopril Sodium
see MONOPRIL

Fulvicin
see GRIS-PEG

Furosemide
see LASIX

Gantrisin

Generic name: Sulfisoxazole

Gantrisin is a sulfa drug and an antibiotic. It inhibits the growth of bacteria by chemically interfering with their ability to survive.

℞ QUICK FACTS

Purpose

Used to treat severe, repeated, or long-lasting urinary tract infections. Also used to treat bacterial meningitis, and as a preventive measure for people exposed to meningitis. May also be used in combination with other medications to treat: some middle ear infections, toxoplasmosis (parasite from cats, cat feces, or uncooked meat), malaria, eye infections, bacterial disease of the lungs, skin, and brain (nocardiosis), and chancroid (venereal disease of the groin).

Dosage

Drink lots of liquids to avoid crystals in the urine and stone formation. Shake suspension well before each use; use marked measuring spoon from your pharmacist. Take at evenly spaced intervals to keep level of this medication constant.

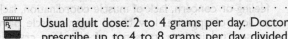

Usual adult dose: 2 to 4 grams per day. Doctor may prescribe up to 4 to 8 grams per day divided into 4 to 6 doses.

Usual child dose: *for children 2 months or older—* *Starting dose*—75 milligrams per 2.2 pounds of body weight divided into 4 to 6 doses in 24 hours. *Regular dose*—120 to 150 milligrams per 2.2 pounds of body weight divided into 4 to 6 doses in 24 hours. Not for children under 2 years *except to treat toxoplasmosis.* Maximum dose is 6 grams per day.

 Missed dose: take as soon as possible, unless almost time for next dose. In that case, do not take missed dose; go back to regular schedule. *Do not double doses.*

Side Effects

 Overdose symptoms: blood or sediment in urine, blue tinge to the skin, colic, dizziness, drowsiness, fever, headache, lack of or loss of appetite, nausea, unconsciousness, vomiting, yellowing of skin and eyes. If you suspect an overdose, immediately seek medical attention.

 Side effects: abdominal bleeding, abdominal pain, allergic reactions, anemia and other blood disorders, angioedema (swelling of the face, lips, tongue, and throat), anxiety, bluish tinge to the skin, chills, colitis, convulsions, cough, dark or tarry stools, depression, diarrhea, disorientation, dizziness, drowsiness, enlarged salivary glands, enlarged thyroid gland, exhaustion, fainting, fatigue, fever, flushing, gas, hallucinations, headache, hearing loss, hepatitis, hives, inability to fall or stay asleep, inability to urinate, increased urination, inflammation of the mouth or tongue, itching, joint pain, kidney failure, lack of feeling or concern, lack of muscle coordination, lack or loss of appetite, low blood sugar, muscle pain, nausea, palpitations, presence of blood or crystals in urine, rapid heartbeat, reddish or purplish skin spots, retention of urine, ringing in the ears, sensitivity to light, serum sickness (fever, painful joints, enlarged lymph nodes, skin rash), severe skin welts or swelling, shortness of breath, skin eruptions, skin rash, swelling due to fluid retention, tingling or pins and needles, vertigo, vomiting, weakness, yellow eyes and skin.

 No known less common or rare side effects.

Interactions

 Inform your doctor before combining Gantrisin with: blood thinners such as Coumadin; methotrexate, an anticancer medication; oral contraceptives; oral diabetes medications such as Micronase.

 No known food/other substance interactions.

Special Cautions

 If pregnant or planning to become pregnant, inform your doctor immediately. Appears in breast milk; could affect a nursing infant. Should not take near the end of pregnancy or when nursing a baby under 2 months.

 No special precautions apply to seniors.

 Follow doctor's instructions carefully for children.

 Severe and fatal reactions have occurred with sulfa medications such as Gantrisin. Monitor for: sudden and severe liver damage, agranulocytosis (severe blood disorder), aplastic anemia (lack of red and white blood cells due to bone marrow disorder), and Stevens-Johnson syndrome (severe blistering).

Doctor should take blood counts and urine and kidney function analysis frequently.

Immediately contact your doctor if you experience reactions such as: skin rash, sore throat, fever, joint pain, cough, shortness of breath or other breathing problems, abnormal skin paleness, reddish or purplish spots, yellowing of skin or eyes, or diarrhea.

. . . .

Should not take if sensitive to or allergic to this or other sulfa medications.

. . . .

Inform your doctor and use with caution if you have impaired kidney or liver function, severe allergies, or bronchial asthma.

Garamycin Ophthalmic

Generic name: Gentamicin sulfate

Other brand names: Cidomycin, Gentacidin

Garamycin Ophthalmic is an aminoglycoside antibiotic. It inhibits the growth of bacteria in the eyes by chemically interfering with their ability to survive.

℞ QUICK FACTS

Purpose

℞ Used to treat conjunctivitis (pink eye) and other eye infections.

Dosage

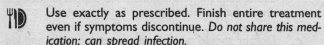 Use exactly as prescribed. Finish entire treatment even if symptoms discontinue. *Do not share this medication; can spread infection.*

. . . .

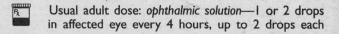 Usual adult dose: *ophthalmic solution*—1 or 2 drops in affected eye every 4 hours, up to 2 drops each

hour. *Ophthalmic ointment*—apply ⅓-inch strip to affected eye 2 or 3 times per day.

 Usual child dose: follow doctor's instructions carefully for children.

 Missed dose: apply as soon as possible, unless almost time for next dose. In that case, do not apply
missed dose; go back to regular schedule.

Side Effects

 Overdose symptoms: no specific information available. If you suspect an overdose, immediately seek
medical attention.

 Side effects: *eye solution*—eye irritation with itching,
redness, and swelling. *Ointment*—burning or stinging
in the eye.

 No known less common or rare side effects.

Interactions

 No drug interactions reported.

 No known food/other substance interactions.

Special Cautions

 If pregnant or planning to become pregnant, inform
your doctor.

 No special precautions apply to seniors.

 Follow doctor's instructions carefully for children.

STOP Vision may blur briefly after application of ointment.

Should not take if sensitive to or allergic to this or other antibiotics such as Amikin and Tobrex.

Ongoing use may cause bacteria or fungi to develop resistance to this medication; contact your doctor if this occurs.

Ointment may slow healing of the cornea.

Gemfibrozil
see LOPID

Gentamicin Sulfate
see GARAMYCIN OPHTHALMIC

Glipizide
see GLUCOTROL

Glucotrol

Generic name: Glipizide

Glucotrol is an oral antidiabetic. It works by inducing the pancreas to secrete more insulin.

℞ QUICK FACTS

Purpose

℞ Used to treat Type II (non-insulin-dependent) diabetes.

Dosage

 Take 30 minutes prior to eating or according to your doctor's specific instructions.

 Usual adult dose: 5 milligrams taken before breakfast; doctor may increase in increments up to 2.5 to 5 milligrams. Maximum daily dose is 40 milligrams, daily doses over 15 milligrams are usually divided into 2 equal doses. *Seniors or individuals with liver disease—2.5 milligrams taken before breakfast.*

 Usual child dose: not generally prescribed for children.

 Missed dose: take as soon as possible, unless almost time for next dose. In that case, do not take missed dose; go back to regular schedule. *Do not double doses.*

Side Effects

 Overdose symptom: low blood sugar. Signs of mild low blood sugar—blurred vision, cold sweats, dizziness, fatigue, headache, hunger, light-headedness, nausea, nervousness, rapid heartbeat. Symptoms of more severe low blood sugar—coma, disorientation, pale skin, seizures, shallow breathing. If you suspect an overdose, immediately seek medical attention.

 More common side effects: constipation, diarrhea, dizziness, drowsiness, headache, hives, itching, low blood sugar, nausea, sensitivity to light, skin rash and eruptions, stomach pain.

Less common or rare side effects: anemia and other blood disorders, yellow eyes and skin.

Interactions

 Inform your doctor before combining Glucotrol with: airway-opening medications such as Sudafed; antacids such as Mylanta; aspirin; chloramphenicol (Chloromycetin); cimetidine (Tagamet); clofibrate (Atromid-S); corticosteroids such as prednisone (Deltasone); diuretics such as HydroDIURIL; estrogens such as Premarin; fluconazole (Diflucan); gemfibrozil (Lopid); heart medications (beta-blockers such as Tenormin and Lopressor); heart medications (calcium channel blockers such as Cardizem and Procardia XL); isoniazid (Nydrazid); itraconazole (Sporanox); MAO inhibitors such as Nardil; major tranquilizers such as Thorazine and Mellaril; miconazole (Monistat); nicotinic acid (Nicobid); nonsteroidal anti-inflammatory medications such as Motrin; oral contraceptives; phenytoin (Dilantin); probenecid (Benemid); rifampin (Rifadin); sulfa medications such as Bactrim; thyroid medications such as Synthroid; warfarin (Coumadin).

 Alcohol use may cause low blood sugar; use carefully.

Special Cautions

 If pregnant or planning to become pregnant, inform your doctor immediately. Not known if Glucotrol appears in breast milk; however, other oral diabetes medications do. If taking during pregnancy, doctor will advise you to stop during the 8th month. To avoid hypoglycemia in nursing infants, doctor may advise you to stop Glucotrol or stop nursing.

 Seniors may be prescribed a lower dose.

Not generally prescribed for children.

 Doctor will stop Glucotrol therapy if you experience diabetic ketoacidosis (life-threatening emergency caused by insufficient insulin).

Glucotrol is not oral insulin and should not be substituted for insulin.

Should not use in place of a sound diet and exercise.

If allergic to Glucotrol, should not take.

Consult with your doctor before starting Glucotrol if you have a heart condition; may worsen condition.

Doctor should monitor glucose levels in blood and urine during therapy.

Doctor may switch you from Glucotrol to insulin if you experience injury, infection, surgery, or fever, leading to loss of control of diabetes.

Effectiveness may decrease over time.

Glyburide
see MICRONASE

Glyceryl Trinitrate
see NITROGLYCERIN

Griseofulvin

see GRIS-PEG

Gris-PEG

Generic name: Griseofulvin

Other brand names: Fulvicin P/G, Fulvicin U/F, Grifulvin V, Grisactin

Gris-PEG is an antifungal. It destroys and prevents the growth of fungi.

℞ QUICK FACTS

Purpose

℞ Used to treat ringworm infections, including: athlete's foot, and ringworm of the body, groin and thigh, nails, and scalp.

Dosage

 Take with food or whole milk to avoid stomach irritation and assist your body in absorbing this medication. Inform your doctor if you are on a low-fat diet. Practice good oral hygiene to prevent and control infection. May observe relief in a few days; must take for an extended period.

 Usual adult dose: *for ringworm of the body, groin, thigh, and scalp*—375 milligrams per day as a single dose or divided into smaller doses. *For athlete's foot and ringworm of the nails*—750 milligrams per day divided into smaller doses. *Treatment periods*—ringworm of the scalp: 4 to 6 weeks; ringworm of the body: 2 to 4 weeks; ringworm of the fingernails: 4 months; ringworm of the toenails: 6 months; and athlete's foot: 4 to 8 weeks.

 Usual child dose: *for ringworm of the scalp*—3.3 milligrams per pound of body weight per day in a single dose. Not prescribed for children 2 years and under.

 Missed dose: take as soon as possible, unless almost time for next dose. In that case, do not take missed dose; go back to regular schedule. *Do not double doses.*

Side Effects

 Overdose symptoms: no specific information available. If you suspect an overdose, immediately seek medical attention.

 More common side effects: hives, skin rashes.

 Less common side effects: confusion, diarrhea, dizziness, fatigue, headache, impairment of performance of daily routine, inability to fall or stay asleep, nausea, oral thrush (mouth inflammation), upper abdominal pain, vomiting. Rare side effects: swelling and itching of areas of skin, tingling sensation in hands and feet.

Interactions

 Inform your doctor before combining Gris-PEG with: blood thinners such as Coumadin, barbiturates such as phenobarbital, oral contraceptives. May decrease effectiveness of birth control pills.

 Use alcohol with caution, may cause fast heartbeat and flushed skin; Gris-PEG may intensify the effects of alcohol.

Special Cautions

 Do not take if pregnant. If you become pregnant during Gris-PEG therapy, immediately contact your doctor; is potentially hazardous to the fetus. Consult with your doctor if breastfeeding.

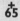 No special precautions apply to seniors.

 Follow doctor's instructions carefully for children. Not prescribed for children 2 years and under.

 Do not take if you have liver damage or porphyria.

Should not take if sensitive to or allergic to this or similar medications, or penicillin.

Minimize exposure to intense natural or artificial sunlight.

If you develop lupus erythematosus or a lupus-like condition (arthritis, red butterfly rash over the nose and cheeks, tiredness, weakness, sensitivity to sunlight, skin eruptions), immediately contact your doctor.

Doctor should monitor kidneys, liver, and blood cell production if taking this medication over an extended period.

Gris-PEG does not prevent fungal infections.

Guaifenesin with Phenylpropanolamine Hydrochloride

see ENTEX LA

Guanabenz Acetate

see WYTENSIN

Guanfacine Hydrochloride

see TENEX

Gyne-Lotrimin

Generic name: Clotrimazole

Other brand names: Femcare, Lotrimin, Mycelex

Gyne-Lotrimin is an antifungal. It destroys and prevents the growth of fungi.

℞ QUICK FACTS

Purpose

℞ Used to treat fungal infections.

Dosage

  Avoid getting into eyes. If taking lozenges, let dissolve in your mouth; do not swallow or chew. To avoid reinfection, use condoms during sexual intercourse. *Do not use tampons if using vaginal medication; will absorb medication. Do not douche unless specifically instructed by your doctor.*

  Usual adult dose: *Lotrimin*—wash hands before and after use. Apply morning and evening to affected areas; massage into skin. *Gyne-Lotrimin cream*—insert I applicatorful vaginally at bedtime for 7 consecutive days. *Mycelex troche*—I troche slowly dissolved orally 5 times per day for 14 consecutive days. For prevention of recurrence, I troche 3 times per day.

 Usual child dose: *Lotrimin*—wash hands before and after use. Apply morning and evening to affected areas; massage into skin.

 Missed dose: take as soon as possible, unless almost time for next dose. In that case, do not take missed dose; go back to regular schedule.

Side Effects

 Overdose symptoms: no specific information available; overdose unlikely. However, if you suspect an overdose, immediately seek medical attention.

 Side effects: blistering, burning, hives, irritated skin, itching, peeling, reddened skin, stinging, swelling due to fluid retention. Side effects of vaginal preparation: abdominal/stomach cramps and pain, burning and irritation of penis of sexual partner, headache, pain during sexual intercourse, skin rash or hives, vaginal burning and/or itching, soreness during sexual intercourse, unpleasant mouth sensation.

 No known less common or rare side effects.

Interactions

 No drug interactions reported.

 No known food/other substance interactions.

Special Cautions

 Do not use during pregnancy without specific instructions from your doctor. Not known whether Gyne-Lotrimin appears in breast milk.

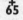 No special precautions apply to seniors.

 Follow doctor's instructions carefully for children.

 If allergic to this medication, should not use.

Notify your doctor if you experience increased skin irritations such as redness, itching, burning, blistering, swelling, or oozing.

If symptoms do not subside after 2 to 4 weeks, contact your doctor.

If you experience abdominal pain, bad-smelling vaginal discharge, or fever, notify your doctor immediately.

Special Cautions

- Do not use during pregnancy without specific instructions from your doctor. It is not known whether Lotrimin appears in breast milk.

- No special precautions apply to seniors.

- Follow doctor's instructions carefully for children.

- If allergic to this medication, should not use.

- Notify your doctor if you experience increased skin irritations such as redness, itching, burning, blistering, swelling or oozing.

- If symptoms do not subside after 2 to 4 weeks, contact your doctor.

- If you experience abdominal pain, trailsmelling vaginal discharge, or fever, notify your doctor immediately.

H

Habitrol

see NICODERM

Halcion

Generic name: Triazolam

Halcion is a benzodiazepine sedative. It selectively reduces the activity of certain brain chemicals.

℞ QUICK FACTS

Purpose

 Used to treat insomnia on a short-term basis.

Dosage

 Take exactly as prescribed; adhere to dosage schedule strictly. May take with food to avoid stomach upset. To avoid withdrawal symptoms, gradually stop medication as directed by your doctor. *Do not take on airplane flights less than 7 or 8 hours to avoid traveler's amnesia.*

 Usual adult dose: 0.25 milligram before bedtime. Never take more than 0.5 milligram. *Seniors*—0.125 milligram, up to 0.25 milligram.

 Usual child dose: not generally prescribed for children.

Missed dose: should take only as needed.

Side Effects

 Halcion overdose can be fatal. Overdose symptoms: apnea (temporary breathing stoppage), coma, confusion, excessive sleepiness, problems in coordination, seizures, shallow or difficult breathing, slurred speech. If you suspect an overdose, immediately seek medical attention.

 More common side effects: coordination problems, dizziness, drowsiness, headache, light-headedness, nausea and vomiting, nervousness.

 Less common or rare side effects: aggressiveness, agitation, behavior problems, burning tongue, changes in sexual drive, chest pain, confusion, congestion, constipation, cramps or pain, delusions, depression, diarrhea, disorientation, dream abnormalities, drowsiness, dry mouth, exaggerated sense of well-being, excitement, fainting, falling, fatigue, hallucinations, impaired urination, inappropriate behavior, incontinence, inflammation of the tongue and mouth, irritability, itching, loss of appetite, loss of sense of reality, memory impairment, memory loss, menstrual irregularities, morning hangover effects, muscle spasms in the shoulders or neck, nightmares, rapid heart rate, restlessness, ringing in the ears, skin inflammation, sleep disturbances including insomnia, sleepwalking, slurred or difficult speech, stiff awkward movements, taste changes, tingling or pins and needles, tiredness, visual disturbances, weakness, yellowing of the skin and eyes.

Interactions

 Inform your doctor before combining Halcion with: antidepressants including Elavil and MAO inhibitors such as Nardil and Parnate; antihistamines such as Benadryl and Tavist; barbiturates such as phenobarbital and Seconal; cimetidine (Tagamet); erythromycin (E.E.S., PCE, or E-Mycin); isoniazid (Nydrazid); narcotic painkillers such as Mellaril and Thorazine; other tranquilizers such as BuSpar, Valium, and Xanax; oral contraceptives; seizure medications such as Dilantin and Tegretol.

Avoid alcohol when taking Halcion.

Special Cautions

 Should not take if pregnant or breastfeeding; benzodiazepines are associated with damage to a developing fetus.

 Seniors are prescribed lower doses.

 Not generally prescribed for children.

 Inform your doctor if you need Halcion for relief of insomnia for more than 7 to 10 days.

Should not take if allergic to this or similar medications such as Valium.

May develop tolerance (loss of effectiveness) or dependence if used nightly for a few weeks, or at consistently high doses.

Immediately contact your doctor if you experience unusual and disturbing thoughts or behavior.

May observe increased daytime anxiety.

At the beginning of Halcion therapy, may impair your ability to operate machinery or perform potentially hazardous activities; use with extreme caution.

. . . .

Immediately after discontinuing medication completely, may experience rebound insomnia (worse than
before Halcion therapy).

. . . .

May experience anterograde amnesia (memory loss
after an injury).

. . . .

Use with caution if you have liver or kidney problems, lung problems, or sleep apnea.

Haldol

~~~~~~

Generic name: Haloperidol

Haldol is an antipsychotic. It calms some parts of the brain
and allows the other parts to function normally.

℞ Quick Facts

Purpose

℞ Used to treat the symptoms of mental disorders
such as schizophrenia. Also used to control tics (uncontrolled contractions); the unintended verbal outbursts associated with Tourette's syndrome; and to
treat severe behavior problems in children on a
short-term basis. Has also been used to relieve severe nausea and vomiting caused by cancer drugs,
to treat drug problems such as LSD flashback and
PCP intoxication, and to control hemiballismus (involuntary writhing of one side of the body).

Dosage

  May take with food or after a meal. If using liquid
concentrate form of Haldol, mix with milk or water.
Gradually stop medication as directed by your doctor to avoid temporary muscle spasms and twitches.

. . . .

Usual adult dose: *for moderate symptoms*—1 to 6 milligrams per day divided into 2 or 3 smaller doses. *For severe symptoms*—6 to 15 milligrams per day divided into 2 or 3 smaller doses. *Seniors*—generally prescribed doses in the lower range of 1 to 6 milligrams per day.

 Usual child dose *(for children 3 to 12 years): for psychotic disorders*—0.05 to 0.15 milligram per each 2.2 pounds of body weight per day. *For nonpsychotic behavior disorders and Tourette's syndrome*—0.05 to 0.075 milligram per each 2.2 pounds of body weight per day. Not prescribed for children under 3 years.

 Missed dose: take as soon as possible. Take remaining doses for the day at equally spaced intervals. *Do not double doses.*

Side Effects

 Overdose symptoms: catatonic (unresponsive) state, coma, decreased breathing, low blood pressure, rigid muscles, sedation, tremor, weakness. If you suspect an overdose, immediately seek medical attention.

 Side effects: abnormal milk secretion, acne-like skin reactions, agitation, anemia, anxiety, blurred vision, breast pain, breast development in males, cataracts, catatonic (unresponsive) state, chewing movements, confusion, constipation, coughing, deeper breathing, dehydration, depression, diarrhea, dizziness, drowsiness, dry mouth, epileptic seizures, exaggerated feeling of well-being, exaggerated reflexes, excessive perspiration, excessive salivation, hair loss, hallucinations, headache, heat stroke, high fever, high or low blood pressure, high or low blood sugar, impotence, inability to urinate, increased sex drive, indigestion, involuntary movements, irregular menstrual periods, irregular pulse, lack of muscular coordination, liver problems, loss of appetite, muscle spasms, nausea, parkinson-like symptoms, persistent abnormal erections, physical rigidity and stupor, protruding tongue, puckering of mouth, puffing of cheeks, rapid heartbeat, restlessness, rigidity (in arms, feet, head, and muscles), rotation of eyeballs, sensitivity to light, skin rash, skin eruptions, sleeplessness, sluggishness, swelling of breasts, twitching (in the body, neck, shoulders, and face), vertigo, visual problems, vomiting, wheezing, or asthma-like symptoms, yellowing of skin and eyes.

 No known less common or rare side effects.

Interactions

 Inform your doctor before combining Haldol with: anticonvulsants such as Dilantin and Tegretol; antidepressants including Elavil, Tofranil, and Prozac; antispasmodics such as Bentyl and Donnatal; blood thinners such as Coumadin; epinephrine (EpiPen); lithium (Lithonate); methyldopa (Aldomet); propranolol (Inderal); rifampin (Rifadin). If Haldol is taken with narcotics, painkillers, sleeping medications, or other medications that slow the central nervous system, can cause extreme drowsiness and serious side effects.

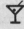 Using alcohol may cause extreme drowsiness and serious side effects. Should not use caffeine during Haldol therapy.

Special Cautions

 If pregnant or planning to become pregnant, inform your doctor immediately. Should not breastfeed during Haldol therapy.

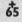 Seniors are generally prescribed doses in the lower ranges.

Follow doctor's instructions carefully for children 3 years and older.

 May cause drowsiness and impair your ability to drive a car or operate machinery. *Do not take part in any activity that requires alertness.*

May cause tardive dyskinesia—involuntary muscle spasms and face and body twitching. Senior women are at higher risk. Talk with your doctor about your risk level.

Should not take if sensitive to or allergic to Haldol, or if you have Parkinson's disease.

Use with caution if you have or ever had: any drug allergies, breast cancer, chest pain, glaucoma, seizures, or severe heart or circulatory disorder.

Use caution in sunlight; may cause skin sensitivity to sunlight.

Interferes with the body's temperature-regulating system; may experience extremely hot or cold body temperatures.

Haloperidol

see HALDOL

Hismanal

Generic name: Astemizole

Hismanal is an antihistamine. Antihistamines block the effects of histamine, a body chemical that causes swelling and itching.

℞ QUICK FACTS

Purpose

 Used to treat hay fever and chronic hives.

Dosage

 Should take on an empty stomach, 1 or 2 hours before meals. Adhere to prescribed dose; higher doses may cause dangerously irregular heartbeats.

 Usual adult dose (and children 12 years and older): 10 milligrams (1 tablet) per day.

 Usual child dose: not generally prescribed for children under 12 years.

 Missed dose: take as soon as possible, unless almost time for next dose. In that case, do not take missed dose; go back to regular schedule. *Do not double doses.*

Side Effects

 Overdose symptoms: cardiac arrest, fainting, irregular heartbeat, seizures. If you suspect an overdose, immediately seek medical attention.

 More common side effects: drowsiness, dry mouth, fatigue, headache, increase in appetite, weight gain.

 Less common side effects: asthma-like symptoms, burning/prickling/tingling skin, depression, diarrhea, dizziness, fluid retention, hepatitis, inflammation of the eyelids, itching, joint pain, muscle pain, nausea, nervousness, nosebleed, palpitations, sensitivity to light, skin rash, sore throat, stomach and intestinal pain. Rare side effect: low blood pressure.

Interactions

 Do not take with erythromycin (PCE or E-Mycin) or ketoconazole (Nizoral); may cause serious heart problems. Inform your doctor before combining Hismanal with: antibiotics such as Flagyl; antifungal drugs such as Diflucan, Nizoral, Monistat, and Sporanox; drugs that affect heart rhythms such as Vascor, Elavil, and Thorazine; macrolide antibiotics such as Zithromax, Biaxin, E-Mycin, and Tao.

 Taking with food reduces effectiveness.

Special Cautions

 If pregnant or planning to become pregnant, inform your doctor immediately. Not known if Hismanal appears in breast milk.

 No special precautions apply to seniors.

 Not generally prescribed for children under 12 years.

 Inform your doctor *before* taking Hismanal if you are currently being treated for lower respiratory tract disease (asthma) or liver or kidney disease.

Should not take if allergic to Hismanal.

Hydergine

Generic name: Ergoloid mesylates

Other brand names: Gerimal, Hydergine-LC

Hydergine is a vasodilator. It dilates the blood vessels, thereby increasing blood flow to the brain.

℞ QUICK FACTS

Purpose

℞ Used to treat symptoms of age-related declining mental capacity.

Dosage

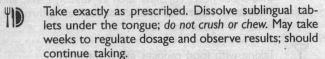 Take exactly as prescribed. Dissolve sublingual tablets under the tongue; *do not crush or chew.* May take weeks to regulate dosage and observe results; should continue taking.

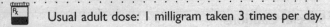 Usual adult dose: 1 milligram taken 3 times per day.

Usual child dose: not generally prescribed for children.

Missed dose: skip missed dose; go back to regular schedule. *Do not double doses.*

Side Effects

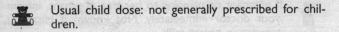 Overdose symptoms: no specific information available. If you suspect an overdose, immediately seek medical attention.

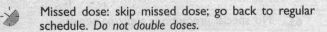 Side effects: irritation below the tongue (if taking sublingual tablets), stomach upset, temporary nausea.

No known less common or rare side effects.

Interactions

No drug interactions reported.

No known food/other substance interactions.

Special Cautions

 Not used by women of childbearing age.

. . . .

 No special precautions apply to seniors.

. . . .

 Not generally prescribed for children.

. . . .

 Do not use if allergic to or sensitive to this medication, or if you have a mental disorder.

Doctor should do a thorough analysis *before* prescribing Hydergine and then closely monitor for any changes.

Hydrochlorothiazide
see HYDRODIURIL

Hydrochlorothiazide with Triamterene
see DYAZIDE

Hydrocodone Bitartrate with Acetaminophen
see VICODIN

Hydrocodone Polistirex with Chlorpheniramine Polistirex

see TUSSIONEX

Hydrocortisone

see ANUSOL-HC

HydroDIURIL

Generic name: Hydrochlorothiazide

Other brand names: Aquazide-H, Diaqua, Esidrix, Ezide, Hydro-Chlor, Hydro-D, Hydromal, Hydro-Par, Hydro-T, Mictrin, Oretic

HydroDIURIL is a thiazide diuretic. It reduces fluid accumulation in the body.

℞ QUICK FACTS

Purpose

℞ Used to treat high blood pressure and conditions requiring elimination of excess body fluid.

Dosage

 Take exactly as prescribed. May take weeks to observe results; must continue to take even if you feel better.

Usual adult dose: *for water retention*—25 to 100 milligrams per day as a single dose or divided into smaller doses. Doctor may suggest day on/day off therapy. *For high blood pressure*—25 milligrams per day as a single dose, up to 50 milligrams as a single dose or divided into 2 doses.

 Usual child dose: 1 milligram per 1 pound of body weight divided into 2 doses per day, up to 50 milligrams per day. *Under 2 years*—Infants under 6 months may be prescribed 1.5 milligrams per 1 pound of body weight per day divided into 2 doses, up to 12.5 to 37.5 milligrams per day maximum. *2 to 12 years*—maximum of 37.5 to 100 milligrams per day divided into 2 doses.

 Missed dose: take as soon as possible, unless almost time for next dose. In that case, do not take missed dose, go back to regular schedule. *Do not double doses.*

Side Effects

 Overdose symptoms: dry mouth, electrolyte imbalance, excessive thirst, muscle pain or cramps, symptoms of low potassium such as dehydration, weak or irregular heartbeat. If you suspect an overdose, immediately seek medical attention.

 More common side effects: abdominal cramping, diarrhea, dizziness when standing up, headache, loss of appetite, low blood pressure, low potassium, stomach irritation or upset, weakness.

 Less common or rare side effects: anemia, blood disorders, changes in blood sugar, constipation, difficulty breathing, dizziness, fever, fluid in lungs, hair loss, high levels of sugar in the urine, hives, hypersensitivity reactions, impotence, inflammation of the lung, inflammation of the pancreas, inflammation of the salivary glands, kidney failure, muscle spasms, nausea, rash, reddish or purplish skin spots, skin disorders such as Stevens-Johnson (severe mouth and eye blisters), skin peeling, tingling or pins and needles, vertigo, vision changes, vomiting, yellow eyes and skin.

Interactions

 Inform your doctor before combining HydroDIURIL with: barbiturates such as phenobarbital; cholestyramine (Questran); colestipol (Colestid); corticosteroids such as Prednisone and adrenocorticotropic hormone (ACTH); diabetes medications such as insulin and Micronase; lithium; narcotics such as Percocet; nonsteroidal anti-inflammatory medications such as Naprosyn; norepinephrine (Levophed); other high blood pressure medications; skeletal muscle relaxants such as Tubocurarine.

 Alcohol may increase sedative effects; *do not drink alcohol when taking this medication.*

Special Cautions

 If pregnant or planning to become pregnant, inform your doctor immediately. Appears in breast milk; could affect a nursing infant.

 No special precautions apply to seniors.

 Follow doctor's instructions carefully for children.

 If you can't urinate, you should not take HydroDIURIL.

Should not take if sensitive to or allergic to this or similar medications, or sulfa/sulfonamide-derived medications. May be at higher risk for allergy if you have a history of allergies or bronchial asthma.

May cause potassium loss; doctor may advise adding foods rich in potassium to your diet or a potassium supplement.

Doctor should assess and monitor kidney function during HydroDIURIL therapy.

Use with caution if you have: diabetes, gout, liver disease, or lupus erythematosus.

If exercising and if in hot weather, use caution not to deplete body fluids; may result in low blood pressure.

Hydromorphone Hydrochloride

see DILAUDID

Hydroxychloroquine Sulfate

see PLAQUENIL

Hydroxyzine Hydrochloride

see ATARAX

Hygroton

ᴧᴧᴧᴧᴧᴧᴧᴧᴧᴧᴧᴧᴧᴧᴧᴧᴧᴧᴧᴧᴧᴧᴧᴧᴧᴧᴧᴧᴧᴧᴧᴧᴧᴧᴧᴧᴧ

Generic name: Chlorthalidone

Other brand name: Thalitone

Hygroton is a thiazide diuretic. It reduces fluid accumulation in the body.

℞ QUICK FACTS

Purpose

℞ Used to treat high blood pressure and conditions requiring elimination of excess body fluid.

Dosage

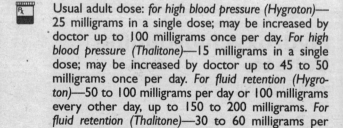

Take exactly as prescribed, with or without food. May take weeks to observe results; you must continue to take even if you feel better. Take in the morning, as it stimulates urination.

Usual adult dose: *for high blood pressure (Hygroton)*—25 milligrams in a single dose; may be increased by doctor up to 100 milligrams once per day. *For high blood pressure (Thalitone)*—15 milligrams in a single dose; may be increased by doctor up to 45 to 50 milligrams once per day. *For fluid retention (Hygroton)*—50 to 100 milligrams per day or 100 milligrams every other day, up to 150 to 200 milligrams. *For fluid retention (Thalitone)*—30 to 60 milligrams per day or 60 milligrams every other day, up to 90 to 120 milligrams.

Usual child dose: not generally recommended for children.

Missed dose: take as soon as possible, unless almost time for next dose. In that case, do not take missed

dose; go back to regular schedule. *Do not double doses.*

Side Effects

Overdose symptoms: confusion, dizziness, nausea, weakness. If you suspect an overdose, immediately seek medical attention.

Side effects: allergic reaction, anemia, changes in blood sugar, change in potassium levels, constipation, cramping, diarrhea, dizziness, dizziness when standing, flaky skin, headache, hives, impotence, inflammation of the pancreas, itching, loss of appetite, low blood pressure, muscle spasms, nausea, rash, restlessness, sensitivity to light, stomach irritation, tingling or pins and needles, vision changes, vomiting, weakness, yellow eyes and skin.

No known less common or rare side effects.

Interactions

Inform your doctor before combining Hygroton with: appetite-control medications such as Tenuate; cholestyramine (Questran); colestipol (Colestid); decongestants; digitalis (Lanoxin); insulin; lithium (Lithonate); oral diabetes medications such as Micronase; other high blood pressure medications such as Catapres and Aldomet; steroids such as prednisone.

Do not drink alcohol while taking Hygroton; increases the risk of dizziness.

Special Cautions

If pregnant or planning to become pregnant, inform your doctor immediately. May appear in breast milk; could affect a nursing infant.

 No special precautions apply to seniors.

 Not generally recommended for children.

 Do not substitute with a generic brand unless specifically directed by your doctor.

If you cannot urinate, should not take Hygroton.

Should not take if sensitive to or allergic to this or similar medications. Inform your doctor if you have kidney or liver disease, gout, or lupus. May be at higher risk for allergy if you have a history of bronchial asthma.

May cause potassium loss; doctor may advise adding foods rich in potassium to your diet or a potassium supplement.

Use caution to avoid dehydration in hot weather. If you experience the following, contact your doctor: excessive thirst, increased heart rate or pulse, muscle pains/cramps, nausea, restlessness, tiredness, or vomiting. Also, avoid long sunlight exposure.

Hyoscyamine Sulfate

see LEVSIN

Hytrin

Generic name: Terazosin hydrochloride

Hytrin is an alpha-blocker/antihypertensive. It lowers blood pressure by relaxing the muscle tissue of the blood vessels.

℞ QUICK FACTS

Purpose

 Used to treat high blood pressure. Also used to treat the symptoms of enlargement of the prostate gland.

Dosage

 Take initial dose at bedtime; *do not take more than your doctor has prescribed.* May take with or without food. May take weeks to observe results if taking for high blood pressure; must continue to take even if you feel better.

 Usual adult dose: 1 milligram at bedtime, up to 5 milligrams per day. Some are prescribed up to 20 milligrams per day. *For enlarged prostate*—1 milligram per day at bedtime, gradually increased up to 10 milligrams per day for 4 to 6 weeks. Some are prescribed 20 milligrams per day.

 Usual child dose: not generally prescribed for children.

 Missed dose: take as soon as possible, unless almost time for next dose. In that case, do not take missed dose, go back to regular schedule. *Do not double doses.*

Side Effects

Overdose symptoms: dizziness, light-headedness, shock. If you suspect an overdose, immediately seek medical attention.

More common side effects: difficult or labored breathing, dizziness, headache, heart palpitations, lightheadedness when standing, nausea, pain in arms and legs, sleepiness, stuffy nose, swollen wrists and ankles, weakness. May require higher dosage if these side effects persist.

 Less common or rare side effects: anxiety, back pain, blurred vision, bronchitis, conjunctivitis (pink eye), constipation, decreased sex drive, depression, diarrhea, dimmed vision, dry mouth, facial swelling, fainting, fever, flu or cold symptoms, fluid retention, frequent urination, gas, gout, impotence, inability to hold urine, increased heart rate, indigestion, inflamed sinuses, insomnia, irregular heartbeat, itching, joint pain and inflammation, low blood pressure, muscle aches, nasal inflammation, nervousness, nosebleed, numbness or tingling pain (in abdomen, chest, neck, or shoulder), rash, ringing in ears, severe allergic reaction, sweating, urinary tract infection, vertigo, vision changes, vomiting, weight gain.

Interactions

 Inform your doctor before combining Hytrin with: nonsteroidal anti-inflammatory painkillers such as Motrin and Naprosyn; other blood pressure medications such as Dyazide, Vasotec, Calan, and Verelan.

 No known food/other substance interactions.

Special Cautions

 If pregnant or planning to become pregnant, inform your doctor immediately. Not known whether Hytrin appears in breast milk.

 No special precautions apply to seniors.

Not generally prescribed for children.

 Do not take if sensitive to or allergic to Hytrin.

May faint due to low blood pressure when taking Hytrin.

Avoid driving and participating in potentially hazardous activities: for 12 hours after the first dose; with each new dosage increase; and when Hytrin is restarted after discontinuance.

If taking for enlarged prostate, it may continue to grow. Can experience prostate cancer with enlarged prostate.

Not generally prescribed for children.

Do not take if sensitive to or allergic to Hytrin.

May take due to low blood pressure when taking Hytrin.

Avoid driving and participating in potentially hazardous activities for 12 hours after the first dose, with each new dosage increase, and when Hytrin is restarted after discontinuance.

In taking for enlarged prostate, it may continue to slow (can experience prostate cancer with enlarged prostate).

Ibuprofen

see ADVIL

Imdur

Generic name: Isosorbide mononitrate

Other brand names: Ismo, Monoket

Imdur is an anti-anginal agent. It works by relaxing muscles of the veins and arteries.

℞ QUICK FACTS

Purpose

℞ Used to prevent angina pectoris—crushing chest pain; does not relieve already present angina attacks.

Dosage

 Take exactly as prescribed—once per day in the morning. May take with or without food, swallowed whole with half a glass of liquid. *Do not substitute brands unless specifically directed by your doctor. Do not abruptly discontinue use; consult doctor for gradual tapering off of medication. Do not change dose to relieve headache; headache stopping may be sign of Imdur losing its effectiveness.*

 Usual adult dose: 20 milligrams taken 2 times per day.

Usual child dose: not generally prescribed for children.

 Missed dose: take as soon as possible, unless almost time for next dose. In that case, do not take missed dose; go back to regular schedule. *Do not double doses.*

Side Effects

 Overdose symptoms: air hunger, bloody diarrhea, coma, confusion, difficulty breathing, fainting, fever, nausea, palpitations, paralysis, pressure in the head, profuse sweating, seizures, skin that is cold and clammy or flushed, slow heartbeat, throbbing headache, vertigo, visual disturbances, vomiting. If you suspect an overdose, immediately seek medical attention.

 Most common side effects: dizziness, headache.

 Less common or rare side effects: abdominal pain, abnormal hair texture, abnormal heart sounds, abnormal or terrifying dreams, abnormal vision, acne, anemia, anxiety, back pain, bacterial infection, black stools, breast pain, bronchitis, confusion, constipation, coughing, decrease in sex drive, depression, diarrhea, difficult or labored breathing, difficulty concentrating, diminished sense of touch, drooping eyelid, dry mouth, earache, excessive amount of urine, fatigue, fever, fluid retention and swelling, flu-like symptoms, flushing, frozen shoulder, gas, general feeling of illness, heart attack, heart failure, heart murmur, hemorrhoids, high blood pressure, hot flashes, impotence, inability to fall sleep, increased mucus from the lungs, increased sweating, indigestion, inflamed eyes, inflammation of the tongue, inflammation of the vagina, intolerance of light, irregular heartbeat, itching, joint pain, kidney stones, leg ulcer, loose stools, low blood pressure, migraine, muscle and/or bone pain, muscle weakness, nasal or sinus inflammation, nausea, nervousness, palpitations, paralysis, perforated eardrum, pneumonia, purple or red skin spots, rapid heartbeat, rash, ringing in ears, severe pain in calf muscles during walking, sleepiness, slow heartbeat, sore throat, stomach ulcer with or without bleeding, stuffy nose, tingling or pins and needles, tremor, twisted neck, urinary tract infection, vomiting, weakness, wheezing, worsening of angina pectoris, yeast infection.

Interactions

 Inform your doctor before combining Imdur with: calcium blockers such as Calan, Cardizem, and Procardia.

 Alcohol may cause swift blood pressure decrease, possibly resulting in light-headedness.

Special Cautions

 If pregnant or planning to become pregnant, inform your doctor immediately. Not known if Imdur appears in breast milk.

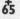 No special precautions apply to seniors.

 Not generally prescribed for children.

 Be extremely cautious if you are driving or participating in other potentially hazardous activities.

Inform your doctor of any medical conditions *before* Imdur therapy.

Use with caution; may cause severe low blood pressure.

. . . .

Should not take if allergic to this or other heart medications containing nitrates or nitrites, or if you have recently had a heart attack or congestive heart failure.

. . . .

May aggravate angina caused by other heart conditions.

Imipramine Hydrochloride

see TOFRANIL

Imitrex Injection

Generic name: Sumatriptan succinate

Imitrex is an anti-migraine. It is thought to work by slowing nerve activity in the brain.

℞ QUICK FACTS

Purpose

℞ Used to treat severe migraines. Will not prevent or reduce migraine attacks.

Dosage

 Inject just below skin as soon as migraine appears; also may be injected during an attack. *Do not use intravenously, may cause heart irregularity.*

. . . .

 Usual adult dose: single dose of 6 milligrams injected under the skin, up to 2 injections in a 24-hour period taken at least 1 hour apart. Doctor may administer first dose and monitor your reaction.

 Usual child dose: not generally prescribed for children.

 Missed dose: *do not take on a regular basis. Take only during an attack.*

Side Effects

 Overdose symptoms: bluish tinge to skin, convulsions, dilated pupils, inactivity, lack of coordination, paralysis, redness in arms and legs, skin changes at injection site, slow breathing, tremor. If you suspect an overdose, immediately seek medical attention.

 More common side effects: burning sensation, dizziness or vertigo, feeling of heaviness, feeling of tightness, flushing, mouth and tongue discomfort, muscle weakness, neck pain and stiffness, numbness, pressure sensation, redness at injection site, sore throat, tingling, warm/hot sensation.

 Less common or rare side effects: abdominal discomfort, anxiety, changes in heart rhythm, cold sensation, difficulty swallowing, drowsiness or calmness, fatigue, feeling strange, general feeling of illness, headache, jaw discomfort, muscle cramps, muscle pain or tenderness, pressure in chest, rise in blood pressure (temporary), sinus or nasal discomfort, sweating, tight feeling in head, tightness in chest, vision changes.

Interactions

 Inform your doctor before combining Imitrex Injection with: ergotamine (Cafergot); other ergot-containing medications such as Ergostat.

No known food/other substance interactions.

Special Cautions

 If pregnant or planning to become pregnant, inform your doctor immediately. May appear in breast milk; could affect a nursing infant.

 No special precautions apply to seniors.

 Not generally prescribed for children.

 If sensitive or allergic to this or similar medications, should not use.

Should not use if you have: heart disease, including angina, history of heart attack, irregular heartbeat, shortness of breath; uncontrolled blood pressure; or if taking a medication containing ergotamine.

Use with caution if you have liver or kidney disease.

Imodium

Generic name: Loperamide hydrochloride

Other brand names: Imodium A-D, Kaopectate II, Maalox Anti-Diarrheal, Pepto Diarrheal Control

Imodium is an antidiarrheal. It decreases the passing of water and other substances into the bowel and slows intestinal tract movement.

℞ QUICK FACTS

Purpose

℞ Used to treat diarrhea associated with inflammatory bowel disease, not diarrhea caused by a specific germ. Also used to reduce discharge from an ileostomy. May also be used to treat traveler's diarrhea.

Dosage

 Do not take more than prescribed. Drink plenty of fluids to avoid dehydration while you have diarrhea.

 Usual adult dose: *for severe diarrhea*—2 capsules (4 milligrams), then 1 capsule (2 milligrams) after each loose stool, up to 8 capsules (16 milligrams) per day. Should see improvement within 48 hours. *For long-lasting or frequently recurring diarrhea*—2 capsules (4 milligrams), then 1 capsule (2 milligrams) after each loose stool until diarrhea is under control. Dosage then adjusted to meet individual needs. Average maintenance dose is 2 to 4 capsules per day, up to 8 capsules. Contact your doctor if no improvement after 10 days.

 Usual child dose: *for children 2 to 5 years or 44 pounds or less*—use nonprescription Imodium A-D liquid. *For children 6 to 12 years*—use capsules (2 milligrams each) or liquid (1 milligram per teaspoon). Dosage schedule: *children 2 to 5 (28–44 pounds)*—1 milligram (1 teaspoonful of liquid) taken 3 times per day. *Children 6 to 8 (45–66 pounds)*—2 milligrams taken 2 times per day. *Children 8 to 12 years (67 pounds and over)*—2 milligrams taken 3 times per day. Not generally prescribed for children under 2 years.

Missed dose: *if taking on a regular schedule*—take as soon as possible, then take remaining doses at evenly spaced intervals. Skip dose if you do not have diarrhea.

Side Effects

 Overdose symptoms: constipation, depression, drowsiness, lethargy, nausea. If you suspect an overdose, immediately seek medical attention.

 Side effects: abdominal distention, abdominal pain or discomfort, allergic reactions including skin rash, constipation, dizziness, drowsiness, dry mouth, nausea and vomiting, tiredness.

 No known less common or rare side effects.

Interactions

 No reported drug interactions.

 No known food/other substance interactions.

Special Cautions

 If pregnant or planning to become pregnant, inform your doctor immediately. Not known if Imodium appears in breast milk.

 No special precautions apply to seniors.

 Not generally prescribed for children under 2 years. Follow doctor's instructions carefully for children 2 to 12 years. Use caution administering to young children; unpredictable responses may occur.

 Do not take if your body cannot tolerate being constipated.

May cause drowsiness and impair your ability to drive a car or operate machinery. *Do not take part in any activity that requires alertness.*

Immediately contact your doctor if diarrhea continues beyond a few days, fever develops, or you observe blood in your stools.

If sensitive or allergic to this medication, should not take.

Not to be used for acute dysentery (caused by bacteria, viruses, or parasites).

Doctor should monitor for central nervous system reactions (drowsiness, convulsions) in the case of liver disease.

Discontinue use of Imodium and contact your doctor if you experience abdominal distention, colitis, or intestinal blockage.

Indapamide

see LOZOL

Inderal

Generic name: Propranolol hydrochloride

Other brand name: Inderal LA

Inderal is a beta-adrenergic blocking agent (beta-blocker). It slows the heart rate and reduces high blood pressure.

℞ Quick Facts

Purpose

 Used to treat high blood pressure, chest pain, changes in heart rhythm, hereditary tumors, hypertrophic subaortic stenosis, and adrenal gland tumors. Also used to prevent of migraines and recurring heart attacks.

Dosage

 Take exactly as prescribed. If you miss doses, may worsen condition. Best if taken before meals. May take weeks to observe results if taking for high blood pressure; must continue to take even if you begin to feel better. Medication should not be stopped suddenly; gradually taper.

. . . .

 Usual adult dose: *for high blood pressure*—40 milligrams taken 2 times per day, increased to 120 to 240 or in some cases 640 milligrams per day for maintenance. May take days or weeks for maximum results. Doctor may prescribe taking 3 times per day. *For chest pain*—80 to 320 milligrams divided into 2, 3, or 4 smaller doses. *For irregular heartbeat*—10 to 30 milligrams taken 3 or 4 times per day before meals and at bedtime. *For heart attack*—180 to 240 milligrams divided into smaller doses. *For migraine*—80 milligrams per day divided into smaller doses; may be increased by your doctor to between 160 to 240 milligrams per day. Should see relief in 4 to 6 weeks, otherwise doctor will gradually taper you off medication. *For tremors*—40 milligrams, 2 times per day to start; may be increased up to 320 milligrams maximum per day. *For hypertrophic subaortic stenosis*—20 to 40 milligrams taken 3 to 4 times per day before meals and at bedtime. *Before adrenal gland therapy*—60 milligrams per day divided into smaller doses for 3 days prior to surgery. *For inop-*

erable tumors—30 milligrams per day divided into smaller doses. *Seniors*—dosage is according to individual needs.

 Usual child dose: individualized for each child. Doses range from 2 to 4 milligrams per 2.2 pounds of body weight daily, divided into 2 equal doses, up to 16 milligrams per 2.2 pounds of body weight per day. When discontinuing this medication, it should be tapered off over a 7 to 14 day period.

 Missed dose: take as soon as possible, unless within 8 hours of next dose. In that case, do not take missed dose; go back to regular schedule. *Do not double doses.*

Side Effects

 Overdose symptoms: extremely slow heartbeat, irregular heartbeat, low blood pressure, severe congestive heart failure, seizures, wheezing. If you suspect an overdose, immediately seek medical attention.

 Side effects: abdominal cramps, colitis, congestive heart failure, constipation, decreased sexual ability, depression, diarrhea, difficulty breathing, disorientation, dry eyes, fever with sore throat, hair loss, hallucinations, headache, light-headedness, low blood pressure, lupus erythematosus, nausea, rash, reddish or purplish skin spots, short-term memory loss, slow heartbeat, tingling, prickling in hands, tiredness, trouble sleeping, upset stomach, visual changes, vivid dreams, vomiting, weakness, worsening of certain heartbeat irregularities.

 No known less common or rare side effects.

Interactions

Inform your doctor before combining Inderal with: aluminum hydroxide gel (Amphojel); calcium blockers such as Cardizem, Procardia, and Calan; high blood pressure medications (Diupres and Ser-Ap-Es); chlorpromazine (Thorazine); cimetidine (Tagamet); epinephrine (EpiPen); haloperidol (Haldol); insulin; lidocaine (Xylocaine); nonsteroidal anti-inflammatory medications such as Motrin and Naprosyn; oral diabetes medications such as Micronase; phenobarbital; phenytoin (Dilantin); rifampin (Rifadin); theophylline (Theo-Dur); thyroid medications such as Synthroid.

No known food/other substance interactions.

Special Cautions

If pregnant or planning to become pregnant, inform your doctor immediately. Appears in breast milk, could affect a nursing infant.

Dosage for seniors is according to individual needs.

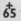

Follow doctor's instructions carefully for children.

Should not take or use with extreme caution if you have: bronchial asthma, certain types of irregular heartbeat, inadequate blood supply to the circulatory system, kidney or liver disease, severe congestive heart failure, or slow heartbeat. Doctor will decide whether to prescribe based on your condition.

May want to monitor pulse for low heartbeat; check with your doctor.

Inform your doctor if you are diabetic; medication may cover the symptoms of low blood sugar or alter blood sugar levels.

Inform your doctor or dentist prior to surgery or dental treatment.

Inderal with Hydrochlorothiazide

see INDERIDE

Inderide

Generic ingredients: Inderal (propranolol hydrochloride) with hydrochlorothiazide

Other brand name: Inderide LA

Inderide is a thiazide diuretic and beta-blocker combination. It slows the heart rate and eliminates urine, thereby reducing high blood pressure.

℞ QUICK FACTS

Purpose

℞ Used to treat high blood pressure.

Dosage

  Take exactly as prescribed. If you miss doses, may worsen condition. Best if taken before meals. May take weeks to observe results if taking for high blood pressure; must continue to take even if you

begin to feel better. Do not stop medication suddenly; gradually taper.

Usual adult dose: 1 tablet taken 2 times per day.

Usual child dose: not generally prescribed for children.

Missed dose: take as soon as possible, unless within 8 hours of next dose. In that case, do not take missed dose; go back to regular schedule. *Do not double doses.*

Side Effects

Overdose symptoms: coma, extremely slow heartbeat, heart failure, increased urination, irritation and overactivity of stomach and intestines, low blood pressure, sluggishness, stupor, wheezing. If you suspect an overdose, immediately seek medical attention.

Side effects: allergic reactions (fever, rash, aching and sore throat), anemia, blood disorders, blurred vision, constipation, congestive heart failure, cramps, decreased mental clarity, depression, diarrhea, difficulty breathing, difficulty sleeping, disorientation, dizziness, dizziness upon standing, dry eyes, emotional changeability, exhaustion, fatigue, hair loss, hallucinations, headache, high blood sugar, hives, increased skin sensitivity to sunlight, inflammation of the large intestine or the pancreas, inflammation of the salivary glands, light-headedness, loss of appetite, low blood pressure, lupus erythematosus, male impotence, muscle spasms, nausea, restlessness, short-term memory loss, slow heartbeat, stomach irritation, sugar in urine, tingling or pins and needles, upset stomach, vertigo, visual disturbances, vivid dreams, vomiting, weakness, wheezing, yellow eyes and skin.

No known less common or rare side effects.

Interactions

 Inform your doctor before combining Inderide with: ACTH (adrenocorticotropic hormone); aluminum hydroxide gel (Mylanta); calcium blockers such as Calan, Cardizem, and Procardia XL; certain blood pressure medications such as Diupres and Ser-Ap-Es; chlorpromazine (Thorazine); corticosteroids such as prednisone; digitalis (Lanoxin); epinephrine (EpiPen); haloperidol (Haldol); insulin; lidocaine (Xylocaine); nonsteroidal anti-inflammatory medications such as Motrin; norepinephrine (Levophed); oral diabetes medications such as Micronase; phenobarbital; phenytoin (Dilantin); rifampin (Rifadin); theophylline (Theo-Dur); thyroid medications such as Synthroid.

 Avoid alcohol while taking Inderide.

Special Cautions

 If pregnant or planning to become pregnant, inform your doctor immediately. Appears in breast milk; could affect a nursing infant.

 No special precautions apply to seniors.

 Not generally prescribed for children.

 Do not take if unable to urinate or sensitive to or allergic to this medication or sulfa medications.

Should not take or should use with extreme caution if you have: bronchial asthma, certain types of irregular heartbeat, inadequate blood supply to the circulatory system, kidney or liver disease, seasonal allergies or other bronchial conditions, severe congestive heart failure, or slow heartbeat. Doctor will decide whether to prescribe depending on your condition.

. . . .

Inform your doctor if you are diabetic; medication may cover the symptoms of low blood sugar or alter blood sugar levels.

. . . .

May interfere with glaucoma screening; eye pressure may increase when Inderide is stopped.

. . . .

Inform your doctor or dentist prior to surgery or dental treatment, or during a medical emergency.

. . . .

May cause potassium loss; if so, doctor will advise you to add potassium-rich foods to your diet or to take a potassium supplement.

Indocin

Generic name: Indomethacin

Other brand name: Indocin SR

Indocin is a nonsteroidal anti-inflammatory medicine. It works by blocking the production of prostaglandins, which may trigger pain.

℞ QUICK FACTS

Purpose

℞ Used to treat inflammation, swelling, stiffness, and joint pain associated with moderate to severe rheumatoid arthritis and osteoarthritis, and ankylosing spondylitis. Also used to treat bursitis, tendinitis, acute gouty arthritis, and other kinds of pain.

Dosage

Take with food or an antacid, and a full glass of water, not on an empty stomach. Take exactly as prescribed, and on a regular basis for arthritis. Shake liquid form well before using. *Do not lie down for ½ hour after taking this medication; may lead to swallowing problems.*

Usual adult dose: *for moderate to severe rheumatoid arthritis, osteoarthritis, and ankylosing spondylitis—* 25 milligrams taken 2 or 3 times per day, up to between 150 to 200 milligrams per day. Doctor may prescribe single 75-milligram dose per day of Indocin SR in place of regular Indocin. *For bursitis or tendinitis—*75 to 150 milligrams per day divided into 3 or 4 smaller doses, for 1 to 2 weeks. *For acute gouty arthritis—*50 milligrams taken 3 times per day until pain is under control, usually 3 to 5 days. *Seniors—*dosage adjusted as needed. In all cases, doctor should prescribe lowest dose effective.

Usual child dose: not generally prescribed for children under 14 years.

Missed dose: take as soon as possible, unless almost time for next dose. In that case, do not take missed dose; go back to regular schedule. *Do not double doses.*

Side Effects

Overdose symptoms: convulsions, disorientation, dizziness, intense headache, lethargy, mental confusion, nausea and vomiting, numbness, tingling or pins and needles. If you suspect an overdose, immediately seek medical attention.

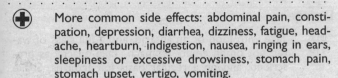

More common side effects: abdominal pain, constipation, depression, diarrhea, dizziness, fatigue, headache, heartburn, indigestion, nausea, ringing in ears, sleepiness or excessive drowsiness, stomach pain, stomach upset, vertigo, vomiting.

Less common or rare side effects: anemia, anxiety, asthma, behavior disturbances, bloating, blurred vision, breast changes, changes in heart rate, chest pain, coma, congestive heart failure, convulsions, decrease in white blood cells, fever, fluid in lungs, fluid retention, flushing, gas, hair loss, hepatitis, high or low blood pressure, hives, itching, increase in blood sugar, insomnia, kidney failure, labored breathing, light-headedness, loss of appetite, mental confusion, muscle weakness, nosebleed, peptic ulcer, problems in hearing, rash, rectal bleeding, Stevens-Johnson syndrome (skin peeling), stomach or intestinal bleeding, unusual redness of skin, vaginal bleeding, weight gain, worsening of epilepsy, yellow eyes and skin.

Interactions

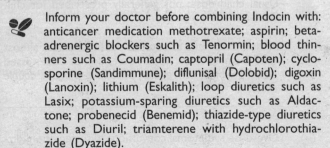

Inform your doctor before combining Indocin with: anticancer medication methotrexate; aspirin; beta-adrenergic blockers such as Tenormin; blood thinners such as Coumadin; captopril (Capoten); cyclosporine (Sandimmune); diflunisal (Dolobid); digoxin (Lanoxin); lithium (Eskalith); loop diuretics such as Lasix; potassium-sparing diuretics such as Aldactone; probenecid (Benemid); thiazide-type diuretics such as Diuril; triamterene with hydrochlorothiazide (Dyazide).

No known food/other substance interactions.

Special Cautions

 If pregnant or planning to become pregnant, inform your doctor immediately. Appears in breast milk, could affect a nursing infant.

 Dosage adjusted as needed for seniors.

 Not generally prescribed for children under 14 years.

 Do not use suppositories with current or history of rectal bleeding.

May cause drowsiness and impair your ability to drive a car or operate machinery. *Do not take part in any activity that requires alertness.*

Doctor should monitor frequently for internal bleeding or ulcers.

Should not take if sensitive to or allergic to Indocin, aspirin or similar medications, or if these medications have caused asthma attacks.

Be aware that Indocin prolongs bleeding time.

Use cautiously if you have kidney or liver disease.

May increase water retention if high blood pressure or heart disease is present.

Existing infections may be masked when taking Indocin.

Indomethacin

see INDOCIN

Insulin

Generic name: Insulin injection or suspension

Other brand names: *Regular*—Beef Regular
Iletin II, Concentrated Regular Iletin II (Pork only),
Humulin, Humulin R, Novolin R, Novolin R
PenFill, Pork Regular Iletin II, Regular Iletin I,
Regular Insulin, Regular Purified Pork Insulin,
Velosulin, Velosulin Human. *Insulin Zinc
Suspension (Lente)*—Humulin L, Lente Iletin I,
Lente Iletin II, Lente Insulin, Lente Purified Pork
Insulin, Novolin L. *Insulin Zinc Suspended,
Extended (Ultralente)*—Humulin U Ultralente,
Ultralente Iletin I, Ultralente Insulin. *Insulin Zinc
Suspension, Prompt (Semilente)*—Semilente Iletin I,
Semilente Insulin. *Isophane Insulin Suspension and
Insulin Injection*—Humulin 70/30, Mixtard,
Mixtard Human 70/30, Novolin 70/30,
Novolin 70/30 PenFill. *Isophane Insulin
Suspension (NPH)*—NPH Iletin II, Humulin N,
Insulatard NPH (Human), Insulatard NPH (Pork),
Novolin N, Novolin N PenFill, NPH Iletin I,
NPH Insulin, NPH Purified, Pork NPH Iletin II.
Protamine Zinc Insulin Suspension (PZI)—
Protamine Zinc and Iletin I (Beef and Pork),
Protamine Zinc and Iletin II (Beef), Protamine Zinc
and Iletin II (Pork)

Insulin is an antidiabetic. It is the hormone that regulates blood sugar levels.

℞ QUICK FACTS

Purpose

℞   Used to treat diabetes mellitus.

Dosage

 Take exactly as prescribed. Always carry a food product containing sugar to counter low blood sugar symptoms. Use disposable needles and syringes or sterilize reusable ones carefully. *Carefully follow dietary instructions from your doctor and take insulin as prescribed; otherwise may result in serious or fatal complications.*

 Usual adult dose: determined by individual needs.

 Usual child dose: determined by individual needs.

 Missed dose: follow doctor's instructions if you miss a dose or a meal. Keep extra insulin and syringes/needles on hand.

Side Effects

 Overdose symptoms: low blood sugar (hypoglycemia)—depressed mood, dizziness, drowsiness, fatigue, headache, hunger, inability to concentrate, irritability, nausea, nervousness, personality changes, rapid heartbeat, restlessness, sleep disturbances, slurred speech, sweating, tingling, tremor, unsteady movements. More severe symptoms—coma, disorientation, low blood pressure, pale skin, perspiration, rash over entire body, seizures, shortness of breath, shallow breathing or wheezing. If you suspect an overdose, immediately seek medical attention.

 Side effects are rare; allergic reactions or low blood sugar may occur. Mild allergic reactions—swelling, itching, or redness at injection site. More serious allergic reactions—low blood pressure, pale skin, perspiration, rash over entire body, seizures, shortness of breath, shallow breathing, wheezing. Low blood sugar symptoms: abnormal behavior; anxiety; blurred vision; depressed mood; dizziness; drowsiness; fatigue; headache; hunger; inability to concentrate; light-headedness; nausea; nervousness; personality changes; rapid heartbeat, restlessness; sleep disturbances; slurred speech; sweating; tingling in the hands, feet, lips, or tongue; tremor; unsteady movement. Severe low blood sugar symptoms—coma, disorientation. Symptoms of insufficient insulin—drowsiness, flushing, fruity breath, heavy breathing, loss of appetite, rapid pulse, thirst. *Insufficient insulin may lead to loss of consciousness or death.*

 No known less common or rare side effects.

Interactions

 Inform your doctor before combining insulin with: anabolic steroids; appetite suppressants such as Tenuate; aspirin in large doses; beta-blockers such as Tenormin and Lopressor; diuretics such as Lasix, Dyazide, and HydroDIURIL; epinephrine (EpiPen); estrogens (Premarin); MAO inhibitors (Nardil or Parnate); nicotine products such as Nicoderm, Habitrol; phenytoin (Dilantin); steroid medications such as prednisone; thyroid medications (Synthroid or Proloid); triamterene (Dyrenium).

 Do not drink alcohol unless your doctor approves use.

Special Cautions

 If pregnant or planning to become pregnant, inform your doctor immediately. Insulin therapy is safe for pregnant mothers, although managing the diabetes is more difficult. Does not appear in breast milk. Strictly adhere to dietary and prescribing instructions.

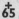 No special precautions apply to seniors.

Follow doctor's instructions carefully for children.

 Only on the instructions of your doctor should you change the Insulin type or brand of syringe or needle.

Wear ID stating you are diabetic and whether or not you are Insulin dependent.

Immediately inform your doctor if you experience nausea and vomiting; doctor should perform a urine test. You should continuously monitor your glucose levels with home blood and urine testing. Immediately contact your doctor if you have above normal sugar levels with the blood test or sugar in the urine.

Intal

∿∿∿∿∿∿∿∿∿∿∿∿∿∿∿∿∿∿∿∿∿∿∿∿∿∿∿∿∿∿∿∿∿∿∿∿∿

Generic name: Cromolyn sodium

Other brand names: Gastrocrom Capsules, Nasalcrom, Opticrom 4%

Intal is an anti-allergenic and anti-asthmatic. It prevents the release of the chemicals in the body that cause the symptoms of allergies and asthma.

℞ QUICK FACTS

Purpose

℞ Used to treat bronchial asthma, prevent asthma attacks, and prevent and treat seasonal and chronic allergies.

Dosage

 Take exactly as prescribed. May take several weeks to observe full effect. Use Spinhaler turbo-inhaler for caplets; should not be swallowed. If you accidentally inhale powder from the capsules, rinse your mouth or drink water before and after using the Spinhaler. Replace Spinhaler and metered spray device every 6 months. Use power-operated nebulizer with face mask, not hand-operated nebulizers. *Do not suddenly stop capsules or nasal solution without consulting your doctor.*

 Usual adult dose: *capsules and inhalation solution—bronchial asthma*—20 milligrams (1 capsule or ampule) inhaled 4 times per day. Must take regularly. Use only when an attack is controlled and you can properly inhale. *Acute asthma attack following exercise or exposure to cold, dry air or environmental irritants*—1 capsule or ampule inhaled no more than 1 hour prior to exposure to irritant. May repeat inhalation during extended exposure. *Aerosol spray—Bronchial asthma*—2 metered sprays taken 4 times per day. Use only when an attack is controlled and you can properly inhale. *Acute asthma attack prevention*—2 metered sprays before exposure to irritant. *Nasalcrom Nasal Solution—Allergy prevention and treatment*—1 spray per nostril 3 to 4 times per day, up to 6 times per day as prescribed by your doctor.

 Usual child dose: *capsules and inhalation solution*—same as adult dose for children 2 years and over. *Aerosol spray*—same as adult dose for children 5 years and over. *Nasalcrom Nasal Solution*—same as adult dose for children 6 years and over.

Missed dose: take as soon as possible; then take remaining doses at equally spaced intervals. *Do not double doses.*

Side Effects

 Overdose symptoms: difficulty breathing, heart failure, low blood pressure, slow heartbeat. If you suspect an overdose, immediately seek medical attention.

 More common side effects: cough, nasal congestion or irritation, nausea, sneezing, throat irritation, wheezing.

 Less common or rare side effects: angioedema (swelling of face around lips, tongue, and throat; swollen arms and legs; difficulty swallowing); bad taste in mouth; dizziness; ear problems; headache; hives; joint swelling and pain; nosebleed; painful urination or frequent urination; postnasal drip; rash; severe allergic reaction; swollen glands; swollen throat; teary eyes; tightness in throat.

Interactions

 Inform your doctor before combining Intal with any prescription or nonprescription medications you are currently taking.

 No known food/other substance interactions.

Special Cautions

 If pregnant or planning to become pregnant, inform your doctor immediately. Not known if Intal appears in breast milk.

 No special precautions apply to seniors.

Follow doctor's instructions carefully for children.

 If sensitive to or allergic to this or similar medications or lactose, should not take.

If dose is reduced or stopped, asthma symptoms may reappear. Intal does not work once an acute asthma attack has begun. Obtain medical help if you experience a severe attack.

Doctor may reduce or discontinue medication if you have liver or kidney problems.

Ipratropium Bromide

see ATROVENT

Isometheptene Mucate with Dichloralphenazone and Acetaminophen

see MIDRIN

Isordil

Generic name: Isosorbide dinitrate

Other brand names: Dilatrate-SR, Iso-Bid, Isordil Sublingual, Isordil Tembids, Isordil Titradose, Sorbitrate, Sorbitrate SA

Isordil is an anti-anginal agent. It works by relaxing muscles of the veins and arteries.

℞ Quick Facts

Purpose

 Used to treat or prevent angina pectoris (crushing chest pain).

Dosage

 Take capsules and tablets on an empty stomach. May crush tablets, *not* sustained release products. When stopping medication, gradually taper off according to doctor's instructions. *If taking sublingual tablet—when it is dissolving, do not eat, drink, smoke, or use tobacco.*

 Usual adult dose: *sublingual (treatment of angina pectoris)*—2.5 to 5 milligrams. *Sublingual (prevention of angina pectoris attack)*—5 or 10 milligrams taken every 2 to 3 hours. *For prevention of chronic stable angina pectoris (immediately released Isordil)*—5 to 20 milligrams, up to 10 to 40 milligrams taken every 6 hours. *For prevention of chronic stable angina pectoris (controlled-release Isordil)*—40 milligrams, up to 80 milligrams taken every 8 to 12 hours.

 Usual child dose: not generally prescribed for children.

 Missed dose: take as soon as possible, unless within 2 hours of next dose, or 6 hours of next dose for controlled-release tablets and capsules. In that case, do not take missed dose; go back to regular schedule. *Do not double doses.*

Side Effects

☠ *Severe overdose can be fatal.* Overdose symptoms: bloody diarrhea, coma, confusion, convulsions, fainting, fever, flushed and perspiring skin followed by cold and blue skin, nausea, palpitations, paralysis, rapid decrease in blood pressure, rapid then difficult and slow breathing, slow pulse, throbbing headache, vertigo, visual disturbances, vomiting. If you suspect an overdose, immediately seek medical attention.

 Most common side effect: headache. Other common side effects: dizziness, low blood pressure, weakness.

 Less common or rare side effects: collapse, fainting, flushed skin, nausea, pallor, perspiration, rash, restlessness, skin inflammation and flaking, vomiting.

Interactions

 Inform your doctor before combining Isordil with other high blood pressure medications such as Cardizem and Procardia.

 Alcohol use may immediately decrease blood pressure, thereby causing dizziness and fainting.

Special Cautions

 If pregnant or planning to become pregnant, inform your doctor immediately. Not known if Isordil appears in breast milk.

 No special precautions apply to seniors.

 Not generally prescribed for children.

 Can cause severe low blood pressure, especially if standing up or sitting quickly. Use with caution if you are taking diuretics, or if you have: anemia, glaucoma, heart disease, low blood pressure, previous head injury or heart attack, or thyroid disease.

. . . .
If allergic to this medication or other nitrates or nitrites, should not take.
. . . .
Inform your doctor if you notice this medication is
losing its effectiveness.

Isosorbide Dinitrate
see ISORDIL

Isosorbide Mononitrate
see IMDUR

Isotretinoin
see ACCUTANE

Isradipine
see DYNACIRC

Itraconazole
see SPORANOX

J

Janimine
see TOFRANIL

Keflex

Generic name: Cephalexin hydrochloride

Other brand names: Keflet, Keftab

Keflex is a cephalosporin antibiotic. It prevents bacteria from multiplying and growing.

℞ QUICK FACTS

Purpose

℞ Used to treat bacterial infections of the respiratory tract including: middle ear, bone, skin, and the reproductive and urinary systems.

Dosage

 May take with or without meals. Take at evenly spaced intervals, per your doctor's instructions. Finish all of the medication even if symptoms subside. Tablets are for adults only. *Do not use with other people or for other infections without advice from your doctor.*

 Usual adult dose: *for throat, skin, and urinary tract infections*—500 milligrams taken every 12 hours. Bladder infection therapy is for 7 to 14 days. *For other infections*—250 milligrams taken every 6 hours.

 Usual child dose: *only capsules and oral suspension are prescribed for children, not tablets.* 25 to 50 milligrams per each 2.2 pounds of body weight per day, divided into smaller doses. *For strep throat in children over 1*

year and for skin infections—2 doses taken every 12 hours. Should take for 10 days in the case of strep throat. *For middle ear infection*—75 to 100 milligrams per each 2.2 pounds of body weight per day, divided into smaller doses.

Missed dose: take as soon as possible. *If taking 2 times per day*—take next dose in 5 to 6 hours. *If taking 3 or more times per day*—take next dose 2 to 4 hours later. Then go back to regular schedule.

Side Effects

Overdose symptoms: blood in urine, diarrhea, nausea, upper abdominal pain, vomiting. If you suspect an overdose, immediately seek medical attention.

Most common side effect: diarrhea.

Less common or rare side effects: abdominal pain, agitation, colitis, confusion, dizziness, fatigue, fever, genital and rectal itching, hallucinations, headache, hepatitis, hives, indigestion, inflammation of joints, inflammation of stomach, joint pain, nausea, rash, seizures, severe allergic reaction, skin peeling, skin redness, swelling due to fluid retention, vaginal discharge, vaginal inflammation, vomiting, yellow skin and eyes.

Interactions

Inform your doctor before combining Keflex with: diarrhea medications such as Lomotil, oral contraceptives.

No known food/other substance interactions.

Special Cautions

 If pregnant or planning to become pregnant, inform your doctor immediately. Appears in breast milk; could affect a nursing infant.

 No special precautions apply to seniors.

 Follow doctor's instructions carefully for children.

 May cause false results in tests for sugar in the urine. Inform your doctor that you are taking Keflex. *Do not alter your diet or dosage of diabetes medications without instructions from your doctor.*

Inform your doctor *before* Keflex therapy if allergic to penicillin or cephalosporin antibiotics in any form, or if you have any drug allergies. *Allergic reaction can be extremely severe.*

Tell your doctor *before* starting the medication if you have a history of stomach or intestinal disease, especially colitis; or kidney disorder.

Consult with your doctor *before* using diarrhea medications; some interact with Keflex.

If used on a long-term basis, may cause a secondary infection not treatable with Keflex.

Inform your doctor if symptoms do not improve within a few days or get worse.

Ketoconazole
see NIZORAL

Ketoprofen
see ORUDIS

Ketorolac Tromethamine
see TORADOL

Klonopin
∧∧

Generic name: Clonazepam

Klonopin is a benzodiazepine anticonvulsant. It selectively reduces overstimulation in the brain.

℞ QUICK FACTS

Purpose

℞ Used to treat epilepsy and other convulsive disorders.

Dosage

 Take exactly as prescribed; is important to keep a constant amount in the bloodstream for maximum effectiveness. Consult with your doctor *before* discontinuing or changing doses.

 Usual adult dose: 1.5 milligrams per day divided into 3 doses. Doctor may increase in increments of 0.5 to 1 milligram every 3 days until seizures are controlled, or side effects increase. Maximum dose is 20 milligrams per day.

 Usual child dose (for children 10 years and older and up to 66 pounds): 0.01 to 0.03 milligram per

2.2 pounds of body weight per day, up to 0.05 milligram per 2.2 pounds of body weight. Doctor may increase in increments of 0.25 to 0.5 milligram every 3 days until seizures are controlled or side effects increase. If doses cannot be divided into 3 equal doses, take largest dose at bedtime. *Maintenance dose—0.1 to 0.2 milligram per 2.2 pounds of body weight per day.*

 Missed dose: *if within 1 hour after missed time*—take as soon as possible. Otherwise, do not take missed dose; go back to regular schedule. *Do not double doses.*

Side Effects

 Overdose symptoms: coma, confusion, sleepiness, slowed reaction time. If you suspect an overdose, immediately seek medical attention.

 More common side effects: behavior problems, drowsiness, lack of muscular coordination.

 Less common or rare side effects: abnormal eye movements, anemia, bedwetting, chest congestion, coated tongue, coma, confusion, constipation, dehydration, depression, diarrhea, double vision, dry mouth, excess hair, fever, fluttery or throbbing heartbeat, "glassy-eyed" appearance, hair loss, headache, hallucinations, inability to fall or stay asleep, inability to urinate, increased sex drive, involuntary rapid movement of the eyeballs, loss of or increased appetite, loss of voice, memory loss, muscle and bone pain, muscle weakness, nausea, nighttime urination, painful or difficult urination, partial paralysis, runny nose, shortness of breath, skin rash, slowed breathing, slurred speech, sore gums, speech difficulties, stomach inflammation, swelling of ankles and face, tremor, uncontrolled body movement or twitching, vertigo, weight loss or gain. Side effects from rapid decrease or abrupt discontinuance of Klonopin: abdominal and muscle cramps, behavior disorders, convulsions, depressed feeling, hallucinations, restlessness, sleeping difficulties, tremors.

Interactions

Inform your doctor before combining Klonopin with: anti-anxiety medications (Valium); antidepressants such as Elavil, Nardil, Parnate, and Tofranil; barbiturates such as phenobarbital; major tranquilizers such as Haldol, Navane, and Thorazine; narcotics such as Demerol and Percocet; other anticonvulsants such as Dilantin, Depakene, and Depakote; sedatives (Halcion).

Do not drink alcohol while taking Klonopin; central nervous system is slowed by alcohol and the side effects of Klonopin may be intensified.

Special Cautions

If pregnant or planning to become pregnant, inform your doctor immediately. Appears in breast milk; could affect a nursing infant.

No special precautions apply to seniors.

Follow doctor's instructions carefully for children.

May cause drowsiness and impair your ability to drive a car or operate machinery. *Do not take part in any activity that requires alertness.*

If sensitive to or allergic to this or similar medications such as Librium and Valium, should not take.

If you have glaucoma or severe liver disease, should not take.

. . . .
Monitor for dependency; can be habit-forming. May also build a tolerance, losing effectiveness of medication.
. . . .
If prior to Klonopin therapy you experience seizures, this medication may increase possibility of grand mal seizures.

L

Labetalol Hydrochloride

see NORMODYNE

Lactulose

see CHRONULAC SYRUP

Lanacort

see ANUSOL-HC

Lanoxin

Generic name: Digoxin

Other brand name: Lanoxicaps

Lanoxin is a cardiac glycoside. It strengthens the heartbeat and improves the rhythm and contraction of the heart by working on the heart muscle.

℞ QUICK FACTS

Purpose

℞   Used to treat congestive heart failure, irregular heartbeat, and other heart problems.

Dosage

Take at the same time each day and on an empty stomach. Avoid high-bran/high-fiber foods. If using liquid form, use dropper that comes with the prescription. Medication should not be stopped unless your doctor advises you. Abrupt discontinuance may cause serious heart problems. Most patients taking Lanoxin do so for an extended period of time or for the rest of their lives. *Do not switch brands unless directed by your doctor.*

Usual adult dose: 0.125 milligram or 0.25 milligram tablet one time per day. Exact dose is based on your individual needs.

Usual child dose: *Infants and young children*—daily dose is divided into smaller doses. *Children ages 10 and over*—prescribed adult doses in proportion to body weight.

Missed dose: take as soon as possible, if within 12 hours of scheduled dose. Otherwise, do not take missed dose; go back to regular schedule. If you miss doses for 2 or more days, consult your doctor. *Do not double doses.*

Side Effects

Overdose symptoms: abdominal pain, diarrhea, irregular heartbeat, loss of appetite, nausea, very slow pulse, vomiting. If you suspect an overdose, immediately seek medical attention.

Side effects: apathy, blurred vision, breast development in males, change in heartbeat, diarrhea, dizziness, headache, loss of appetite, lower stomach pain, nausea, psychosis, rash, vomiting, weakness, yellow vision.

No known less common or rare side effects.

Interactions

 Inform your doctor before combining Lanoxin with: airway-opening medications such as Proventil and Ventolin; alprazolam (Xanax); amiloride (Midamor); amiodarone (Cordarone); antacids such as Maalox and Mylanta; anti-arrhythmic medications (Quinidex); antibiotics such as neomycin and tetracycline; beta-blockers such as Tenormin and Inderal; calcium (injectable); calcium blockers such as Calan SR, Cardizem, Procardia; certain anticancer medications (Neosar); cholestyramine (Questran); colestipol (Colestid); cyclosporine (Sandimmune); diphenoxylate (Lomotil); disopyramide (Norpace); diuretics (Lasix); indomethacin (Indocin); itraconazole (Sporanox); kaolin-pectin; metoclopramide (Reglan); propafenone (Rythmol); propantheline (Pro-Banthine); rifampin (Rifadin); steroids such as Decadron and Deltasone; succinylcholine (Anectine); sucralfate (Carafate); sulfasalazine (Azulfidine); thyroid hormones (Synthroid).

Unless directed by your doctor; avoid over-the-counter medications such as antacids; laxatives; cough, cold, and allergy medications; and diet products.

Special Cautions

 If pregnant or planning to become pregnant, inform your doctor immediately. Appears in breast milk; could affect a nursing infant.

 No special precautions apply to seniors.

 Follow doctor's instructions carefully for children.

Monitor pulse rate while taking Lanoxin. Effective dosage level is close to level that causes serious overdose problems.

. . . .

If sensitive to or allergic to this or other digitalis preparations, should not take.

. . . .

Should not be used if you have ventricular fibrillation, or for weight reduction; *may cause irregular heartbeat or death.*

. . . .

Notify your doctor that you are taking this medication in the event of a medical emergency, surgery, or dental treatment.

Lasix

Generic name: Furosemide

Other brand name: SK-Furosemide

Lasix is a loop diuretic. It increases the elimination of sodium and water through the kidneys.

℞ QUICK FACTS

Purpose

 Used to treat high blood pressure and other conditions requiring elimination of excess fluid, including congestive heart failure, cirrhosis of the liver, and kidney disease.

Dosage

 Take exactly as prescribed—on a regular basis for maximum effectiveness. May take several weeks to observe the full effects. Continue taking even if symptoms subside.

 Usual adult dose: *For fluid retention*—single dose of 20 to 80 milligrams, which may be repeated in 6 to 8 hours. Doctor may raise dose by 20 or 40 milligrams 6 to 8 hours after each successive dose. Maximum daily dose is 600 milligrams. *For high blood pressure*—80 milligrams per day divided into 2 doses. *Seniors*—dose determined by individual needs.

 Usual child dose: 2 milligrams per 2.2 pounds of body weight. Doctor may raise dose by 1 to 2 milligrams per 2.2 pounds. Doses are 6 to 8 hours apart, not to exceed 6 milligrams per 2.2 pounds.

 Missed dose: take as soon as possible, unless almost time for next dose. In that case, do not take missed dose; go back to regular schedule. *Do not double doses.*

Side Effects

 Overdose symptoms: dehydration, dry mouth, excessive thirst, low blood pressure, muscle pain or cramps, weak or irregular heartbeat. If you suspect an overdose, immediately seek medical attention.

 Side effects: anemia, blood disorders, blurred vision, constipation, cramping, diarrhea, dizziness, dizziness upon standing, fever, headache, hearing loss, high blood sugar, hives, itching, loss of appetite, low potassium, muscle spasms, nausea, rash, reddish or purplish skin spots, restlessness, ringing in ears, sensitivity to light, skin eruptions, skin inflammation and flaking, stomach or mouth irritation, tingling or pins and needles, vertigo, vision changes, vomiting, weakness, yellow eyes and skin.

No known less common or rare side effects.

Interactions

 Inform your doctor before combining Lasix with: aminoglycoside antibiotics such as Garamycin; aspirin; barbiturates such as phenobarbital; ethacrynic acid (Edecrin); indomethacin (Indocin); lithium (Lithonate); muscle relaxants such as Tubocurarine; narcotics such as Darvon and Percocet; nonsteroidal anti-inflammatory medications such as Advil and Naprosyn; norepinephrine (Levophed); other high blood pressure medications such as Vasotec and Aldomet; skeletal muscle relaxants such as succinylcholine (Anectine); sucralfate (Carafate).

 No known food/other substance interactions.

Special Cautions

 If pregnant or planning to become pregnant, inform your doctor immediately. Appears in breast milk; could affect a nursing infant.

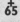 For seniors, dose determined by individual needs.

 Follow doctor's instructions carefully for children.

 If sensitive to or allergic to this or other diuretics, or if unable to urinate, should not take.

May cause potassium loss; symptoms include muscle weakness and rapid or irregular heartbeat. Doctor may prescribe potassium supplements or eating potassium-rich foods such as bananas, prunes, raisins, orange juice, and whole and skim milk.

. . . .

Inform your doctor and use Lasix with caution if you have: diabetes, gout, kidney disease, liver disease, or lupus erythematosus.

. . . .

Allergies to sulfa drugs may indicate allergy to Lasix.

. . . .

Avoid nonprescription medications such as cold remedies and appetite suppressants if you have high blood pressure.

. . . .

May experience sensitivity to sunlight.

Lescol

Generic name: Fluvastatin sodium

Lescol is an antihyperlipidemic. It interferes with the enzyme that synthesizes cholesterol, thereby decreasing the low-density lipoprotein (LDL) in the blood.

℞ QUICK FACTS

Purpose

 Used to lower cholesterol levels.

Dosage

 Take at bedtime, either with or without food. Adhere to diet and exercise program; Lescol supplements these measures.

. . . .

 Usual adult dose: 20 milligrams per day taken in one dose at bedtime, up to 40 milligrams per day as a single dose. Doctor may alter initial dosage after 4 weeks. If taking with other cholesterol medications, take the other medications at least 2 hours prior to taking Lescol.

 Usual child dose: not prescribed for children under 18 years.

 Missed dose: take as soon as possible, unless almost time for next dose. In that case, do not take missed dose, go back to regular schedule. *Do not double doses.*

Side Effects

 Overdose symptoms: no specific information available. If you suspect an overdose, immediately seek medical attention.

 More common side effects: abdominal pain, accidental injury, back pain, diarrhea, fatigue, flu-like symptoms, headache, indigestion, joint disease, muscle pain, nasal inflammation, nausea, sore throat, upper respiratory infection.

 Less common side effects: allergy, bronchitis, constipation, coughing, dizziness, dental problems, gas, inflamed sinuses, insomnia, rash.

Interactions

 Inform your doctor before combining Lescol with: cholestyramine (Questran); cimetidine (Tagamet); clofibrate (Atromid-S); cyclosporine (Sandimmune); digoxin (Lanoxin); erythromycin (E-Mycin or E.E.S.); gemfibrozil (Lopid); ketoconazole (Nizoral); omeprazole (Prilosec); ranitidine (Zantac); rifampin (Rifadin); spironolactone (Aldactone or Aldactazide).

 No known food/other substance interactions.

Special Cautions

 Do not take if pregnant or nursing. Lescol lowers cholesterol needed by a developing baby, and it appears in breast milk.

 No special precautions apply to seniors.

 Not prescribed for children under 18 years.

 Lescol therapy usually starts after doctor structures a cholesterol-lowering diet.

Avoid if you have liver problems or are/have been a heavy drinker.

Should not take if sensitive to or allergic to Lescol.

Doctor may order test to check liver enzyme levels *prior* to taking medication; there is some risk for liver damage with Lescol. Monitoring will continue once Lescol therapy begins.

Inform your doctor if you experience: unexplained muscle pain, tenderness, weakness, fever, or if you feel sick at the start of taking this medication; may be signs of muscle tissue damage.

If factors increasing risk of muscle and/or kidney damage appear, doctor may temporarily discontinue this medication.

Inform your doctor of any medical conditions present *before* starting medication.

Levobunolol Hydrochloride
see BETAGAN

Levodopa with Carbidopa

see SINEMET CR

Levothroid

see SYNTHROID

Levothyroxine

see SYNTHROID

Levsin

Generic name: Hyoscyamine sulfate

Other brand names: Anaspaz, Cystospaz, Cystospaz-M, Neoquess

Levsin is an antispasmodic. It slows the action of the bowel and production of stomach acid, thereby relaxing the muscles and relieving spasms.

℞ QUICK FACTS

Purpose

℞   Used to treat stomach, intestinal, and urinary tract disorders involving cramps, colic, or other painful muscle contractions. Also used before anesthesia to dry excess secretions or a runny nose. Also used to: control excess secretions and reduce pain in the case of pancreas inflammation; reduce muscle rigidity and tremors and control drooling and excess sweating in the case of Parkinson's disease; and as preparation for certain diagnostic X-rays.

Dosage

Sublingual tablets may be dissolved under the tongue, chewed, or swallowed. Regular tablets can be dissolved under tongue or swallowed.

Usual adult dose (and children 12 years and older): *Levsin/SL and Levsin Tablets*—1 to 2 tablets every 4 hours as needed; swallow or place under tongue; tablets may be chewed. *Do not take more than 12 tablets in 24 hours. Levsin Elixir*—1 to 2 teaspoonfuls every 4 hours as needed, not to exceed 12 teaspoonfuls in 24 hours. *Levsin Drops*—1 to 2 milliliters every 4 hours as needed, not to exceed 12 milliliters in 24 hours. *Levsinex Timecaps*—1 to 2 Timecaps every 12 hours; doctor may adjust to 1 Timecap every 8 hours. *Do not exceed more than 4 Timecaps in 24 hours.*

Usual child dose (children 2 to 12 years): *Levsin/SL and Levsin Tablets*—½ to 1 tablet every 4 hours as needed; *do not exceed 6 tablets in 24 hours. Levsin Elixir*—¼ to 1 teaspoonful every 4 hours as needed; *do not exceed more than 6 teaspoonfuls in 24 hours. Levsin Drops*—¼ to 1 milliliter every 4 hours as needed; *do not exceed more than 6 milliliters in 24 hours.* Children under 2 years—dosage determined by body weight. *Levsinex Timecaps*—1 Timecap every 12 hours; *do not exceed more than 2 Timecaps in 24 hours.*

Missed dose: take as soon as possible, unless almost time for next dose. In that case, do not take missed dose; go back to regular schedule. *Do not double doses.*

Side Effects

Overdose symptoms: blurred vision, central nervous system stimulation, dilated pupils, dizziness, dry mouth, headache, hot and/or dry skin, nausea, swallowing difficulty, vomiting. If you suspect an overdose, immediately seek medical attention.

Side effects: allergic reactions, bloating, blurred vision, confusion, constipation, decreased sweating, dilated pupils, dizziness, drowsiness, dry mouth, excitement, headache, hives, impotence, inability to urinate, insomnia, itching, heart palpitations, lack of coordination, loss of sense of taste, nausea, nervousness, rapid heartbeat, skin reactions, speech problems, vomiting, weakness.

No known less common or rare side effects.

Interactions

Inform your doctor before combining Levsin with: amantadine (Symmetrel); antidepressants such as Elavil, Nardil, Parnate, and Tofranil; antihistamines such as Benadryl; major tranquilizers such as Thorazine and Haldol; other antispasmodics such as Bentyl; potassium supplements such as Slow-K.

Avoid taking simultaneously with antacids; take Levsin 1 hour before or 2 hours after a meal.

Special Cautions

If pregnant or planning to become pregnant, inform your doctor immediately. Not known if Levsin appears in breast milk.

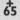

No special precautions apply to seniors.

Follow doctor's instructions carefully for children.

 Do not take if sensitive to or allergic to Levsin.

May cause dizziness, drowsiness, blurred vision, or impair your ability to drive a car or operate machinery. *Do not take part in any activity that requires alertness.*

Doctor should not prescribe this medication if you have: bowel or digestive tract obstruction or paralysis, diarrhea (especially if with an ileostomy or colostomy), glaucoma, myasthenia gravis, severe bowel inflammation, or urinary obstruction.

Avoid high temperatures such as sauna, very hot baths, or being outside on hot days; may be at risk for heatstroke when taking Levsin.

Use with caution if you have: congestive heart failure, heart disease, high blood pressure, irregular heartbeats, kidney disease, or overactive thyroid.

May experience: agitation, an exaggerated sense of well-being, coma, confusion, decreased anxiety, difficulty speaking, disorientation, fatigue, hallucinations, lack of coordination, short-term memory loss, sleeplessness—which should disappear 12 to 48 hours after you stop taking Levsin.

Librax

Generic ingredients: Chlordiazepoxide hydrochloride with clidinium bromide

Other brand names: Clindex, Clinoxide, Clipoxide, Lidox

Librax is a benzodiazepine anti-anxiety and anticholinergic. It slows gastrointestinal tract action by reducing stomach acid production, and it relieves anxiety by depressing the central nervous system.

℞ QUICK FACTS

Purpose

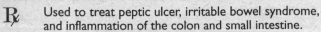

℞ Used to treat peptic ulcer, irritable bowel syndrome, and inflammation of the colon and small intestine.

Dosage

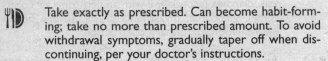

Take exactly as prescribed. Can become habit-forming; take no more than prescribed amount. To avoid withdrawal symptoms, gradually taper off when discontinuing, per your doctor's instructions.

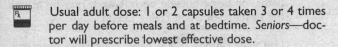

Usual adult dose: 1 or 2 capsules taken 3 or 4 times per day before meals and at bedtime. *Seniors*—doctor will prescribe lowest effective dose.

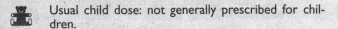

Usual child dose: not generally prescribed for children.

Missed dose: take as soon as possible, unless almost time for next dose. In that case, do not take missed dose; go back to regular schedule. *Do not double doses.*

Side Effects

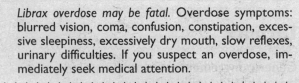

Librax overdose may be fatal. Overdose symptoms: blurred vision, coma, confusion, constipation, excessive sleepiness, excessively dry mouth, slow reflexes, urinary difficulties. If you suspect an overdose, immediately seek medical attention.

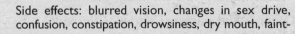

Side effects: blurred vision, changes in sex drive, confusion, constipation, drowsiness, dry mouth, fainting, lack of coordination, liver problems, minor menstrual irregularities, nausea, skin eruptions, swelling due to fluid retention, urinary difficulties, yellowing of skin and eyes.

 No known less common or rare side effects.

Interactions

 Inform your doctor before combining Librax with: antidepressants such as Nardil and Parnate; blood thinners such as Coumadin; diarrhea medications such as Donnagel and Kaopectate; ketoconazole (Nizoral); major tranquilizers such as Stelazine and Thorazine; potassium supplements such as Micro-K. Benadryl and Valium taken with Librax may cause excessive drowsiness or other potentially dangerous side effects.

 Alcohol may cause excessive drowsiness or other potentially dangerous side effects.

Special Cautions

 If pregnant or planning to become pregnant, inform your doctor immediately. Increased risk of birth defects if taken during the first trimester of pregnancy.

 Doctor will prescribe lowest effective dose for seniors to reduce side effects such as confusion, excessive drowsiness, and uncoordinated movements.

 Not generally prescribed for children.

 May cause drowsiness and impair your ability to drive a car or operate machinery. *Do not take part in any activity that requires alertness.*

Should not take if you have: bladder obstruction, enlarged prostate, glaucoma, or if sensitive to or allergic to this medication or any of its ingredients.

Use with extreme caution if you have had drug or alcohol abuse problems.

Doctor may test blood and liver functions if taking Librax for an extended period.

Librium

Generic name: Chlordiazepoxide

Other brand names: Libritabs, Lipoxide, Mitran

Librium is a benzodiazepine sedative. It relieves anxiety by depressing the central nervous system.

℞ QUICK FACTS

Purpose

℞ Used to treat anxiety disorders. Also used to provide short-term relief for symptoms of anxiety, alcohol withdrawal in the case of alcoholism, and apprehension prior to surgery.

Dosage

Take exactly as prescribed. Never increase dose; can be habit-forming and cause dependence. To avoid withdrawal symptoms, gradually taper off when discontinuing, per your doctor's instructions.

 Usual adult dose: *For mild or moderate anxiety*—5 or 10 milligrams taken 3 or 4 times per day. *For severe anxiety*—20 to 25 milligrams taken 3 or 4 times per day. *For apprehension prior to surgery*—5 to 10 milligrams taken 3 or 4 times per day for days preceding surgery. *For alcohol withdrawal*—50 to 100 milligrams orally, repeated up to a maximum of 300 milligrams per day until anxiety is controlled. Dose then reduced to smallest possible level. *Seniors*—5 milligrams taken 2 to 4 times per day.

 Usual child dose (for children 6 years and older): 5 milligrams taken 2 to 4 times per day. Not recommended for children under 6 years.

 Missed dose: take as soon as possible, unless within an hour of next dose. In that case, do not take missed dose; go back to regular schedule. *Do not double doses.*

Side Effects

 Overdose symptoms: coma, confusion, slow reflexes, sleepiness. If you suspect an overdose, immediately seek medical attention.

 Side effects: confusion, constipation, drowsiness, fainting, increased or decreased sex drive, liver problems, lack of muscle coordination, minor menstrual irregularities, nausea, skin rash or eruptions, swelling due to fluid retention, yellow eyes and skin. Side effects due to abrupt decrease or withdrawal: abdominal and muscle cramps, convulsions, exaggerated feeling of depression, sleeplessness, sweating, tremors, vomiting.

 No known less common or rare side effects.

Interactions

 Inform your doctor before combining Librium with: antacids such as Maalox and Mylanta, antidepressants such as Nardil and Parnate, barbiturates such as phenobarbital, blood thinners such as Coumadin, cimetidine (Tagamet), disulfiram (Antabuse), levodopa (Laradopa), major tranquilizers such as Stelazine and Thorazine, narcotic pain relievers such as Demerol and Percocet, oral contraceptives.

Do not drink alcohol when taking Librium; may intensify effects of alcohol.

Special Cautions

Do not take Librium if pregnant or planning to become pregnant. Increased risk of birth defects. May appear in breast milk.

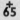

Seniors are prescribed reduced doses.

Follow doctor's instructions carefully for children. May decrease alertness. Notify your doctor if you observe contrary reactions such as excitement, stimulation, or acute rage. Not prescribed for children under 6 years.

May cause drowsiness and impair your ability to drive a car or operate machinery. *Do not take part in any activity that requires alertness.*

Inform your doctor before starting Librium if you are severely depressed or have a history of severe depression, or if you have porphyria or liver or kidney disease.

If sensitive to or allergic to this or similar tranquilizers, should not take.

Librium is not to be used for everyday stress, tension, or anxiety.

Lidex

~~~~~~

Generic name: Fluocinonide

Other brand names: FAPG, Lidex-E Cream, Fluonex Cream

Lidex is an adrenocorticosteroid hormone. It interferes with the natural body mechanisms that produce rash, itching, or inflammation.

℞ QUICK FACTS

Purpose

 Used to treat inflammatory and itchy symptoms of skin disorders.

Dosage

 Use only on the skin; keep out of eyes. Bandage treated areas only under the direction of your doctor. *Do not use more than or longer than prescribed dose.*

 Usual adult dose: apply thin film to affected areas 2 to 4 times per day.

 Usual child dose: apply smallest effective dose.

 Missed dose: apply as soon as possible, unless almost time for next dose. In that case, do not apply missed dose, go back to regular schedule.

Side Effects

Overdose symptoms (of steroid medications): abnormal sugar levels in urine; excessive blood sugar levels; symptoms of Cushing's syndrome (easily bruised skin, increased blood pressure, mood swings, water retention, weak muscles, weight gain).

Lidex absorbed in large amounts can temporarily affect the adrenal, hypothalamic, and pituitary glands. If you suspect an overdose, immediately seek medical attention.

Side effects: acne-like eruptions, burning, dryness, excessive hair growth, infection of skin, irritation, itching, lack of skin color, prickly heat, skin inflammation from contact with watch band, skin loss, stretch marks.

No known less common or rare side effects.

Interactions

No drug interactions reported.

No known food/other substance interactions.

Special Cautions

If pregnant or planning to become pregnant, inform your doctor immediately. Pregnant women should not use large amounts for prolonged periods of time. Steroids do appear in breast milk.

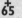

No special precautions apply to seniors.

Follow doctor's instructions carefully for children. Should not use plastic pants or diapers if Lidex is applied to diaper area. Children may absorb greater amount of this medication and experience such effects as: bulges on the head, delayed weight gain, headache, slow growth.

Should not use if allergic to Lidex.

Doctor will stop Lidex therapy and prescribe another treatment if irritation develops.

Long-term treatment can cause skin to waste away in the short term, on the face and areas of the body that bend.

Lisinopril

see ZESTRIL

Lisinopril with Hydrochlorothiazide

see ZESTORETIC

Lithium Carbonate

see LITHONATE

Lithonate

Generic name: Lithium carbonate

Other brand names: Cibalith-S (lithium citrate), Eskalith Capsules, Eskalith-CR, Lithane, Lithobid, Lithotabs

Lithium is an antimanic and antipsychotic. It calms certain parts of the brain while allowing the rest of the brain to function properly.

℞ QUICK FACTS

Purpose

℞ Used to treat the manic episodes of manic depression, including: aggressiveness, elation, fast or urgent talking, frenetic physical activity, grandiose or unrealistic ideas, hostility, little need for sleep, poor judgment. Continued at lower dosage to prevent or reduce intensity of future manic episodes. Also used to treat premenstrual tension, eating disorders such as bulimia, certain movement disorders, and sexual addictions.

Dosage

 Take after meals or with food or milk to avoid stomach irritation. Drink 10 to 12 glasses of water or fluid per day, eat a balanced diet which includes some salt. If taking Cibalith-S, dilute with fruit juice or other flavored beverages; use measuring spoon provided by pharmacist. Long-acting forms should be swallowed whole; do not chew, crush, or break. *Do not change brands unless directed by your doctor.*

 Usual adult dose: *for acute episodes*—total of 1,800 milligrams per day. Immediate-release forms taken in 3 or 4 doses; long-acting forms taken in 2 doses per day. Syrup dose—2 teaspoons taken 3 times per day. Doctor will monitor blood levels when Lithonate is first prescribed and then regularly thereafter. *For long-term control*—total of between 900 to 1,200 milligrams per day. Immediate-release forms taken in 3 or 4 doses per day; long-acting forms taken in 2 doses per day. Syrup dose—1 teaspoon taken 3 or 4 times per day. Blood levels should be checked every 2 months. *Seniors*—usually prescribed lower doses.

Usual child dose: not prescribed for children under 12 years.

 Missed dose: take as soon as possible, unless within 2 hours of next dose (6 hours for controlled-release). In that case, do not take missed dose; go back to regular schedule. *Do not double doses.*

Side Effects

 Overdose symptoms: diarrhea, drowsiness, lack of coordination, vomiting, weakness. Stop taking medication if you observe any of these symptoms—harmful levels and treatment levels are close. If you suspect an overdose, immediately seek medical attention.

 Side effects: blackout spells, blurred vision, coma, confusion, dehydration, diarrhea, dizziness, drowsiness, drying, thinning hair, dry mouth, dry skin, fatigue, general discomfort, giddiness, goiter (enlarged thyroid gland), grimace, hair loss, headache, inability to hold urine or feces, involuntary eyeball movement, irregular heartbeat, itching, jerky movements, lack of coordination, lack of sensation in skin, large amounts of urine, lethargy, little or no urine, loss of appetite, low blood pressure, metallic taste, mild thirst, nausea, restlessness, ringing in ears, seizures, skin ulcers, sleepiness, slight hand tremor, slow reactions, slurred speech, stupor, swollen ankles or wrists, temporary blind spot in eye, tendency to sleep, tremor, twitching, vertigo, vomiting, weakness, weight gain, weight loss, worsening of psoriasis.

 No known less common or rare side effects.

Interactions

 Inform your doctor before combining Lithonate with: ACE inhibitors such as Capoten and Vasotec; acetazolamide (Diamox); amphetamines such as Dexedrine; anti-inflammatory medications such as Indocin and Feldene; bicarbonate of soda; caffeine (No-Doz); calcium blockers such as Calan and Cardizem; carbamazepine (Tegretol); diuretics such as Lasix or HydroDIURIL; fluoxetine (Prozac); iodine-containing preparations such as potassium iodine (Quadrinal); major tranquilizers such as Haldol and Thorazine; methyldopa (Aldomet); metronidazole (Flagyl); tetracyclines such as Achromycin V; theophylline (Theo-Dur or Quibron). Lithonate can intensify certain anesthesia medications; inform your surgeon and anesthesiologist that you are taking Lithonate before surgery.

🍸 No known food/other substance interactions.

Special Cautions

 If pregnant or planning to become pregnant, inform your doctor immediately. May cause birth defects; not recommended for use during pregnancy. Does appear in breast milk and can harm a nursing infant.

 Seniors are usually prescribed lower doses.

 Not prescribed in children under 12 years.

 Do not take if sensitive to or allergic to Lithonate.

 May cause drowsiness and impair your ability to drive a car or operate machinery. *Do not take part in any activity that requires alertness.*

Use extra care if you are in hot weather, and avoid activities that cause you to sweat profusely. Avoid drinking large amounts of coffee, tea, or cola, which can promote dehydration through increased urination. *Do not change eating habits dramatically or go on a weight loss diet without consulting your doctor; loss of water and salt may lead to lithium poisoning.*

To establish appropriate dosage level, doctor will do frequent blood tests. Too low a dosage has no effect; too high a dosage can cause poisoning. Ongoing monitoring of any new symptoms should be immediately reported to your doctor.

Doctor may reduce or temporarily discontinue Lithonate if you develop an infection with a fever.

Use with extra caution if you have heart or kidney disease, are weak, run-down, or dehydrated.

Inform your doctor if you have: diabetes, epilepsy, thyroid problems, Parkinson's disease, or difficulty urinating.

Lithotabs

see LITHONATE

Lodine

Generic name: Etodolac

Lodine is a nonsteroidal anti-inflammatory. It works by blocking the production of prostaglandins, which may trigger pain.

℞ QUICK FACTS

Purpose

 Used to treat the inflammation, swelling, stiffness, and joint pain associated with acute and long-term treatment of osteoarthritis.

Dosage

 Take with food or an antacid and a full glass of water, not on an empty stomach. Follow doctor's instructions carefully. Should take on a regular basis for arthritis.

 Usual adult dose: *For general pain relief*—200 to 400 milligrams every 6 to 8 hours as needed; *do not exceed 1,200 milligrams per day.* Individuals weighing less than 132 pounds are prescribed a maximum of 20 milligrams per 2.2 pounds. *For osteoarthritis*—800 to 1,200 milligrams per day divided in smaller doses initially, then 600 to 1,200 milligrams per day divided in 2 or 3 doses per day. Individuals weighing less than 132 pounds are prescribed a maximum of 20 milligrams per 2.2 pounds. Doctor will prescribe lowest effective dose.

 Usual child dose: not generally prescribed for children.

 Missed dose: take as soon as possible, unless within an hour of next dose. In that case, do not take missed dose; go back to regular schedule. *Do not double doses.*

Side Effects

 Overdose symptoms: drowsiness, lethargy, nausea, stomach pain, vomiting. If you suspect an overdose, immediately seek medical attention.

More common side effects: abdominal pain, black stools, blurred vision, chills, constipation, depression, diarrhea, dizziness, fever, gas, increased frequency of urination, indigestion, itching, nausea, nervousness, rash, ringing in ears, painful or difficult urination, vomiting, weakness.

 Less common or rare side effects: abdominal bleeding, abnormal intolerance of light, anemia, asthma, blood disorders, congestive heart failure, dry mouth, fainting, flushing, hepatitis, high blood pressure, high blood sugar in some diabetics, hives, inability to sleep, inflammation of mouth, kidney problems including kidney failure, loss of appetite, peptic ulcer, rapid heartbeat, rash, skin disorders including increased pigmentation, sleepiness, Stevens-Johnson syndrome (peeling skin), sweating, swelling (fluid retention), thirst, visual disturbances, yellowed skin and eyes.

Interactions

 Do not take aspirin or other anti-inflammatory medications during Lodine therapy. Inform your doctor before combining Lodine with: blood thinners such as Coumadin, cyclosporine (Sandimmune), diuretics such as HydroDIURIL, digoxin (Lanoxin), lithium (Lithobid), methotrexate, phenylbutazone (Butazolidin).

 No known food/other substance interactions.

Special Cautions

 If pregnant or planning to become pregnant, inform your doctor immediately. Appears in breast milk; could affect a nursing infant.

 No special precautions apply to seniors.

Not generally prescribed for children.

 Lodine increases risk for sudden ulcers and internal bleeding; doctor should provide ongoing check-ups.

If sensitive to or allergic to this medication, aspirin, or similar medications, should not take. If you have experienced asthma attacks from aspirin or similar medications, should not take.

Use with caution if you have kidney or liver disease (can cause liver inflammation), or heart disease or high blood pressure (may increase water retention).

Doctor will monitor for anemia if taking Lodine for an extended period.

Lomefloxacin Hydrochloride

see MAXAQUIN

Lomotil

Generic ingredients: Diphenoxylate hydrochloride with atropine sulfate

Other brand names: Lofene, Logen Tablets, Lomanate Liquid, Lonox Tablets, Low-Quel

Lomotil is an antidiarrheal. It slows the movement of the gastrointestinal tract.

℞ QUICK FACTS

Purpose

Used to treat diarrhea.

Dosage

Take exactly as prescribed as this medication can be habit-forming. Drink plenty of liquids and eat bland food such as cooked cereals, breads, and crackers.

Usual adult dose: 2 tablets 4 times per day or 2 regular teaspoonfuls (10 milliliters) of liquid 4 times per day. Doctor may reduce dose to 5 milligrams (2 tablets or 10 milliliters of liquid) once diarrhea is controlled. Should see improvement after 48 hours. If no improvement after taking 20 milligrams daily for 10 days, Lomotil is unlikely to be effective.

Usual child dose (for children 2 to 13 years): 0.3 to 0.4 milligram per 2.2 pounds of body weight divided into 4 equal doses per day. Use Lomotil liquid *only* and use pharmacist-supplied dropper. Approximate initial doses: *2 years (24–31 pounds)*—1.5 to 3.0 milliliters 4 times per day; *3 years (26–35 pounds)*—2.0 to 3.0 milliliters 4 times per day; *4 years (31–44 pounds)*—2.0 to 3.0 milliliters 4 times per day; *5 years (35–51 pounds)*—2.5 to 4.5 milliliters 4 times per day; *6 to 8 years (38–71 pounds)*—2.5 to 5.0 milliliters 4 times per day; *9 to 12 years (51–121 pounds)*—3.5 to 5.0 milliliters 4 times per day. Doctor may reduce dose as soon as diarrhea is controlled. If symptoms do not improve within 48 hours, Lomotil is unlikely to be effective. Not generally prescribed for children under 2 years.

Missed dose: take as soon as possible, unless within an hour of next dose. In that case, do not take missed dose; go back to regular schedule. *Do not double doses.*

Side Effects

Lomotil overdose can be fatal. Overdose symptoms: coma, dry skin and mucous membranes, enlarged pupils of the eyes, extremely high body temperature, flushing, involuntary eyeball movement, lower-than-normal muscle tone, pinpoint pupils, rapid heartbeat, restlessness, sluggishness, suppressed breathing (which may happen 30 hours after an overdose). If you suspect an overdose, immediately seek medical attention.

Side effects: abdominal discomfort, confusion, depression, difficulty urinating, dizziness, dry mouth and skin, exaggerated feeling of elation, fever, flushing, general feeling of not being well, headache, hives, intestinal blockage, itching, loss of appetite, nausea, numbness of arms and legs, rapid heartbeat, restlessness, sedation/drowsiness, severe allergic reaction, sluggishness, swelling due to fluid retention, swollen gums, vomiting.

No known less common or rare side effects.

Interactions

Inform your doctor before combining Lomotil with: barbiturates such as phenobarbital, MAO inhibitors such as Nardil and Parnate, tranquilizers such as Valium and Xanax.

Avoid alcohol when taking Lomotil; may intensify the effects of alcohol.

Special Cautions

 If pregnant or planning to become pregnant, inform your doctor immediately. Appears in breast milk; could affect a nursing infant.

 No special precautions apply to seniors.

 Follow doctor's instructions carefully for children. Use with caution as side effects may appear with prescribed dosage levels—especially in the case of Down's syndrome. Not generally prescribed for children under 2 years.

 Do not take if you have obstructive jaundice, diarrhea associated with inflammation of the intestines, or an infection with enterotoxin-producing bacteria unless directed by your doctor.

May cause drowsiness and impair your ability to drive a car or operate machinery. *Do not take part in any activity that requires alertness.*

Use very cautiously if you have kidney or liver disease, or if your liver is not properly functioning.

Diarrhea caused by antibiotics can be worsened if you use Lomotil; consult with your doctor before using Lomotil with antibiotics.

Should not take if sensitive to or allergic to any of the ingredients of Lomotil.

May slow digestion and build up fluid in the intestine, contributing to dehydration and imbalance in body salts.

Inform your doctor if you experience an enlarged abdomen, which may be preceded by inflammation of the intestines.

Loniten

Generic name: Minoxidil, oral

Loniten in its oral form is an antihypertensive. It lowers blood pressure by dilating blood vessels throughout the body.

℞ QUICK FACTS

Purpose

℞ Used to treat high blood pressure.

Dosage

 May take with food, water, or milk, or on an empty stomach. Take at the same time each day. Do not suddenly stop taking Loniten unless directed by your doctor; may worsen blood pressure.

 Usual adult dose: initially—5 milligrams per day, which doctor may increase to 40 milligrams, not to exceed 100 milligrams per day. Usually combined with a diuretic and a beta-blocker. For people on dialysis—lower doses may be prescribed.

 Usual child dose: for children 12 years and older—same as adult dose. For children under 12 years—0.1 milligram per 1 pound of body weight. Doctor may increase up to 0.5 milligram per 1 pound of body weight, not to exceed 50 milligrams per day total.

Missed dose: take as soon as possible, unless almost time for next dose. In that case, do not take missed dose; go back to regular schedule. *Do not double doses.*

Side Effects

 Overdose symptoms: chest pain; difficulty breathing; dizziness; elevated pulse; fainting; headache; severe indigestion; skin flushing; unusual swelling of arms, legs, face, or stomach. If you suspect an overdose, immediately seek medical attention.

 More common side effects: abnormal hair growth, bronchitis, changes in heart rhythm, darkening of skin, difficult or painful urination, fatigue, flushing, nausea, rapid weight gain, unusual bleeding or bruising, vomiting, water and sodium retention.

 No known less common or rare side effects.

Interactions

 Inform your doctor before combining Loniten with: guanethidine (Ismelin); oral contraceptives; over-the-counter cough, cold, asthma, sinus, or diet medications.

 No known food/other substance interactions.

Special Cautions

 May cause birth defects. If pregnant or planning to become pregnant, inform your doctor immediately. May appear in breast milk; could affect a nursing infant.

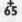 Seniors should use caution when taking Loniten in oral form.

Follow doctor's instructions carefully for children.

 Inform your doctor before starting Loniten if you have or recently had: angina (crushing chest pain), heart attack, congestive heart failure, kidney disease, stroke.

Doctor should monitor blood pressure and levels of sodium and water retention.

Should not take if sensitive to or allergic to Loniten or if you have pheochromocytoma (rare tumor which creates extra body stimulants).

Loperamide Hydrochloride

see IMODIUM

Lopid

Generic name: Gemfibrozil

Lopid is an antihyperlipidemic (lipid-lowering medication). It is thought to work by reducing the body's production of certain fats.

℞ QUICK FACTS

Purpose

 Used to treat high levels of fatty substances in the blood in people at risk for inflammation of the pancreas, who do not respond to a strict diet. Is prescribed along with a special diet. Also used to reduce risk of coronary heart disease where diet, exercise, and other medications have failed.

Dosage

 Take exactly as prescribed. Strictly adhere to diet and exercise plan developed by your doctor.

 Usual adult dose: 1,200 milligrams divided into 2 doses—30 minutes before morning and evening meals. *Seniors*—use with caution.

 Usual child dose: not generally prescribed for children.

 Missed dose: if within 4 hours of next dose, do not take missed dose; go back to regular schedule. *Do not double doses.*

Side Effects

 Overdose symptoms: no reported cases of overdose. However, if you suspect an overdose, immediately seek medical attention.

 More common side effects: abdominal pain, acute appendicitis, constipation, diarrhea, eczema, fatigue, headache, indigestion, nausea/vomiting, rash, vertigo.

 Less common or rare side effects: anemia, blood disorders, blurred vision, confusion, convulsions, decreased male fertility, decreased sex drive, depression, dizziness, fainting, hives, impotence, inflammation of colon, irregular heartbeat, itching, joint pain, laryngeal swelling, muscle disease, muscle pain, muscle weakness, painful extremities, sleepiness, tingling sensation, weight loss, yellow eyes and skin.

Interactions

 Inform your doctor before combining Lopid with: blood thinners such as Coumadin, colestipol (Colestid), glyburide (Micronase), lovastatin (Mevacor), pravastatin (Pravachol).

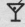 Doctor may advise you to stop drinking alcohol during Lopid therapy, as it may lead to high levels of fats in the body.

Special Cautions

 If pregnant or planning to become pregnant, inform your doctor immediately. May appear in breast milk; could affect a nursing infant.

 Seniors should use with caution.

 Not generally prescribed for children.

 Slight risk of developing: malignancy, gallbladder disease, abdominal pain leading to appendectomy, *or other serious or fatal abdominal disorders; should not be used if you have mildly elevated cholesterol levels.*

Do not take if you are taking medication for severe kidney or liver disorders or gallbladder disease, unless directed by your doctor.

Inform your doctor *before* Lopid therapy if you are being treated for diseases that increase blood cholesterol, including: overactive thyroid, diabetes, kidney and blood vessel disorder, excess protein in the blood, or obstructive liver disease.

Lopid is a supplement to other weight loss measures, not a substitute.

If sensitive to or allergic to this or similar medications, should not take.

Doctor may advise you to lose weight before start-ing Lopid therapy as excess weight may lead to un-usually high levels of fats in the body.

Doctor should monitor blood levels during first year of Lopid therapy due to risk of blood diseases. Will also periodically test your liver function due to risk of liver disorders with Lopid.

If cholesterol is not lowered in first 3 months of Lopid therapy, doctor will discontinue medication.

May increase risk for myositis, muscle inflammation. Inform your doctor if you experience muscle pain, tenderness, or weakness.

Lopressor

Generic name: Metoprolol tartrate

Other brand name: Toprol XL

Lopressor is a beta-blocker. It slows the heart rate and reduces high blood pressure.

℞ QUICK FACTS

Purpose

℞ Used to treat high blood pressure, angina pectoris (crushing chest pain), and heart attack. Also occa-sionally used to treat aggressive behavior, prevent migraines, and relieve temporary anxiety.

Dosage

Take with food or immediately after a meal. Con-tinue to take, even if symptoms subside; must take regularly for this medication to be effective. *Do not abruptly stop this medication; follow doctor's instructions for gradual reduction.*

 Usual adult dose: *For hypertension*—total of 100 milligrams per day taken in 1 or 2 doses, up to 400 milligrams per day. *For angina pectoris*—total of 100 milligrams per day taken in 2 doses, up to 400 milligrams per day. *For heart attack*—dosage determined for each individual.

 Usual child dose: not generally prescribed for children.

 Missed dose: if within 4 hours of next dose, do not take missed dose, go back to regular schedule. *Do not double doses.*

Side Effects

 Overdose symptoms: asthma-like symptoms, heart failure, low blood pressure, slow heartbeat. If you suspect an overdose, immediately seek medical attention.

 More common side effects: depression, diarrhea, dizziness, itching, rash, shortness of breath, slow heartbeat, tiredness.

 Less common or rare side effects: blurred vision, cold hands and feet, confusion, congestive heart failure, constipation, difficult or labored breathing, dry eyes, dry mouth, gas, hair loss, headache, heart attack, heartburn, low blood pressure, muscle pain, nausea, nightmares, rapid heartbeat, ringing in the ears, short-term memory loss, stomach pain, swelling due to fluid retention, trouble sleeping, wheezing, worsening of heart irregularities.

Interactions

Inform your doctor before combining Lopressor with: certain high blood pressure medications such as reserpine (Ser-Ap-Es). Other medications that might interact with Lopressor include: albuterol (Proventil or Ventolin); amiodarone (Cordarone); barbiturates such as phenobarbital; calcium channel blockers such as Calan and Cardizem; cimetidine (Tagamet); ciprofloxacin (Cipro); clonidine (Catapres); epinephrine (EpiPen); hydralazine (Apresoline); Insulin; nonsteroidal anti-inflammatory medications such as Motrin and Indocin; oral diabetes medications such as Glucotrol and Micronase; prazosin (Minipress); quinidine (Quinaglute); ranitidine (Zantac); rifampin (Rifadin).

No known food/other substance interactions.

Special Cautions

If pregnant or planning to become pregnant, inform your doctor immediately. Appears in breast milk; could affect a nursing infant.

No special precautions apply to seniors.

Not generally prescribed for children.

May cause drowsiness and impair your ability to drive a car or operate machinery. *Do not take part in any activity that requires alertness.*

Should not take Lopressor if you have: slow heartbeat, certain heart irregularities, low blood pressure, inadequate output from the heart, or heart failure.

Use with caution if you have: asthma, congestive heart failure, other bronchial conditions, or liver disease.

Ask your doctor if it is necessary to monitor your pulse during Lopressor therapy.

Inform your doctor if you are diabetic; Lopressor may mask low blood sugar symptoms.

Contact your doctor if you have difficulty breathing.

Inform your doctor or dentist that you are on Lopressor therapy during a medical emergency, or before you have surgery or dental treatment.

Loprox

Generic name: Ciclopirox olamine

Loprox is an antifungal. It destroys and prevents the growth of fungi.

℞ QUICK FACTS

Purpose

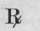

Used to treat fungal skin infections including: athlete's foot; jock itch; fungal infection of non-hairy parts of the skin; candidiasis (yeast fungal infection of the skin, nails, mouth, vagina, and lungs); tinea versicolor (skin infection with brown or tan patches on the trunk).

Dosage

 Use entire prescription even if symptoms subside. Notify your doctor if symptoms have not improved after 4 weeks. Shake lotion well before each use. Never use airtight coverings on the affected areas. For external use only, *do not use in the eyes.*

 Usual adult dose: apply lotion or cream to affected area and surrounding skin 2 times per day, in the morning and night. Should see improvement after one week.

 Usual child dose: not generally prescribed for children under 10 years.

 Missed dose: apply as soon as possible, unless almost time for next dose. In that case, do not apply missed dose; go back to regular schedule.

Side Effects

 Overdose symptoms: no specific information available. However, if you suspect an overdose, immediately seek medical attention.

 More common side effects: rarely causes side effects.

 Rare side effects: burning, itching, redness, worsening of infection symptoms.

Interactions

 No drug interactions reported.

 No known food/other substance interactions.

Special Cautions

 If pregnant or planning to become pregnant, inform your doctor immediately. Not known if Loprox appears in breast milk.

 No special precautions apply to seniors.

 Not generally prescribed for children under 10 years.

 If you experience irritation in the affected area, contact your doctor.

If sensitive to or allergic to this or similar medications, should not use.

Lopurin

see ZYLOPRIM

Lorabid

Generic name: Loracarbef

Lorabid is a cephalosporin antibiotic. It interferes with the production of certain biochemicals necessary for bacteria to sustain life.

℞ QUICK FACTS

Purpose

 Used to treat mild to moderate bacterial infections of the lungs, ears, throat, sinuses, skin, urinary tract, and kidneys.

Dosage

 Take 1 hour prior to eating or 2 hours after. *Do not stop medication even if symptoms subside; symptoms may return if you do not finish prescription.* Important to keep a constant level of Lorabid in your system.

 Usual adult dose (for adults and children 13 years and older): *For bronchitis*—200 to 400 milligrams every 12 hours for 7 days. *For pneumonia*—400 milligrams every 12 hours for 14 days. *For sinusitis*—400 milligrams every 12 hours for 10 days. *For skin and soft tissue infections*—200 milligrams every 12 hours for 7 days. *For strep throat and tonsillitis*—200 milligrams every 12 hours for 10 days. *For bladder infections*—200 milligrams every 24 hours for 7 days. *For kidney infections*—400 milligrams every 12 hours for 14 days.

 Usual child dose (for children under 13 years): *For middle ear infection*—30 milligrams of liquid per 2.2 pounds of body weight per day divided into 2 doses for 10 days. Use suspension, *do not use pulvules. For strep throat and tonsillitis*—15 milligrams per 2.2 pounds of body weight per day divided into 2 doses for at least 10 days. *For impetigo*—15 milligrams per 2.2 pounds of body weight per day divided into 2 doses for at least 10 days.

 Missed dose: take as soon as possible, unless almost time for next dose. In that case, do not take missed dose; go back to regular schedule. *Do not double doses.*

Side Effects

 Overdose symptoms: diarrhea, nausea, stomach upset, vomiting. If you suspect an overdose, immediately seek medical attention.

More common side effects *in children:* diarrhea; inflamed, runny nose; vomiting. More common side effects *in adults:* diarrhea, headache.

 Less common or rare side effects *in children:* headache, loss of appetite, rash, sleepiness. Less common side effects *in adults:* abdominal pain, nausea, rhinitis, skin rashes, vaginitis, vomiting, yeast infection. Rare side effects *in adults:* blood disorders, dizziness, hives, insomnia, itching, loss of appetite, nervousness, red bumps on skin, sleepiness, vasodilation (blood vessel expanding). Side effects for other drugs of this class: allergic reactions (sometimes severe); anemia; blood disorders; hemorrhage; kidney problems; serum sickness (fever, skin rash, joint pain, swollen lymph nodes); skin peeling.

Interactions

 Inform your doctor before combining Lorabid with: diuretics such as Lasix and Bumex, probenecid (Benemid).

 No known food/other substance interactions.

Special Cautions

 If pregnant or planning to become pregnant, inform your doctor immediately. Not known if Lorabid appears in breast milk.

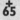 No special precautions apply to seniors.

 Follow doctor's instructions carefully for children.

 Immediately notify your doctor if you develop diarrhea; Lorabid can inflame the bowel, which may be mild *or life-threatening. Do not take diarrhea medications unless directed by your doctor.*

May develop secondary infection from prolonged use. *Do not use leftover Lorabid for any later infections.*

Inform your doctor if sensitive to or allergic to this medication, penicillin, cephalosporins, or any other medication; you are at risk for a severe reaction.

Doctor should perform blood tests to check your urine and kidney function before and during Lorabid therapy.

Loracarbef
see LORABID

Loratadine
see CLARITIN

Lorazepam
see ATIVAN

Lorelco

Generic name: Probucol

Lorelco is an antihyperlipidemic (lipid-lowering medication). It is thought to work by reducing the body's production of certain fats.

℞ QUICK FACTS

Purpose

 Used to lower cholesterol levels in people with primary hypercholesterolemia. May reduce both low-density lipoprotein (LDL or "bad cholesterol") and high-density lipoprotein (HDL or "good cholesterol").

Dosage

 Take with meals, exactly as prescribed. Strictly adhere to diet and exercise plan developed by your doctor; Lopid is a supplement to other weight loss measures, not a substitute.

 Usual adult dose: 1,000 milligrams per day divided into 2 doses taken in the morning and at night. *Seniors*—should use with caution.

 Usual child dose: not generally prescribed for children.

 Missed dose: take as soon as possible, unless almost time for next dose. In that case, do not take missed dose; go back to regular schedule. *Do not double doses.*

Side Effects

 Overdose symptoms: diarrhea, nausea, stomach upset, vomiting. If you suspect an overdose, immediately seek medical attention.

 Side effects at the onset of treatment: brief loss of consciousness or fainting, chest pain, dizziness, nausea, rapid or strong heartbeat, vomiting. Side effects during treatment: abdominal pain, blurred vision, bruising, diarrhea, diminished sense of taste and smell, dizziness, excessive nighttime urination, excessive perspiration, fainting, gas, headache, impotence, inability to fall or stay asleep, indigestion, inflammation of the eyelid, irregular heartbeat, itching, loss of appetite, nausea, rash, ringing in the ears, stomach or intestinal bleeding, swelling due to fluid retention, tearing, tingling sensation, vomiting.

 No known less common or rare side effects.

Interactions

 Inform your doctor before combining Lorelco with: certain antidepressants such as Elavil and Norpramin, Clofibrate (Atromid-S), major tranquilizers such as Mellaril and Thorazine, medications for irregular heartbeat such as Norpace and Quinidex.

 No known food/other substance interactions.

Special Cautions

 If pregnant or planning to become pregnant, inform your doctor immediately. May appear in breast milk; could affect a nursing infant. Doctors advise women taking Lorelco to delay pregnancy for 6 months after discontinuing Lorelco therapy.

 Seniors should use with caution.

 Not generally prescribed for children.

 Do not take if you have: recent heart damage, progressive heart disease, serious abnormal heart rhythm, or unexplained fainting spells or other dangerous conditions, unless directed by your doctor.

Inform your doctor *before* Lorelco therapy if you are being treated for diseases that increase blood cholesterol, including: overactive thyroid, diabetes, kidney and blood vessel disorder, or obstructive liver disease.

. . . .

If cholesterol is not lowered in first 3 months of Lorelco therapy, doctor will discontinue medication.

. . . .

If sensitive to or allergic to this or similar medications, should not take.

Lortab

see VICODIN

Lotensin

Generic name: Benazepril hydrochloride

Lotensin is an angiotensin-converting enzyme (ACE) inhibitor. It works to reduce blood pressure by preventing angiotensin I from converting into a more potent enzyme that increases salt and water retention.

℞ QUICK FACTS

Purpose

Used to treat high blood pressure.

Dosage

Take with or without food; *do not use salt substitutes that contain potassium.* Adhere to prescription schedule; abrupt discontinuance can increase blood pressure. Must take regularly for Lotensin to be effective.

. . . .

Usual adult dose: *If not using a diuretic*—10 milligrams one time per day, initially. Ongoing dose—20 to 40 milligrams per day taken in a single dose or divided into 2 equal doses, up to 80 milligrams per day maximum. *If using a diuretic*—5 milligrams per day. If patient can tolerate not taking diuretic, should be stopped 2 to 3 days before starting Lotensin therapy. *For reduced kidney function*—5 milligrams per day, up to 40 milligrams per day maximum. If using kidney dialysis, doctor may prescribe a different medication. *Seniors*—should use with caution.

 Usual child dose: not generally prescribed for children.

 Missed dose: take as soon as possible, unless almost time for next dose. In that case, do not take missed dose; go back to regular schedule. *Do not double doses.*

Side Effects

 Overdose symptom: sudden drop in blood pressure. If you suspect an overdose, immediately seek medical attention.

 More common side effects: cough, dizziness, fatigue, headache, high potassium levels, nausea. *Immediately contact your doctor if you experience: swelling of the face around the lips, tongue, or throat; swelling of arms and legs; sore throat; fever and chills; or difficulty swallowing; may be an emergency situation.*

 Less common or rare side effects: allergic reactions; anxiety; arthritis; asthma; bronchitis; chest pain; constipation; dark tarry stool with blood; decreased sex drive; difficulty sleeping; dizziness upon standing; fainting; fluid retention; flushing; impotence; infection; inflammation of the skin; inflammation of the stomach; itching; joint pain; low blood pressure; muscle pain; nervousness; pounding heartbeat; rash; sensitivity to light; shortness of breath; sinus inflammation; sweating; swelling of arms, legs, face; tingling or pins and needles; urinary infection; vomiting; weakness.

Interactions

 Inform your doctor before combining Lotensin with: diuretics such as Dyazide and Lasix, lithium (Lithonate), potassium supplements such as Slow-K, potassium-sparing diuretics such as Moduretic.

 No known food/other substance interactions.

Special Cautions

 If taken during 2nd and 3rd trimesters can cause death to developing babies and newborns. If pregnant or planning to become pregnant, inform your doctor immediately. Small amounts appear in breast milk; could affect a nursing infant.

 Seniors should use with caution.

 Not generally prescribed for children.

 Do not take if sensitive to or allergic to this or other ACE *inhibitors.*

Immediately contact your doctor if you experience sore throat or fever.

Doctor should assess kidney function prior to and during Lotensin therapy; may prescribe different medication if you are on kidney dialysis.

If you feel light-headed or faint in first few days, may be due to low blood pressure. Immediately contact your doctor.

Use with caution if you have congestive heart failure.

Be aware that excessive sweating, dehydration, severe diarrhea, or vomiting can deplete your body's fluids and cause low blood pressure.

Lotrisone

Generic ingredients: Clotrimazole with betamethasone dipropionate

Lotrisone is a steroid and antifungal combination. It destroys and prevents the growth of fungi and it interferes with the natural body mechanisms that produce rash, itching, or inflammation.

℞ QUICK FACTS

Purpose

℞ Used to treat skin infections caused by fungus such as athlete's foot, jock itch, and ringworm of the body.

Dosage

 Before and after application of Lotrisone, wash your hands. Use full prescription even if symptoms subside. Avoid using large amounts over wide areas. *Do not cover areas with airtight dressings unless directed by your doctor. Do not get cream into eyes or swallow. Do not use for more than 4 weeks, and only for the prescribed condition.*

Usual adult dose (and for children over 12 years): *For jock itch or fungal skin infections*—apply to affected and surrounding areas 2 times per day in the morning and evening for 2 weeks. Apply sparingly to groin area. Inform doctor if not improved after 1 week. *For athlete's foot*—apply to affected and surrounding areas 2 times per day in the morning and evening. Inform doctor if not improved after 2 weeks.

 Usual child dose: not generally prescribed for children under 12 years. Children may absorb proportionately larger amounts than adults and are more sensitive than adults.

 Missed dose: apply as soon as possible, unless almost time for next dose. In that case, do not apply missed dose; go back to regular schedule.

Side Effects

 Overdose is unlikely with Lotrisone. However, if you suspect an overdose, immediately seek medical attention.

 More common side effects: blistering, hives, infection, irritated skin, itching, peeling, reddened skin, skin eruptions and rash, stinging, swelling due to fluid retention, tingling sensation.

 Less common side effects: acne, burning, dryness, excessive hair growth, inflamed hair follicles, inflamed skin, irritated skin around mouth, loss of skin color, softening of the skin, streaks in the skin.

Interactions

 No drug interactions reported.

 No known food/other substance interactions.

Special Cautions

 If pregnant or planning to become pregnant, inform your doctor immediately. Not known if Lotrisone appears in breast milk. Large amounts should not be used over an extended period by pregnant women.

 No special precautions apply to seniors.

 Follow doctor's instructions carefully for children 12 years and older. Not generally prescribed for children under 12 years. *Not for use on diaper rash.*

 If sensitive to the ingredients of this medication or similar medications, should not take.

May affect the adrenal, hypothalamic, and pituitary glands, and temporarily produce sugar in the urine and excessive blood sugar levels, resulting in Cushing's syndrome (easily bruised skin, increased blood pressure, mood swings, water retention, weak muscles, weight gain).

Lovastatin

see MEVACOR

Lozol

∿∿

Generic name: Indapamide

Lozol is a thiazide diuretic. It promotes the loss of salt and water in the body, and increases the diameter of the blood vessels, thereby lowering blood pressure.

℞ QUICK FACTS

Purpose

℞ Used to treat high blood pressure. Also used to reduce salt and fluid retention. May be prescribed to reduce fluid retention in pregnant women.

Dosage

 Take exactly as prescribed. Never stop this medication abruptly; may cause condition to worsen. Must take regularly for Lozol to be effective; may take several weeks before you observe full effects. Continue to take even if you feel well.

. . . .

 Usual adult dose: *For high blood pressure*—1.25 milligrams as a single dose taken in the morning. Doctor may increase gradually up to 5 milligrams per day if initial dose is ineffective. *For fluid buildup in congestive heart failure*—2.5 milligrams as a single daily dose taken in the morning. Doctor may increase gradually up to 5 milligrams per day if initial dose is ineffective.

. . . .

 Usual child dose: not generally prescribed for children.

. . . .

 Missed dose: take as soon as possible, unless almost time for next dose. In that case, do not take missed dose; go back to regular schedule. *Do not double doses.*

. . . .

Side Effects

 Overdose symptoms: electrolyte imbalance, nausea, stomach disorders, vomiting, weakness. If you suspect an overdose, immediately seek medical attention.

 More common side effects: agitation, anxiety, back pain, dizziness, headache, infection, irritability, muscle cramps or spasms, nasal inflammation, nervousness, numbness in hands and feet, pain, tension, weakness, fatigue, loss of energy or tiredness.

 Less common or rare side effects: abdominal pain or cramps, blurred vision, chest pain, conjunctivitis, constipation, cough, depression, diarrhea, dizziness when standing up quickly, drowsiness, dry mouth, excessive urination at night, fluid retention, flu-like symptoms, flushing, fluttering heartbeat, frequent urination, hives, impotence or reduced sex drive, indigestion, insomnia, irregular heartbeat, itching, light-headedness, loss of appetite, nausea, nervousness, premature heart contractions, production of large amounts of pale urine, rash, runny nose, sore throat, stomach irritation, tingling in hands and feet, vertigo, vomiting, weakness, weak or irregular heartbeat, weight loss.

Interactions

 Inform your doctor before combining Lozol with: lithium (Eskalith), norepinephrine, other high blood pressure medications such as Aldomet and Tenormin. Taking Lozol with lithium increases the risk of lithium poisoning.

 No known food/other substance interactions.

Special Cautions

 If pregnant or planning to become pregnant, inform your doctor immediately. May appear in breast milk; could affect a nursing infant.

 Senior women are particularly susceptible to salt and potassium loss. Doctor may advise potassium-rich diet or potassium supplement.

 Not generally prescribed for children.

 Should not use if you are unable to urinate; have an allergic reaction to Lozol; or are sensitive to other sulfa-containing medications.

Risk of potassium loss increases as dose is increased if you have cirrhosis, are using corticosteroids, or adrenocorticotropic hormone (ACTH).

Doctor should regularly do blood tests if you have irregular heartbeat or are taking heart medications.

Use with caution if you have: gout or high uric acid levels, liver disease, diabetes, lupus erythematosus, or kidney disease. Doctor should have kidney assessment and continual monitoring.

Luride

Generic name: Sodium fluoride

Other brand names: ACT, Fluorigard, Fluorinse, Gel 11, Karigel, Listermint with Fluoride, Lozi-Tabs, PediaFlor, Phos-Flur, Point Two, PreviDent, Thera-Flur

Luride is a dental caries (cavity) prophylactic. It encourages remineralization and inhibits the cariogenic microbial process.

℞ QUICK FACTS

Purpose

℞   Used to strengthen children's teeth against decay while they are still developing. Prescribed when water fluoride level is 0.7 parts per million or less. Also used for adults with calcium, vitamin D, or estrogen therapy.

Dosage

🍴   Administer exactly as prescribed, preferably at bedtime after teeth brushing. Child may chew or swallow tablet or suck on it until it dissolves. Liquid can be mixed with water or fruit juice.

. . . .

💊   Usual adult dose: *Rinse*—10 milliliters once per day after brushing teeth. *Tablet*—30 to 100 milligrams per day.

. . . .

🧸   Usual child dose: *For infants under 2 years*—0.25 milligram tablet or 2 drops. *2 years*—0.5 milligram tablet or 4 drops. *3 to 12 years*—1 milligram tablet or 8 drops. In areas where fluoride content is between 0.3 and 0.7 parts per million, halve these dosages. *Do not give full strength 1 milligram tablets to children under 3 years.*

. . . .

   Missed dose: take as soon as possible, unless almost time for next dose. In that case, do not take missed dose; go back to regular schedule. *Do not double doses.*

. . . .

Side Effects

 Overdose symptom: teeth discoloration—brown, black, or white spots on the teeth. If you suspect an overdose, immediately seek medical attention.

 More common side effects: none reported.

 Less common or rare side effects: allergic rash or other unexpected effect.

Interactions

 No reported drug interactions.

 Dairy products should be avoided when using Luride.

Special Cautions

 If pregnant or planning to become pregnant, consult your doctor before using.

 No special precautions apply to seniors.

 Follow doctor's instructions carefully for children.

 Doctor should know fluoride level in the water *before* prescribing Luride.

Should not take if child has past sensitivity to or allergy to Luride.

Macrodantin

Generic name: Nitrofurantoin

Other brand names: Furadantin, Furalan, Furan, Furanite, Macrobid, Nitrofan

Macrodantin is a urinary antibiotic. It inhibits the growth of bacteria by chemically interfering with their ability to survive.

℞ QUICK FACTS

Purpose

℞ Used to treat urinary tract infections caused by bacteria.

Dosage

 Take with food to stimulate absorption. Entire prescription should be finished, even if symptoms subside. Works best if your urine is acidic; talk with your doctor about how to ensure this. Urine may turn brown.

 Usual adult dose: *Macrodantin*—50 to 100 milligrams taken 4 times per day. Long-term use dosage may be reduced to 50 to 100 milligrams taken once at bedtime. Treatment duration is for 3 days to 1 week after an infection-free urine specimen is obtained. *Macrobid*—one 100 milligram capsule taken every 12 hours for 7 days.

Usual child dose: *Macrodantin—For children over one month to 12 years*—5 to 7 milligrams per 2.2 pounds of body weight divided into 4 doses in 24 hours. Long-term use—1 milligram per 2.2 pounds of body weight taken in 1 or 2 doses per day. *Macrobid—For children over 12 years*—one 100 milligram capsule taken every 12 hours for 7 days. Not prescribed for children under 12 years.

 Missed dose—take as soon as possible. Take remaining doses for the day at equal intervals.

Side Effects

 Overdose symptom: vomiting. If vomiting does not happen after an excessive dose, induce vomiting. If you suspect an overdose, immediately seek medical attention.

 More common side effects: lack or loss of appetite, nausea, vomiting.

 Less common or rare side effects: abdominal pain or discomfort, chills, confusion, cough, chest pain, depression, diarrhea, difficulty breathing, dizziness, drowsiness, exaggerated sense of well-being, fever, hair loss, headache, hepatitis, hives, inflammation of nerves causing numbness, involuntary eye movement, itching, itchy red skin patches, joint pain, muscle pain, peeling skin, psychotic reactions, rash, severe allergic reactions, skin inflammation with flaking, skin swelling or welts, tingling pain or muscle weakness, vertigo, yellowing of skin and eyes, weakness.

Interactions

 Inform your doctor before combining Macrodantin or Macrobid with: antispasmodics such as Bentyl and

Donnatal, magnesium trisilicate (Gaviscon), urico-
suric medications such as Benemid.

 No known food/other substance interactions.

Special Cautions

 If pregnant or planning to become pregnant, inform your doctor immediately. Should not take at term of pregnancy or during labor and delivery. Not known if Macrodantin and Macrobid appear in breast milk.

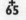 No special precautions apply to seniors.

 Follow doctor's instructions carefully for children.

 Death has occurred from peripheral neuropathy (disease of the nerves) during Macrodantin therapy. Use very cautiously if you have kidney disorder, anemia, diabetes, a debilitating disease, or vitamin B deficiency—these conditions increase the risk of peripheral neuropathy.

Doctor should closely monitor changes in liver function for signs of hepatitis. *Hepatitis has caused death during long-term treatment with this medication.*

Do not take if you have a kidney disorder, are unable to produce urine, or produce only a small amount.

Monitor for breathing disorders. *Pulmonary fibrosis (abnormal increase in fibrous tissue in the lungs) develops gradually and can be fatal.*

Allergic reactions may occur with no warning. Reactions are rare and happen with long-term therapy (6 months or more). Lung reactions often occur in the first week of therapy and disappear when therapy is stopped.

. . . .
May be at risk for below normal hemoglobin content in the blood as a result of red blood cell destruction.
. . . .
If sensitive to or allergic to this or similar medications, should not take.
. . . .
Notify your doctor of any unusual symptoms.
. . . .
Can develop a secondary infection not curable by this medication if using Macrodantin for an extended period.

Materna

see STUARTNATAL PLUS

Maxaquin

Generic name: Lomefloxacin hydrochloride

Maxaquin is a fluoroquinolone antibiotic. It inhibits the growth of bacteria by chemically interfering with their ability to survive.

℞ QUICK FACTS

Purpose

℞   Used to treat lower respiratory infections including bronchitis, and urinary tract infections. Also used prior to bladder surgery to prevent infection.

Dosage

    Finish entire medication, otherwise symptoms may return. May take with or without food; take with a full 8-ounce glass of water. Drink lots of liquids during Maxaquin therapy.

 Usual adult dose: *for chronic bronchitis*—400 milligrams once per day for 10 days. *For cystitis*—400 milligrams once per day for 10 days. *For urinary tract infections*—400 milligrams once per day for 14 days. *For impaired renal function or cirrhosis*—doctor will adjust dose. *For dialysis patients*—400 milligrams followed by daily maintenance doses of 200 milligrams taken once per day.

 Usual child dose: not generally prescribed for children under 18 years.

 Missed dose: take as soon as possible, unless almost time for next dose. In that case, do not take missed dose; go back to regular schedule. *Do not double doses.*

Side Effects

 Overdose symptoms: no specific information available. If you suspect an overdose, immediately seek medical attention.

 More common side effects: headache, nausea.

 Less common side effects: diarrhea, dizziness, sensitivity to light. Rare side effects: abdominal pain, abnormal or terrifying dreams, abnormal vision, agitation, allergic reaction, altered taste, angina pectoris (crushing chest pain), anxiety, back pain, bleeding between menstrual periods, bleeding in stomach and intestines, blood clots in the lungs, blood in the urine, blue skin color, chest pain, chills, coma, confusion, conjunctivitis (pink eye), constipation, convulsions, cough, decreased heat tolerance, depression, difficult or labored breathing, difficulty swallowing, dry mouth, earache, eye pain, facial swelling, fainting, fatigue, fluid retention and swelling, flu-like symptoms, flushing, gas, general feeling of illness, gout, heart attack, heart failure, high blood pressure, hives, inability to sleep, increased appetite, increased mucus from the lungs, increased sweating, indigestion, inflammation in male genital area, inflammation of stomach and intestines, inflammation of vagina, irregular heartbeat, itching, joint pain, lack of urine, leg cramps, loss of appetite, loss of sense of identity, low blood pressure, low blood sugar, lung infection or other problems, muscle pain, nervousness, nosebleed, overactivity, pain in the genital-rectal area, problems with urination, purple or red skin spots, rapid heartbeat, rash, ringing in ears, skin disorders, skin eruptions or peeling, sleepiness, slow heartbeat, thirst, tingling or pins and needles, tongue discoloration, tremor, vaginal yeast infection, vertigo, vomiting, weakness, wheezing, white or yellow vaginal discharge.

Interactions

Inform your doctor before combining Maxaquin with: antacids containing magnesium or aluminum such as Maalox and Tums, caffeine, cimetidine (Tagamet), cyclosporine (Sandimmune), probenecid (Benemid), sucralfate (Carafate), theophylline (Theo-Dur), warfarin (Coumadin), vitamins or products containing iron or zinc.

No known food/other substance interactions.

Special Cautions

If pregnant or planning to become pregnant, inform your doctor immediately. Not known if Maxaquin appears in breast milk.

No special precautions apply to seniors.

Not generally prescribed for children under 18 years.

 Severe or fatal reactions have on rare occasion been experienced after one dose. Immediately seek medical help if you experience: confusion, convulsions, difficulty breathing, hallucinations, hives, itching, light-headedness, loss of consciousness, rash, restlessness, swelling in the face or throat, tingling, or trembling.

Can cause mild to life-threatening bowel inflammation. Inform your doctor if you have experienced diarrhea from other antibiotics.

May cause drowsiness and impair your ability to drive a car or operate machinery. *Do not take part in any activity that requires alertness.*

May cause sensitivity if exposed to sunlight or sunlamps even if sunblock is used. Should avoid exposure even to indirect sunlight during and for several days after therapy is completed.

If sensitive to or allergic to this or similar medications, should not take.

Use cautiously if you have: epilepsy, hardening of brain arteries, or other conditions that cause seizures.

Maxzide

Generic ingredients: Triamterene with hydrochlorothiazide

Maxzide is a thiazide and potassium-sparing diuretic. Diuretics promote the loss of salt and water in the body and increase the diameter of the blood vessels, thereby lowering blood pressure.

℞ QUICK FACTS

Purpose

 Used to treat high blood pressure and other conditions requiring elimination of excess fluid.

Dosage

 Take regularly to be effective against high blood pressure, and can take several weeks before full effects are observed. Continue to take even if feeling well. Abruptly stopping this medication can cause condition to get worse.

· ·

 Usual adult dose: *Maxzide-25*—1 or 2 tablets in a single dose. *Maxzide*—1 tablet daily. Maxzide cannot be interchanged with Dyazide; they contain the same ingredients in different amounts.

· ·

 Usual child dose: not generally prescribed for children.

· ·

 Missed dose: take as soon as possible, unless almost time for next dose. In that case, do not take missed dose; go back to regular schedule. *Do not double doses.*

Side Effects

 Overdose symptoms: no specific information on Maxzide. Symptoms of triamterene overdose: dehydration, nausea, vomiting, weakness. Symptoms of hydrochlorothiazide overdose: dehydration, sluggishness possibly leading to coma, stomach and intestinal irritation. If you suspect an overdose, immediately seek medical attention.

Side effects: abdominal cramps, anemia, anxiety, change in potassium levels, change in taste, chest pain, constipation, decreased sexual performance, depression, diarrhea, difficulty breathing, difficulty sleeping, discolored urine, dizziness, dizziness when standing, drowsiness, dry mouth, fatigue, fever, headache, hives, hypersensitivity reaction, inflammation of the pancreas, inflammation of salivary glands, kidney stones, loss of appetite, muscle cramps, muscle weakness, nausea, rapid heartbeat, rash, reddish or purplish skin spots, restlessness, sensitivity to light, shortness of breath, stomach irritation, tingling or pins and needles, vertigo, vision changes, vomiting, yellow eyes and skin.

 No known less common or rare side effects.

Interactions

 Use with extreme caution if you are taking other ACE-inhibitor medications such as Vasotec. Inform your doctor before combining Maxzide with: amantadine (Symmetrel); barbiturates such as phenobarbital; beta-blockers such as Inderal; cholestyramine (Questran); fluconazole (Diflucan); indomethacin (Indocin); lithium (Lithonate); narcotics such as Percocet; norepinephrine (Levophed); oral diabetes medications such as Micronase; other diuretics that minimize potassium loss such as Midamor; other high blood pressure medications such as Aldomet; potassium-containing salt substitutes; Tubocurarine.

 Effects of alcohol may be increased while taking this medication; avoid alcohol use during Maxzide therapy. Alcohol also decreases the antihypertensive effects of Maxzide. Also avoid potassium-containing salt substitutes, potassium supplements, and potassium-enriched diets.

Special Cautions

 If pregnant or planning to become pregnant, inform your doctor immediately. Appears in breast milk; could affect a nursing infant.

 No special precautions apply to seniors.

 Not generally prescribed for children.

 Use with caution if you have: gout, liver disease, or lupus erythematosus.

Should not take if you are unable to urinate or have serious kidney disease, you have high potassium levels, or if you are taking other medications preventing potassium loss.

If sensitive to or allergic to this or other sulfa medications, should not take. History of bronchial asthma may increase risk for allergic reaction.

Doctor should do continual monitoring of kidneys if you have kidney disease.

Closely monitor dehydration, excessive sweating, diarrhea, or vomiting, and use caution in hot weather—may induce low blood pressure.

In the event of medical emergency or surgery, inform your doctor or dentist that you are taking Maxzide.

Meclizine Hydrochloride
see ANTIVERT

Medipren

see ADVIL

Medrol

~~~~~~

Generic name: Methylprednisolone

Medrol is an anti-inflammatory corticosteroid. It works by stimulating the synthesis of enzymes needed to decrease the inflammatory response.

℞ QUICK FACTS

Purpose

℞ Used to treat inflammation and improve symptoms of rheumatic arthritis, acute gouty arthritis, and severe asthma. Also used to treat primary or secondary adrenal cortex insufficiency. Also prescribed to treat: severe allergic conditions, blood disorders, certain cancers, skin diseases, connective tissue diseases (lupus), digestive tract diseases (ulcerative colitis), high serum levels of calcium associated with cancer, fluid retention due to kidney damage, various eye diseases, lung diseases such as tuberculosis.

Dosage

 Take as prescribed; may take every other day depending on condition for which you are being treated. To avoid upset stomach, take with food. *Do not stop taking suddenly; should be gradually tapered off.* Take single and alternate day doses in the morning with food.

Usual adult dose: 4 to 48 milligrams depending on condition for which you are being treated. Dose is decreased once a satisfactory response is achieved.

 Usual child dose: follow doctor's instructions.

 Missed dose: *for one daily dose*—take as soon as possible, unless it is the next day. In that case, do not take missed dose; go back to regular schedule. *Do not double doses. For more than one dose per day*—take as soon as possible, unless almost time for next dose. In that case, do not take missed dose; go back to regular schedule. *Do not double doses. For alternate day dose*—take dose if it is the same morning; go back to regular schedule. If it is the afternoon, skip the next morning; return to regular schedule.

Side Effects

 Overdose symptoms: acid indigestion, excessive sweating, fatigue, muscle weakness, swelling of arms and legs, upset stomach. If you suspect an overdose, immediately seek medical attention.

 Side effects: abdominal swelling; allergic reactions; bone fractures; bruising; congestive heart failure; cataracts; convulsions; Cushingoid symptoms (moon face, weight gain, high blood pressure, emotional disturbances, growth of facial hair in women); facial redness; fluid and salt retention; high blood pressure; increased eye pressure; increased sweating; increase in amounts of insulin or hypoglycemic medications needed; inflammation of upper digestive tract; inflammation of the pancreas; irregular menstruation; muscle wasting and weakness; poor healing of wounds; protrusion of eyes; stomach ulcer; suppression of growth in children; symptoms of diabetes; thin, fragile skin; tiny red or purplish skin spots; vertigo.

No known less common or rare side effects.

Interactions

 Inform your doctor before combining Medrol with: aspirin; barbiturates such as phenobarbital; carbamazapine (Tegretol); cholestyramine (Questran); cyclosporine (Sandimmune); diuretics such as Lasix and HydroDIURIL; Estrogens such as Premarin; indomethacin (Indocin); insulin; ketoconazole (Nizoral); oral diabetes medications such as Glucotrol; phenytoin (Dilantin); rifampin (Rifadin). Avoid vaccinations and immunizations, especially in high doses; may prevent antibody production to build up immunities, causing nervous system problems. Aspirin use should be monitored if you have a blood-clotting disorder.

 No known food/other substance interactions.

Special Cautions

 If pregnant or planning to become pregnant, inform your doctor immediately. May appear in breast milk; could affect a nursing infant. Babies born to mothers taking steroids are at risk for adrenal problems. Prolonged use may slow growth and development of infants and children.

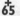 No special precautions apply to seniors.

 Follow doctor's instructions carefully for children.

 Should not use if you have a fungal infection, or are sensitive to or allergic to steroids.

May experience lowered resistance to infections, or the drug may mask the signs of infection.

. . . .

May alter your body's reaction to unusual stress; higher dosage may be prescribed by your doctor. Higher dose may also be necessary if you are injured, need surgery, or develop an acute illness.

. . . .

Ingredient used to color medication (tartrazine) has on rare occasions caused allergic reactions.

. . . .

Ongoing use may cause cataracts, glaucoma, and eye infections.

. . . .

High doses can cause: high blood pressure, salt and water retention, and potassium and calcium loss.

. . . .

Dormant tuberculosis may be activated by Medrol. Your doctor should prescribe antituberculosis medication if taking Medrol for a prolonged period.

. . . .

Use with caution if you have underactive thyroid, liver cirrhosis, or herpes simplex eye infection.

. . . .

May cause or aggravate existing emotional problems; notify your doctor if you experience mood changes.

. . . .

Use cautiously if you have diverticulitis or other intestinal disorders, high blood pressure, kidney disease, myasthenia gravis, osteoporosis, peptic ulcer, or ulcerative colitis.

. . . .

Immediately inform your doctor if you are exposed to measles or chicken pox.

Medroxyprogesterone Acetate

see PROVERA

Mefenamic Acid

see PONSTEL

Mellaril

Generic name: Thioridazine hydrochloride

Other brand names: Apo-Thioridazine, Millazine, Novoridazine, PMS Thioridazine

Mellaril is an antipsychotic. It calms certain areas of the brain and allows the rest of the brain to function normally.

℞ QUICK FACTS

Purpose

Used to treat symptoms of psychotic disorders such as schizophrenia, depression, and anxiety in adults. Also used to treat agitation, fears, sleep disturbances, tension, depression, anxiety in elderly people, and certain behavior problems in children.

Dosage

If taking liquid concentrate, dilute with liquid such as water or juice. *Do not change brands without the supervision of your doctor.*

Usual adult dose: *for psychotic disorders*—150 to 300 milligrams per day, divided into 3 equal doses. May be increased by doctor up to 800 milligrams. *For depression and anxiety*—75 milligrams per day divided into 3 equal doses; dose may range from 20 to 200 milligrams per day. *For seniors (depression, anxiety, and sleep disturbances*—prescribed doses in lower ranges.

Usual child dose: *for behavior problems*—0.5 to 3 milligrams per 2.2 pounds of body weight. Usual beginning dose is 20 to 30 milligrams per day divided into 2 or 3 doses.

Missed dose: *for 1 dose per day*—take as soon as possible, unless it is the next day. In that case, do not take missed dose; go back to regular schedule. *Do not double doses.* For 2 or more doses per day— take as soon as possible, unless within one hour of next dose. In that case, do not take missed dose; go back to regular schedule. *Do not double doses.*

Side Effects

Overdose symptoms: agitation, coma, convulsions, dry mouth, extreme drowsiness, extreme low blood pressure, fever, intestinal blockage, irregular heart rate, restlessness. If you suspect an overdose, immediately seek medical attention.

Side effects: abnormal and excessive milk secretion, agitation, anemia, asthma, blurred vision, body spasm, breast development in males, changed mental state, changes in sex drive, chewing movement, confusion (especially at night), constipation, diarrhea, discolored eyes, drowsiness, dry mouth, excitement, eyeball rotation, fever, fluid accumulation and swelling, headache, inability to hold urine, inability to urinate, inhibition of ejaculation, intestinal blockage, involuntary movements, irregular blood pressure and pulse, irregular heartbeat, irregular or missed menstrual periods, jaw spasm, loss of appetite, loss of muscle movement, mouth puckering, muscle rigidity, nasal congestion, nausea, overactivity, painful muscle spasm, paleness, pinpoint pupils, protruding tongue, psychotic reactions, puffing of cheeks, rapid heartbeat, redness of the skin, restlessness, rigid and masklike face, sensitivity to light, skin pigmentation and rash, sluggishness, stiff or twisted neck, strange dreams, sweating, swelling in the throat, swelling or filling of breasts, swollen glands, tremors, vomiting, weight gain, yellowing of skin and eyes.

 No known less common or rare side effects.

Interactions

 Inform your doctor before combining Mellaril with: epinephrine (EpiPen), phosphorus insecticides, pindolol (Visken), propranolol (Inderal). Central nervous system depressants such as narcotics, painkillers, and sleeping medications may cause extreme drowsiness or other serious side effects.

 Alcohol may cause extreme drowsiness and other serious side effects.

Special Cautions

 If pregnant or planning to become pregnant, inform your doctor immediately. Pregnant women should use only if it is necessary. May cause false positive results in pregnancy tests.

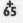 Seniors are prescribed doses in lower ranges due to risk of tardive dyskinesia.

 Follow doctor's instructions carefully for children.

 Do not take if you have heart disease or severe high blood pressure.

May cause drowsiness and impair your ability to drive a car or operate machinery. *Do not take part in any activity that requires alertness.*

. . . .
Check with your doctor about your risk for tardive dyskinesia.
. . . .
Alert your doctor if you have ever had breast cancer.

Meperidine Hydrochloride
see DEMEROL

Meprobamate
see MILTOWN

Mesalamine
see ROWASA

Metaproterenol Sulfate
see ALUPENT

Methazolamide
see NEPTAZANE

Methenamine with Methylene Blue, Phenyl Salicylate, Benzoic Acid, Atropine Sulfate, and Hyoscyamine

see URISED

Methergine

Generic name: Methylergonovine maleate

Methergine is an oxytocic, a blood-vessel constrictor. It increases uterine contractions which impede uterine blood flow.

℞ QUICK FACTS

Purpose

 Used to control or prevent excessive bleeding after childbirth.

Dosage

 Take exactly as prescribed.

 Usual adult dose: 0.2 milligram tablet 3 or 4 times per day for up to 1 week.

 Usual child dose: not prescribed for children.

 Missed dose: *do not take missed dose; do not double doses; go back to regular schedule.*

Side Effects

 Overdose symptoms: abdominal pain, coma, convulsions, elevated blood pressure, hypothermia (drop in body temperature), lowered blood pressure, nausea, numbness, slowed breathing, tingling of arms and legs, vomiting. If you suspect an overdose, immediately seek medical attention.

 More common side effects: high blood pressure, low blood pressure.

 Less common or rare side effects: bad taste, blood clots, blood in urine, chest pains (temporary), diarrhea, difficult or labored breathing, dizziness, edema, hallucinations, leg cramps, nasal congestion, nausea, palpitations, ringing in ears, sweating, vomiting.

Interactions

 Inform your doctor before combining Methergine with: other blood-vessel constrictors such as EpiPen, other ergot-derived medications such as Ergotrate.

 No known food/other substance interactions.

Special Cautions

 Should not take if pregnant. If pregnant or planning to become pregnant, inform your doctor immediately. Appears in breast milk; could affect a nursing infant.

 No special precautions apply to seniors.

 Not prescribed for children.

 Inform your doctor of any existing blood-vessel disorders, infections, or liver or kidney problems.

Should not take if you have high blood pressure or toxemia (poisons circulating in the blood).

Methocarbamol

see ROBAXIN

Methotrexate (MTX)

Generic name: Methotrexate

Other brand names: Folex, Mexate, Rheumatrex

Methotrexate is an antineoplastic and antipsoriatic. It slows cellular growth rate.

℞ QUICK FACTS

Purpose

℞ Used to treat lymphoma and certain forms of leukemia. Also used to treat cancers of the uterus, breast, lung, head, neck, and ovary. Used to treat rheumatoid arthritis and very severe psoriasis.

Dosage

 Take exactly as prescribed. Is prescribed at high doses for cancer. After high-dose therapy, leucovorin may be prescribed to limit toxic effects of methotrexate.

Usual adult dose: dosage is specifically individualized to prevent under- or overdosage. *When taking for psoriasis or rheumatoid arthritis, take once a week, not*

*once a day—taking dosage on a daily basis can lead to
fatal overdose.*

 Usual child dose: dosage is specifically individualized
to prevent under- or overdosage.

 Missed dose: skip missed dose and return to regular
schedule. *Do not double doses.*

Side Effects

 *May cause serious and fatal damage to liver, kidneys,
bone marrow, lungs, or other parts of the body.* Overdose symptoms: lung or breathing problems, mouth
ulcers, or diarrhea. Also, if you experience dry
cough or fever, immediately inform your doctor. If
you suspect an overdose, immediately seek medical
attention.

 More common side effects: abdominal pain and
upset, chills and fever, decreased resistance to infection, dizziness, fatigue, general feeling of illness,
mouth ulcers, nausea. Side effects associated with
taking methotrexate for psoriasis: burning sensation
at psoriasis sites; hair loss and/or sun sensitivity.

 Less common side effects: abortion, acne, anemia,
birth defects, black or tarry stool, blurred vision,
boils, bruises, changes in skin coloration, convulsions, diarrhea, drowsiness, fatigue, hair loss, headaches, hives, inability to speak, infection of hair
follicles, infertility, inflammation of the gums or
mouth, intestinal inflammation, kidney failure, loss of
appetite, lung disease, menstrual problems, partial
or complete paralysis, rash or itching, red patches
on skin, sensitivity to light, sore throat, stomach and
intestinal ulcers and bleeding, stomach pain, vaginal
discharge, vomiting, vomiting blood. Rare side effects: diabetes, impotence, infection, joint pain, loss
of sexual desire, muscular pain, osteoporosis, ringing

in the ears, severe allergic reaction, shortness of breath, sleepiness, sudden death, sweating.

Interactions

 Do not take aspirin or other nonsteroidal painkillers (Advil or Naprosyn) while taking methotrexate for (high-dose) cancer therapy; can make this medication more toxic. Inform your doctor before combining methotrexate with the following medications, which may increase toxic effects: cisplatin (Platinol), phenylbutazone (Butazolidin), phenytoin (Dilantin), probenecid (Benemid), sulfa medications such as Bactrim and Gantrisin. Certain antibiotics, such as Achromycin and chloramphenicol (Chloromycetin), and vitamin preparations containing folic acid may reduce effectiveness of this medication.

 No known food/other substance interactions.

Special Cautions

 Methotrexate causes birth defects and miscarriages. Must not be taken during pregnancy except in the case of cancer, where the potential benefit outweighs risk to fetus. For those wanting to conceive a child after methotrexate therapy, men should wait at least 3 months, and women should complete at least one menstrual cycle. Appears in breast milk; could affect a nursing infant.

 Seniors are susceptible to the toxic effects from methotrexate.

 Follow doctor's instructions carefully for children.

🛑 *Do not take if sensitive to or allergic to this medication.*

Doctor should perform regular blood tests to monitor any serious damage to the body.

Inform your doctor of any new symptoms that develop during methotrexate therapy.

Should not be taken if you have psoriasis or rheumatoid arthritis and any of the following: abnormal blood count, cirrhosis of the liver or other chronic liver disease, alcoholism, anemia, immune-system deficiency.

Doctor should do a chest X-ray before starting this medication. If you experience cough or chest pain, chest X-ray will be repeated.

Doctor will prescribe with extreme caution if you have: active infection, liver disease, peptic ulcer, ulcerative colitis.

Methyldopa
see ALDOMET

Methylergonovine Maleate
see METHERGINE

Methylphenidate Hydrochloride
see RITALIN

Methylprednisolone

see MEDROL

Metoclopramide Hydrochloride

see REGLAN

Metolazone

see ZAROXOLYN

Metoprolol Tartrate

see LOPRESSOR

Metronidazole

see FLAGYL

Mevacor

Generic name: Lovastatin

Mevacor is an antihyperlipidemic (lipid-lowering medication). It is thought to work by reducing the body's production of certain fats.

℞ Quick Facts

Purpose

℞ Used to lower cholesterol levels in people with primary hypercholesterolemia. May reduce both low-density lipoprotein (LDL or "bad cholesterol") and high-density lipoprotein (HDL or "good cholesterol"). Prescribed when diet alone does not sufficiently lower cholesterol levels.

Dosage

 Take exactly as prescribed, with meals. To get full benefit of Mevacor, adhere to diet and exercise program.

 Usual adult dose: 20 milligrams once per day, taken with the evening meal, up to 80 milligrams maximum. If taking with immunosuppressive drugs, 10 milligrams per day is prescribed, up to 20 milligrams per day. Doctor should monitor cholesterol levels.

 Usual child dose: not generally prescribed for children.

 Missed dose: take as soon as possible, unless almost time for next dose. In that case, do not take missed dose; go back to regular schedule. *Do not double doses.*

Side Effects

 Overdose symptoms: no reported cases, however, if you suspect an overdose, immediately seek medical attention.

 Side effects: abdominal pain or cramps, altered sense of taste, blurred vision, constipation, diarrhea, dizziness, gas, headache, heartburn, indigestion, itching, muscle cramps, muscle pain, nausea, rash, weakness.

Mevacor side effects are usually mild and last for a short period of time, if they appear.

 No known less common or rare side effects.

Interactions

 Inform your doctor before combining Mevacor with: blood thinners such as Coumadin; cyclosporine (Sandimmune) and other immunosuppressive medications; erythromycin (E.E.S. or PCE); gemfibrozil (Lopid); nicotine acid or niacin (Nicobid).

 No known food/other substance interactions.

Special Cautions

 Do not take if pregnant or nursing; may cause damage to fetus or nursing infant. If pregnant or planning to become pregnant, inform your doctor immediately.

 No special precautions apply to seniors.

 Not generally prescribed for children.

 Do not take if being treated for acute muscle disease or liver disease, or if you are at risk for developing kidney failure due to muscle tumors.

Inform your doctor *before* starting Mevacor if you are being treated for any disease that contributes to increased blood cholesterol—hypothyroidism, diabetes, kidney and blood vessel disorder, excess protein in the blood, or liver disease.

Doctor should perform liver function tests before treatment; every 6 weeks (for 3 months) after Mevacor therapy begins; every 8 weeks during the rest of the first year; then at 6-month intervals.

. . . .

If sensitive to or allergic to this or similar medications, should not take.

. . . .

Use with caution if you have past history of liver disease or consume large amounts of alcohol.

. . . .

Monitor for signs and symptoms of muscle pain, tenderness, or weakness with fever or general bodily discomfort, especially during the starting months of therapy and whenever dose is increased.

Mexiletine Hydrochloride

see MEXITIL

Mexitil

~~~~~~

Generic name: Mexiletine hydrochloride

Mexitil is an anti-arrhythmic. It alleviates cardiac arrhythmias by alternating nerve impulses in the heart.

℞ QUICK FACTS

Purpose

 Used to treat severe irregular heartbeat.

Dosage

 Take with food or antacid, exactly as prescribed.

. . . .

 Usual adult dose: 200 milligrams every 8 hours, adjusted by your doctor by 50 or 100 milligrams up or down every 2 to 3 days. Doctor may increase dosage to up to 1,200 milligrams per day. *For fast*

relief—400 milligrams followed by 200 milligrams in 8 hours. Effects will be apparent within 30 minutes to 2 hours. *For severe kidney disease*—usually prescribed lower doses. At dosage level of 300 milligrams or less, and if medication is tolerated well, doctor will prescribe 12-hour dosage schedule. *For seniors*—dosage adjusted according to individual needs. Mexitil treatment usually starts in the hospital.

Usual child dose: not generally prescribed for children.

Missed dose: take as soon as possible, up to 4 hours past regular schedule. Otherwise, do not take missed dose; go back to regular schedule. *Do not double doses.*

Side Effects

Overdose may be fatal. Overdose symptoms: low blood pressure, nausea, seizures, slow heartbeat, tingling or pins and needles. If you suspect an overdose, immediately seek medical attention.

More common side effects: blurred vision, changes in sleep habits, chest pain, constipation, depression, diarrhea, difficult or labored breathing, dizziness, headache, heartburn, light-headedness, nausea, nervousness, numbness, poor coordination, rash, swelling due to fluid retention, throbbing heartbeat, tingling or pins and needles, tremors, upset stomach, vision changes, vomiting.

Less common or rare side effects: abdominal pain or cramps, angina (crushing chest pain), appetite changes, behavior changes, bleeding from the stomach, confusion, congestive heart failure, decreased sex drive, depression, difficulty swallowing, difficulty urinating, dry mouth, dry skin, excessive perspiration, fainting, fatigue, fever, hallucinations, hair loss, hepatitis, hiccups, high blood pressure, hot flashes, impotence, joint pain, loss of consciousness, low blood pressure, peptic ulcer, ringing in the ears, seizures, short-term memory loss, skin inflammation and flaking, skin peeling, slow heartbeat, sore throat, speech difficulties, taste changes, vague feeling of discomfort, weakness, worsening of irregular heartbeat.

Interactions

 Inform your doctor before combining Mexitil with: antacids such as Maalox, caffeine products such as No-Doz, cimetidine (Tagamet), other anti-arrhythmic medications such as Norpace and Quinidex, phenobarbital, phenytoin (Dilantin), rifampin (Rifadin), theophylline (Theo-Dur).

 No known food/other substance interactions.

Special Cautions

 If pregnant or planning to become pregnant, inform your doctor immediately. Appears in breast milk; could affect a nursing infant.

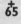 Dosage adjusted according to individual needs for seniors. Elderly patients should be monitored during Mexitil therapy.

 Not generally prescribed for children.

 Doctor will monitor heartbeat to assure Mexitil is having desired effect.

Should not be used if you have heart failure, heart block that has not been corrected with a pacemaker, structural heart disease, or a recent heart attack.

May be prescribed with a heart block condition and pacemaker, with ongoing monitoring.

Prescribed with caution if you have liver disease or abnormal liver function due to congestive heart failure.

Talk with your doctor about your diet—changing pH (acid or alkaline content) of your urine can change the Mexitil excretion from your body.

Doctor should monitor for blood disorders; you are at risk while taking Mexitil.

Use cautiously if you have a seizure disorder.

Micatin
see MONISTAT

Miconazole Nitrate
see MONISTAT

Micro-K

Generic name: Potassium chloride

Other brand names: Cena-K, K+10, Kaochlor, KAON-CL, K-DUR, Kay Ciel, Kato, Klor-Con, K-Lease, Klorvess, Klotrix, K-Lyte, K-Norm, K-Tab, Rum-K, Slow-K, Ten-K

Micro-K is a potassium replacement.

℞ QUICK FACTS

Purpose

 Used to treat or prevent low potassium levels when taking digoxin (Lanoxin) and non-potassium-sparing diuretics such as Diuril and Dyazide, and certain diseases. Prescribed when potassium chloride in liquid or effervescent forms cannot be tolerated.

Dosage

 Take with meals and with water or other liquid. Should not crush, chew, or suck capsule. If you have trouble swallowing capsule, doctor may advise sprinkling contents onto a spoonful of soft food. *Do not change brands unless directed by your doctor.*

 Usual adult dose: *to treat low potassium levels—* ranges from 4 to 12 tablets or capsules per day, depending on brand. Doctor will specify exact dose. *To prevent low potassium levels—*ranges from 2 to 3 tablets or capsules per day, depending on brand. Doctor will specify exact dose. If taking more than 2 tablets or capsules per day, will be divided into smaller doses.

 Usual child dose: not generally prescribed for children.

 Missed dose: take as soon as possible, up to 2 hours past regular schedule. Otherwise, do not take missed dose, go back to regular schedule. *Do not double doses.*

Side Effects

 Overdose can be fatal. Overdose symptoms: blood in stools, cardiac arrest, irregular heartbeat, muscle paralysis, muscle weakness. Early stages of overdose may not show noticeable symptoms. If you suspect an overdose, immediately seek medical attention.

 Side effects: abdominal pain or discomfort, diarrhea, nausea, stomach and intestinal ulcers and bleeding, blockage or perforation, vomiting.

 No known less common or rare side effects.

Interactions

 Inform your doctor before combining Micro-K with: antispasmodics such as Bentyl, ACE inhibitors such as Vasotec and Capoten, digoxin (Lanoxin), potassium-sparing diuretics such as Midamor and Aldactone.

 Inform your doctor if you are using salt substitutes.

Special Cautions

 Generally considered safe during pregnancy or breastfeeding.

 No special precautions apply to seniors.

 Not generally prescribed for children.

 Inform your doctor *before* Micro-K therapy if you have ever had: acute dehydration, heat cramps, adrenal insufficiency, diabetes, heart disease, kidney disease, liver disease, ulcers, or severe burns.

Immediately contact your doctor if you experience black or tarry stools.

If taking medication or have a condition that stops or slows Micro-K as it goes through intestinal tract, should not take.

Avoid use if you have high potassium levels.

Micronase

Generic name: Glyburide

Other brand names: DiaBeta, Glynase

Micronase is an oral antidiabetic. It stimulates the pancreas to produce more insulin.

℞ QUICK FACTS

Purpose

℞   Used to treat Type II (non-insulin-dependent) diabetes.

Dosage

 Take with breakfast or first main meal of the day. To avoid mild hypoglycemia (low blood sugar), strictly adhere to the diet and exercise plan prescribed by your doctor. Keep quick-acting sugar or sugar-based product with you at all times.

 Usual adult dose: 2.5 to 5 milligrams per day. Maintenance therapy—1.25 to 20 milligrams per day. With doses 10 milligrams per day and above, may be divided into 2 doses. *Seniors, malnourished, or those with impaired kidney and liver function*—may be prescribed lower doses.

 Usual child dose: not generally prescribed for children.

 Missed dose: take as soon as possible, unless almost time for next dose. In that case, do not take missed

dose; go back to regular schedule. *Do not double doses.*

Side Effects

Overdose may cause low blood sugar (hypoglycemia). Symptoms of mild hypoglycemia: cold sweat, drowsiness, fast heartbeat, headache, nausea, nervousness. Symptoms of more severe hypoglycemia: coma, pale skin, seizure, shallow breathing. If you suspect an overdose, immediately seek medical attention.

More common side effects: bloating, heartburn, nausea.

Less common or rare side effects: anemia and other blood disorders, blurred vision, changes in taste, headache, hepatic porphyria, hepatitis, hives, itching, joint pain, muscle pain, reddening of the skin, skin rash, skin eruptions.

Interactions

Inform your doctor before combining Micronase with: adrenal corticosteroids such as prednisone; airway-opening medications such as Proventil and Ventolin; anabolic steroids such as testosterone and Danazol; antacids such as Mylanta; beta-blockers such as Inderal and Tenormin; calcium channel blockers such as Cardizem and Procardia; certain antibiotics such as Cipro; chloramphenicol (Chloromycetin); cimetidine (Tagamet); clofibrate (Atromide-S); estrogens such as Premarin; fluconazole (Diflucan); Furosemide (Lasix); gemfibrozil (Lopid); isoniazid; itraconazole (Sporanox); major tranquilizers such as Stelazine and Mellaril; MAO inhibitors such as Nardil and Parnate; miconazole (Monistat); niacin (Nicolar or Nicobid); nonsteroidal anti-inflammatory medications such as Advil, aspirin, Motrin, Naprosyn, and Voltaren; oral contraceptives;

phenytoin (Dilantin); probenecid (Benemid or Col-
BENEMID); sulfa medications such as Septra; Synthroid; thiazide diuretics such as Diuril and HydroDIURIL; warfarin (Coumadin).

 Alcohol may increase risk of hypoglycemia.

Special Cautions

 If pregnant or planning to become pregnant, inform
your doctor immediately. Not known if Micronase
appears in breast milk, although other similar medications do. Should be prescribed if benefit outweighs risk to fetus. Doctor may prescribe insulin
injections during pregnancy as maintaining blood
sugar levels is important.

 Seniors may be prescribed lower doses.

 Not generally prescribed for children.

 Micronase is not an oral form of insulin and cannot
be substituted for Insulin.

Should not take if allergic to this medication.

If you have diabetic ketoacidosis, should not take
Micronase.

Risk of hypoglycemia also increased by: missed meals,
other medications, fever, trauma, infection, surgery,
kidney or liver problems, lack of adrenal or pituitary
hormone; or if you are run-down, hungry, or too
much exercise.

May increase risk of heart problems.

Should monitor blood or urine on an ongoing basis
for abnormal sugar (glucose) levels.

Effectiveness may decrease over time, due to either decreased responsiveness to medication or worsening of diabetes.

Midrin

Generic ingredients: Isometheptene mucate with dichloralphenazone and acetaminophen

Other brand names: Amidrine, I.D.A., Iso-Acetazone, Isocom, Midchlor, Migrapap, Migratine, Migrazone, Migrend, Migrex, Misquin, Mitride

Midrin is a combination analgesic/sedative/vascular headache suppressant. It causes blood vessels in the head to constrict or become narrower, and it relieves pain.

℞ QUICK FACTS

Purpose

 Used to treat tension headaches. Also used to treat vascular headaches such as migraines.

Dosage

 Take at the onset of headache. *Do not take more than the dose prescribed.*

 Usual adult dose: *for migraine*—2 capsules at once, 1 capsule every hour until there is relief. *Do not take more than 5 capsules in a 12-hour period. For tension headache*—1 or 2 capsules every 4 hours up to 8 capsules per day maximum.

 Usual child dose: not generally prescribed for children.

Missed dose: take only as needed.

Side Effects

 Overdose symptoms: no specific information available. However, if you suspect an overdose, immediately seek medical attention.

 Side effects: short period of dizziness, skin rash.

 No known less common or rare side effects.

Interactions

 Inform your doctor before combining Midrin with: acetaminophen-containing medications such as Tylenol; antihistamines such as Benadryl; central nervous system depressants such as Halcion, Valium, and Xanax. *Do not take MAO inhibitor antidepressant medications (Nardil or Parnate) unless specifically instructed by your doctor.*

 Avoid alcohol while taking Midrin.

Special Cautions

 If pregnant, planning to become pregnant, or breast-feeding, inform your doctor.

 No special precautions apply to seniors.

 Not generally prescribed for children.

 Do not take if you have: glaucoma, severe kidney disease, high blood pressure, physical heart defect, or liver disease unless specifically instructed by your doctor.

Midrin does *not* prevent headaches.

Photo Identification Guide

To assist in confirming that the medication you have is the correct one your doctor prescribed, we have included photographs of some of the most commonly prescribed drugs—both generic and brand names, and at different dosage levels—in this book. Although numerous photos are included here, note that not all the drugs referenced in this book are shown in photographs.

Note also that the size or color of the photos may differ slightly from the actual pills as a result of the printing process. In addition, although the photographs of prescription pills are approximately life size, the photos of inhalers, liquid solutions, ointments and suppositories are not. Brand Name drugs are listed in ALL CAPS, while generic drug names are in lower case.

For those pills with two distinct sides, we've made every attempt to include photos of both sides. This is why you will find multiple photos for some drugs. If you look closely, you will see distinctions between the photos such as the drug manufacturer's name, the dosage strength, and/or any drug code numbers.

Do not rely solely on these photographs to identify a particular drug. If you have any questions about why your particular medication varies from a specific picture, check with your pharmacist or doctor for clarification. This book is meant to supplement the information your doctor and pharmacist have provided. It should not be used to substitute a doctor's care and medical advice, or for self-medication purposes.

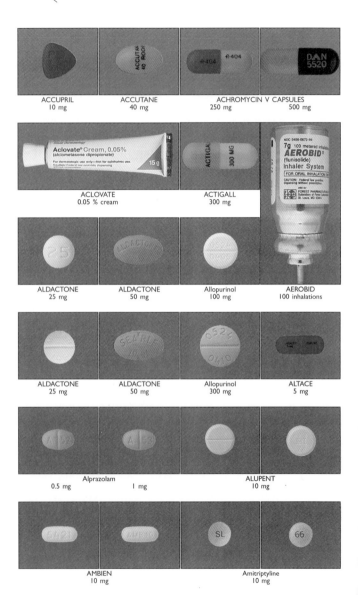

ACCUPRIL 10 mg	ACCUTANE 40 mg	ACHROMYCIN V CAPSULES 250 mg	ACHROMYCIN V CAPSULES 500 mg

ACLOVATE 0.05 % cream	ACTIGALL 300 mg	AEROBID 100 inhalations

ALDACTONE 25 mg	ALDACTONE 50 mg	Allopurinol 100 mg	AEROBID 100 inhalations

ALDACTONE 25 mg	ALDACTONE 50 mg	Allopurinol 300 mg	ALTACE 5 mg

Alprazolam 0.5 mg	Alprazolam 1 mg	ALUPENT 10 mg	ALUPENT 10 mg

AMBIEN 10 mg	AMBIEN 10 mg	Amitriptyline 10 mg	Amitriptyline 10 mg

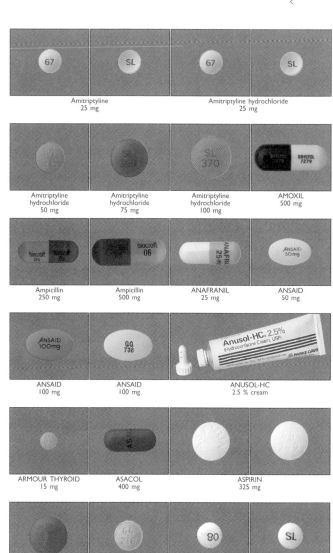

Amitriptyline
25 mg

Amitriptyline hydrochloride
25 mg

Amitriptyline
hydrochloride
50 mg

Amitriptyline
hydrochloride
75 mg

Amitriptyline
hydrochloride
100 mg

AMOXIL
500 mg

Ampicillin
250 mg

Ampicillin
500 mg

ANAFRANIL
25 mg

ANSAID
50 mg

ANSAID
100 mg

ANSAID
100 mg

ANUSOL-HC
2.5 % cream

ARMOUR THYROID
15 mg

ASACOL
400 mg

ASPIRIN
325 mg

ASPIRIN
325 mg

ASPIRIN, CHEWABLE
81 mg

ATARAX
white tablet
25 mg

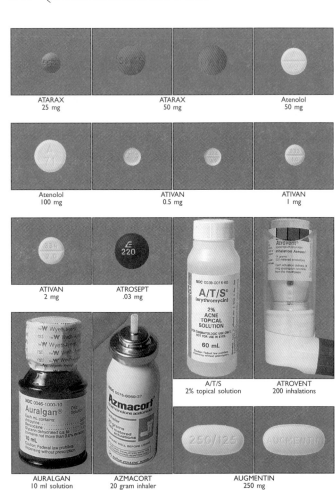

ATARAX
25 mg

ATARAX
50 mg

Atenolol
50 mg

Atenolol
100 mg

ATIVAN
0.5 mg

ATIVAN
1 mg

ATIVAN
2 mg

ATROSEPT
.03 mg

A/T/S
2% topical solution

ATROVENT
200 inhalations

AURALGAN
10 ml solution

AZMACORT
20 gram inhaler

AUGMENTIN
250 mg

AUGMENTIN
500 mg

AZULFIDINE
500 mg

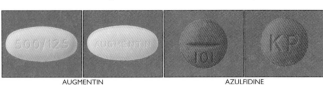

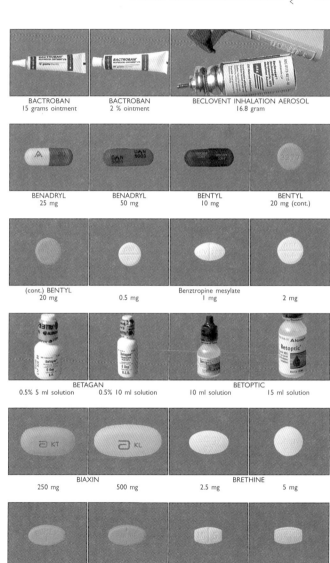

BACTROBAN
15 grams ointment

BACTROBAN
2 % ointment

BECLOVENT INHALATION AEROSOL
16.8 gram

BENADRYL
25 mg

BENADRYL
50 mg

BENTYL
10 mg

BENTYL
20 mg (cont.)

(cont.) BENTYL
20 mg

0.5 mg

Benztropine mesylate
1 mg

2 mg

BETAGAN
0.5% 5 ml solution

0.5% 10 ml solution

BETOPTIC
10 ml solution

15 ml solution

BIAXIN
250 mg

500 mg

BRETHINE
2.5 mg

5 mg

BUMEX
1 mg

BUSPAR
5 mg

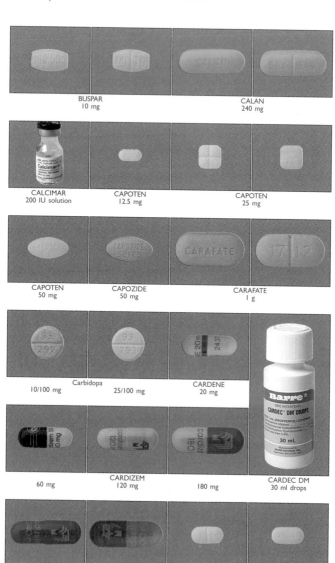

BUSPAR
10 mg

CALAN
240 mg

CALCIMAR
200 IU solution

CAPOTEN
12.5 mg

CAPOTEN
25 mg

CAPOTEN
50 mg

CAPOZIDE
50 mg

CARAFATE
1 g

Carbidopa
10/100 mg

25/100 mg

CARDENE
20 mg

CARDEC DM
30 ml drops

60 mg

CARDIZEM
120 mg

180 mg

CARDIZEM
240 mg

CARDIZEM
300 mg

CARDURA
1 mg

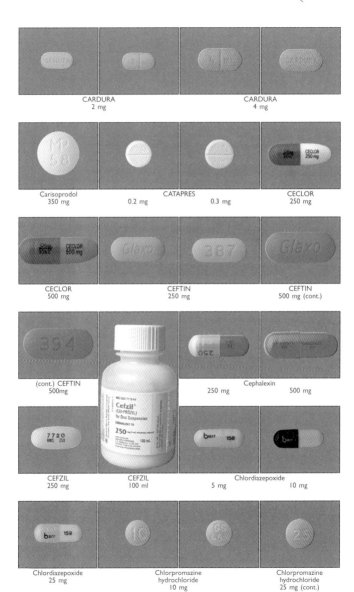

CARDURA
2 mg

CARDURA
4 mg

Carisoprodol
350 mg

CATAPRES
0.2 mg

0.3 mg

CECLOR
250 mg

CECLOR
500 mg

CEFTIN
250 mg

CEFTIN
500 mg (cont.)

(cont.) CEFTIN
500mg

Cephalexin
250 mg

500 mg

CEFZIL
250 mg

CEFZIL
100 ml

Chlordiazepoxide
5 mg

10 mg

Chlordiazepoxide
25 mg

Chlorpromazine
hydrochloride
10 mg

Chlorpromazine
hydrochloride
25 mg (cont.)

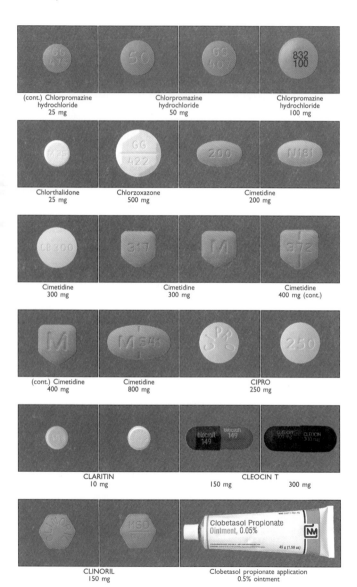

(cont.) Chlorpromazine
hydrochloride
25 mg

Chlorpromazine
hydrochloride
50 mg

Chlorpromazine
hydrochloride
100 mg

Chlorthalidone
25 mg

Chlorzoxazone
500 mg

Cimetidine
200 mg

Cimetidine
300 mg

Cimetidine
300 mg

Cimetidine
400 mg (cont.)

(cont.) Cimetidine
400 mg

Cimetidine
800 mg

CIPRO
250 mg

CLARITIN
10 mg

CLEOCIN T

150 mg

300 mg

CLINORIL
150 mg

Clobetasol propionate application
0.5% ointment

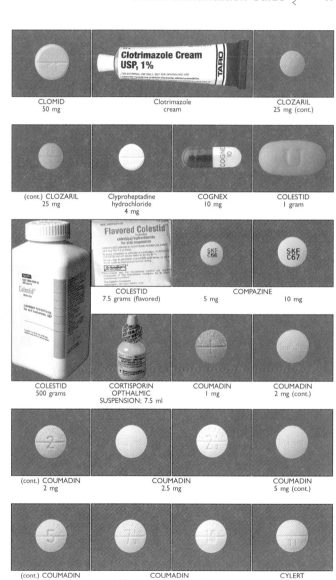

CLOMID
50 mg

Clotrimazole
cream

CLOZARIL
25 mg (cont.)

(cont.) CLOZARIL
25 mg

Clyproheptadine
hydrochloride
4 mg

COGNEX
10 mg

COLESTID
I gram

COLESTID
500 grams

COLESTID
7.5 grams (flavored)

COMPAZINE
5 mg   10 mg

CORTISPORIN
OPTHALMIC
SUSPENSION; 7.5 ml

COUMADIN
I mg

COUMADIN
2 mg (cont.)

(cont.) COUMADIN
2 mg

COUMADIN
2.5 mg

COUMADIN
5 mg (cont.)

(cont.) COUMADIN
5 mg

COUMADIN
7.5 mg   10 mg

CYLERT
37.5 mg (cont.)

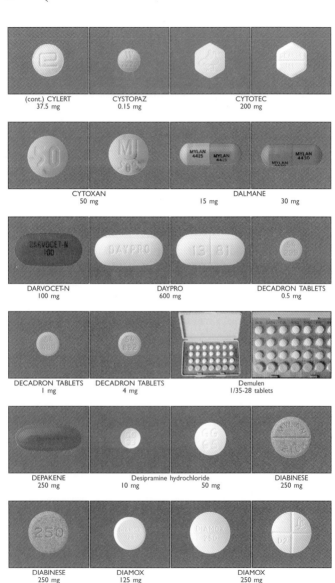

(cont.) CYLERT
37.5 mg

CYSTOPAZ
0.15 mg

CYTOTEC
200 mg

CYTOXAN
50 mg

DALMANE
15 mg   30 mg

DARVOCET-N
100 mg

DAYPRO
600 mg

DECADRON TABLETS
0.5 mg

DECADRON TABLETS
1 mg

DECADRON TABLETS
4 mg

Demulen
1/35-28 tablets

DEPAKENE
250 mg

Desipramine hydrochloride
10 mg   50 mg

DIABINESE
250 mg

DIABINESE
250 mg

DIAMOX
125 mg

DIAMOX
250 mg

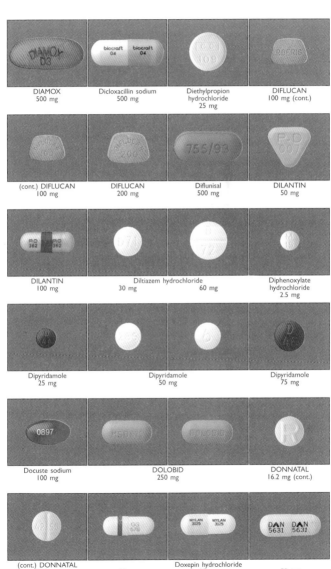

DIAMOX
500 mg

Dicloxacillin sodium
500 mg

Diethylpropion
hydrochloride
25 mg

DIFLUCAN
100 mg (cont.)

(cont.) DIFLUCAN
100 mg

DIFLUCAN
200 mg

Diflunisal
500 mg

DILANTIN
50 mg

DILANTIN
100 mg

Diltiazem hydrochloride
30 mg

60 mg

Diphenoxylate
hydrochloride
2.5 mg

Dipyridamole
25 mg

Dipyridamole
50 mg

Dipyridamole
75 mg

Docuste sodium
100 mg

DOLOBID
250 mg

DONNATAL
16.2 mg (cont.)

(cont.) DONNATAL
16.2 mg

10 mg

Doxepin hydrochloride
25 mg

50 mg

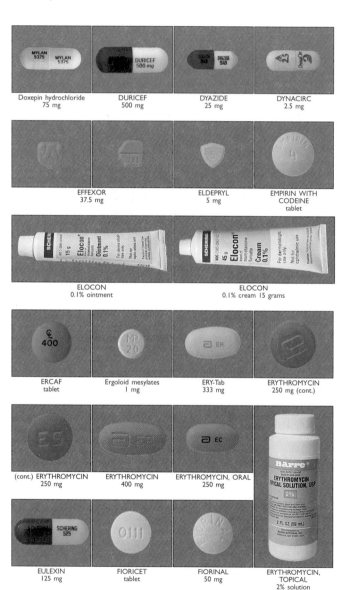

Doxepin hydrochloride
75 mg

DURICEF
500 mg

DYAZIDE
25 mg

DYNACIRC
2.5 mg

EFFEXOR
37.5 mg

ELDEPRYL
5 mg

EMPIRIN WITH
CODEINE
tablet

ELOCON
0.1% ointment

ELOCON
0.1% cream 15 grams

ERCAF
tablet

Ergoloid mesylates
1 mg

ERY-Tab
333 mg

ERYTHROMYCIN
250 mg (cont.)

(cont.) ERYTHROMYCIN
250 mg

ERYTHROMYCIN
400 mg

ERYTHROMYCIN, ORAL
250 mg

ERYTHROMYCIN,
TOPICAL
2% solution

EULEXIN
125 mg

FIORICET
tablet

FIORINAL
50 mg

ERYTHROMYCIN,
TOPICAL
2% solution

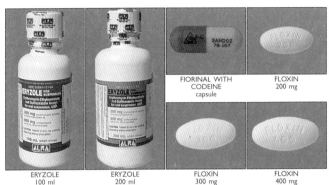

ERYZOLE
100 ml

ERYZOLE
200 ml

FIORINAL WITH
CODEINE
capsule

FLOXIN
200 mg

FLOXIN
300 mg

FLOXIN
400 mg

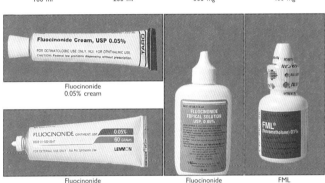

Fluocinonide
0.05% cream

Fluocinonide
0.05% 60 grams

Fluocinonide
0.05% topical solution
60 ml

FML
0.1% liquifilm

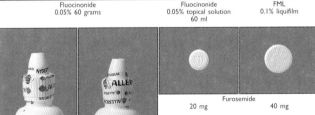

Furosemide
20 mg   40 mg

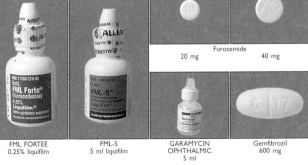

FML FORTEE
0.25% liquifilm

FML-S
5 ml liquifilm

GARAMYCIN
OPHTHALMIC
5 ml

Gemfibrozil
600 mg

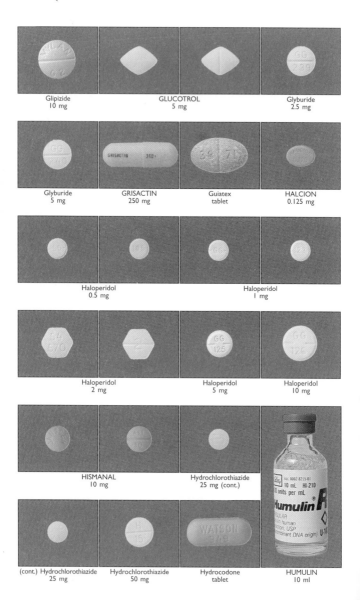

Glipizide
10 mg

GLUCOTROL
5 mg

Glyburide
2.5 mg

Glyburide
5 mg

GRISACTIN
250 mg

Guiatex
tablet

HALCION
0.125 mg

Haloperidol
0.5 mg

Haloperidol
1 mg

Haloperidol
2 mg

Haloperidol
5 mg

Haloperidol
10 mg

HISMANAL
10 mg

Hydrochlorothiazide
25 mg (cont.)

(cont.) Hydrochlorothiazide
25 mg

Hydrochlorothiazide
50 mg

Hydrocodone
tablet

HUMULIN
10 ml

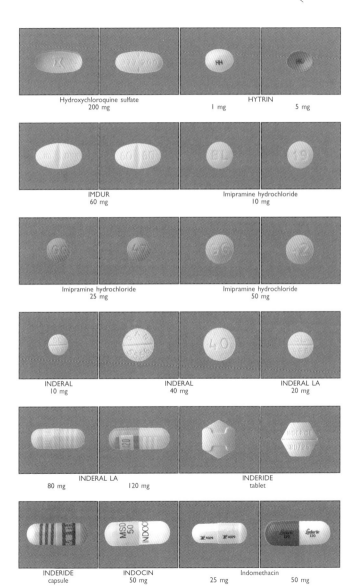

Hydroxychloroquine sulfate
200 mg

HYTRIN
1 mg

5 mg

IMDUR
60 mg

Imipramine hydrochloride
10 mg

Imipramine hydrochloride
25 mg

Imipramine hydrochloride
50 mg

INDERAL
10 mg

INDERAL
40 mg

INDERAL LA
20 mg

INDERAL LA
80 mg   120 mg

INDERIDE
tablet

INDERIDE
capsule

INDOCIN
50 mg

Indomethacin
25 mg   50 mg

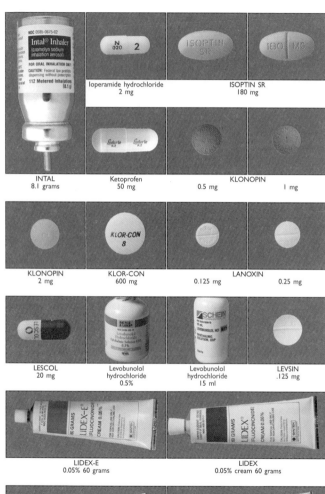

INTAL
8.1 grams

loperamide hydrochloride
2 mg

ISOPTIN SR
180 mg

Ketoprofen
50 mg

KLONOPIN
0.5 mg

KLONOPIN
1 mg

KLONOPIN
2 mg

KLOR-CON
600 mg

LANOXIN
0.125 mg

LANOXIN
0.25 mg

LESCOL
20 mg

Levobunolol
hydrochloride
0.5%

Levobunolol
hydrochloride
15 ml

LEVSIN
.125 mg

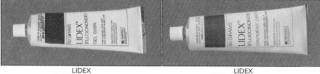

LIDEX-E
0.05% 60 grams

LIDEX
0.05% cream 60 grams

LIDEX
0.05% gel 60 grams

LIDEX
0.05% ointment (cont.)

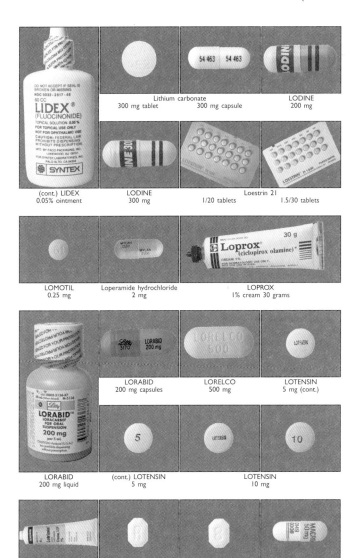

LIDEX® (FLUOCINONIDE)
SYNTEX

Lithium carbonate
300 mg tablet

300 mg capsule

54 463   54 463

LODINE
200 mg

(cont.) LIDEX
0.05% ointment

LODINE
300 mg

Loestrin 21
1/20 tablets

1.5/30 tablets

LOMOTIL
0.25 mg

Loperamide hydrochloride
2 mg

LOPROX
1% cream 30 grams

LORABID
200 mg liquid

LORABID
200 mg capsules

LORELCO
500 mg

LOTENSIN
5 mg (cont.)

(cont.) LOTENSIN
5 mg

LOTENSIN
10 mg

LOTRIMIN
1% cream 45 grams

LOZOL
2.5 mg

MACRODANTIN
50 mg

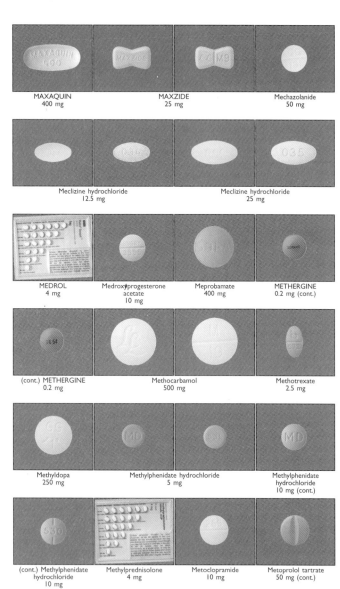

MAXAQUIN
400 mg

MAXZIDE
25 mg

Mechazolanide
50 mg

Meclizine hydrochloride
12.5 mg

Meclizine hydrochloride
25 mg

MEDROL
4 mg

Medroxyprogesterone
acetate
10 mg

Meprobamate
400 mg

METHERGINE
0.2 mg (cont.)

(cont.) METHERGINE
0.2 mg

Methocarbamol
500 mg

Methotrexate
2.5 mg

Methyldopa
250 mg

Methylphenidate hydrochloride
5 mg

Methylphenidate
hydrochloride
10 mg (cont.)

(cont.) Methylphenidate
hydrochloride
10 mg

Methylprednisolone
4 mg

Metoclopramide
10 mg

Metoprolol tartrate
50 mg (cont.)

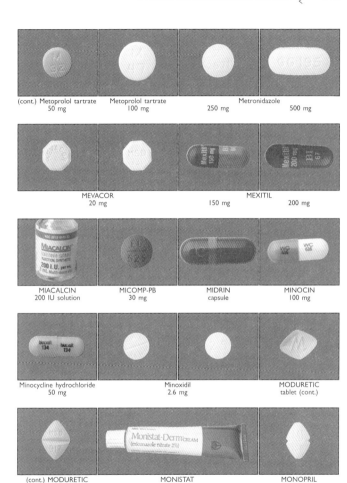

(cont.) Metoprolol tartrate
50 mg

Metoprolol tartrate
100 mg

Metronidazole
250 mg

500 mg

MEVACOR
20 mg

MEXITIL
150 mg

200 mg

MIACALCIN
200 IU solution

MICOMP-PB
30 mg

MIDRIN
capsule

MINOCIN
100 mg

Minocycline hydrochloride
50 mg

Minoxidil
2.6 mg

MODURETIC
tablet (cont.)

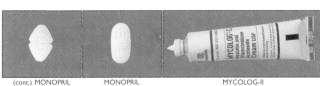

(cont.) MODURETIC
tablet

MONISTAT
2% cream

MONOPRIL
tablet, 20 mg (cont.)

(cont.) MONOPRIL
tablet, 20 mg

MONOPRIL
tablet, 20 mg

MYCOLOG-II
1 mg cream

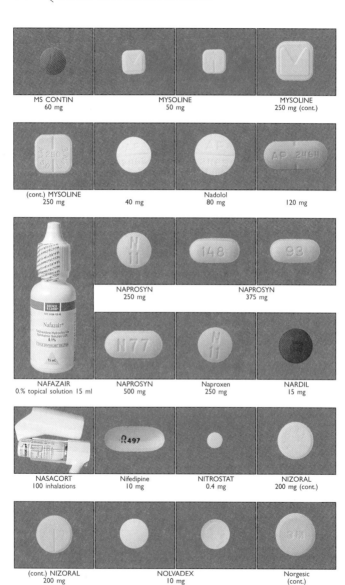

MS CONTIN
60 mg

MYSOLINE
50 mg

MYSOLINE
250 mg (cont.)

(cont.) MYSOLINE
250 mg

40 mg

Nadolol
80 mg

120 mg

NAFAZAIR
0.% topical solution 15 ml

NAPROSYN
250 mg

NAPROSYN
375 mg

NAPROSYN
500 mg

Naproxen
250 mg

NARDIL
15 mg

NASACORT
100 inhalations

Nifedipine
10 mg

NITROSTAT
0.4 mg

NIZORAL
200 mg (cont.)

(cont.) NIZORAL
200 mg

NOLVADEX
10 mg

Norgesic
(cont.)

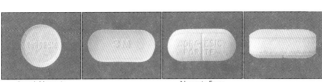

(cont.) Norgesic
tablet

Norgesic Forte
tablets

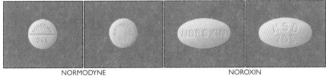

NORMODYNE
100 mg

NOROXIN
400 mg

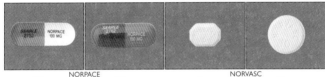

NORPACE

100 mg   150 mg

NORVASC

5 mg   10 mg

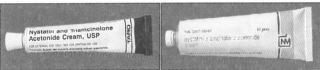

Nystatin
cream

Nystatin
cream

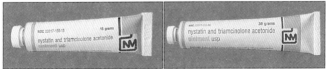

Nystatin
cream

Nystatin
cream

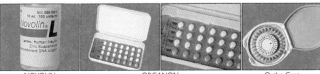

NOVOLIN
10ml

ORGANON
birth control packet

Ortho-Cept
birth control packet
(cont.)

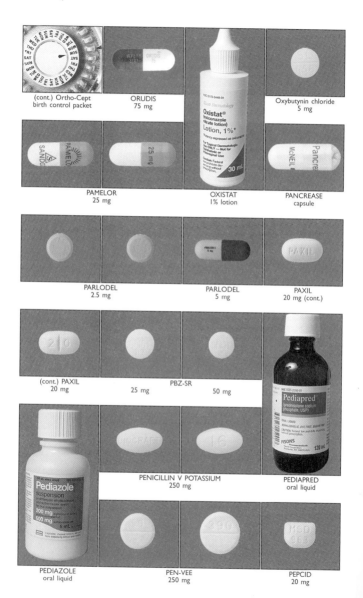

(cont.) Ortho-Cept
birth control packet

ORUDIS
75 mg

OXISTAT
1% lotion

Oxybutynin chloride
5 mg

PAMELOR
25 mg

PANCREASE
capsule

PARLODEL
2.5 mg

PARLODEL
5 mg

PAXIL
20 mg (cont.)

(cont.) PAXIL
20 mg

PBZ-SR
25 mg

50 mg

PENICILLIN V POTASSIUM
250 mg

PEDIAPRED
oral liquid

PEDIAZOLE
oral liquid

PEN-VEE
250 mg

PEPCID
20 mg

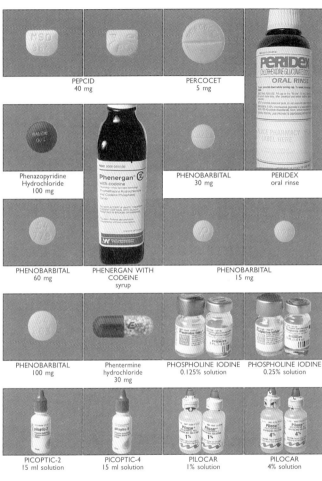

PEPCID
40 mg

PERCOCET
5 mg

PERIDEX
CHLORHEXIDINE GLUCONATE 0.12%
ORAL RINSE

Phenazopyridine
Hydrochloride
100 mg

Phenergan
with codeine

PHENOBARBITAL
30 mg

PERIDEX
oral rinse

PHENOBARBITAL
60 mg

PHENERGAN WITH
CODEINE
syrup

PHENOBARBITAL
15 mg

PHENOBARBITAL
100 mg

Phentermine
hydrochloride
30 mg

PHOSPHOLINE IODINE
0.125% solution

PHOSPHOLINE IODINE
0.25% solution

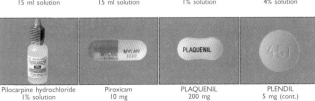

PICOPTIC-2
15 ml solution

PICOPTIC-4
15 ml solution

PILOCAR
1% solution

PILOCAR
4% solution

Pilocarpine hydrochloride
1% solution

Piroxicam
10 mg

PLAQUENIL
200 mg

PLENDIL
5 mg (cont.)

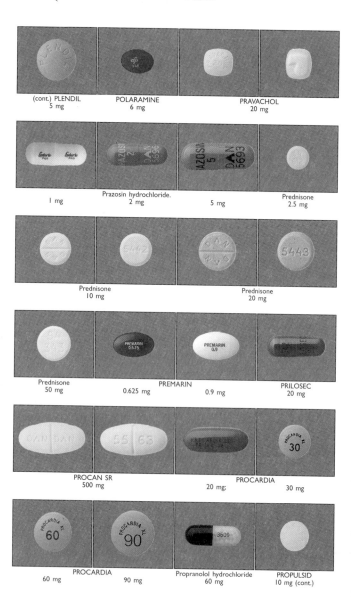

(cont.) PLENDIL
5 mg

POLARAMINE
6 mg

PRAVACHOL
20 mg

1 mg

Prazosin hydrochloride.
2 mg

5 mg

Prednisone
2.5 mg

Prednisone
10 mg

Prednisone
20 mg

Prednisone
50 mg

PREMARIN
0.625 mg

0.9 mg

PRILOSEC
20 mg

PROCAN SR
500 mg

PROCARDIA
20 mg;

30 mg

PROCARDIA
60 mg

90 mg

Propranolol hydrochloride
60 mg

PROPULSID
10 mg (cont.)

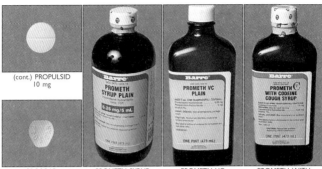

(cont.) PROPULSID
10 mg

PROSCAR
5 mg (cont.)

PROMETH SYRUP
6.25 mg

PROMETH VC
syrup

PROMETH WITH
CODEINE

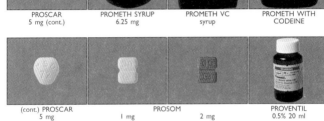

(cont.) PROSCAR
5 mg

PROSOM
1 mg

2 mg

PROVENTIL
0.5% 20 ml

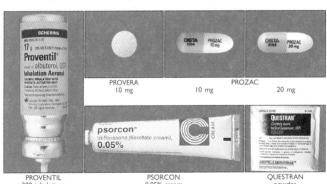

PROVENTIL
200 inhalations

PROVERA
10 mg

PROZAC
10 mg

PROZAC
20 mg

PSORCON
0.05% cream

QUESTRAN
powder,
168 grams

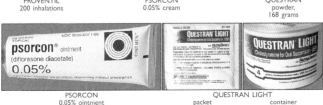

PSORCON
0.05% ointment

QUESTRAN LIGHT
packet   container

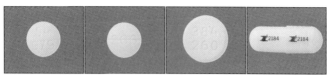

Quinidine sulfate
200 mg

Quinidine sulfate
260 mg   325 mg

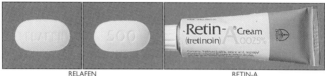

RELAFEN
500 mg

RETIN-A
0.025% cream

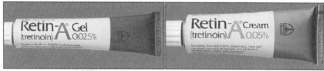

(cont.) RETIN-A
0.025% gel

RETIN-A
0.05% cream

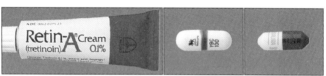

(cont.) RETIN-A
0.1% cream

RETROVIR
100 mg

RIDAURA
1 mg

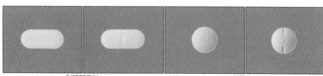

RISPERDAL
1 mg

RITALIN
10 mg

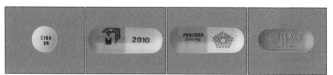

RITALIN
20 mg

ROWASA
250 mg

RYNATAN
15 mg

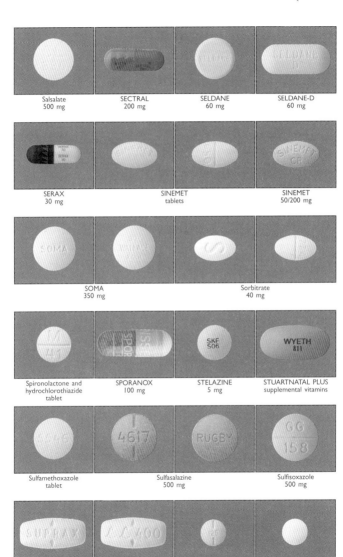

Salsalate
500 mg

SECTRAL
200 mg

SELDANE
60 mg

SELDANE-D
60 mg

SERAX
30 mg

SINEMET
tablets

SINEMET
50/200 mg

SOMA
350 mg

Sorbitrate
40 mg

Spironolactone and
hydrochlorothiazide
tablet

SPORANOX
100 mg

STELAZINE
5 mg

STUARTNATAL PLUS
supplemental vitamins

Sulfamethoxazole
tablet

Sulfasalazine
500 mg

Sulfisoxazole
500 mg

SUPRAX
400 mg

SYNTHROID
0.125 mg

SYNTHROID
50 mg (cont.)

BBB ⦃ **Photo Identification Guide**

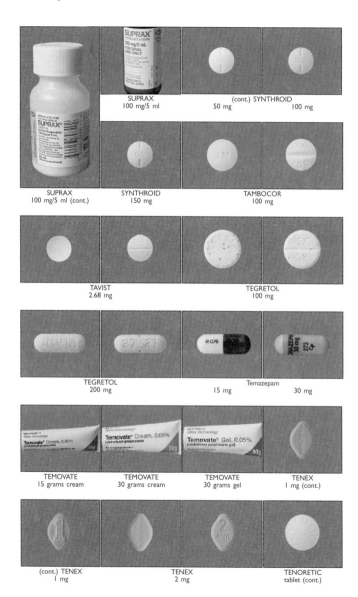

SUPRAX
100 mg/5 ml

(cont.) SYNTHROID
50 mg   100 mg

SUPRAX
100 mg/5 ml (cont.)

SYNTHROID
150 mg

TAMBOCOR
100 mg

TAVIST
2.68 mg

TEGRETOL
100 mg

TEGRETOL
200 mg

Temazepam
15 mg   30 mg

TEMOVATE
15 grams cream

TEMOVATE
30 grams cream

TEMOVATE
30 grams gel

TENEX
1 mg (cont.)

(cont.) TENEX
1 mg

TENEX
2 mg

TENORETIC
tablet (cont.)

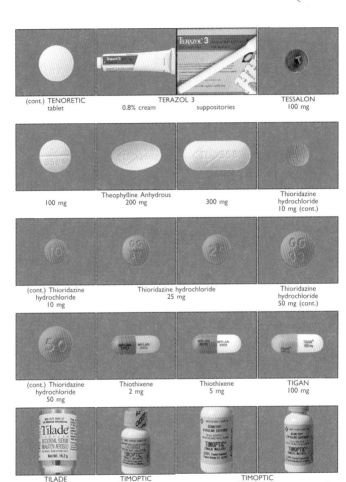

(cont.) TENORETIC
tablet

TERAZOL 3
0.8% cream   suppositories

TESSALON
100 mg

100 mg

Theophylline Anhydrous
200 mg

300 mg

Thioridazine
hydrochloride
10 mg (cont.)

(cont.) Thioridazine
hydrochloride
10 mg

Thioridazine hydrochloride
25 mg

Thioridazine
hydrochloride
50 mg (cont.)

(cont.) Thioridazine
hydrochloride
50 mg

Thiothixene
2 mg

Thiothixene
5 mg

TIGAN
100 mg

TILADE
104 inhalations

TIMOPTIC
5 ml solution

TIMOPTIC
15 ml solution

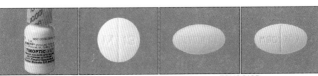

TIMOPTIC-XE
5 ml solution

Tolbutamide
500 mg

TONOCARD
400 mg

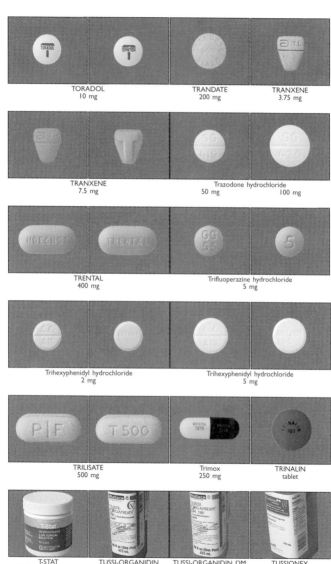

TORADOL
10 mg

TRANDATE
200 mg

TRANXENE
3.75 mg

TRANXENE
7.5 mg

Trazodone hydrochloride
50 mg   100 mg

TRENTAL
400 mg

Trifluoperazine hydrochloride
5 mg

Trihexyphenidyl hydrochloride
2 mg

Trihexyphenidyl hydrochloride
5 mg

TRILISATE
500 mg

Trimox
250 mg

TRINALIN
tablet

T-STAT
2.0% topical, 60 pads

TUSSI-ORGANIDIN
473 ml
16 fluid oz.

TUSSI-ORGANIDIN DM
473 ml
16 fluid oz.

TUSSIONEX
473 ml

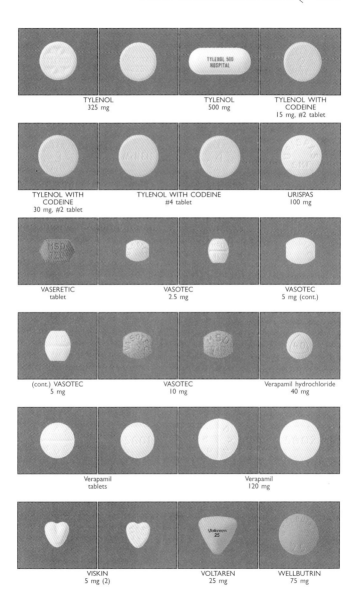

TYLENOL
325 mg

TYLENOL
500 mg

TYLENOL WITH
CODEINE
15 mg, #2 tablet

TYLENOL WITH
CODEINE
30 mg, #2 tablet

TYLENOL WITH CODEINE
#4 tablet

URISPAS
100 mg

VASERETIC
tablet

VASOTEC
2.5 mg

VASOTEC
5 mg (cont.)

(cont.) VASOTEC
5 mg

VASOTEC
10 mg

Verapamil hydrochloride
40 mg

Verapamil
tablets

Verapamil
120 mg

VISKIN
5 mg (2)

VOLTAREN
25 mg

WELLBUTRIN
75 mg

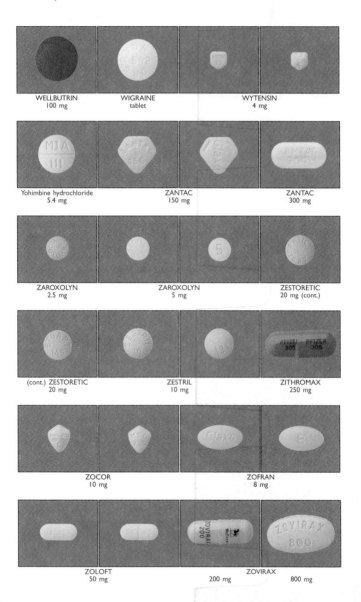

WELLBUTRIN
100 mg

WIGRAINE
tablet

WYTENSIN
4 mg

Yohimbine hydrochloride
5.4 mg

ZANTAC
150 mg

ZANTAC
300 mg

ZAROXOLYN
2.5 mg

ZAROXOLYN
5 mg

ZESTORETIC
20 mg (cont.)

(cont.) ZESTORETIC
20 mg

ZESTRIL
10 mg

ZITHROMAX
250 mg

ZOCOR
10 mg

ZOFRAN
8 mg

ZOLOFT
50 mg

ZOVIRAX

200 mg   800 mg

Use with caution if you have any abnormal condition of blood vessels outside the heart, or have recently had a heart attack or stroke.

Miltown

Generic name: Meprobamate

Other brand names: Equanil, Meprospan, Neuramate

Miltown is a minor tranquilizer. It calms certain areas of the brain and allows the rest of the brain to function normally.

℞ QUICK FACTS

Purpose

 Used to treat anxiety disorders and provide short-term relief for anxiety.

Dosage

 Take exactly as prescribed. Follow doctor's instructions for reducing or discontinuing medication.

Usual adult dose: *Miltown 200 and 400*—1,200 to 1,600 milligrams per day divided into 3 or 4 doses, not to exceed 2,400 milligrams per day. *Miltown 600*—one tablet 2 times per day, not to exceed 2,400 milligrams per day. *Seniors*—prescribed lowest possible dose.

 Usual child dose: *for children 6 to 12 years—Miltown 200 and 400*—200 to 600 milligrams per day divided into 2 or 3 doses. Not recommended for children under 6 years.

Missed dose: take as soon as possible, up to 1 hour past regular schedule. Otherwise, do not take missed dose; go back to regular schedule. *Do not double doses.*

Side Effects

 Overdose symptoms: coma, drowsiness, lack or loss of muscle control, shock, sluggishness and unresponsiveness. If you suspect an overdose, immediately seek medical attention.

 More common side effects: bruises, diarrhea, dizziness, drowsiness, exaggerated feeling of well-being, fainting, fast or throbbing heartbeat, fever, headache, inappropriate excitement, itchy rash, loss of muscle coordination, nausea, rapid or irregular heartbeat, skin eruptions, slurred speech, small or purplish skin spots, swelling due to fluid retention, tingling sensation, vertigo, vision problems, vomiting, weakness.

 Less common or rare side effects: breathing difficulty, chills, high fever, inflammation of the mouth, little or no urine, redness and swelling of skin, severe allergic reaction, skin inflammation and flaking, Stevens-Johnson syndrome (peeling skin). Side effects due to sudden decrease in dose or withdrawal: anxiety, confusion, convulsions, hallucinations, inability to fall or stay asleep, lack or loss of appetite, lack or loss of coordination, muscle twitching, tremors, vomiting. Withdrawal symptoms appear 12 to 48 hours after discontinuation and should disappear in another 12 to 48 hours.

Interactions

 Inform your doctor before combining Miltown with: barbiturates such as Seconal and phenobarbital, major tranquilizers such as Thorazine and Mellaril, narcotics such as Percocet and Demerol, MAO inhibitors such as Nardil and Parnate.

· · · · · · · · · ·

 Do not drink alcohol during Miltown therapy; it intensifies the effects of alcohol.

Special Cautions

 Do not take if pregnant or planning to become pregnant; *increased risk of birth defects.* Appears in breast milk; could affect a nursing infant.

· · · · · · · · · ·

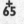 Seniors are prescribed lowest possible dose to avoid oversedation.

· · · · · · · · · ·

 Follow doctor's instructions carefully for children. Not recommended for children under 6 years.

· · · · · · · · · ·

 May cause drowsiness and impair your ability to drive a car or operate machinery. *Do not take part in any activity that requires alertness.*

· · · · · · · · · ·

Inform your doctor *before* starting Miltown if you have liver or kidney disorders.

If you already experience seizures, Miltown may prompt them.

Monitor for tolerance of and dependence on this medication.

Should not take if sensitive to or allergic to this or similar medications. Contact your doctor if you experience such allergic reactions as skin rash, sore throat, fever, shortness of breath.

Miltown is not prescribed for everyday anxiety or tension.

Minipress

‹‹‹

Generic name: Prazosin hydrochloride

Minipress is an antihypertensive. It is thought to act on the central nervous system to prevent the release of chemicals responsible for maintaining high blood pressure.

℞ QUICK FACTS

Purpose

℞   Used to treat high blood pressure. Also used to treat benign prostatic hyperplasia (BPH), enlargement of the prostate gland.

Dosage

 Take with or without food. May take weeks to observe results if taking for high blood pressure; must continue to take even if you feel better. Adhere to schedule; if not taken regularly, blood pressure will increase.

 Usual adult dose: *initial dose*—1 milligram taken 2 or 3 times per day. *Regular dose*—6 to 15 milligrams per day divided into smaller doses, up to 40 milligrams maximum.

 Usual child dose: not generally prescribed for children.

 Missed dose: take as soon as possible, unless almost time for next dose. In that case, do not take missed dose; go back to regular schedule. *Do not double doses.*

Side Effects

 Overdose symptoms: extreme drowsiness, low blood pressure. If you suspect an overdose, immediately seek medical attention.

 More common side effects: dizziness, drowsiness, headache, lack of energy, nausea, palpitations, weakness.

 Less common side effects: blurred vision; constipation; depression; diarrhea; dizziness upon standing; dry mouth; fainting; fluid retention; frequent urination; nasal congestion; nervousness; nosebleeds; rash; red eyes; shortness of breath; vertigo; vomiting. Rare side effects: abdominal discomfort or pain; excessive perspiration; fever; hair loss; hallucinations; impotence; inability to hold urine; inflammation of the pancreas; itching; itchy purple spots on wrists, forearms, and thighs; joint pain; persistent, painful erection; rapid heartbeat; ringing in ears; tingling or pins and needles.

Interactions

 Inform your doctor before combining Minipress with: beta-blockers such as Inderal; dextroamphetamine (Dexedrine); diuretics such as Dyazide; ibuprofen (Motrin or Advil); other high blood pressure medications; verapamil (Calan or Verelan).

 Avoid alcohol; may intensify its effects.

Special Cautions

 If pregnant or planning to become pregnant, inform your doctor immediately. Appears in breast milk; could affect a nursing infant.

 No special precautions apply to seniors.

Not generally prescribed for children.

 May cause dizziness when first starting medication. Avoid any hazardous activities such as driving for 24 hours after first dose, and after each dose increase. At risk for dizziness in hot weather, during exercise, or standing for long periods.

Minocin

Generic name: Minocycline hydrochloride

Other brand name: Dynacin

Minocin is a tetracycline antibiotic. It is used to prevent bacteria from multiplying and growing. It is an alternative drug for those who are allergic to penicillin.

℞ QUICK FACTS

Purpose

 Used to treat infections, including: acne, amebic dysentery, anthrax (rare skin infection), cholera, gonorrhea, plague, respiratory infections such as pneumonia, Rocky Mountain spotted fever, syphilis, urinary tract infections caused by certain microbes.

Dosage

 Take the entire prescription, even if you feel better after a few days. Adhere to schedule to keep a constant level of the medication in the body. May take with or without food; drink plenty of fluids.

 Usual adult dose: 200 milligrams followed by 100 milligrams every 12 hours. Doctor may increase dose to two or four 50-milligram capsules followed by one 50-milligram capsule 4 times per day.

Usual child dose: *for children 8 years and older—4 milligrams per 2.2 pounds of body weight, followed by 2 milligrams per 2.2 pounds of body weight every 12 hours.*

Missed dose: take as soon as possible; then take remaining doses at evenly spaced intervals for that day. *Never double doses.*

Side Effects

Overdose symptoms: no specific information available. However, if you suspect an overdose, immediately seek medical attention.

Side effects: aching or inflamed joints, anal or genital sores with fungus infection, anaphylaxis (life-threatening allergic reaction), anemia, appetite loss, blurry vision, bulging of soft spots on infants' heads, decreased hearing, diarrhea, difficulty swallowing, discoloration of children's teeth, fluid retention, headache, hepatitis, hives, inflammation of head of penis, inflammation of intestines, inflammation of tongue, nausea, rash, sensitivity to light, skin coloration, skin inflammation and peeling, throat irritation, vomiting.

No known less common or rare side effects.

Interactions

Inform your doctor before combining Minocin with: blood thinners such as Coumadin, oral contraceptives, penicillin (Pen•Vee K).

Avoid using antacids containing aluminum, calcium, or magnesium, such as Maalox, and iron preparations such as Feosol, or take 2 to 3 hours before or after taking Minocin.

Special Cautions

 If pregnant or planning to become pregnant, inform your doctor immediately. May cause discoloration of baby's teeth if taken in 2nd half of pregnancy. Minocin may cause other harm to a developing baby, so should take only if it cannot be replaced with a non-tetracycline antibiotic. Appears in breast milk; could affect a nursing infant.

 No special precautions apply to seniors.

 Follow doctor's instructions carefully for children 8 years and older. Not generally prescribed for children under 8 years.

 Do not take if allergic to tetracycline antibiotics.

Should not be used to treat meningococcal meningitis; is used only to kill the meningococcal bacteria in people who are carriers.

Not for use in treating a staph infection.

If you have a kidney disorder, normal dosage levels will trigger overdose. Doctor should frequently test your blood for overdosage.

May cause dizziness when first starting medication. Avoid any hazardous activities such as driving until you know how the medication affects you.

Use care in sunlight; may cause sensitivity and easy sunburning. If you experience red and/or hot skin, immediately stop taking Minocin.

Contact your doctor immediately if you develop a fungus infection, such as a yeast infection.

Monitor for signs of fluid buildup in the skull—adults (headache, blurry vision); and infants ("soft spots," or fontanels, on the head). Immediately stop taking, contact your doctor.

Minocycline Hydrochloride

see MINOCIN

Minoxidil

see ROGAINE, TOPICAL

Minoxidil, Oral

see LONITEN

Misoprostol

see CYTOTEC

Moduretic

Generic ingredients: Amiloride with hydrochlorothiazide

Moduretic is a thiazide and potassium-sparing diuretic. It promotes the loss of salt and water in the body, and increases the diameter of the blood vessels, thereby lowering blood pressure, and it helps minimize potassium loss.

℞ QUICK FACTS

Purpose

℞ Used to treat high blood pressure and congestive heart failure.

Dosage

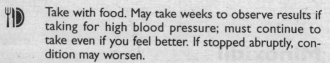 Take with food. May take weeks to observe results if taking for high blood pressure; must continue to take even if you feel better. If stopped abruptly, condition may worsen.

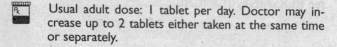 Usual adult dose: 1 tablet per day. Doctor may increase up to 2 tablets either taken at the same time or separately.

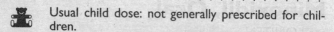 Usual child dose: not generally prescribed for children.

Missed dose: take as soon as possible, unless almost time for next dose. In that case, do not take missed dose; go back to regular schedule. *Do not double doses.*

Side Effects

Overdose symptom: no specific information available; may experience dehydration. However, if you suspect an overdose, immediately seek medical attention.

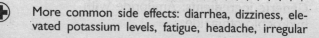 More common side effects: diarrhea, dizziness, elevated potassium levels, fatigue, headache, irregular

heartbeat, itching, leg pain, loss of appetite, nausea, rash, shortness of breath, stomach and intestinal pain, weakness.

 Less common or rare side effects: anemia, appetite changes, back pain, bad taste, breast development in males, changes in liver function, changes in potassium levels leading to dry mouth, excessive thirst, weak or irregular heartbeat, muscle pain or cramps, chest pain, constipation, cough, decreased sex drive, dehydration, depression, dermatitis, dizziness upon standing up, dry mouth, excessive perspiration, excessive night urination, fainting, fever, fluid in lungs, flushing, frequent urination, fullness in abdomen, gas, gout, hair loss, heartburn, hiccups, hives, impotence, incontinence, indigestion, insomnia, itching, joint pain, mental confusion, muscle cramps, nasal congestion, neck and shoulder ache, nervousness, numbness, painful or difficult urination, rapid heartbeat, ringing in ears, sensitivity to light, sleepiness, Stevens-Johnson syndrome (peeling skin), stomach and intestinal bleeding, stupor, sugar in blood or urine, thirst, tingling or pins and needles, tremors, vague feeling of bodily discomfort, vertigo, vision changes, vomiting, yellow eyes and skin.

Interactions

Inform your doctor before combining Moduretic with: ACE inhibitors such as Vasotec; barbiturates such as Phenobarbital; cholestyramine (Questran); colestipol (Colestid); corticosteroids such as prednisone; insulin; lithium (Lithonate); muscle relaxants such as Tubocurarine; narcotics such as Percocet; nonsteroidal anti-inflammatory medications such as Naprosyn; oral diabetes medications such as Micronase and DiaBeta; other high blood pressure medications. Use Moduretic with extreme caution if taking ACE inhibitors such as Vasotec.

Avoid alcohol; may intensify its effects. Limit intake of potassium-rich foods, and avoid potassium supplements or potassium-containing salt substitutes, and other diuretics.

Special Cautions

 If pregnant or planning to become pregnant, inform your doctor immediately. Appears in breast milk; could affect a nursing infant.

 No special precautions apply to seniors.

 Not generally prescribed for children.

 Should not take if you are unable to urinate, have serious kidney disease, or have high potassium levels in your blood.

If sensitive or allergic to this or similar medications, or sulfonamide-derived medications, should not take. May be at risk for allergic reaction if you have bronchial asthma or history of allergies.

Use cautiously if you have liver disease, diabetes, gout, or lupus erythematosus.

Doctor should completely assess kidneys, and continue to monitor during Moduretic therapy.

Use caution to not deplete your fluids—may cause blood pressure to become too low. Monitor severe diarrhea or vomiting, excessive sweating, or exercising.

Inform your doctor or dentist that you are taking Moduretic in the case of an emergency or surgery.

Mometasone Furoate

see ELOCON

Monistat

Generic name: Miconazole nitrate

Other brand name: Micatin

Monistat is an antifungal. It destroys and prevents the growth of fungi.

℞ QUICK FACTS

Purpose

Used to treat fungal infections. Monistat 3 and 7 are used for vaginal yeast infections. Monistat-Derm is used to treat skin infections such as athlete's foot, ringworm, jock itch, yeast infection on the skin, and tinea versicolor.

Dosage

Take exactly as prescribed. *If using vaginal form, do not douche unless directed to by your doctor. Do not scratch—causes more irritation and may spread infection.* Continue taking prescription even if symptoms disappear; not finishing prescription may cause infection to return. Use even if your menstrual period starts.

Usual adult dose: *vaginal cream*—1 applicatorful inserted vaginally at bedtime for 7 consecutive days. *Vaginal suppositories*—1 suppository inserted vaginally at bedtime for 7 consecutive days. *Monistat-Derm*—apply thin layer over affected area morning and night. For tinea versicolor, apply thin layer over affected area once per day.

 Usual child dose: follow doctor's instructions carefully for children.

 Missed dose: take as soon as possible, unless almost time for next dose. In that case, do not take missed dose; go back to regular schedule.

Side Effects

 Overdose symptoms: none reported. However, if you suspect an overdose, immediately seek medical attention.

 Side effects: burning sensation, cramping, headaches, hives, irritation, rash, vulval or vaginal itching.

 No known less common or rare side effects.

Interactions

 No known drug interactions.

 No known food/other substance interactions.

Special Cautions

 Do not use if first trimester of pregnancy; is absorbed in small amounts from the vagina. If pregnant or planning to become pregnant, inform your doctor immediately. Not known if Monistat appears in breast milk.

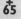 No special precautions apply to seniors.

 Follow doctor's instructions carefully for children. *Do not give to girls under 12 years.*

Avoid use if you have: fever above 100°F (using an oral thermometer); foul-smelling vaginal discharge; pain in the lower abdomen, back, or either shoulder. If these symptoms develop during Monistat use, stop treatment and contact your doctor.

Contact your doctor if the infection has not improved within 3 days or relief is not complete within 7 days, or if symptoms return within 2 months.

If sensitive to or allergic to this medication, should not use.

Inform your doctor of any irritation, or if symptoms persist.

Vaginal cream or suppositories may interact with latex used in vaginal diaphragms and condoms.

Avoid sexual intercourse if using suppositories, or use a condom.

Monopril

Generic name: Fosinopril sodium

Monopril is an angiotensin-converting enzyme (ACE) inhibitor. It works to reduce blood pressure by preventing angiotensin I from converting into a more potent enzyme that increases salt and water retention.

℞ QUICK FACTS

Purpose

℞ Used to treat high blood pressure.

Dosage

 Take one hour before meals or with food if you experience stomach irritation. May take weeks to observe results if taking for high blood pressure; must continue to take even if you feel better. If stopped abruptly, may cause increase in blood pressure.

 Usual adult dose: 10 milligrams taken once per day. After blood pressure adjusts, 20 to 40 milligrams per day in a single dose. Diuretics should be stopped prior to Monopril therapy; otherwise, doctor may give initial dose of 10 milligrams. *Seniors*—dose prescribed according to individual needs.

 Usual child dose: not generally prescribed for children.

 Missed dose: take as soon as possible, unless almost time for next dose. In that case, do not take missed dose; go back to regular schedule.

Side Effects

 Overdose symptom: sudden drop in blood pressure. If you suspect an overdose, immediately seek medical attention.

 More common side effects: cough, diarrhea, dizziness, fatigue, headache, nausea, vomiting.

 Less common or rare side effects: abdominal pain, anaphylaxis (severe allergic reaction), changes in appetite and weight, changes in sexual performance, confusion, constipation, decreased sex drive, drowsiness, dry mouth, excessive sweating, eye irritation, gas, heartburn, itching, kidney failure, liver failure, muscle cramps, rash, ringing in ears, skin sensitivity to sunlight, sleep disturbances, tremors, vertigo, vision disturbances, weakness, yellow eyes and skin.

Interactions

Inform your doctor before combining Monopril with: antacids such as Maalox and Mylanta, Lithium, potassium preparations such as K-Ten and K-Lyte, potassium-sparing diuretics such as Moduretic and Aldactone, thiazide diuretics such as Esidrix and Diuril.

Avoid using potassium-containing salt substitutes unless directed by your doctor.

Special Cautions

ACE inhibitors have caused damage and death of fetus if used in 2nd or 3rd trimesters. If pregnant, discontinue use of this medication as soon as possible. If planning to become pregnant, discuss hazards of this medication. Appears in breast milk, could affect a nursing infant.

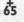

Dose prescribed according to individual needs for seniors.

Not generally prescribed for children.

Swelling of the face, lips, tongue or throat, or arms and legs or difficulty swallowing may indicate the need for emergency treatment. Immediately contact your doctor.

If you faint during first few days of therapy, stop taking and notify your doctor at once.

Use with caution if on dialysis, at risk for extreme allergic reactions.

If sensitive to or allergic to this or similar medications, should not take.

Inform your doctor immediately if you develop a sore throat or fever.

Tell your doctor if you have kidney or liver problems, or connective tissue disease. With connective disease, may need blood tests.

When taken with a diuretic in high doses, may cause very low blood pressure.

If you have congestive heart failure, doctor should closely monitor you for the first 2 weeks, and whenever the dosage is increased.

Use caution to not deplete your fluids—may cause blood pressure to become dangerously low. Monitor severe diarrhea or vomiting, excessive sweating, or exercising.

Morphine Sulfate

see MS CONTIN

Motrin

see ADVIL

MS Contin

Generic name: Morphine sulfate

Other brand names: Astramorph, Duramorph, MSIR, Oramorph SR, RMS, Roxanol, Roxanol SR

MS Contin is a narcotic analgesic. It relieves pain and gives a feeling of well-being.

℞ QUICK FACTS

Purpose

℞ Used to relieve moderate to severe pain. For people needing a morphine painkiller for more than a few days.

Dosage

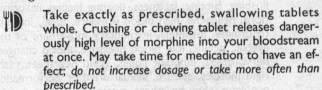 Take exactly as prescribed, swallowing tablets whole. Crushing or chewing tablet releases dangerously high level of morphine into your bloodstream at once. May take time for medication to have an effect; *do not increase dosage or take more often than prescribed.*

 Usual adult dose: based on individual needs due to high potency of this medication.

 Usual child dose: not generally prescribed for children.

 Missed dose: take as soon as possible, unless almost time for next dose. In that case, do not take missed dose; go back to regular schedule. *Do not double doses.*

Side Effects

 Overdose can be fatal. Overdose symptoms: cold and clammy skin, flaccid muscles, lowered blood pressure, pinpoint pupils, sleepiness leading to stupor and coma, slowed breathing, slow pulse rate. If you

suspect an overdose, immediately seek medical attention.

 Most dangerous potential side effect: respiratory depression (dangerously slow breathing). More common side effects: constipation, depressed or irritable mood, dizziness, exaggerated sense of well-being, light-headedness, nausea, sedation, sweating, vomiting. Some side effects may be reduced by lying down.

Less common side effects: agitation, appetite loss, apprehension, blurred vision, chills, constipation, cramps, depression, diarrhea, difficult urination, disorientation, double vision, dreams, dry mouth, facial flushing, fainting, faintness, floating feeling, hallucinations, headache, high blood pressure, hives, inability to urinate, insomnia, involuntary movement of the eyeball, itching, low blood pressure, mood changes, nervousness, pinpoint pupils, rapid heartbeat, rash, rigid muscles, seizure, sexual drive or performance problems, slow heartbeat, sweating, swelling due to fluid retention, taste alterations, throbbing heartbeat, tingling or pins and needles, tremor, uncoordinated muscle movements, vision disturbances, weakness. Withdrawal symptoms after long use of MS Contin: dilated pupils, goose bumps, restlessness, restless sleep, runny nose, sweating, tearing, yawning. Withdrawal symptoms after 72 hours: abdominal and leg pains, abdominal and muscle cramps, anxiety, diarrhea, hot and cold flashes, inability to fall or stay asleep, increase in body temperature, increase in blood pressure and breathing, increase in heart rate, kicking movements, loss of appetite, nasal discharge, nausea, severe backache, sneezing, twitching and muscle spasms, vomiting, weakness. Withdrawal symptoms after 1 to 2 weeks: aching muscles, insomnia, and irritability lasting for 2 to 6 months.

Interactions

 Inform your doctor before combining MS Contin with: certain analgesics such as Talwin, Nubain, Stadol, and Buprenex; major tranquilizers such as Thorazine and Phenergan; muscle relaxants such as Flexeril and Valium; sedatives such as Dalmane and Halcion; tranquilizers such as Librium and Xanax.

 Do not drink alcohol while taking MS Contin.

Special Cautions

 If pregnant or planning to become pregnant, inform your doctor immediately. If taken during close to birth of baby, baby may experience breathing problems, and may also suffer withdrawal symptoms. Appears in breast milk, *do not take while breastfeeding, baby may experience withdrawal symptoms when you stop taking MS Contin.*

 Seniors may be at risk for respiratory depression.

 Not generally prescribed for children.

 Do not take if sensitive to or allergic to morphine, or if you have bronchial asthma.

May cause drowsiness and impair your ability to drive a car or operate machinery. *Do not take part in any activity that requires alertness.*

Use with extreme caution if you have: alcoholism, coma, curvature of the spine, delirium tremens (severe alcohol withdrawal), drug-related psychosis, enlarged prostate or constricted urinary canal, kidney disorder, liver disorder, low adrenaline levels, lung disorder, swallowing difficulty.

Can increase risk of seizure if epileptic.

May be at risk for respiratory depression if you have a lung or breathing problem.

If you have abnormally slow breathing, should not take unless there is access to resuscitation equipment.

Should not take if you have intestinal blockage, brain injury, or abdominal problem requiring surgery.

Use cautiously if you are having biliary tract surgery; may worsen condition.

May experience dizziness upon standing, due to lowered blood pressure.

Mupirocin

see BACTROBAN

Mycolog-II

Generic ingredients: Nystatin with triamcinolone acetonide

Other brand names: Myco-Triacet II, Mytrex

Mycolog-II is an antifungal and steroid combination. It destroys and prevents the growth of fungi, and interferes with the natural body mechanisms that produce rash, itching, or inflammation.

℞ Quick Facts

Purpose

 Used to treat candidiasis of the skin.

Dosage

 Use entire amount prescribed, even if symptoms disappear. If applying to groin area, use very little and wear clothes that fit loosely. *Do not bandage affected area unless directed by your doctor. Do not use more often or longer than prescribed.* Keep affected area cool and dry. Avoid eye contact.

 Usual adult dose: *cream*—applied to affected areas 2 times per day in the morning and evening. If symptoms persist after 25 days, doctor will stop treatment. *Ointment*—applied to affected areas 2 times per day in the morning and evening. If symptoms persist after 25 days, doctor will stop treatment.

 Usual child dose: follow doctor's instructions for dosage.

 Missed dose: apply as soon as possible, unless almost time for next dose. In that case, do not apply missed dose; go back to regular schedule.

Side Effects

 Overdose symptoms: long-term use may cause reactions throughout the body due to steroid excess, including weight gain, reddening and rounding of the face and neck, growth of excess body and facial hair, high blood pressure, emotional disturbances, increased blood sugar, urinary excretion of glucose. If you suspect an overdose, immediately seek medical attention.

Side effects: blistering, burning, dryness, eruptions resembling acne, excessive discoloring of skin, excessive growth of hair (especially facial hair), hair loss (especially scalp), inflammation around mouth, inflammation of hair follicles, irritation, itching, peeling, prickly heat, reddish-purple lines on skin, secondary infection, severe inflammation of skin, softening of skin, stretch marks, stretching or thinning of skin.

 No known less common or rare side effects.

Interactions

 No drug interactions reported.

 No known food/other substance interactions.

Special Cautions

 If pregnant or planning to become pregnant, inform your doctor. Not known if Mycolog-II appears in breast milk.

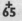 No special precautions apply to seniors.

 Follow doctor's instructions carefully for children. Avoid using tight-fitting diapers or plastic pants if diaper area is being treated.

 Do not use for any condition other than the prescribed condition.

If sensitive to or allergic to this or other antifungals or steroids, should not take.

Inform your doctor if an irritation develops.

. . . .

Contact your doctor if there is no improvement or condition worsens after 2 to 3 weeks.

Mykrox

see ZAROXOLYN

Mysoline

Generic name: Primidone

Other brand names: Myidone, Sertan

Mysoline is an anticonvulsant. It acts as a central nervous system depressant.

℞ QUICK FACTS

Purpose

℞ Used to treat epileptic and other seizures.

Dosage

 Take exactly as prescribed. *Do not change brands unless directed by your doctor. Should not stop abruptly; may cause seizures.* If using suspension form, shake well before each use. May take several weeks to observe full effects of medication.

 Usual adult dose: *for children 8 years and older and adults who are being treated for the first time—Day 1 to Day 3—100 to 125 milligrams at bedtime. Day 4 to Day 6—100 to 125 milligrams taken 2 times per day. Day 7 to Day 9—100 to 125 milligrams taken 3 times per day. Day 10 to maintenance—250 milligrams taken 3 to 4 times per day. For patients already using*

anticonvulsants—starting dose of 100 to 125 milligrams at bedtime, and gradually increased to a maintenance level.

 Usual child dose: *for children under 8 years—Day 1 to Day 3*—50 milligrams at bedtime. *Day 4 to Day 6*—50 milligrams taken 2 times per day. *Day 7 to Day 9*—100 milligrams taken 2 times per day. *Day 10 to maintenance*—125 to 150 milligrams taken 3 times per day, up to 250 milligrams taken 3 times per day, or 10 to 25 milligrams per 2.2 pounds of body weight per day.

 Missed dose: take as soon as possible, unless within 1 hour of next dose. In that case, do not take missed dose; go back to regular schedule. *Do not double doses.*

Side Effects

 Overdose symptoms: no specific information available. However, if you suspect an overdose, immediately seek medical attention.

 More common side effects: lack of muscle coordination, vertigo.

 Less common side effects: double vision, drowsiness, emotional disturbances, excessive irritability, fatigue, impotence, loss of appetite, nausea, skin eruptions resembling measles, uncontrolled eyeball movements, vomiting.

Interactions

 Inform your doctor before combining Mysoline with: blood thinners such as Coumadin; doxycycline (Doryx or Vibramycin); estrogen-containing oral contraceptives such as Ortho-Novum and Triphasil; griseofulvin (Fulvisin-U/F or Grifulvin V); MAO inhibitors such as Nardil and Parnate; steroid medications such as Decadron.

 Avoid alcohol during Mysoline therapy.

Special Cautions

 If pregnant or planning to become pregnant, inform your doctor immediately. Increased risk of birth defects in infants born to epileptic women taking anticonvulsants. Appears in breast milk; could affect a nursing infant.

 No special precautions apply to seniors.

 Follow doctor's instructions carefully for children.

 Should not take if you have porphyria (inherited metabolic disorder), or if you are sensitive to or allergic to phenobarbital.

Doctor should check your blood count every 6 months.

Mytrex
see MYCOLOG-II

Nabumetone
see RELAFEN

Nadolol
see CORGARD

Nadolol with Bendroflumethiazide
see CORZIDE

Napamide
see NORPACE

Naphazoline Hydrochloride with Pheniramine Maleate
see NAPHCON-A

Naphcon-A

Generic ingredients: Naphazoline hydrochloride with pheniramine maleate

Other brand names: Ak-Con, Albalon, Allerest, Clear Eyes, Comfort Eye Drops, Degest 2, I-Naphline, Muro's Opcon, Privine Hydrochloride, VasoClear, Vasocon

Naphcon-A is a decongestant and vasoconstrictor. It constricts nasal and sinus blood vessels, opening up air passages.

℞ QUICK FACTS

Purpose

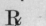 Used to relieve eye irritation and allergic eye conditions.

Dosage

 Remove contact lens before administering. *Do not use if solution clouds or changes color.*

 Usual adult dose: 1 or 2 drops in each eye every 3 to 4 hours or less.

 Usual child dose: *do not give to infants or children; may cause stupor or coma, or severe drop in body temperature.*

 Missed dose: use on an as needed basis only.

Side Effects

 Overdose: may have serious consequences. If you suspect an overdose, immediately seek medical attention.

Side effects: dilated pupils, drowsiness, high blood pressure, high blood sugar, increased pressure inside eyeball, irregular heartbeat.

 No known less common or rare side effects.

Interactions

 Do not use with MAO inhibitors such as Nardil or Parnate. May cause sudden and dangerous elevation of blood pressure.

 No known food/other substance interactions.

Special Cautions

 If pregnant or planning to become pregnant, inform your doctor immediately. Not known if Naphcon-A appears in breast milk.

 No special precautions apply to seniors.

 Not generally prescribed for children.

 Do not take if sensitive to or allergic to any ingredients of this medication.

Do not use if you have glaucoma.

May blur vision temporarily; use caution when driving or performing other hazardous activities.

Use with caution if you have: severe heart disease (including heartbeat irregularity), high blood pressure that is not under control, or diabetes, especially if prone to ketoacidosis.

Naprosyn

Generic name: Naproxen

Naprosyn is a nonsteroidal anti-inflammatory drug (NSAID). It works by blocking the production of prostaglandins, which may trigger pain.

℞ QUICK FACTS

Purpose

Used to relieve inflammation, swelling, stiffness, and joint pain associated with rheumatoid arthritis, juvenile arthritis, osteoarthritis, ankylosing spondylitis (spinal arthritis), tendinitis, bursitis, and acute gout. Also used to relieve menstrual cramps and mild to moderate pain.

Dosage

Take with food or antacid and a full glass of water to avoid stomach irritation. If taking for arthritis, take on regular basis, as prescribed.

Usual adult dose: *for rheumatoid arthritis, osteoarthritis, and ankylosing spondylitis*—250 milligrams (10 milliliters or 2 teaspoons of suspension), 375 milligrams (15 milliliters or 3 teaspoons), or 500 milligrams (20 milliliters or 4 teaspoons) 2 times per day in the morning and evening. *For acute gout*—750 milligrams (30 milliliters or 6 teaspoons), followed by 250 milligrams (10 milliliters or 2 teaspoons) every 8 hours until symptoms are relieved. *For mild to moderate pain, menstrual cramps, acute tendinitis and bursitis*—500 milligrams (20 milliliters or 4 teaspoons), followed by 250 milligrams (10 milliliters or

2 teaspoons) every 6 to 8 hours as needed. Maximum dose is 1,250 milligrams (50 milliliters or 10 teaspoons).

 Usual child dose: *for juvenile arthritis*—10 milligrams per 2.2 pounds of body weight, taken 2 times per day. Follow doctor's instructions carefully for children. Not prescribed for children under 2 years.

 Missed dose: *if on a regular schedule*—take as soon as possible, unless almost time for next dose. In that case; do not take missed dose, go back to regular schedule. *Do not double doses.*

Side Effects

 Overdose symptoms: drowsiness, heartburn, indigestion, nausea, vomiting. If you suspect an overdose, immediately seek medical attention.

 More common side effects: abdominal pain, bruising, constipation, difficult or labored breathing, dizziness, drowsiness, headache, heartburn, itching, nausea, ringing in ears, skin eruptions, swelling due to fluid retention.

 Less common or rare side effects: abdominal bleeding, black stools, blood in urine, changes in liver function, chills and fever, colitis, congestive heart failure, depression, diarrhea, dream abnormalities, general feeling of illness, hair loss, hearing disturbances or loss, inability to sleep, indigestion, inflammation of lungs, inflammation of mouth, kidney disease or failure, light-headedness, menstrual disorders, muscle pain and weakness, peptic ulcer, red or purple spots on skin, severe allergic reaction, skin inflammation due to sensitivity to light, skin rashes, sweating, thirst, throbbing heartbeat, vertigo, visual disturbances, vomiting of blood, yellow skin and eyes.

Interactions

 Inform your doctor before combining Naprosyn with: aspirin, beta-blockers such as Tenormin, blood thinners such as Coumadin, furosemide (Lasix), lithium (Lithonate), methotrexate, naproxen sodium (Anaprox), phenytoin (Dilantin), probenecid (Benemid), sulfa medications such as Bactrim and Septra, oral diabetes medications such as Diabinese and Micronase.

 No known food/other substance interactions.

Special Cautions

 If pregnant or planning to become pregnant, inform your doctor immediately. Appears in breast milk; could affect a nursing infant.

 No special precautions apply to seniors.

 Follow doctor's instructions carefully for children.

 May cause drowsiness and impair your ability to drive a car or operate machinery. *Do not take part in any activity that requires alertness.*

You should not take Naprosyn if you have had any reactions to this medication, Anaprox, or similar drugs; or if you have had asthma or nasal inflammation or tumors caused by aspirin or similar medications.

Ulcers or internal bleeding can occur without warning; doctor should monitor.

Use with caution if you have heart disease, high blood pressure, or kidney or liver disease.

May cause vision problems or changes in vision; monitor closely, and report any changes to your doctor.

Use with caution if you are taking a blood-thinning medication.

Can increase water retention, use cautiously if you have high blood pressure or heart disease.

Inform your doctor if you are on a low-sodium diet.

Naproxen

see NAPROSYN

Naproxen Sodium

see ANAPROX

Nardil

Generic name: Phenelzine sulfate

Nardil is a monoamine oxidase (MAO) inhibitor antidepressant. It restores normal mood states by inhibiting MAO from breaking down certain neurotransmitters in the brain.

℞ QUICK FACTS

Purpose

 Used to treat depression and anxiety or phobias mixed with depression.

Dosage

 Take with or without food, as prescribed by your doctor; *see list of food interactions.* May take up to 4 weeks before you observe effects of the medication. *Carry a card or wear a Medic Alert bracelet stating that you are taking Nardil.* Abruptly stopping medication may lead to withdrawal symptoms such as nightmares, agitation, strange behavior, and convulsions.

. . . .

 Usual adult dose: 15 milligrams (1 tablet) 3 times per day, up to 90 milligrams per day maximum dose. Doctor may reduce maximum dose gradually once desired results are achieved.

. . . .

 Usual child dose: not generally prescribed for children under 16 years.

. . . .

 Missed dose: take as soon as possible, unless within 1 hour of next dose. In that case, do not take missed dose; go back to regular schedule. *Do not double doses.*

Side Effects

 Overdose can be fatal. Overdose symptoms: agitation, backward arching of head and neck, backward arching of back, cool and clammy skin, coma, convulsions, difficult breathing, dizziness, drowsiness, faintness, hallucinations, high blood pressure, high fever, hyperactivity, irritability, jaw muscle spasms, low blood pressure, pain in the heart area, rapid and irregular pulse, severe headache, sweating. If you suspect an overdose, immediately seek medical attention.

 More common side effects: constipation, disorders of the stomach and intestines, dizziness, drowsiness, dry mouth, excessive sleeping, fatigue, headache, insomnia, low blood pressure (especially when standing up), muscle spasms, muscle twitchings, sexual difficulties, strong reflexes, swelling due to fluid retention, tremors, weakness, weight gain.

 Less common or rare side effects: anxiety, blurred vision, coma, convulsions, delirium, exaggerated feeling of well-being, fever, glaucoma, inability to urinate, involuntary eyeball movements, jitteriness, lack of coordination, liver damage, mania, muscular rigidity, onset of schizophrenia, rapid breathing, rapid heart rate, repetitious use of words and phrases, skin rash, sweating, swelling in the throat, tingling sensation, yellowed skin and eyes.

Interactions

 Inform your doctor before combining Nardil with blood pressure medications including diuretics and beta-blockers. *Avoid taking Nardil with the following medications, and for 2 weeks after therapy; may cause fatal high blood pressure:* amphetamines; appetite suppressants such as Tenuate; antidepressants and related medications such as Prozac, Elavil, Triavil, Tegretol, and Flexeril; asthma inhalants such as Proventil and Ventolin; bupropion (Wellbutrin); buspirone (BuSpar); cocaine; cold and cough preparations such as Robitussin DM; guanethidine (Ismelin); Dextromethorphan; hay fever medications such as Contac, Dristan, and Sudafed; L-dopa; L-tryptophan-containing products; L-tyrosine; meperidine (Demerol); methyldopa (Aldomet); narcotics; nasal decongestants; phenylalanine; Ritalin; sinus medications; weight loss medications.

Avoid the following foods while taking Nardil and for 2 weeks after therapy; may cause fatally high blood pressure: beer (including alcohol-free or reduced alcohol); caffeine in excessive amounts; cheese (except cottage and cream cheeses); chocolate in excessive amounts; dry sausage (including Genoa salami, hard salami, pepperoni, and Lebanon bologna); fava bean pods; liver; meat extract; pickled herring; picked, fermented, aged, or smoked meat, fish, or dairy products; sauerkraut; spoiled or improperly stored meat, fish, or dairy products; wine (including alcohol-free or reduced-alcohol); yeast extract (including large amounts of brewer's yeast); yogurt.

Special Cautions

 If pregnant or planning to become pregnant, inform your doctor immediately. Not known if Nardil appears in breast milk.

 No special precautions apply to seniors.

 Not generally prescribed for children under 16 years.

 Promptly report headache or other unusual symptoms.

Should not take if you have pheochromocytoma (tumor of adrenal gland), congestive heart failure, history of liver disease, or if you have had an allergic reaction to Nardil.

Doctor will prescribe with caution if you are diabetic.

Inform your doctor you are taking Nardil before elective surgery.

Nasacort

Generic name: Triamcinolone acetonide

Nasacort is a corticosteroid inhaler. It works to control inflammation of the mucosal lining of the bronchi, making it easier to breathe.

℞ QUICK FACTS

Purpose

℞ Used to relieve the symptoms of hay fever and other nasal allergies. Also used to treat nasal polyps.

Dosage

🍴 Take exactly as prescribed, on a regular daily basis. For oral inhalation only. *Do not use Nasacort canister after 100 inhalations.*

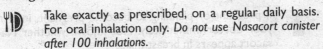 Usual adult dose: *for children 12 and over and adults*—220 micrograms a day, taken as 2 sprays in each nostril once per day. Doctor may increase up to 440 micrograms a day taken once, twice, or 4 times per day. Once desired effect is achieved, doctor may lower to 110 micrograms per day.

Usual child dose: *for children 6 to 12 years*—not generally prescribed.

Missed dose: take as soon as possible, unless almost time for next dose. If so, skip missed dose; go back to regular schedule. *Do not double doses.*

Side Effects

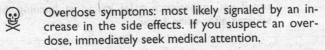 Overdose symptoms: most likely signaled by an increase in the side effects. If you suspect an overdose, immediately seek medical attention.

Most common side effect: headache.

 Less common side effects: dryness of membranes lining nose, mouth and throat; nasal irritation; nasal and sinus congestion; nosebleeds; sneezing; throat discomfort.

Interactions

 Inform your doctor before combining Nasacort with alternate-day prednisone treatment.

 No known food/other substance interactions.

Special Cautions

 If pregnant or planning to become pregnant, inform your doctor immediately. Not known whether Nasacort appears in breast milk.

 No specific precautions apply to seniors.

 Follow doctor's instructions carefully for children. Children are more susceptible to infection; try to avoid exposure to chicken pox and measles.

 Tell your doctor if you experience depression, fungal infection in the mouth and throat, joint or muscular pain, light-headedness, weariness, or weight loss.

Use with caution if you have nasal ulcers that are not fully healed, or nose injury.

If symptoms do not improve or if they worsen after 3 weeks, notify your doctor. Also inform your doctor if you experience nasal irritation, burning, or stinging after using spray.

Nasalide
see AEROBID

Natalins
see STUARTNATAL PLUS

Navane

Generic name: Thiothixene

Navane is an antipsychotic. It calms certain areas of the brain while allowing the rest of the brain to function normally.

℞ QUICK FACTS

Purpose

℞ Used to treat psychotic disorders.

Dosage

 May take in liquid or capsule form. Use dropper supplied with medication if taking liquid form.

 Usual adult dose: *milder conditions*—6 milligrams per day total, divided into 3 equal doses. Doctor may increase up to 15 milligrams per day total. *For more severe conditions*—10 milligrams per day total, divided into 2 equal doses. Doctor may prescribe up to 60 milligrams per day total. *Seniors*—usually prescribed lower doses to avoid low blood pressure.

Usual child dose: not generally prescribed for children under 12 years.

 Missed dose: take as soon as possible, unless within 2 hours of next dose. If so, skip missed dose; go back to regular schedule. *Do not double doses.*

Side Effects

 Overdose symptoms: central nervous system depression, coma, difficulty swallowing, dizziness, drowsiness, head tilted to the side, low blood pressure, muscle twitching, rigid muscles, salivation, tremors, walking disturbances, weakness. If you suspect an overdose, immediately seek medical attention.

 Side effects: abnormal muscle rigidity, abnormal milk secretion, abnormalities in movements and posture, agitation, anemia, blurred vision, breast development in males, chewing movements, constipation, diarrhea, dizziness, drowsiness, dry mouth, excessive thirst, eyeball rotation or state of fixed gaze, fainting, fatigue, fluid accumulation and swelling, headache, high fever, high or low blood sugar, hives, impotence, insomnia, intestinal blockage, involuntary movements of arms and legs, irregular menstrual periods, itching, light-headedness, loss or increase of appetite, low blood pressure, narrow or dilated pupils of the eye, nasal congestion, nausea, painful muscle spasm, protruding tongue, puckering of mouth, puffing of cheeks, rapid heartbeat, rash, restlessness, salivation, sedation, seizures, sensitivity to light, severe allergic reaction, skin inflammation and peeling, strong reflexes, sweating, swelling of breasts, tremors, twitching (in the body, neck, shoulders, and face), visual problems, vomiting, weakness, weight increase, worsening of psychotic symptoms.

No known less common or rare side effects.

Interactions

 Inform your doctor before combining Navane with: antihistamines such as Benadryl; barbiturates such as phenobarbital; medications containing atropine such as Donnatal. Painkillers, narcotics, or sleeping medications may cause extreme drowsiness.

 Alcohol may cause extreme drowsiness.

Special Cautions

 If pregnant or planning to become pregnant, inform your doctor immediately. Not known whether Navane appears in breast milk; doctor may have you discontinue breastfeeding during Navane therapy.

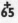 Senior women at higher risk for tardive dyskinesia—involuntary muscle spasms and twitches in face and body. Seniors are generally at risk for developing low blood pressure; lower doses are prescribed as a result.

 Not generally prescribed for children under 12 years.

 Do not administer to comatose patients.

Do not take if hypersensitive to this medication.

May cause drowsiness and impair your ability to drive a car or operate machinery. *Do not take part in any activity that requires alertness.*

. . . .

Should not take if you have slowed central nervous system activity due to sleeping medication, circulatory system collapse, or abnormal bone marrow or blood condition.

. . . .

May mask symptoms of brain tumor or intestinal obstruction. If you have or had: brain tumor, breast cancer, convulsive disorders, glaucoma, intestinal blockage, or heart disease, or were exposed to extreme heat, or are recovering from alcohol addiction, doctor will prescribe cautiously.

. . . .

May cause tardive dyskinesia—involuntary muscle spasms and twitches in face and body, which can be permanent.

Nedocromil Sodium

see TILADE

NeoDecadron Ophthalmic Ointment and Solution

Generic ingredients: Dexamethasone sodium phosphate with neomycin sulfate

NeoDecadron is a steroid and antibiotic combination. It works by stimulating the synthesis of enzymes needed to decrease the inflammatory response, and it kills bacteria.

℞ QUICK FACTS

Purpose

 Used to treat inflammatory eye conditions with a bacterial infection or the possibility of bacterial infection.

Dosage

 Wash hands thoroughly before and after application of medication.

. . . .

 Usual adult dose: *ophthalmic ointment*—apply thin coating 3 or 4 times per day. As condition clears, doctor will reduce to 2, and later to 1, application per day. *Ophthalmic solution*—1 or 2 drops in conjunctival sac every hour during the day and every 2 hours at night.

. . . .

 Usual child dose: not generally prescribed for children.

. . . .

 Missed dose: take as soon as possible, unless almost time for next dose. If so, skip missed dose, go back to regular schedule. *Do not double doses.*

Side Effects

 Overdose symptoms: no specific information available. However, if you suspect an overdose, immediately seek medical attention.

. . . .

 Side effects: allergic skin reactions; cataracts; delay in healing of wounds; development of additional eye infections; increased eye pressure with possible glaucoma and optic nerve damage.

. . . .

 No known less common or rare side effects.

Interactions

 No drug interactions reported.

 No known food/other substance interactions.

Special Cautions

 If pregnant or planning to become pregnant, inform your doctor immediately. No information known about safety of this medication during pregnancy and breastfeeding.

 No special precautions apply to seniors.

 Not generally prescribed for children.

 Do not use if sensitive to or allergic to any of the ingredients in this medication. May cause allergic reaction in people susceptible to sulfites.

Immediately contact your doctor if exposed to measles or chicken pox while taking NeoDecadron; may be fatal in adults.

If you develop a skin rash or allergic reaction, stop using medication and immediately contact your doctor.

May experience temporary blurring of vision or stinging.

Doctor will reexamine your eyes before renewing prescription.

Doctor should monitor eye pressure if using this medication for more than 10 days.

Avoid if you have: inflammation of the cornea (lens); other bacterial, fungal, or viral eye infections; or if you have recently had a foreign object removed from your cornea.

Neptazane

~~~~~~

Generic name: Methazolamide

Neptazane is a carbonic anhydrase inhibitor. It decreases the formation of the watery fluid of the eye, thereby lowering intraocular pressure.

℞ QUICK FACTS

Purpose

℞ Used to treat chronic open-angle glaucoma. Also used in acute angle-closure glaucoma when eye pressure must be lowered before surgery.

Dosage

 Take exactly as prescribed; doctor may prescribe other medications with Neptazane.

 Usual adult dose: 50 to 100 milligrams taken 2 to 3 times per day.

 Usual child dose: not generally prescribed for children.

 Missed dose: take as soon as possible, unless almost time for next dose. If so, skip missed dose; go back to regular schedule. *Do not double doses.*

Side Effects

 Overdose symptoms: no specific information available. However, if you suspect an overdose, immediately seek medical attention.

 More common side effects: confusion; depression; diarrhea; dizziness; drowsiness; excessive urination; fatigue; fever; general feeling of not being well; headache; hearing problems; loss of appetite; nausea and vomiting; rash; ringing in ears; severe allergic reaction; taste changes; temporary nearsightedness; tingling in fingers, toes, hands, or feet.

 Rare side effects: black or tarry stools, blood in urine, convulsions, hives, increased sensitivity to light, kidney stones, paralysis.

Interactions

 Inform your doctor before combining Neptazane with high doses of aspirin taken at the same time; can cause loss of appetite, rapid breathing, lethargy, coma, and even death. Using with steroids may lower potassium levels.

 No known food/other substance interactions.

Special Cautions

 If pregnant or planning to become pregnant, inform your doctor immediately. Appears in breast milk; could affect a nursing infant.

 No special precautions apply to seniors.

 Not generally prescribed for children.

 May cause allergic reactions including fever, rash, redness and peeling of skin, hives, difficulty breathing, seri-

ous skin and blood disorders, and even death. Doctor should monitor blood during Neptazane therapy. Immediately contact your doctor if you experience any of these symptoms.

· ·

Should not use if you have kidney or liver disease, adrenal gland disorders, or low sodium or potassium levels.

· ·

May aggravate acidosis (too much acid in the blood).

· ·

Doctor will prescribe with caution if you have emphysema or lung blockage.

Nicardipine Hydrochloride

see CARDENE

Nicoderm

Category: Nicotine patches

Other brand names: Habitrol, Nicotrol, Prostep

Nicoderm is a stop-smoking agent.

℞ QUICK FACTS

Purpose

  Used to assist in quitting smoking by reducing the craving for tobacco.

Dosage

Carefully follow doctor's detailed guidelines to avoid side effects and addiction to Nicoderm. Any single patch should not be worn for more than 16 to 24

hours; apply fresh patch according to your dosage
schedule. *Do not change brands unless directed by your
doctor. Do not remove patches from wrapping until
ready for immediate use.*

 Usual adult dose: 1 high-strength patch per day. If
you weigh less than 100 pounds or smoke less than a
½ pack of cigarettes per day or have heart disease,
doctor may prescribe lower-dose patch. Habitrol
patches are round and come in 3 strengths; are
worn 24 hours a day. Nicoderm patches are rectangular and come in 3 strengths; are worn 24 hours
per day. Nicotrol patches are rectangular and come
in 3 strengths; must be removed at bedtime. Prostep
patches are round and come in 2 strengths; are
worn 24 hours a day.

 Usual child dose: not generally prescribed for children.

 Missed dose: apply patch as soon as possible. *Never
use 2 patches at one time.*

Side Effects

 Overdose symptoms: abdominal pain, blurred vision,
breathing abnormalities, cold sweat, confusion, diarrhea, dizziness, drooling, fainting, hearing difficulties,
heart palpitations, low blood pressure, nausea, pallor, salivation, severe headaches, sweating, tremor,
upset stomach, vision problems, vomiting, weakness.
Large overdose may cause prostration and respiratory failure. If you suspect an overdose, immediately
seek medical attention.

 More common side effects: itching and burning at
application site, rash, redness of skin.

 Less common side effects: abnormal dreaming, allergic reactions, back pain, chest pain, constipation,

cough, diarrhea, dizziness, drowsiness, dry mouth, headache, high blood pressure, impaired concentration, indigestion, inflammation of sinuses, menstrual irregularities, nausea, nervousness, numbness, pain, pins and needles sensation, sleeplessness, sore throat, stomach pain, sweating, taste changes, tingling, vomiting, weakness.

Interactions

 Inform your doctor before combining Nicoderm with: acetaminophen-containing medications; caffeine-containing medications such as No-Doz; certain airway-opening medications such as Isuprel; Dristan; certain blood pressure medications such as Minipress, Trandate, and Normodyne; cimetidine (Tagamet); haloperidol (Haldol); imipramine (Tofranil); insulin; lithium (Lithonate); oxazepam (Serax); pentazocine (Talwin); propranolol (Inderal); theophylline (Theo-Dur).

 Do not smoke any form of tobacco during Nicoderm therapy; may result in overdose. Nicotine from patch is still in your skin and passing into the bloodstream for several hours after removing patch.

Special Cautions

 Should not use if pregnant or nursing. Immediately contact your doctor if you become pregnant during Nicoderm therapy.

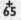 Seniors should use with caution.

 Not generally prescribed for children.

 Do not take if sensitive to or allergic to nicotine, nicotine patches, or adhesive material.

Carefully dispose of patches; contain enough nicotine to poison a child or a pet.

Nicoderm should be part of a comprehensive stop-smoking program including behavior modification, counseling, and support with the goal of complete smoking cessation, not cutting down on smoking.

If after 4 weeks of Nicoderm therapy you are unable to stop smoking, most likely the patch will not work for you.

Nicorette

Generic name: Nicotine polacrilex

Nicorette is a stop-smoking agent. It acts on the adrenal gland to overcome physical dependence on nicotine.

℞ QUICK FACTS

Purpose

℞ Used as a temporary aid for cigarette smokers who are trying to stop smoking. Most effective when used with a behavior modification program.

Dosage

 Carefully follow doctor's detailed guidelines to avoid side effects and addiction to Nicorette.

Usual adult dose: *Nicorette 2-milligram*—chew 1 piece every 1 to 2 hours; *do not use more than 30 pieces per day.* Most adults use 9 to 12 pieces per day. After 2 to 3 months, doctor will gradually reduce dose. *Nicorette DS-4 milligram*—chew 1 piece every 1 to 2 hours; *do not use more than 20 pieces*

per day. Most adults use 9 to 12 pieces per day. After 2 to 3 months, doctor will gradually reduce dose.

 Usual child dose: not generally prescribed for children and adolescents who smoke.

 Missed dose: *do not take missed dose, and do not double doses.*

Side Effects

 Overdose symptoms (similar to acute nicotine poisoning): abdominal pain, blurred vision, cold sweat, diarrhea, difficulty breathing, disturbed hearing, dizziness, exhaustion, fainting, headache, low blood pressure, mental confusion, nausea, paleness, rapid and irregular pulse, salivation, tremor, upset stomach, vomiting, weakness. If you suspect an overdose, immediately seek medical attention. Large overdose may cause prostration and respiratory failure.

 More common side effects: bleeding gums, excessive saliva in mouth, hiccups, indigestion, inflammation of the mouth, injury to teeth or cheeks, nausea, stomach and intestinal discomfort, throat soreness, tingling or pins and needles.

 Less common or rare side effects: diarrhea; dry mouth; inflammation of the gums, tongue, throat; mouth sores; muscle pain; rash; sweating; tongue sores.

Interactions

 Inform your doctor before combining Nicorette with: acetaminophen (Tylenol), caffeine, furosemide (Lasix), glutethimide (Doriden), imipramine (Tofranil), insulin, isoproterenol (Isuprel), labetalol (Normodyne), oxazepam (Serax), pentazocine (Talwin), phenacetin, phenylephrine (Entex), prazosin

(Minipress), propoxyphene (Darvon), propranolol (Inderal), theophylline (Theo-Dur).

 No known food/other substance interactions.

Special Cautions

 Should not use if pregnant or nursing. Immediately contact your doctor if you become pregnant during Nicorette therapy.

 Seniors should use with caution.

 Not generally prescribed for children and adolescents who smoke.

 Do not use if sensitive to or allergic to nicotine or other ingredients of Nicorette. Stop using, and immediately contact your doctor if you develop an allergic reaction.

Inform your doctor *before* Nicorette therapy if you have ever had: angina (severe chest pain), Buerger's disease (disease of the arteries), diabetes or other endocrine diseases, dental problems, difficulty swallowing, drug allergies, heartburn, heart disease, high blood pressure, kidney or liver disease, peptic ulcer, throat or mouth inflammation, overactive thyroid, or TMJ (disorder of joint of jaw).

Use cautiously if you have had a heart attack or seriously irregular heartbeat.

Nicotine is an addictive and toxic substance.

May stick to dentures, if so stop chewing and notify your doctor.

Nicotine Polacrilex
see NICORETTE

Nifedipine
see PROCARDIA

Nitro-Bid
see NITROGLYCERIN

Nitrofurantoin
see MACRODANTIN

Nitroglycerin

Generic name: Glyceryl trinitrate

Brand names: Ang-O-Span, Deponit, Klavikordal, N-G-C, Niong, Nitro-Bid, Nitro-Dur, Nitroglyn, Nitroguard, Nitrolingual Spray, Nitronet, Nitrong, Nitrostat Tablets, NTS, Transderm-Nitro

Nitroglycerin is an anti-anginal agent, or vasodilator. It increases the amount of oxygen that reaches the heart muscle.

℞ QUICK FACTS

Purpose

℞ Used to prevent and treat angina pectoris (crushing chest pain).

Dosage

 Follow doctor's instructions carefully for the brand prescribed; *never interchange brands*. If used excessively, at risk for acute headaches or tolerance. However, daily headaches indicate the drug's activity; *do not reduce dosage unless instructed by your doctor. Do not open sublingual tablet container until you need a dose. Do not put cotton plug or objects into container. Keep sublingual tablets accessible at all times.*

· ·

 Usual adult dose: *sublingual or buccal tablets*—at onset of chest pain, dissolve 1 tablet under tongue or inside cheek. May repeat every 5 minutes until pain subsides. If pain does not subside after 15 minutes or 3 tablets, immediately contact your doctor. May take tablets 5 to 10 minutes prior to activities that may cause chest pain. *Patch*—applied to skin for 12 to 14 hours, off for 10 to 12 hours, then new patch applied, per doctor's instructions. *Spray*—at onset of chest pain, spray 1 or 2 premeasured doses onto or under tongue. If pain does not subside after 15 minutes or 3 doses, immediately contact your doctor. May use spray 5 to 10 minutes prior to activities that may cause chest pain. *Ointment*—total of 1 inch of ointment per day, ½ inch in the morning and ½ inch 6 hours later. Chest is the site with highest absorption. Must have 10-to-12-hour period with no ointment on skin. *Sustained release capsules or tablets*—doctor will prescribe smallest amount to take 2 or 3 times per day at 8-to-12-hour intervals. *Seniors*—lower doses are prescribed.

· ·

Usual child dose: not generally prescribed for children.

 Missed dose: *skin patch or ointment*—apply as soon as possible, unless almost time for next dose. If so, skip missed dose, go back to regular schedule. *Do not apply 2 skin patches at the same time. Oral tablets or capsules*—take as soon as possible, unless within 2 hours of next dose. If so, skip missed dose; go back to regular schedule. *Do not double doses.*

Side Effects

 Severe overdose can result in death. Overdose symptoms: bluish skin, clammy skin, colic, coma, confusion, diarrhea (possibly bloody), difficulty and/or slow breathing, dizziness, fainting, fever, flushed skin, headache (persistent and throbbing), increased pressure within skull, irregular pulse, loss of appetite, nausea, palpitations, paralysis, rapid decrease in blood pressure, seizures, slow pulse/heartbeat, sweating, vertigo, visual disturbances, vomiting. If you suspect an overdose, immediately seek medical attention.

 More common side effects: dizziness, flushed neck and face, headache, light-headedness, worsened angina.

 Less common or rare side effects: diarrhea, fainting, heart pounding, low blood pressure, nausea, numbness, pallor, restlessness, skin rashes, sweating, vertigo, vomiting, weakness.

Interactions

 Inform your doctor before combining nitroglycerin with: blood vessel dilators such as Loniten; calcium channel blockers such as Calan and Procardia; Dihydroergotamine (D.H.E.); high blood pressure medications (may cause extremely low blood pressure); isorbide mononitrate (Ismo); isosorbide dinitrate (Sorbitrate or Isordil); Tenormin.

 Avoid alcohol; may cause sudden drop in blood pressure resulting in dizziness and fainting.

Special Cautions

 If pregnant or planning to become pregnant, inform your doctor immediately. Not known if nitroglycerin appears in breast milk.

 To avoid low blood pressure and headaches, lower doses are prescribed for seniors.

 Not generally prescribed for children.

 May cause drowsiness and impair your ability to drive a car or operate machinery. *Do not take part in any activity that requires alertness.*

Should not use if you have: head injury or condition causing increased fluid pressure in the head; severe anemia; recent heart attack; kidney, liver, or thyroid disease. Avoid using capsule form if you have closed-angle glaucoma or suffer from dizziness when standing.

Immediately stop taking this medication and inform your doctor if you experience blurred vision or dry mouth.

Use with caution if you have low systolic blood pressure (less than 90 mm Hg).

Nitroglycerin increases risk of severe low blood pressure, slowed heart rate, and increased chest pain.

> Should not use if sensitive to or allergic to nitro-
> glycerin or adhesive used in the patch.

Nizatidine

see AXID

Nizoral

Generic name: Ketoconazole

Nizoral is an antifungal. It destroys and prevents the growth of fungi.

℞ QUICK FACTS

Purpose

℞ Used to treat a variety of fungal infections, including oral thrush and candidiasis.

Dosage

 Take exactly as prescribed. Continue prescription if symptoms subside; otherwise infection may return. May take with food to avoid stomach irritation.

 Usual adult dose: single daily dose of 200 milligrams. May be increased to 400 milligrams for serious infections.

 Usual child dose: is infrequently prescribed for children in a single daily dose of 3.3 to 6.6 milligrams per 2.2 pounds of body weight. Not prescribed for children under 2 years.

Missed dose: take as soon as possible, unless almost time for next dose. If so, skip missed dose, go back to regular schedule. *Do not double doses.*

Side Effects

 Overdose symptoms: no specific information available. If you suspect an overdose, immediately seek medical attention.

 More common side effects: nausea, vomiting.

 Less common side effects: abdominal pain, itching. Rare side effects: breast swelling in men, bulging fontanel (soft areas on baby's scalp), depression, diarrhea, dizziness, drowsiness, fever and chills, headache, hives, impotence, light sensitivity, rash.

Interactions

 Inform your doctor before combining Nizoral with: anticoagulants such as Coumadin; antiulcer medications such as Axid, Pepcid, Tagamet, Zantac; astemizole (Hismanal)—*has caused fatal reactions involving the heart;* corticosteroids such as prednisone and Medrol; cyclosporine (Sandimmune); isoniazid (Nydrazid); phenytoin (Dilantin); rifampin (Rifadin, Rifamate, Rimactane); terfenadine (Seldane)—*has caused fatal reactions involving the heart;* theophylline (Theo-24, Slo-Phyllin, Theo-Dur).

 Avoid alcohol and antacids during Nizoral therapy. If necessary, take antacids 2 or 3 hours *after* taking medication.

Special Cautions

 If pregnant or planning to become pregnant, inform your doctor immediately. Most likely appears in breast milk; could affect a nursing infant.

No special precautions apply to seniors.

 Infrequently prescribed for children 2 years and over.

 Do not take if sensitive to or allergic to Nizoral. Do not take with Seldane or Hisminal.

At risk of serious or fatal liver damage when taking Nizoral. Doctor will monitor your liver through blood tests. Immediately contact your doctor if you experience: unusual fatigue, loss of appetite, nausea or vomiting, jaundice, dark urine, pale stools.

Cases of anaphylaxis (life-threatening allergic reaction) have been reported after the first dose of Nizoral.

May cause drowsiness and impair your ability to drive a car or operate machinery. *Do not take part in any activity that requires alertness.*

Nolamine

Generic ingredients: Phenindamine tartrate with chlorpheniramine maleate and phenylpropanolamine hydrochloride

Nolamine is an antihistamine and decongestant combination. It works by blocking the effects of histamine, a body chemical that narrows air passages, reducing swelling and itching, and drying secretions.

℞ QUICK FACTS

Purpose

 Used to treat stuffiness caused by the common cold, inflamed sinuses, hay fever, or other allergies.

Dosage

 Take exactly as prescribed.

 Usual adult dose: 1 tablet every 8 hours. In mild cases, 1 tablet every 10 to 12 hours.

 Usual child dose: not generally prescribed for children.

 Missed dose: take as soon as possible, unless almost time for next dose. If so, skip missed dose; go back to regular schedule. *Do not double doses.*

Side Effects

 Overdose symptoms: no reports of Nolamine overdose. However, if you suspect an overdose, immediately seek medical attention.

 Side effects: difficulty sleeping, dizziness, drowsiness, nervousness, tremors.

 No known less common or rare side effects.

Interactions

 Inform your doctor before combining Nolamine with: bromocriptine (Parlodel); central nervous system depressants such as Valium, Demerol, and Dalmane; MAO inhibitors such as Nardil and Parnate; methyldopa (Aldomet).

 Avoid alcohol during Nolamine therapy.

Special Cautions

 No special warnings for pregnant or breastfeeding women.

 No special precautions apply to seniors.

 Not generally prescribed for children.

 May cause drowsiness and impair your ability to drive a car or operate machinery. *Do not take part in any activity that requires alertness.*

Should not take if sensitive to or allergic to any ingredients of Nolamine, or if taking MAO inhibitors.

Use with caution if you have: high blood pressure, heart disease, diabetes, overactive thyroid gland, glaucoma, or enlarged prostate gland.

Nolvadex

Generic name: Tamoxifen citrate

Nolvadex is an anti-estrogenic antineoplastic. It prevents the growth of rapidly dividing cells such as cancer cells.

℞ QUICK FACTS

Purpose

 Used to treat breast cancer in women, is most effective in stopping the type of breast cancer that thrives on estrogen. Also used to treat cancer that has spread to other parts of the body.

Dosage

 Take exactly as prescribed. *Do not discontinue use unless directed by your doctor.* May need to take Nolvadex for several years. Birth control methods other than the Pill are recommended during Nolvadex therapy.

 Usual adult dose: 1 or 2 10-milligram tablets in the morning and evening.

 Usual child dose: not generally prescribed for children.

 Missed dose: *do not try to make up missed dose.* Go back to regular schedule.

Side Effects

 Overdose symptoms: dizziness, overactive reflexes, tremor, unsteady gait. If you suspect an overdose, immediately seek medical attention.

 More common side effects: hot flashes, nausea, vomiting.

 Less common or rare side effects: bone pain, diarrhea, menstrual irregularities, skin rash, tumor pain, vaginal bleeding, vaginal discharge. Rare side effects: depression, distaste for food, dizziness, hair thinning or partial loss, headache, light-headedness, liver disorders, swelling of arms or legs, vaginal itching, visual problems.

Interactions

 Inform your doctor before combining Nolvadex with: blood thinners such as Coumadin; bromocriptine (Parlodel); phenobarbital.

No known food/other substance interactions.

Special Cautions

 Important to avoid pregnancy during Nolvadex therapy; can harm fetus. If you become pregnant, immediately inform your doctor. Appears in breast milk; can cause serious harm to a nursing infant.

 No special precautions apply to seniors.

 Not generally prescribed for children.

 Do not take if sensitive to or allergic to this medication.

Doctor should perform routine gynecological exams. Immediately report any abnormal vaginal bleeding.

Immediately inform your doctor if you experience visual problems.

May be a link between Nolvadex therapy and blood cell abnormalities such as too few white blood cells or platelets.

Doctor should monitor cholesterol levels; may raise cholesterol and triglyceride levels.

May cause abnormally high level of calcium in the blood.

Norfloxacin
see NOROXIN

Norgesic

Generic ingredients: Orphenadrine citrate with aspirin and caffeine

Other brand names: Norgesic Forte, Orphengesic

Norgesic is an analgesic and muscle relaxant combination. It blocks pain impulses from generating.

℞ QUICK FACTS

Purpose

 Used to treat mild to moderate pain of severe muscle disorders, in combination with rest and physical therapy.

Dosage

 Take with food to avoid stomach irritation.

 Usual adult dose: *Norgesic*—1 to 2 tablets taken 3 or 4 times per day. *Norgesic Forte*—½ to 1 tablet taken 3 or 4 times per day. *Seniors*—dose is lowered if confusion is experienced.

 Usual child dose: not generally prescribed for children under 12 years.

 Missed dose: take as soon as possible, unless within an hour of next dose. If so, skip missed dose, go back to regular schedule. *Do not double doses.*

Side Effects

Overdose symptoms: no specific information available. However, if you suspect an overdose, immediately seek medical attention.

Side effects: blurred vision, constipation, difficulty urinating, dilation of pupils, dizziness, drowsiness, dry mouth, fainting, hallucinations, headache, hives, lightheadedness, nausea, palpitations, rapid heart rate, skin diseases, stomach and intestinal bleeding, vomiting, weakness.

. . . .

 No known less common or rare side effects.

Interactions

 Inform your doctor before combining Norgesic with propoxyphene (Darvon)—can cause confusion, anxiety, and tremors.

. . . .

 No known food/other substance interactions.

Special Cautions

 If pregnant or planning to become pregnant, inform your doctor immediately. May appear in breast milk; could affect a nursing infant.

. . . .

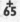 Some seniors experience confusion when taking Norgesic; dosage is lowered in these cases.

. . . .

 Not generally prescribed for children under 12 years.

. . . .

 Do not use if chicken pox or flu is present; may cause Reye's syndrome.

. . . .

May cause drowsiness and impair your ability to drive a car or operate machinery. *Do not take part in any activity that requires alertness.*

. . . .

Do not take if sensitive to or allergic to ingredients in Norgesic, or if you have: glaucoma, stomach or intestinal blockage, enlarged prostate, bladder obstruction, achalasia (failure of stomach or intestinal muscles to relax), or myasthenia gravis (muscle weakness and fatigue).

. . . .

Doctor should monitor blood, urine, and liver function with long-term Norgesic therapy.

. . . .

Use with caution if you have a peptic ulcer or blood-clotting problems.

Normodyne

Generic name: Labetalol hydrochloride

Other brand name: Trandate

Normodyne is an alpha/beta-adrenergic blocking agent. It works by blocking impulses along certain nerve pathways.

℞ QUICK FACTS

Purpose

℞ Used to treat high blood pressure.

Dosage

 Can take with or without food; level of Normodyne absorbed into the bloodstream is increased by food. Take exactly as prescribed, even if symptoms disappear. Adhere to dosage schedule for Normodyne to be effective; missing doses may worsen symptoms. May take several weeks to observe full effects of medication.

. . . .

 Usual adult dose: 100 milligrams taken 2 times per day, alone or with a diuretic medication. Initial dose may be given in doctor's office, with 1-to-3-hour observation period. Doctor may increase dose after 2

or 3 days of monitoring blood pressure. Regular dose ranges—200 to 400 milligrams taken 2 times per day. *Seniors*—dose determined based on individual needs.

 Usual child dose: not generally prescribed for children.

 Missed dose: take as soon as possible, unless almost time for next dose. If so, skip missed dose; go back to regular schedule. *Do not double doses.*

Side Effects

 Overdose symptoms: dizziness when standing up, severely low blood pressure, severely slow heartbeat. If you suspect an overdose, immediately seek medical attention.

 More common side effects: dizziness, fatigue, indigestion, nausea, stuffy nose.

 Less common or rare side effects: anaphylaxis (severe allergic reaction); angioedema (swelling of face, lips, tongue, and throat; difficulty swallowing); change in taste; depression; diarrhea; difficulty urinating; dizziness upon standing up; drowsiness; dry eyes; ejaculation failure; fainting; fluid retention; hair loss; headache; heart block; hives; impotence; increased sweating; itching; low blood pressure; lupus erythematosus; muscle cramps; rash; shortness of breath; slow heartbeat; tingling or pins and needles; tingling scalp; vertigo; vision changes; weakness; wheezing; vomiting; yellow eyes and skin.

Interactions

 Inform your doctor before combining Normodyne with: airway-opening medications such as Proventil and Ventolin; antidepressants such as Elavil; cimetidine (Tagamet); diabetes medications such as Micronase; epinephrine (EpiPen); insulin; nitroglycerin products such as Transderm-Nitro; nonsteroidal anti-inflammatory medications such as Advil and Motrin; ritrodrine (Yutopar); verapamil (Calan).

 No known food/other substance interactions.

Special Cautions

 If pregnant or planning to become pregnant, inform your doctor immediately. Appears in breast milk; could affect a nursing infant.

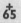 Use with caution; dose based on individual needs.

 Not generally prescribed for children.

 If you stop medication abruptly, can cause chest pain or heart attack.

Should not take if you have: bronchial asthma, congestive heart failure, heart block, inadequate blood supply to the circulatory system, severely slow heartbeat, or other conditions causing severe and continued low blood pressure.

In rare cases has caused severe liver damage; symptoms include: itching, dark urine, continuing loss of appetite, yellow eyes and skin, unexplained flu-like symptoms.

Use with caution if you have a history of: asthma, chronic bronchitis, congestive heart failure, emphysema, kidney or liver disease.

If susceptible to severe allergic reactions, may experience severe reaction to Normodyne.

Symptoms of low blood sugar may be masked, or blood sugar levels may be altered during Normodyne therapy.

Inform your dentist or doctor in the event of a medical emergency or before surgery or dental treatment.

Noroxin

Generic name: Norfloxacin

Noroxin is a fluoroquinolone antibiotic. It inhibits the growth of bacteria.

℞ QUICK FACTS

Purpose

℞   Used to treat infections of the urinary tract, including cystitis; certain sexually transmitted diseases such as gonorrhea; and prostatis.

Dosage

    Take with a glass of water 1 hour *before* or 2 hours *after* eating a meal; should drink lots of water during Noroxin therapy. *Do not increase dosage unless specifically directed by your doctor.* Finish prescription; otherwise infection may reappear.

    Usual adult dose: *for uncomplicated urinary tract infections*—800 milligrams per day total, taken as 400 milligrams 2 times per day, for 3 to 10 days, depending on type of infection. *For complicated urinary tract infections*—800 milligrams total, taken as 400 milligrams 2 times per day, for 10 to 21 days. *For sexually transmitted diseases*—one single dose of 800 milligrams for 1 day. *For prostatitis*—800 milligrams per day total, taken as 400 milligrams every 12 hours for 28 days.

 Usual child dose: not generally prescribed for children under 18 years.

 Missed dose: take as soon as possible, unless almost time for next dose. If so, skip missed dose; go back to regular schedule. *Do not double doses.*

Side Effects

 Overdose symptoms: no specific information available. However, if you suspect an overdose, immediately seek medical attention.

 More common side effects: dizziness, fatigue, headache, nausea.

 Other side effects: abdominal cramping; arthritis; back pain; bitter taste; blood abnormalities; confusion; constipation; convulsions; dead skin; depression; diarrhea; dizziness; dry mouth; double vision; extreme sleepiness; fever; flushing or reddish skin; gas; hallucinations; headache; heartburn; hives; indigestion; insomnia; itching; joint pain; kidney failure (symptoms—reduced amount of urine, drowsiness, nausea, vomiting, and coma); lack of coordination; light-headedness; loss of appetite; low blood sugar; muscle pain; nausea; peeling skin; psychotic reactions; rash on skin and mucous membranes; reduced blood platelets causing bleeding disorders; restlessness; severe blisters and bleeding in genitals and in mucous membranes of eyes, lips, mouth, and nasal passages; severe skin reaction to sun; shock; shortness of breath; stomach pain; sweating; temporary hearing loss; tingling or pins and needles; vomiting; weakness; yellow eyes and skin.

Interactions

 Inform your doctor before combining Noroxin with: calcium supplements, cyclosporine (Sandimmune), multivitamins and other products containing iron or zinc, nitrofurantoin (Macrodantin or Macrobid), oral anticoagulants such as warfarin (Coumadin), probenecid (Benemid), sucralfate (Carafate), theophylline (Theo-Dur).

 Check with your doctor before using: antacids such as Maalox and Tums, and caffeine during Noroxin therapy.

Special Cautions

 If pregnant or planning to become pregnant, inform your doctor immediately. *Do not take while nursing an infant.*

 No special precautions apply to seniors.

 Not generally prescribed for children.

 On occasion, severe or fatal reactions have been experienced after the first dose with medications similar to Noroxin. Reactions may include: confusion, convulsions, difficulty breathing, hallucinations, heart collapse, hives, increased pressure in the head, itching, light-headedness, loss of consciousness, psychosis, rash, restlessness, shock, swelling in face or throat, tingling, tremors. If you experience any of these symptoms, stop taking Noroxin and immediately seek medical help.

May cause dizziness and impair your ability to drive a car or operate machinery. *Do not take part in any activity that requires alertness.*

. . . .

Not prescribed for syphilis. If prescribed for gonorrhea, may mask syphilis symptoms; doctor may test
for syphilis at the same time you are diagnosed with
gonorrhea, and after Noroxin therapy.

. . . .

Should not take if you have: epilepsy, severe cerebral arteriosclerosis, and other conditions causing
seizures.

. . . .

Avoid excessive exposure to sunlight. If you have a
severe reaction to sunlight, immediately discontinue
Noroxin and call your doctor.

Norpace

Generic name: Disopyramide phosphate

Other brand names: Napamide, Norpace CR

Norpace is an anti-arrhythmic. It corrects irregular heartbeats and helps produce a more normal rhythm by altering nerve impulses in the heart.

℞ QUICK FACTS

Purpose

℞ Used to treat severe irregular heartbeat.

Dosage

 Take exactly as prescribed. Comes in immediate and
suspended release forms. *Do not discontinue use unless directed by your doctor; can cause serious changes
in heart function.*

. . . .

 Usual adult dose: ranges from 400 to 800 milligrams
per day divided into smaller doses. *For those weighing
less than 110 pounds—400 milligrams per day di-*

vided into smaller doses. *For those with severe heart disease*—100 milligrams of immediate release every 6 to 8 hours. *For those with moderately reduced kidney or liver function*—400 milligrams per day divided into smaller doses. *For those with severe kidney impairment*—100 milligrams per day. Not recommended if you have severe kidney disease.

Usual child dose: *for children under 18 years*—based on body weight, and divided into equal doses taken orally every 6 hours or at intervals prescribed for the individual's specific needs.

Missed dose: take as soon as possible, if next dose is more than 4 hours away. Otherwise, skip missed dose; go back to regular schedule. *Do not double doses.*

Side Effects

Overdose may be fatal. Overdose symptoms: apnea (no breathing), loss of consciousness, loss of spontaneous respiration. If you suspect an overdose, immediately seek medical attention.

More common side effects: abdominal pain; bloating and gas; aches and pains; blurred vision; constipation; dizziness; dry eyes, nose, mouth, and throat; fatigue; headache; inability to urinate; increased urinary frequency and urgency; muscle weakness; nausea; vague feeling of bodily discomfort.

Less common or rare side effects: breast development in males, chest pain, congestive heart failure, depression, diarrhea, difficulty breathing, difficulty sleeping, fainting, fever, itching, impotence, low blood pressure, low blood sugar (hypoglycemia), nervousness, numbness or tingling, painful urination, rash, psychosis, shortness of breath, skin diseases, swelling due to fluid retention, vomiting, weight gain, yellow eyes and skin.

Interactions

Inform your doctor before combining Norpace with: heart-regulating medications such as lidocaine (Xylocaine), procainamide (Procan SR), propranolol (Inderal), quinidine (Quinidex), and verapramil (Calan); phenytoin (Dilantin). Doctor will prescribe other heart-regulating medications such as quinidine, procainamide, encainide, flecainide, propafenone, and propranolol with Norpace if the irregular rhythm is considered life-threatening; or if other anti-arrhythmic medications have not worked.

Avoid alcohol during Norpace therapy.

Special Cautions

If pregnant or planning to become pregnant, inform your doctor immediately. Appears in breast milk; could affect a nursing infant.

No special precautions apply to seniors.

Follow doctor's instructions carefully for children.

Should not use if the output of your heart is inadequate, or if sensitive to or allergic to Norpace.

Your doctor will advise usage based on a specific type of irregular heartbeat.

Use with extreme caution if you have: structural heart disease, inflammation of the heart muscle, or other heart disorders; glaucoma; myasthenia gravis; or difficulty urinating.

Doctor should check potassium levels *before* Norpace therapy begins; if you have low levels, medication may be ineffective; with high levels, may be toxic.

. . . .

May worsen or cause congestive heart failure; doctor will monitor your heart if you have a history of heart failure.

. . . .

At risk for low blood sugar if you have: congestive heart failure, poor nutrition, kidney or liver diseases, if you are taking beta-blockers, or if you drink alcohol during Norpace therapy.

Norpramin

Generic name: Desipramine hydrochloride

Other brand name: Pertofrane

Norpramin is a tricyclic antidepressant. It is thought to relieve depression by increasing the concentration of certain chemicals responsible for brain nerve transmissions.

℞ QUICK FACTS

Purpose

℞ Used to treat depression. Also used to treat bulimia, attention deficit disorders, and help with cocaine withdrawal.

Dosage

 Take exactly as prescribed. *Do not discontinue if there is not an immediate effect; can take up to 3 weeks to observe any effects of the medication. Stopping medica-*

tion abruptly may result in nausea, headache, and uneasiness.

 Usual adult dose: ranges from 100 to 200 milligrams per day taken in 1 dose or divided into smaller doses. Doctor may increase dose up to 300 milligrams per day maximum if needed. *Seniors*—ranges from 25 to 100 milligrams per day, up to a maximum of 150 milligrams.

 Usual child dose: adolescents—ranges from 25 to 100 milligrams per day, up to a maximum of 150 milligrams.

 Missed dose: *if taking several doses per day*—take as soon as possible, then take remaining doses for the day at evenly spaced intervals. *If taking once per day at bedtime*—skip missed dose, go back to regular schedule. *Do not double doses.*

Side Effects

 Overdose symptoms: agitation, coma, confusion, delirium, difficult breathing, dilated pupils, extremely low blood pressure, fever, inability to urinate, irregular heart rate, kidney failure, restlessness, rigid muscles, seizures, shock, stupor, vomiting. If you suspect an overdose, immediately seek medical attention.

 Side effects: abdominal cramps; agitation; anxiety; black tongue; black, red, or blue spots on skin; blurred vision; breast development in males; breast enlargement in females; confusion; constipation; delusions; diarrhea; dilated pupils; disorientation; dizziness; drowsiness; dry mouth; excessive or spontaneous flow of milk; fatigue; fever; flushing; frequent urination or difficulty or delay in urinating; hallucinations; headache; heart attack; heartbeat irregularities; hepatitis; high or low blood pressure; high or low blood sugar; hives; impotence; increased or decreased sex drive; inflammation of the mouth; insomnia; intestinal blockage; lack of coordination; light-headedness (especially when standing up); loss of appetite; loss of hair; mild elation; nausea; nightmares; odd taste in mouth; painful ejaculation; palpitations; purplish spots on skin; rapid heartbeat; restlessness; ringing in ears; seizures; sensitivity to light; skin itching and rash; sore throat; stomach pain; stroke; sweating; swelling due to fluid retention (especially in face or tongue); swelling of testicles; swollen glands; tingling; numbness and pins and needles in hands and feet; tremors; urinating at night; visual problems; vomiting; weakness; weight gain or loss; worsening of psychosis; yellowed skin and eyes.

No known less common or rare side effects.

Interactions

At risk for fatal reaction if taking MAO inhibitors such as Nardil or Parnate; do not take Norpramin within 2 weeks of taking any of these medications. Inform your doctor before combining Norpramin with: cimetidine (Tagamet), fluoxetine (Prozac), guanethidine (Ismelin), medications to improve breathing such as Proventil, medications that relax certain muscles such as Bentyl, sedatives such as Valium and Halcion, thyroid medications (Synthroid). Extreme drowsiness may occur if combining Norpramin with other depressants including narcotic painkillers such as Percocet and Demerol, sleeping medications such as Halcion and Nembutal, and tranquilizers such as Valium and Xanax.

Alcohol may cause extreme drowsiness.

Special Cautions

 If pregnant or planning to become pregnant, inform your doctor immediately. Not known if Norpramin appears in breast milk.

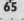 Seniors are prescribed lower doses.

 Not generally prescribed for children younger than adolescent age.

 May cause dizziness and impair your ability to drive a car or operate machinery. *Do not take part in any activity that requires alertness.*

Inform your doctor *before* Norpramin therapy if you have: heart or thyroid disease, seizure disorder, history of being unable to urinate, or glaucoma.

Alert your doctor *before* elective surgery that you are taking Norpramin.

Should not take if hypersensitive to this medication or if you recently had a heart attack.

Sensitivity to sunlight may be increased. Overexposure may lead to rash, itching, redness, or sunburn.

Inform your doctor if you experience fever and sore throat during Norpramin therapy; doctor may perform blood tests.

Nortriptyline Hydrochloride
see PAMELOR

Norvasc

Generic name: Amlodipine besylate

Norvasc is a calcium channel blocker. It increases the amount of oxygen that reaches the heart muscle.

℞ QUICK FACTS

Purpose

℞ Used to treat angina (crushing chest pain). Also used to treat high blood pressure.

Dosage

 Requires taking on regular schedule to be effective. May take several weeks to observe full effects of medication. Continue taking even if symptoms disappear. Dosage should be gradually reduced under the direction of your doctor.

 Usual adult dose: *for angina*—5 to 10 milligrams 1 time per day. *In the case of liver disease*—5 milligrams once per day. *Seniors with angina*—5 milligrams taken once per day. *High blood pressure*—5 milligrams taken once per day. *If taking with other blood pressure medications*—2.5 milligrams once per day. *In the case of liver disease*—5 milligrams once per day. *Seniors with high blood pressure*—2.5 milligrams once per day.

 Usual child dose: not generally prescribed for children.

 Missed dose: take as soon as possible, if next dose is more than 4 hours away. Otherwise, skip missed dose; go back to regular schedule. *Do not double doses.*

Side Effects

 Overdose symptoms: drop in blood pressure and faster heartbeat. If you suspect an overdose, immediately seek medical attention.

 More common side effects: dizziness, fatigue, flushing, fluid retention and swelling, headache, palpitations.

 Less common side effects: abdominal pain, nausea, sleepiness. Rare side effects: abnormal dreams, agitation, altered sense of smell or taste, anxiety, apathy, back pain, chest pain, cold and clammy skin, conjunctivitis (pink eye), constipation, coughing, depression, diarrhea, difficult or labored breathing, difficult or painful urination, difficulty swallowing, dizziness when standing, double vision, dry mouth, dry skin, excessive urination, eye pain, fainting, frequent urination, gas, general feeling of illness, hair loss, heart failure, hives, hot flashes, inability to sleep, increased appetite, increased sweating, indigestion, irregular heartbeat, irregular pulse, itching, joint pain or problems, lack of coordination, lack of sensation, loose stools, loss of appetite, loss of memory, loss of sense of identity, low blood pressure, migraine, muscle cramps or pain, muscle weakness, nasal inflammation, nervousness, nosebleed, pain, purple or red spots on skin, rapid heartbeat, rash, ringing in ears, sexual problems, skin discoloration, skin inflammation, slow heartbeat, stomach inflammation, thirst, tingling or pins and needles, tremor, twitching, urinating at night, urinating problems, vertigo, vision problems, vomiting, weakness, weight gain.

Interactions

 No drug interactions reported.

No known food/other substance interactions.

Special Cautions

 If pregnant or planning to become pregnant, inform your doctor immediately. May appear in breast milk; could affect a nursing infant.

 Seniors are prescribed lower dosage levels.

 Not generally prescribed for children.

 Do not take if sensitive to or allergic to this medication.

Norvasc will be prescribed cautiously if you have certain heart conditions or liver disease.

In rare cases, may experience increase in frequency and length of angina attacks, or you may have a heart attack when starting Norvasc or when dosage is increased.

Nystatin with Triamcinolone Acetonide

see MYCOLOG-II

~~~~~~

Ofloxacin

see FLOXIN

Ogen

~~~~~~

Generic name: Estropipate

Other brand name: Ortho-Est 1.25

Ogen is an estrogen replacement. It mimics the action of naturally produced estrogen.

℞ QUICK FACTS

Purpose

Used to reduce symptoms of menopause, including warmth in face, neck and chest, and hot flashes. Also prescribed for teenagers who do not mature at the usual rate. Also prescribed for dry, itchy external genitals and vaginal irritation; and to prevent osteoporosis.

Dosage

Take exactly as prescribed, adhering to cycle your doctor establishes. Vaginal cream is for short-term use.

Usual adult dose: *for hot flashes and night sweats—Ogen tablets*—dose ranges from one 0.625 tablet to two 2.5 tablets per day. *Ortho-Est 1.25 tablets*—

½ tablet to 4 tablets per day. *For vaginal inflammation and dryness: Ogen tablets*—dose ranges from one 0.625 tablet to two 2.5 tablets per day. *Orth-Est 1.25 tablets*—½ tablet to 4 tablets per day. *Ogen vaginal cream*—2 to 4 grams. *For estrogen hormone deficiency*—*Ogen tablets*—ranges from one 1.25 tablet to three 2.5 tablets per day taken for 3 weeks, and off medication for 8 to 10 days. *Ortho-Est 1.25 tablets*—ranges from 1 to 6 tablets per day taken for 3 weeks, and off medication for 8 to 10 days. *For hysterectomy or ovarian failure*—*Ogen tablets*—ranges from one 1.25 tablet to three 2.5 tablets per day for 3 weeks, and off medication for 8 to 10 days. *Ortho-Est 1.25 tablets* —ranges from 1 to 6 tablets per day taken for 3 weeks, and off medication for 8 to 10 days. *For prevention of osteoporosis*—*Ogen tablets*—one 0.625 tablet per day for 25 days of a 31-day cycle.

. . . .

 Usual child dose: prescribed for children in limited circumstances; dosage is individualized.

. . . .

 Missed dose—take as soon as possible, unless almost time for next dose. In that case, do not take missed dose; go back to regular schedule. *Do not double doses.*

Side Effects

 Overdose symptoms: nausea, vomiting, withdrawal bleeding. If you suspect an overdose, immediately seek medical attention.

. . . .

 Side effects: abdominal cramps; bloating; breakthrough bleeding; breast enlargement; breast tenderness; change in amount of cervical secretion; change in menstrual flow; changes in sex drive; changes in vaginal bleeding patterns; chorea (irregular, rapid jerky movements, usually in face and limbs); depression; dizziness; enlargement of benign tumors (fibroids); excessive hairiness; fluid retention; hair loss; headache; inability to use contact lenses; lack of menstruation; migraine; nausea; painful menstruation; secretion from breasts; spotting; spotty darkening of skin, especially around face; skin eruptions, especially on arms and legs; skin irritation; vaginal yeast infection; vision problems; vomiting; weight gain or loss; yellow eyes and skin.

 No known less common or rare side effects.

Interactions

 Inform your doctor before combining Ogen with: barbiturates such as phenobarbital, blood thinners such as Coumadin, epilepsy medications such as Tegretol and Dilantin, insulin, tricyclic antidepressants such as Elavil and Tofranil, rifampin (Rifadin).

 No known food/other substance interactions.

Special Cautions

 Do not use Ogen if pregnant. If you become pregnant during Ogen therapy, inform your doctor immediately. May appear in breast milk; could affect a nursing infant.

 No special precautions apply to seniors.

 Follow doctor's instructions carefully for children.

 Do not use if abnormal, undiagnosed genital bleeding is present, or if you have blood clots, a blood-clotting disorder, or a history of blood-clotting disorders.

Immediately contact your doctor if you experience: abdominal pain, tenderness or swelling, abnormal vaginal bleeding, breast lumps, coughing up blood, pain in chest or calves, severe headache, dizziness or faintness, sudden shortness of breath, vision changes, yellowing of skin.

. . . .

Use cautiously if you have: asthma, epilepsy, migraine, heart or kidney disease.

. . . .

Postmenopausal women at risk for endometrial cancer; inform your doctor of any unusual vaginal bleeding.

. . . .

Should not use if breast cancer or other cancers promoted by estrogen are known or suspected to be present.

. . . .

If sensitive to or allergic to vaginal cream, should not use.

. . . .

Increased risk of uterine cancer when Ogen is used for a long period of time.

. . . .

Increased risk of gallbladder disease in postmenopausal women.

. . . .

May cause fluid retention.

Olsalazine Sodium
see DIPENTUM

Omeprazole
see PRILOSEC

Omnipen

Generic name: Ampicillin

Other brand names: D-Amp, Polycillin, Principen, Totacillin

Omnipen is a penicillin antibiotic. Antibiotics inhibit the growth of bacteria.

℞ QUICK FACTS

Purpose

℞ Used to treat a wide variety of infections, including gonorrhea and other genital and urinary infections, and gastrointestinal infections.

Dosage

 Capsules to be taken with a full glass of water ½ hour *before* or 2 hours *after* a meal. Shake oral suspension well before use. Take exactly as prescribed; try not to miss doses. For best results must maintain a constant level in the body. Must take entire amount prescribed (especially in the case of strep throat); otherwise you may get other infections, such as kidney infection or rheumatic fever.

 Usual adult dose: *for infections of genital, urinary, or gastrointestinal tracts*—500 milligrams taken 4 times per day. *For gonorrhea*—3.5 grams in a single oral dose, with 1 gram of probenecid. *For respiratory tract infections*—250 milligrams taken 4 times per day.

 Usual child dose: *for children weighing over 44 pounds*—follow adult schedule. *For children weighing under 44 pounds*—Infections of genital, urinary or gastrointestinal tracts—100 milligrams for each 2.2 pounds of body weight divided into 4 doses for capsules and 3 to 4 doses for suspension. *Respiratory*

tract infections—50 milligrams for each 2.2 pounds of body weight per day, divided into 3 to 4 doses.

Missed dose—*If taking 2 doses per day*—take as soon as possible; take next dose 5 to 6 hours later. Then go back to regular schedule. *If taking 3 or more doses per day*—take as soon as possible; take next dose 2 to 4 hours later. Then go back to regular schedule. *Do not double doses.*

Side Effects

Overdose symptoms: no specific information available. If you suspect an overdose, immediately seek medical attention.

Side effects: anemia; colitis (inflammation of the bowel); diarrhea; fever; hives; itching; nausea; hives; rash; skin redness, peeling or flaking; sore or inflamed tongue or mouth; vomiting.

No known less common or rare side effects.

Interactions

Inform your doctor before combining Omnipen with: allopurinol (Zyloprim); atenolol (Tenormin); chloroquine (Aralen); mefloquine (Lariam); other antibiotics such as chloramphenicol, tetracycline, erythromycin, and sulfonamides; oral contraceptives; probenecid (Benemid). Oral contraceptives may have a reduced effect with Omnipen.

No known food/other substance interactions.

Special Cautions

If you become pregnant during Omnipen therapy, inform your doctor immediately. Appears in breast milk; could affect a nursing infant.

 No special precautions apply to seniors.

 Follow doctor's instructions carefully for children.

 Inform your doctor *before* taking Omnipen if you are allergic to penicillin or cephalosporin antibiotics in any form; may cause extremely severe reaction.

Stop taking medication and immediately contact your doctor if you feel signs of allergic reaction.

Secondary infection not treatable by this medication (superinfection) may occur if taking Omnipen for an extended period.

Can cause diarrhea; consult your doctor before taking a diarrhea medication.

Has caused false positive urine glucose tests in diabetics.

Ondansetron Hydrochloride

see ZOFRAN

Oral Contraceptives

Generic names: Progestin estrogen

Brand names: Brevicon, Demulen, Desogen, Genora 1/35-28, Levlen, Levonorgestrel Implant, Loestrin, Lo/Ovral, Modicon, Micronor, NEE,

Nelova, Nordette, Norethin, Norinyl, Norlestrin, Norplant, Nor-Q.D., Ortho-Cept, Ortho-Cyclen, Ortho-Novum, Ortho Tri-Cyclen, Ovcon, Ovral, Ovrette, Progestasert, Progesterone Intrauterine Insert, Tri-Levlen, Tri-Norinyl, Triphasil

Oral contraceptives prevent egg production and ovulation, alter the uterine lining, and thicken cervical mucus—to prevent conception and egg implantation.

℞ QUICK FACTS

Purpose

℞ Used to prevent pregnancy.

Dosage

 Take every day, ideally at the same time. Pills should be taken no more than 24 hours apart.

 Usual adult dose: take on 21-day or 28-day schedule. Follow doctor's instructions carefully before taking medication.

 Usual child dose: not generally prescribed for children.

 Missed dose: take as soon as possible if you miss one pill; return to regular schedule. If you miss more than 1 tablet, *do not take missed tablet; return to regular schedule, but use another form of birth control during this medication cycle.*

Side Effects

 Overdose symptoms: nausea, withdrawal bleeding in women. If you suspect an overdose, immediately seek medical attention.

Side effects: abdominal cramps; acne; appetite changes; bladder infection; bleeding in spots during menstrual period; bloating; blood clots; breast tenderness or enlargement; cataracts; chest pain; contact lens discomfort; decreased flow of milk when given immediately after birth; depression; difficulty breathing; dizziness; fluid retention; gallbladder disease; growth of face, back, chest, or stomach hair; hair loss; headache; heart attack; high blood pressure; inflammation of large intestine; kidney trouble; lack of menstrual periods; liver tumors; lumps in breast; menstrual pattern changes; migraine; muscle, joint, or leg pain; nausea; nervousness; premenstrual syndrome (PMS); secretion of milk; sex drive changes; skin infection; skin rash or discoloration; stomach cramps; stroke; swelling; temporary infertility; unexplained bleeding in the vagina; vaginal discharge; vaginal infections (and/or burning and itching); visual disturbances; vomiting; weight gain or loss; yellow skin or eyes.

 No known less common or rare side effects.

Interactions

 Inform your doctor before combining oral contraceptives with: amitriptyline (Elavil or Endep), ampicillin (Polycillin or Principen), barbiturates (phenobarbital), carbamazepine (Tegretol), chloramphenicol (Chloromycetin), clomipramine (Anafranil), diazepam (Valium), doxepin (Sinequan), glipzide (Glucotrol), griseofulvin (Fulvicin or Grisactin), imipramine (Tofranil or Janimine), lorazepam (Ativan), metoprolol (Lopressor), oxazepam (Serax), penicillin (Veetids or Pen•Vee K), phenylbutazone (Butazolidin), phenytoin (Dilantin), prednisolone (Delta-Cortef or Prelone), prednisone (Deltasone), primidone (Mysoline), propranolol (Inderal), rifampin (Rifadin or Rimactane), sulfonamides (Bactrim or

Septra), tetracycline (Achromycin V), theophylline (Theo-Dur), warfarin (Coumadin).

 No known food/other substance interactions.

Special Cautions

 Should not use oral contraceptives during pregnancy. If you become pregnant, inform your doctor immediately. Appears in breast milk; may cause jaundice and enlarged breasts in nursing infants.

 No special precautions apply to seniors.

 Not generally prescribed for children.

 At risk for stroke, heart attack, and blood clots if you smoke and use oral contraceptives.

Should not take if sensitive to or allergic to this medication, or if you have ever had breast cancer, cancer of the reproductive organs, liver tumors, pregnancy-related jaundice or jaundice stemming from previous use of oral contraceptives.

Use cautiously if: you are over 40 years; smoke tobacco; have liver, gallbladder, kidney, or thyroid disease; have high blood pressure or cholesterol; diabetes; epilepsy; asthma; porphyria (blood disorder); are obese; have a family history of breast or other cancers. Also use cautiously if you have a personal history of depression, migraine, other headaches, irregular menstrual periods, or visual disturbances.

Doctor may discontinue use of oral contraceptives prior to surgery, to avoid affecting the body's blood-clotting mechanism.

Organidin with Dextromethorphan Hydrobromide

see TUSSI-ORGANIDIN DM

Orinase

Generic name: Tolbutamide

Orinase is an oral antidiabetic medication. It works by inducing the pancreas to secrete more insulin.

℞ QUICK FACTS

Purpose

℞ Used to treat Type II (non-insulin-dependent) diabetes.

Dosage

 Take 30 minutes prior to eating or according to your doctor's specific instructions.

 Usual adult dose: 1 to 2 grams initially. *Maintenance therapy*—ranges from 0.25 to 3 grams per day. *Seniors*—prescribed lower doses.

 Usual child dose: not generally prescribed for children.

 Missed dose: take as soon as possible, unless almost time for next dose. In that case, do not take missed dose; go back to regular schedule. *Do not double doses.*

Side Effects

 Overdose symptom: low blood sugar. Signs of mild hypoglycemia (low blood sugar)—blurred vision, cold sweats, dizziness, fatigue, headache, hunger, light-headedness, nausea, nervousness, rapid heartbeat. Symptoms of more severe hypoglycemia—coma, pale skin, seizures, shallow breathing. If you suspect an overdose, immediately seek medical attention.

 More common side effects: bloating, heartburn, nausea.

 Less common or rare side effects: anemia and other blood disorders; blistering; changes in taste; headache; hepatic porphyria (sensitivity to light, stomach pain, and nerve damage); hives; itching; redness of skin; skin eruptions; skin rash.

Interactions

 Inform your doctor before combining Orinase with: adrenal corticosteroids (prednisone or cortisone), airway-opening medications (Proventil or Ventolin), anabolic steroids (testosterone), barbiturates (Seconal or phenobarbital), beta-blockers such as Inderal and Tenormin, blood thinners such as Coumadin, calcium channel blockers such as Cardizem and Procardia, chloramphenicol (Chloromycetin), cimetidine (Tagamet), clofibrate (Atromid-S), epinephrine (EpiPen), estrogens (Premarin), fluconazole (Diflucan), furosemide (Lasix), isoniazid (Laniazid or Rifamate), itraconazole (Sporanox), major tranquilizers such as Stelazine and Mellaril, MAO inhibitors such as Nardil, methyldopa (Aldomet), miconazole (Monistat), niacin (Nicobid or Nicolar), nonsteroidal anti-inflammatory medications such as Motrin and Naprosyn, oral contraceptives, phenytoin (Dilantin), probenecid (Benemid), rifampin (Rifadin), sulfa medications such as Bactrim and Septra, thiazide and other diuretics such as Diuril and HydroDIURIL, thyroid medications such as Synthroid.

 Alcohol use may cause low blood sugar; use carefully.

Special Cautions

 If pregnant or planning to become pregnant, inform your doctor immediately. Not known if Orinase appears in breast milk; however, other oral diabetes medications do.

 Seniors may be prescribed a lower dose to minimize risk of low blood sugar (hypoglycemia).

 Not generally prescribed for children.

 Should not use in place of a sound diet and exercise.

Orinase is *not* insulin and should not be used as a substitute for insulin.

To help prevent hypoglycemia (low blood sugar), always keep a quick-acting sugar product handy.

Hypoglycemia risk increases by: missed meals, use of other medications, fever, trauma, infection, surgery, excessive exercise. Also at higher risk for hypoglycemia if you have: kidney or liver problems; lack of adrenal or pituitary hormone; are elderly, run-down, malnourished; or are using more than one glucose-lowering medication.

If allergic to Orinase, should not take.

Should not take if you have diabetic ketoacidosis (a life-threatening emergency with symptoms that include excessive thirst, nausea, fatigue, pain below breastbone, fruity breath).

Not to be used as the only therapy for treating Type I (insulin-dependent) diabetes.

Consult with your doctor before starting Orinase if you have a heart condition; may worsen condition.

Doctor should monitor glucose levels in blood and urine during therapy.

Doctor may switch you from Orinase to insulin if you experience injury, infection, surgery, or fever, leading to loss of control of diabetes.

Effectiveness may decrease over time.

Orphenadrine Citrate with Aspirin and Caffeine
see NORGESIC

Orphengesic
see NORGESIC

Ortho-Est 1.25
see OGEN

Orudis

ᴧᴧᴧᴧᴧᴧᴧᴧᴧᴧᴧᴧᴧᴧᴧᴧᴧᴧᴧᴧᴧᴧᴧᴧᴧᴧᴧᴧᴧᴧᴧᴧᴧᴧᴧᴧ

Generic name: Ketoprofen

Other brand name: Oruvail

Orudis is a nonsteroidal anti-inflammatory drug (NSAID). It works by blocking the production of prostaglandins, which may trigger pain.

℞ QUICK FACTS

Purpose

℞ Used to treat the inflammation, swelling, stiffness, and joint pain with rheumatoid arthritis and osteoarthritis. Also used to relieve menstrual pain and mild to moderate pain.

Dosage

 Take with food, antacid, or milk to avoid stomach upset. If taking for arthritis, take regularly.

 Usual adult dose: *for rheumatoid arthritis and osteoarthritis—Orudis—*75 milligrams taken 3 times per day or 50 milligrams taken 4 times per day, maximum 300 milligrams per day. *Oruvail—*200 milligrams taken once per day, maximum 300 milligrams per day. *For mild to moderate pain or menstrual pain—Orudis—*25 to 50 milligrams every 6 to 8 hours as needed for pain. Doctor may adjust dose for smaller individuals or those with liver or kidney disease. *Seniors—*may require a lower dose.

 Usual child dose: not generally prescribed for children.

 Missed dose: *if taking on a regular schedule—*take as soon as possible, unless almost time for next dose.

In that case, do not take missed dose; go back to regular schedule. *Do not double doses.*

Side Effects

Overdose symptoms: no specific information available. If you suspect an overdose, immediately seek medical attention.

More common side effects: abdominal pain, changes in kidney function, constipation, diarrhea, fluid retention, gas, headache, inability to sleep, indigestion, nausea.

Less common or rare side effects: allergic reaction, amnesia, anemia, asthma, belching, blood in urine, bloody or black stools, change in taste, chills, confusion, congestive heart failure, coughing up blood, conjunctivitis (pink eye), depression, difficult or labored breathing, dizziness, dry mouth, eye pain, facial swelling due to fluid retention, general feeling of illness, hair loss, high blood pressure, hives, impaired hearing, impotence, increase in appetite, increased salivation, infection, inflammation of the mouth, irregular or excessive menstrual bleeding, itching, kidney failure, loosening of fingernails, loss of appetite, migraine, muscle pain, nasal inflammation, nosebleed, pain, peptic or intestinal ulcer, rapid heartbeat, rash, rectal bleeding, red or purple spots on skin, ringing in ears, sensitivity to light, skin discoloration, skin eruptions, skin inflammation and flaking, sleepiness, sore throat, stomach inflammation, sweating, swelling of throat, thirst, throbbing heartbeat, tingling or pins and needles, vertigo, visual disturbances, vomiting, vomiting blood, weight gain or loss.

Interactions

Inform your doctor before combining Orudis with: aspirin, blood thinners such as Coumadin, diuretics such as hydrochlorothiazide (HydroDIURIL), lithium (Lithonate), methotrexate, probenecid (Benemid).

 No known food/other substance interactions.

Special Cautions

 If pregnant or planning to become pregnant, inform your doctor immediately. May appear in breast milk, could affect a nursing infant.

 Seniors may require a lower dose.

 Not generally prescribed for children.

 At risk for ulcers or internal bleeding; should have frequent check-ups.

If sensitive to or allergic to Orudis, or if you have asthma attacks, hives, or other allergic reactions caused by aspirin or other NSAIDs, should not take.

Use with caution if you have liver or kidney disease, or heart disease—causes water retention.

Doctor should monitor blood for anemia if you take this medication for a prolonged period.

Oruvail
see ORUDIS

Oxaprozin
see DAYPRO

Oxazepam

see SERAX

Oxiconazole Nitrate

see OXISTAT

Oxistat

〜〜〜〜〜〜〜〜〜〜〜〜〜〜〜〜〜〜〜〜〜〜〜〜〜〜〜〜〜〜〜〜

Generic name: Oxiconazole nitrate

Oxistat is an antifungal. It destroys and prevents the growth of fungi.

℞ QUICK FACTS

Purpose

℞ Used to treat fungal skin diseases such as ringworm (tinea). Also used to treat athlete's foot, jock itch, and ringworm of the entire body.

Dosage

 Use exactly as prescribed. Not for use in or near the eyes or vagina.

. . . .

 Usual adult dose: apply cream or lotion once or twice per day. Athlete's foot is treated for one month. Jock itch and ringworm of the body are treated for 2 weeks.

. . . .

 Usual child dose: same as adult dose.

. . . .

Missed dose: apply cream or lotion as soon as possible, then return to regular schedule.

Side Effects

 Overdose symptoms: none reported. However, if you suspect an overdose, immediately seek medical attention.

 Side effects: allergic skin inflammation; burning; cracks in the skin; eczema; irritation; itching; pain; rash; scaling; skin redness; skin softening; small, firm, raised skin eruptions similar to chicken pox; stinging; tingling.

 No known less common or rare side effects.

Interactions

 No drug interactions reported.

 No known food/other substance interactions.

Special Cautions

 If pregnant or planning to become pregnant, inform your doctor immediately. Appears in breast milk; could affect a nursing infant.

 No special precautions apply to seniors.

 Follow doctor's instructions carefully for children.

 Do not use if sensitive to or allergic to any of the ingredients of this medication.

Inform your doctor if you develop an irritation or sensitivity.

Oxybutynin Chloride
see DITROPAN

Pamelor

Generic name: Nortriptyline hydrochloride

Other brand name: Aventyl

Pamelor is a tricyclic antidepressant. It is thought to relieve depression by increasing the concentration of certain chemicals responsible for brain nerve transmissions.

℞ QUICK FACTS

Purpose

℞ Used to treat depression. Also used to treat chronic hives, premenstrual depression, attention deficit disorder in children, bedwetting.

Dosage

 Take regularly to be effective. *Do not miss doses, even if medication does not relieve symptoms right away. May take several weeks to observe effects.*

. . . .

 Usual adult dose: 25 milligrams taken 3 or 4 times per day, or in a single daily dose. Maximum dose is 150 milligrams per day. *Seniors*—30 to 50 milligrams taken as a single dose or divided into smaller doses.

. . . .

 Usual child dose: *adolescents only*—30 to 50 milligrams per day in a single dose or divided into smaller doses.

. . . .

Missed dose: take as soon as possible, unless almost time for next dose. In that case, do not take missed dose; go back to regular schedule. *Do not double doses. If taking once per day at bedtime, do not take the following morning; may cause disturbing side effects. Do not double doses.*

Side Effects

 Overdose may be fatal. Overdose symptoms: agitation, coma, confusion, congestive heart failure, convulsions, decreased breathing, excessive reflexes, extremely high fever, rapid heartbeat, restlessness, rigid muscles, shock, stupor, vomiting. If you suspect an overdose, immediately seek medical attention.

 Side effects: abdominal cramps; agitation; anxiety; black tongue; blurred vision; breast development; confusion; constipation; delusions; diarrhea; dilation of pupils; disorientation; dizziness; drowsiness; dry mouth; excessive or spontaneous flow of milk; excessive urination at night; fatigue; fever; fluid retention; flushing; frequent urination; hair loss; hallucinations; headache; heart attack; high or low blood pressure; high or low blood sugar; hives; impotence; inability to sleep; inability to urinate; increased or decreased sex drive; inflammation of the mouth; intestinal blockage; itching; loss of appetite; loss of coordination; nausea; nightmares; numbness; panic; perspiration; pins and needles in the arms and legs; rapid, fluttery, or irregular heartbeat; rash; reddish or purplish skin parts; restlessness; ringing in ears; seizures; sensitivity to light; stomach upset; strange taste; stroke; swelling of the testicles; swollen glands; tingling; tremors; vision problems; vomiting; weakness; weight gain or loss; yellow eyes and skin. Side effects due to sudden withdrawal after long-term treatment: headache, nausea, vague feeling of bodily discomfort.

No known less common or rare side effects.

Interactions

 Do not take Pamelor with MAO *inhibitors, can be fatal.*
Inform your doctor before combining Pamelor with:
acetazolamide (Diamox), airway-opening medications such as Ventolin and Proventil, amphetamines
such as Dexedrine, antispasmodics such as Donnatal
and Bentyl, blood pressure medications such as Catapres and Ismelin, cimetidine (Tagamet), levodopa
(Laradopa), other antidepressants such as Prozac,
quinidine (Quinaglute), reserpine (Diupres), thyroid
medications such as Synthroid, vitamin C (in large
doses), warfarin (Coumadin).

 *Do not drink alcohol during Pamelor therapy; may inten-
sify the effects of alcohol.*

Special Cautions

 If pregnant or planning to become pregnant, inform
your doctor immediately. Not known if Pamelor appears in breast milk.

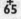 Seniors are prescribed lower doses.

 Follow doctor's instructions carefully for children.

 *Do not take if you have just had a heart attack or are
taking other antidepressant medications.*

May cause drowsiness and impair your ability to
drive a car or operate machinery. *Do not take part
in any activity that requires alertness.*

Inform your doctor *before starting* Pamelor if you are
being treated for schizophrenia, manic depression,
or other severe mental disorders.

If allergic to or sensitive to this or similar medications, should not take.

Use with caution if you have: history of seizures, difficulty urinating, diabetes, glaucoma, heart disease, high blood pressure, overactive thyroid, or are taking thyroid medication.

May cause sensitivity to sunlight.

Inform doctor or dentist before having surgery or dental treatment.

Pancrease

Generic name: Pancrelipase

Other brand names: Cotazym, Ilozyme, Ku-Zyme HP, Pancrease MT, Protilase, Ultrase, Viokase, Zymase

Pancrease is a source of pancreatic enzymes. It enhances the digestion of proteins, starches, and fats.

℞ QUICK FACTS

Purpose

℞ Used to treat pancreatic enzyme deficiency. Often used for people with cystic fibrosis, chronic pancreas inflammation, or blockages of the pancreas or common bile duct caused by cancer. Also prescribed for people who have had their pancreas removed or who have had gastrointestinal bypass surgery.

Dosage

 Take exactly as prescribed. A special diet may be prescribed if you have cystic fibrosis. *Do not change brands unless directed by your doctor.* If unable to swallow capsules, shake contents onto soft food and swallow immediately, without chewing. Should not be mixed with alkaline foods such as ice cream or milk; it may reduce effects of medication. Take with food.

 Usual adult dose: 1 or 2 capsules with each meal and 1 capsule with snacks.

 Usual child dose: not generally prescribed for children.

 Missed dose: take medication with your next meal or snack.

Side Effects

 Overdose symptoms: no specific information available. However, if you suspect an overdose, immediately seek medical attention.

 More common side effects: stomach and intestinal upset.

 Less common side effects: allergic-type reactions.

Interactions

 Inform your doctor before combining Pancrease with ulcer medications such as Pepcid and Zantac.

 Check with your doctor before taking Pancrease with certain antacids such as Tums and milk of magnesia.

Special Cautions

 If pregnant or planning to become pregnant, inform your doctor immediately. Not known if Pancrease appears in breast milk.

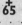 No special precautions apply to seniors.

 Not generally prescribed for children.

 If sensitive to or allergic to pork protein, should not use.

Pancrelipase

see PANCREASE

Parafon Forte DSC

Generic name: Chlorzoxazone

Other brand name: Paraflex

Parafon is a skeletal muscle relaxant. It is thought to modify central perception of pain without eliminating peripheral pain reflexes.

℞ QUICK FACTS

Purpose

℞ Used to treat discomfort associated with severe, painful muscle spasms.

Dosage

 Take exactly as prescribed. *Do not change dosage unless under direction from your doctor.* May turn urine orange or purple red.

 Usual adult dose: 1 caplet taken 3 or 4 times per day. Doctor may increase up to 1½ caplets 3 or 4 times per day.

 Usual child dose: not generally prescribed for children.

 Missed dose: take as soon as possible if within 1 hour of missed dose. Otherwise, do not take missed dose; go back to regular schedule. *Do not double doses.*

Side Effects

 Overdose symptoms: diarrhea, dizziness, drowsiness, headache, light-headedness, nausea, vomiting. Symptoms developing after a period of time: feeling of illness, loss of muscle strength, lowered blood pressure, sluggishness, troubled or rapid breathing. If you suspect an overdose, immediately seek medical attention.

 More common side effects: none reported.

 Uncommon and rare side effects: bruises, dizziness, drowsiness, feeling of illness, fluid retention, light-headedness, overstimulation, red or purple skin spots, severe allergic reaction, skin rashes, stomach or intestinal disturbances or bleeding, urine discoloration.

Interactions

 Inform your doctor before combining Parafon Forte DSC with central nervous system medications such as Percocet, Valium, and Xanax.

 Do not take Parafon Forte DSC with alcohol.

Special Cautions

 If pregnant or planning to become pregnant, inform your doctor immediately. May appear in breast milk; could affect a nursing infant.

 No special precautions apply to seniors.

 Not generally prescribed for children.

 If allergic to any medication or if you have allergies, use with caution. Contact your doctor immediately if you experience hives, redness, or skin itching. If allergic to this medication, inform your doctor.

If you experience any liver problems, inform your doctor.

Parlodel

Generic name: Bromocriptine mesylate

Parlodel is a dopamine agonist and antiparkinsonism agent. It replaces the dopamine that is diminished in the brains of Parkinson's patients, and blocks the action of prolactin, a milk production hormone.

℞ QUICK FACTS

Purpose

Used to treat: infertility in women, menstrual problems such as abnormal stoppage or absence of flow, excessive spontaneous flow of milk, growth hormone overproduction, Parkinson's disease, pituitary gland tumors.

Dosage

Must take with food in your stomach. Take the first dose lying down, as you may experience dizziness or faint. Full effects of this medication become apparent after a few weeks; *do not stop medication unless directed by your doctor.*

Usual adult dose: *to prevent milk production after delivery*—1 tablet 2 times per day for 14 days, up to 21 days maximum. *For excess prolactin hormone (excessive milk production, menstrual problems, pituitary gland tumors)*—½ to 1 tablet daily. Doctor may add a tablet every 3 to 7 days until correct dose is determined (longer term dose ranges from 2.5 to 15 milligrams per day). *For growth hormone overproduction*—½ to 1 tablet with food at bedtime for 3 days (20 to 30 milligrams per day, not to exceed 100 milligrams per day). *For Parkinson's disease*—½ tablet 2 times per day with meals. Doctor may increase dose by 1 tablet every 14 to 28 days. Usually taken with levodopa.

Usual child dose: follow doctor's instructions carefully for children 15 years and older.

Missed dose: take as soon as possible if within 4 hours of missed dose. Otherwise, do not take missed dose; go back to regular schedule. *Do not double doses.*

Side Effects

 Overdose symptoms: no specific information available. If you suspect an overdose, immediately seek medical attention.

 More common side effects: abdominal cramps or discomfort, confusion, constipation, depression, diarrhea, dizziness, drop in blood pressure, drowsiness, dry mouth, fainting, fatigue, hallucinations (especially in Parkinson's patients), headache, inability to sleep, indigestion, light-headedness, loss of appetite, loss of coordination, nasal congestion, nausea, shortness of breath, uncontrolled body movement, vertigo, visual disturbance, vomiting, weakness.

 Less common side effects: abdominal bleeding, anxiety, difficulty swallowing, frequent urination, heart attack, inability to hold urine, inability to urinate, nightmares, nervousness, rash, seizures, splotchy skin, stroke, swelling or fluid retention in feet and ankles, twitching of eyelids. Rare side effects: abnormal heart rhythm, blurred vision or temporary blindness, cold feet, fast or slow heartbeat, hair loss, heavy headedness, increase in blood pressure, lower back pain, muscle cramps, muscle cramps in feet and legs, numbness, pale face, paranoia, prickling or tingling, reduced tolerance to cold, severe or continuous headache, shortness of breath, sluggishness, tingling of ears or fingers.

Interactions

 Inform your doctor before combining Parlodel with: blood pressure medications such as Aldomet and Catapres; erythromycin (E.E.S. or ERYC); metoclopramide (Reglan); oral contraceptives; other ergot derivatives such as Hydergine; progesterone (Provera). Medications used for psychotic conditions such as Haldol and Thorazine and the other phenothiazines inhibit the action of Parlodel.

 Do not drink alcohol during Parlodel therapy; can cause blurred vision, chest pain, headache, confusion, and other problems.

Special Cautions

 If pregnant or planning to become pregnant, inform your doctor immediately. Should not be used by women who are breastfeeding, as it prevents the flow of milk.

 No special precautions apply to seniors.

 Not generally prescribed for children under 15 years. Follow doctor's instructions carefully for children 15 years and older.

 Women not wanting to become pregnant during Parlodel therapy should use a "barrier" method of contraception. *Do not use oral contraceptives; they prevent Parlodel from working properly.*

May cause drowsiness and impair your ability to drive a car or operate machinery. *Do not take part in any activity that requires alertness.*

Should not use if you have: high blood pressure that is not being treated, or toxemia of pregnancy, or if allergic to this or ergot alkaloid medications such as Bellergal-S or Caftergot.

Doctor should check pituitary gland *before* Parlodel therapy.

Inform your doctor before taking Parlodel if you have kidney or liver disease, or abnormal heart rhythm caused by heart attack.

Stopping Parlodel may cause rapid regrowth of tumor related to endocrine problems.

Immediately notify your doctor if you experience hallucinations, confusion, and low blood pressure or severe persistent headache.

If you observe persistent runny nose with watery discharge, contact your doctor.

Paroxetine Hydrochloride

see PAXIL

Pathocil

Generic name: Dicloxacillin sodium

Other brand names: Dycill, Dynapen

Pathocil is a penicillin antibiotic. Antibiotics inhibit the growth of bacteria.

℞ QUICK FACTS

Purpose

℞ Used to treat certain bacterial infections caused by staph (staphylococci).

Dosage

 Take entire amount prescribed even when symptoms subside. Should take 1 to 2 hours before meals or 2 hours after meals unless directed otherwise by your doctor.

 Usual adult dose: *for mild to moderate infections*—125 milligrams every 6 hours. *For severe infections*—250 milligrams every 6 hours.

 Usual child dose: children 88 pounds or more are prescribed adult dose. Children weighing less than 88 pounds—*mild to moderate infections*—12.5 milligrams per 2.2 pounds of body weight per day, divided into equal doses and taken every 6 hours; *severe infections*—25 milligrams per 2.2 pounds of body weight per day, divided into equal doses and taken every 6 hours.

 Missed dose: *for 2 doses per day*—take as soon as possible, take next dose 5 to 6 hours later, then go back to regular schedule. *For 3 or more doses per day*—take as soon as possible, take next dose 2 to 4 hours later, then go back to regular schedule. *Do not double doses.*

Side Effects

 Overdose symptoms: no specific information available. If you suspect an overdose, immediately seek medical attention.

 Side effects: allergic reaction (delayed or immediate), black or hairy tongue, diarrhea, feeling of being sick, fever, gas, hives, itching, loose stools, low blood pressure, nausea, rashes, serum sickness symptoms (joint and muscle pain with fever and hives), stomach pain, vomiting, wheezing.

No known less common or rare side effects.

Interactions

 Do not take if allergic to Penicillin. Inform your doctor before combining Pathocil with: chloramphenicol (Chloromycetin), erythromycin (PCE or E.E.S.), oral contraceptives, probenecid (Benemid), tetracycline medications such as Achromycin V.

 No known food/other substance interactions.

Special Cautions

 If pregnant or planning to become pregnant, inform your doctor immediately. Appears in breast milk; could affect a nursing infant.

 No special precautions apply to seniors.

 Follow doctor's instructions carefully for children.

 Doctor will perform a complete history before prescribing Pathocil; in rare cases fatal allergic reactions have occurred. Immediately contact your doctor if you develop allergy symptoms.

Contact your doctor immediately if you experience: shortness of breath, wheezing, skin rash, mouth irritation, black tongue, sore throat, nausea, vomiting, diarrhea, fever, swollen joints, or unusual bruising or bleeding.

At risk for developing infection which is not treatable by this medication (superinfection) if taking Pathocil for extended periods of time.

Paxil

Generic name: Paroxetine hydrochloride

Paxil is an antidepressant. It increases the concentration of certain chemicals responsible for brain nerve transmission.

℞ QUICK FACTS

Purpose

 Used to treat serious, continuing depression that interferes with the ability to function normally.

Dosage

 Take exactly as prescribed. Let your doctor know of any over-the-counter medications or prescriptions you are taking. Depression may begin to subside in 1 to 4 weeks; continue to take for the length of time your doctor prescribes.

 Usual adult dose: 20 milligrams per day as a single dose in the morning. Doctor may prescribe up to 50 milligrams per day. *Seniors or those with severe kidney or liver disease*—10 milligrams per day up to 40 milligrams per day maximum.

 Usual child dose: not generally prescribed for children.

 Missed dose: skip missed dose, go back to regular schedule. *Do not double doses.*

Side Effects

Overdose symptoms: drowsiness, enlarged pupils, nausea, rapid heartbeat. If you suspect an overdose, immediately seek medical attention.

✚ More common side effects: abdominal pain, amnesia, anxiety, blurred vision, breathing disorders, burning sensation, chills, cold symptoms, constipation, decreased appetite, decreased sex drive, depression, diarrhea, difficulty concentrating, dizziness, drowsiness, dry mouth, emotional instability, fainting, feeling of general discomfort, fluid retention, frequent urination, headache, high blood pressure, increased coughing, inflammation of nose, intestinal gas, itching, male genital disorders, nausea, nervousness, pricking and tingling, rapid heartbeat, sleepiness, sleeplessness, stomach pain, stuffy nose, sweating, tremor, trouble ejaculating, vertigo, weight gain, weight loss, yawning.

✚ Less common side effects: abnormal thinking; abortion; acne; agitation; alcohol abuse; allergic reactions; altered sense of taste; anemia; arthritis; asthma; back pain; belching; blood disorders; boils; breast pain; bronchitis; bruises; cessation of menstruation; chest pain; confusion; convulsions; difficulty swallowing; dilation of pupils; dizziness on standing; drugged feeling; dry skin; ear pain; eczema; excessive menstrual bleeding; excessive muscular activity; excessive urination; eye pain; feeling of persecution; feeling of unreality; female genital disorders; fevers; grinding of teeth; hair loss; hallucinations; high blood sugar; hives; hyperventilation; incoordination; increased appetite; increased salivation; indigestion; infection of hair follicles; infection of middle ear; infection of skin and mucous membranes; inflammation of the bladder, stomach, throat, tongue, urethra, or vagina; joint pain; lack of coordination; lack of emotion; loss of muscle movement; loss of taste; low blood pressure; lump in throat; manic reaction; menstrual difficulties; migraine headache; mouth ulcers; muscle disease; muscle pain; muscle rigidity; muscle twitching; muscle weakness; neck pain; nosebleeds; overactivity; painful or difficult urination; pneumonia; pounding heartbeat; rash; rectal bleeding; red or purple skin spots; respiratory flu; ringing in ears; shortness of breath; sinusitis; slow heartbeat; swelling of arms and legs; swelling of face; thirst; tightness in throat; tumor; urinary urgency; urinating at night; vision problems; vomiting. Rare side effects: abnormal gait; abnormal kidney function; abscesses; antisocial reaction; blood in urine; bloody diarrhea; breast cancer; bulimia; bursitis; cataract; chest pain; congestive heart failure; dark, tarry, bloody stools; decreased reflexes; decreased urination; dehydration; delirium; delusions; diabetes; difficulty performing voluntary movements; difficulty speaking; dimmed vision; double vision; drug dependence; elevated cholesterol; exaggerated feeling of well-being; extreme sensitivity to painful stimuli; eye hemorrhage; glaucoma; gout; grand mal epileptic convulsions; heart attack; hepatitis; hiccups; hostility; hysteria; impacted stool; inability to control bowel movements; increased reflexes; increased sexual appetite; increased sputum; inflammation of the breast, gums, lining of the eyelid, lining of the stomach and intestine; inflammation of the outer ear, skin, or esophagus; intestinal blockage; intolerance of light; irregular heartbeat; jerky movement; kidney pain; kidney stone; low blood sugar; lung cancer; neck rigidity; osteoporosis; paralysis; pelvic pain; peptic or stomach ulcer; protruding eyeballs; red and painful spots on legs; salivary gland enlargement; sensitivity to light; sensitivity to sound; skin discoloration; skin tumor; spasms in arms and legs; stomach ulcer; stomach pain; stroke; stupor; swelling of thyroid; swelling of tongue; tooth cavities; ulcer on cornea; ulcers; yeast infection; varicose veins; vomiting blood; yellowed eyes and skin.

Interactions

Do not take if you have taken MAO inhibitors such as Nardil and Parnate within the past 2 weeks; can cause serious or fatal reaction. Inform your doctor before

combining Paxil with: amitriptyline (Elavil), cimetidine (Tagamet), desipramine (Norpramin), diazepam (Valium), digoxin (Lanoxin), flecainide (Tambocor), fluoxetine (Prozac), imipramine (Tofranil), lithium (Lithonate), nortriptyline (Pamelor), phenobarbital, phenytoin (Dilantin), procyclidine (Kemadrin), propafenone (Rythmol), propranolol (Inderal or Inderide), quinidine (Quinaglute), thioridazine (Mellaril), tryptophan, warfarin (Coumadin).

 Do not drink alcohol during Paxil therapy.

Special Cautions

 If pregnant or planning to become pregnant, inform your doctor immediately. Appears in breast milk; could affect a nursing infant.

 Seniors are prescribed lower doses.

 Not generally prescribed for children.

 May impair your judgment, thinking, or motor skills. *Do not drive or take part in any activity that requires alertness.*

Use with caution if you have: a disease or condition affecting your metabolism or blood circulation, a history of manic disorders, or seizures. Discontinue if you experience seizures.

PBZ-SR

Generic name: Tripelennamine hydrochloride

Other brand name: Pelamine

PBZ-SR is an antihistamine. Antihistamines block the effects of histamine, a body chemical that causes swelling and itching.

℞ QUICK FACTS

Purpose

 Used to relieve nasal stuffiness and inflammation and red, inflamed eyes caused by fever and other allergies. Also used to treat: itching, swelling, and redness from hives and other rashes caused by mild allergic reactions; allergic reactions to blood transfusions; and with other medications, anaphylactic shock (severe allergic reaction).

Dosage

 Take exactly as prescribed, swallowing tablets whole, not crushed or chewed.

 Usual adult dose: one 100-milligram extended-release tablet in the morning and 1 tablet in the evening. Doctor may prescribe 1 tablet every 8 hours, up to a maximum of 600 millgrams per day.

 Usual child dose: children 12 years and older are prescribed adult dose. Under 12 years—2 milligrams per 1 pound of body weight, up to 300 milligrams per day. Older children may be prescribed up to 3 extended-release tablets per day.

 Missed dose: take as soon as possible, unless almost time for next dose. In that case, do not take missed dose, go back to regular schedule. *Do not double doses.*

Side Effects

 Overdose symptoms: cardiovascular collapse, coma, decreased alertness, drowsiness. *For children—*convulsions, dry mouth, excitement, fever, fixed and/or dilated pupils, flushing, hallucinations, involuntary wringing of hands, lack of coordination, stimulation. If you suspect an overdose, immediately seek medical attention.

 More common side effects: disturbed coordination; dizziness; drowsiness; dry mouth, nose, and throat; extreme calm; increased chest congestion; sleepiness; stomach upset.

 Less common or rare side effects: allergic reactions (hives, rash, sensitivity to light, severe allergic reaction); anemia; an exaggerated sense of well-being; blood disorders; blurred vision; chills; confusion; constipation; convulsions; diarrhea; difficulty sleeping; difficulty urinating; double vision; excitement; fatigue; frequent urination; headache; hysteria; inability to urinate; irritability; loss of appetite; low blood pressure; nausea; nervousness; pounding heartbeat; rapid heartbeat; restlessness; ringing in ears; stuffy nose; tightness in chest; vertigo; vomiting; wheezing.

Interactions

 Inform your doctor before combining PBZ-SR with: MAO inhibitors such as Nardil; sedatives such as Nembutal and Seconal; tranquilizers such as Librium, Valium, and BuSpar.

 Do not drink alcohol during PBZ-SR therapy, may increase the effects of alcohol.

Special Cautions

 If pregnant or planning to become pregnant, inform your doctor immediately. Not recommended for mothers who are nursing.

65 No special precautions apply to seniors. Monitor for dizziness and low blood pressure.

Not generally prescribed for children. Can cause drowsiness or excitability in children.

STOP May cause drowsiness and impair your ability to drive a car or operate machinery. *Do not take part in any activity that requires alertness.*

Do not take if you have: narrow-angle glaucoma; peptic ulcer; symptoms of enlarged prostate, or bladder or intestinal obstruction; asthma or other breathing disorders; or if sensitive to or allergic to this or other antihistamines.

Use with caution if you have: overactive thyroid, heart disease, high blood pressure, circulatory problems.

Pediapred

Generic ingredient: Prednisolone sodium phosphate

Other brand names: Hydeltrasol, Key-Pred SP, Predate-S

Pediapred is a corticosteroid. It works by stimulating the synthesis of enzymes needed to decrease the inflammatory response.

℞ Quick Facts

Purpose

 Used to treat inflammation and symptoms of several disorders, including rheumatoid arthritis, acute gouty arthritis, and severe asthma. Also used to treat primary or secondary adrenal cortex insufficiency, and the following conditions: blood disorders such as leukemia, certain cancers, connective tissue diseases such as lupus erythematosus, digestive tract diseases such as ulcerative colitis, eye diseases, fluid retention due to nephrotic syndrome (kidney disorder), high serum levels of calcium associated with cancer, lung diseases such as tuberculosis, severe allergic reactions to medications, skin diseases such as severe psoriasis. High doses have been effective in controlling severe symptoms of multiple sclerosis.

Dosage

 Take with food to avoid stomach irritation. Take exactly as prescribed. Dose is gradually decreased by your doctor; *do not stop medication on your own. Do not use Pediapred for any other condition than which it was prescribed.*

 Usual adult dose: ranges from 5 to 60 milliliters, depending on condition for which it is prescribed. *For acute flare-ups of multiple sclerosis*—200 milligrams per day of Pediapred, followed by 80 milligrams every other day or 4 to 8 milligrams of dexamethasone every other day for 1 month.

 Usual child dose: follow doctor's instructions carefully for children.

 Missed dose: take as soon as possible, unless almost time for next dose. In that case, do not take missed dose; go back to regular schedule. *Do not double doses.*

Side Effects

Overdose symptoms: no specific information available. If you suspect an overdose, immediately seek medical attention.

Side effects: abnormal loss of bony tissue causing fragile bones, abnormal redness of face, backbone break that collapses the spinal column, bruising, cataracts, convulsions, dizziness, fluid retention, fracture of long bones, glaucoma, headache, high blood pressure, increased sweating, loss of muscle mass, menstrual irregularities, mental capacity changes, muscle disease, muscle weakness, peptic ulcer, protrusion of eyeball, salt retention, slow growth in children, slow wound healing, sugar diabetes, swelling of abdomen, thinning of skin, vertigo. Side effects may be intensified if you have underactive thyroid or long-term liver disease.

No known less common or rare side effects.

Interactions

Inform your doctor before combining Pediapred with: amphotericin B; aspirin; barbiturates such as phenobarbital and Seconal; carbamazepine (Tegretol); cyclosporine (Sandimmune); diabetes medications; diuretics such as Lasix; estrogens such as Premarin; isoniazid (Nydrazid); ketoconazole (Nizoral); nonsteroidal anti-inflammatory medications such as Motrin; oral contraceptives; phenytoin (Dilantin); rifampin (Rifadin). Avoid vaccinations during Pediapred therapy, especially smallpox. Use aspirin with caution if you are taking Pediapred and also being treated for a blood-clotting factor deficiency.

No known food/other substance interactions.

Special Cautions

 If pregnant or planning to become pregnant, inform your doctor immediately. May appear in breast milk, could affect a nursing infant.

. . . .

 No special precautions apply to seniors.

. . . .

 Follow doctor's instructions carefully for children.

. . . .

 If you have not had measles or chicken pox, avoid exposure during Pediapred therapy; may cause serious reaction, and in children fatal reaction.

. . . .

Immediately inform your doctor if you experience fever or other signs of infection.

. . . .

Doctor will prescribe with extreme precaution if you have: ulcerative colitis (inflammation of colon and rectum) where there is a possibility of puncture, abscess or other infection; diverticulitis; recent intestinal anastomoses (surgical connection in colon); active or inactive peptic ulcer; unsatisfactory kidney function; high blood pressure; osteoporosis; and myasthenia gravis (fatigue and muscle weakness).

. . . .

As Pediapred lowers resistance to infection, may get a new infection while taking this medication. Signs and symptoms of new infection may be masked.

. . . .

Not for use for fungal infections.

. . . .

Inform your doctor if you experience unusual stress while using Pediapred.

. . . .

Ongoing use may cause posterior subcapsular cataracts or glaucoma or may intensify eye infections due to fungi or viruses.

. . . .

May cause increase in blood pressure, salt and water retention, and loss of potassium.

Use with caution if you have: ocular herpes simplex.

At risk for mood swings, feelings of elation, insomnia, personality changes, severe depression, or severe mental disorders.

Pediazole

Generic ingredients: Erythromycin ethylsuccinate with sulfisoxazole acetyl

Other brand names: EryPed, Eryzole, Wyamycin E

Pediazole is a macrolide and sulfa antibiotic. It is used to treat a variety of bacterial infections.

℞ QUICK FACTS

Purpose

Used to treat severe middle ear and sinus infections in children.

Dosage

Use entire prescription, even if your child feels better after a few days. Maintain regular schedule; medication works best when there is a constant level in the blood. Can give with or without food; should not give immediately after carbonated drinks, fruit juice, or tea. If your child has upset stomach, give Pediazole with crackers or light snack.

Usual adult dose: not generally prescribed for adults.

Usual child dose: *4 doses per day schedule—children less than 18 pounds—determined by doctor; children 18 pounds—¹/₂ teaspoonful; children 35 pounds—1 teaspoonful; children 53 pounds—1¹/₂ teaspoonfuls; children over 70 pounds—2 teaspoonfuls. 3 doses per day schedule—children less than 13 pounds—determined by doctor; children 13 pounds—¹/₂ teaspoonful; children 26 pounds—1 teaspoonful; children 40 pounds—1¹/₂ teaspoonfuls; children 53 pounds—2 teaspoonfuls; children over 66 pounds—2¹/₂ teaspoonfuls.* Not recommended for infants under 2 months.

 Missed dose: give missed dose as soon as possible, then give the rest of the doses at evenly spaced intervals.

Side Effects

 Overdose symptoms: no specific information available. If you suspect an overdose, immediately seek medical attention.

 More common side effects: abdominal cramping and discomfort, diarrhea, lack or loss of appetite, nausea, vomiting.

 Less common or rare side effects: anxiety, blood disorders, blood or stone formation in urine, bluish skin discoloration, chills, colitis, convulsions, cough, dark or tarry stools, depression, difficulty urinating or inability to urinate, disorientation, dizziness, drowsiness, exhaustion, fainting, fatigue, fluid retention, flushing, fever, gas, hallucinations, headache, hepatitis, hives, inability to fall or stay asleep, increased urine, inflammation of mouth, irregular heartbeat, itching, lack of muscle coordination, low blood sugar, palpitations, rapid heartbeat, redness and tongue swelling, ringing in ears, scaling of dead skin due to inflammation, sensitivity to light, severe allergic reactions, severe skin welts or swelling, shortness of breath, skin eruptions, skin rash, Stevens-Johnson syndrome, stomach or intestinal bleeding, swelling around the eye, temporary hearing loss, tingling or pins and needles, vertigo, weakness, yellow eyes and skin.

Interactions

 Inform your doctor before combining Pediazole with: bromocriptine (Parlodel), carbamazepine (Tegretol), cyclosporine (Sandimmune), digoxin (Lanoxin), disopyramide (Norpace), ergotamine (Cafergot), hexobarbital, lovastatin (Mevacor), methotrexate (Rheumatrex), oral antidiabetic medications such as Micronase, phenytoin (Dilantin), terfenadine (Seldane), theophylline (Theo-Dur), triazolam (Halcion), warfarin (Coumadin). Should not use Pediazole if taking Seldane or Hismanal.

No known food/other substance interactions.

Special Cautions

 Not prescribed for adults; should never be taken if pregnant or breastfeeding.

 Not prescribed for adults.

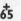 Follow doctor's instructions carefully for children 2 months and older.

 Pediazole is a sulfonamide, which has caused fatalities due to severe reactions such as Stevens-Johnson syndrome, sudden and severe liver damage, severe blood disorder (agranulocytosis), lack of red and white blood cells due to bone marrow disorder. Immediately notify your doctor if you experience: skin rash, sore throat, fever, abnormal skin paleness, darkened urine, reddish or purplish spots on skin, yellowing of eyes or skin.

· ·
If child is sensitive to or allergic to erythromycin, sulfon-amides, or similar medications, do not use Pediazole.
· ·

Use with caution if child has impaired kidney or liver function or history of severe allergies or bronchial asthma.
· ·

Long-term uses may cause new infections not treatable by Pediazole (superinfection).
· ·

Doctor may monitor your child's urine during Pediazole therapy.

Pelamine

see PBZ-SR

Pemoline

see CYLERT

Penetrex

Generic name: Enoxacin

Penetrex is a fluoroquinolone antibiotic/anti-infective. It is used to treat a variety of bacterial infections.

℞ QUICK FACTS

Purpose

℞   Used to treat urinary tract infections, including cystitis (inflammation of inner lining of bladder caused by bacterial infection), and certain sexually transmitted diseases such as gonorrhea.

Dosage

 Take regularly; try not to miss doses to keep constant level in blood and urine—Penetrex will be most effective in this way. Take with a full glass of water either 1 hour before or 2 hours after a meal. *Do not take more than prescribed dose.* Use all of the prescription; otherwise at risk for symptoms returning.

 Usual adult dose: *for uncomplicated urinary tract infections*—200 milligrams taken every 12 hours for 7 days. *Other urinary tract infections*—400 milligrams taken every 12 hours for 14 days. *For sexually transmitted disease (gonorrhea)*—400 milligrams taken in a single dose.

 Usual child dose: not generally prescribed for children.

 Missed dose: take as soon as possible, unless almost time for next dose. In that case, do not take missed dose; go back to regular schedule. *Do not double doses.*

Side Effects

 Overdose symptoms: no specific information available. If you suspect an overdose, immediately seek medical attention.

 More common side effects: nausea, vomiting.

 Less common or rare side effects: abdominal pain, agitation, back pain, bloody stools, chest pain, chills, confusion, constipation, convulsions, cough, depression, diarrhea, difficult or labored breathing, dizziness, dry mouth and throat, emotional changeability, excessive sweating, fainting, fatigue, fever, fluid retention and swelling, fungal infection, gas, general feeling of illness, hallucinations, headache, hives, inability to hold urine, indigestion, inflammation of eyes, inflammation of large intestine, inflammation of mouth, inflammation of stomach, inflammation of vagina, joint pain, kidney failure, lack of coordination, loss of appetite, loss of feeling of identity, loss of memory, mental disorders, muscle pain, nosebleed, overactivity, palpitations, purple or red skin spots, rapid heartbeat, ringing in ears, sensitivity to light, skin eruptions, skin peeling, sleepiness, tingling or pins and needles, tremor, twitching, vaginal yeast infection, vision disturbances, weakness.

Interactions

 Inform your doctor before combining Penetrex with: bismuth subsalicylate (Pepto-Bismol), caffeine, cyclosporine (Sandimmune), digoxin (Lanoxin), ranitidine (Zantac), sucralfate (Carafate), theophylline (Theo-Dur), warfarin (Coumadin).

 Check with your doctor before using antacids containing calcium, magnesium, or aluminum, such as Maalox and Tums, or vitamins or products containing iron or zinc.

Special Cautions

 If pregnant or planning to become pregnant, inform your doctor immediately. May appear in breast milk; could affect a nursing infant.

 No special precautions apply to seniors.

 Not generally prescribed for children.

Has caused severe, fatal reactions, sometimes after first dose. If you develop any of the following symptoms, immediately seek medical help: confusion, convulsions, difficulty breathing, hallucinations, hives, itching, light-headedness, loss of consciousness, rash, restlessness, swelling in face or throat, tingling, or tremors.

Inform your doctor if you have experienced diarrhea when taking other antibacterial medications, or develop diarrhea at the start of Penetrex therapy. May cause bowel inflammation, which could be life-threatening.

May cause drowsiness and impair your ability to drive a car or operate machinery. *Do not take part in any activity that requires alertness.*

Should not take if sensitive to or allergic to this or other quinolone antibiotics such as Cipro and Floxin.

Use with caution if you have epilepsy, severe hardening of the arteries in the brain, and other seizure-inducing conditions.

Avoid overexposure to sunlight. Immediately stop taking Penetrex if you experience a severe reaction such as skin rash.

Penicillin V Potassium

Brand names: Beepen VK, Betapen-VK, Biotic-V Powder, Bopen V-K, Ledercillin VK, Penpar VK, Pen-V, Pen•Vee K, Pfizerpen VK, Robicillin-VK, Uticillin VK, V-cillin K, Veetids

Penicillin V potassium is an antibiotic. It is used to treat a variety of bacterial infections.

℞ QUICK FACTS

Purpose

℞   Used to treat a variety of infections including: dental infection, infections in the heart, middle ear infections, rheumatic fever, scarlet fever, skin infections, upper and lower respiratory tract infections. Is ineffective against fungi, viruses, and parasites.

Dosage

    Take on a full or empty stomach; complete entire course of treatment prescribed. Use spoon from pharmacy for oral solution, shake well before using.

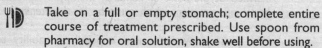   Usual adult dose: *for mild to moderately severe strep infections of the upper respiratory tract and skin, and scarlet fever*—125 to 250 milligrams every 6 to 8 hours for 10 days. *For mild to moderately severe pneumococcal infections of the respiratory tract, including middle ear infections*—250 milligrams every 6 hours until fever subsides for at least 2 days. *For mild staph infections of the skin*—250 milligrams every 6 to 8 hours. *For mild to moderately severe gum infections known as Vincent's gingivitis*—250 milligrams every 6 to 8 hours. *To prevent rheumatic fever and/or chorea*—125 milligrams taken 2 times per day on a continuing basis. *To prevent bacterial endocarditis (inflammation of heart membrane) in people with heart disease who are undergoing dental or surgical procedures*—orally—2 grams ½ hour to 1 hour before surgery, then 500 milligrams every 6 hours for 8 doses.

    Usual child dose: *for children 12 and over*—same as adult dose. *For children under 12*—not generally prescribed.

Missed dose: *for 2 doses per day*—take as soon as possible, take next dose 5 to 6 hours later, then go back to regular schedule. *For 3 or more doses per day*—take as soon as possible, take next dose 2 to 4 hours later, then go back to regular schedule.

Side Effects

 Overdose symptoms: diarrhea, nausea, vomiting. If you suspect an overdose, immediately seek medical attention.

 Side effects: anemia, black or hairy tongue, diarrhea, fever, hives, nausea, skin eruptions, stomach upset or pain, swelling in throat, vomiting.

 No known less common or rare side effects.

Interactions

 Inform your doctor before combining penicillin V with: chloramphenicol (Chloromycetin), cholestyramine (Questran), colestipol (Colestid), oral contraceptives, tetracyclines such as Achromycin V.

 No known food/other substance interactions.

Special Cautions

 If pregnant or planning to become pregnant, inform your doctor immediately. Appears in breast milk; could affect a nursing infant.

 No special precautions apply to seniors.

 Not generally prescribed for children under 12 years. Follow doctor's instructions carefully for children 12 years and older.

STOP Should not use if allergic to penicillin or cephalosporin antibiotics in any form; may experience severe reaction.

If you experience any allergic reaction, stop taking medication and immediately contact your doctor.

If you have rashes, hives, hay fever, asthma, colitis, diabetes, or liver or kidney disease, inform your doctor before taking Penicillin V.

Pentasa
see ROWASA

Pentazocine Hydrochloride with Aspirin
see TALWIN COMPOUND

Pentoxifylline
see TRENTAL

Pepcid

Generic name: Famotidine

Pepcid is an antiulcer agent. It reduces stomach acid by blocking the effects of histamine in the stomach.

Pepcid 689

℞ QUICK FACTS

Purpose

℞ Used to treat active duodenal ulcer (in the upper intestine) for 4 to 8 weeks, and active benign gastric ulcer (in the stomach) for 6 to 8 hours. Also used to treat gastroesophageal reflux disease (GERD), condition in which acid contents of the stomach flow back into the esophagus and inflame it. Also used to treat diseases which result in excessive amounts of acid in the stomach, such as Zollinger- Ellison syndrome.

Dosage

 Shake suspension 5 to 10 seconds before use. May take several days for medication to relieve stomach pain. Can use antacids, but not within 1 hour of a dose of Pepcid. Must take full treatment to cure your ulcer.

 Usual adult dose: *for duodenal ulcer*—40 milligrams or 5 milliliters (1 teaspoonful) once per day at bedtime. Should see results in 4 weeks. Do not take for longer than 6 to 8 weeks. *For benign gastric ulcer*— 40 milligrams or 5 milliliters (1 teaspoonful) once per day at bedtime. *For GERD*—20 milligrams or 2.5 milliliters (½ teaspoonful) 2 times per day for up to 6 weeks. *For esophagus inflammation due to GERD*— 20 or 40 milligrams or 2.5 to 5 milliliters twice per day for up to 12 weeks. *For excess acid conditions*— 20 milligrams every 6 hours. *For people with kidney disease*—doctor will adjust dosage.

 Usual child dose: not generally prescribed for children.

 Missed dose: take as soon as possible, unless almost time for next dose. In that case, do not take missed

dose; go back to regular schedule. *Do not double doses.*

Side Effects

 Overdose symptoms: no specific information available. If you suspect an overdose, immediately seek medical attention.

 Most common side effect: headache.

 Less common or rare side effects: abdominal discomfort; acne; agitation; altered taste; anxiety; changes in behavior; confusion; constipation; decreased sex drive; depression; diarrhea; difficulty sleeping; dizziness; dry mouth; dry skin; facial swelling due to fluid retention; fatigue; fever; flushing; grand mal seizures; hair loss; hallucinations; hives; impotence; irregular heartbeat; itching; loss of appetite; muscle, bone, or joint pain; nausea; pounding heartbeat; prickling, tingling, or pins and needles; rash; ringing in ears; severe allergic reaction; sleepiness; vomiting; weakness; wheezing; yellow eyes and skin.

Interactions

 Inform your doctor before taking Pepcid with: itraconazole (Sporanox), ketoconazole (Nizoral), pancrelipase (Pancrease MT), pentoxifylline (Trental), probenecid (Benemid).

 No known food/other substance interactions.

Special Cautions

 If pregnant or planning to become pregnant, inform your doctor immediately. May appear in breast milk; could affect a nursing infant.

65 No special precautions apply to seniors.

Not generally prescribed for children.

 Should not take if sensitive to or allergic to Pepcid.

Percocet

~~~~~~

Generic ingredients: Acetaminophen with oxycodone hydrochloride

Other brand names: Oxycet, Roxicet, Roxilox, Tylox

Percocet is a narcotic analgesic. It relieves pain and gives the patient a feeling of well-being.

℞ QUICK FACTS

Purpose

℞ Used to treat moderate to moderately severe pain.

Dosage

 May take with meals or milk.

 Usual adult dose: I tablet every 6 hours as needed.

 Usual child dose: not generally established in children.

 Missed dose: *if taking on a regular basis*—take as soon as possible, unless almost time for next dose. In that case, do not take missed dose; go back to regular schedule. *Do not double doses.*

Side Effects

 Overdose symptoms: bluish skin, eyes or skin with yellow tone, cold and clammy skin, decreased or irregular breathing (ceasing in severe overdose), extreme sleepiness progressing to stupor or coma, heart attack, low blood pressure, muscle weakness or softness, nausea, slow heartbeat, sweating, vague bodily discomfort, vomiting. If you suspect an overdose, immediately seek medical attention.

 Most common side effects: dizziness, light-headedness, nausea, sedation, vomiting.

 Less common or rare side effects: constipation, depressed feeling, exaggerated feeling of well-being, itchy skin, skin rash, slowed breathing (at higher doses).

Interactions

 Inform your doctor before combining Percocet with: antidepressants such as Elavil, Nardil, Pamelor, and Parnate; antispasmodics such as Cogentin, Bentyl, and Donnatal; medications for severe mental disorders such as Thorazine; other narcotic painkillers such as Darvon; sedatives such as phenobarbital and Seconal; tranquilizers such as Xanax and Valium.

 Should not drink alcohol while taking Percocet; it increases sedative effects of Percocet.

Special Cautions

 If pregnant or planning to become pregnant, inform your doctor immediately. If taken just before delivery, may cause impaired breathing in newborn. May appear in breast milk; could affect a nursing infant.

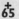 Seniors should take with caution.

Not generally prescribed for children.

 May cause drowsiness and impair your ability to drive a car or operate machinery. *Do not take part in any activity that requires alertness.*

Monitor for physical and psychological dependence if taking for an extended period. Notify your doctor of any alcohol addiction problems.

Should not use if sensitive to Percocet ingredients.

Notify your doctor *before* taking Percocet if you have: a head injury; stomach problems; liver, kidney, or thyroid problems; Addison's disease; difficulty urinating; enlarged prostate; or weakened condition.

Periactin

Generic name: Cyproheptadine hydrochloride

Periactin is an antihistamine. Antihistamines block the effects of histamine, a body chemical that causes swelling and itching.

℞ QUICK FACTS

Purpose

 Used to relieve cold and allergy symptoms such as hay fever, nasal inflammation, stuffy nose, red and inflamed eyes, hives, and swelling. Also used to treat anaphylaxis, a life-threatening allergic reaction. Also prescribed for cluster headaches, and to stimulate appetite in underweight people.

Dosage

Take exactly as prescribed.

Usual adult dose: 4 milligrams (1 tablet or 2 tea-spoonfuls) 3 times per day, initially. Ongoing dose—ranges from 12 to 16 milligrams per day.

Usual child dose: *for ages 2 to 6 years*—2 milligrams (½ tablet or 1 teaspoon) 2 or 3 times per day, up to 12 milligrams per day. *For ages 7 to 14 years*—4 milligrams (1 tablet or 2 teaspoons) 2 or 3 times per day, up to 16 milligrams per day.

Missed dose: take as soon as possible, unless almost time for next dose. In that case, do not take missed dose; go back to regular schedule. *Do not double doses.*

Side Effects

Overdose symptoms: dilated pupils, dry mouth, extreme excitement and agitation, fever, flushing, stomach or bowel distress, stupor or coma. If you suspect an overdose, immediately seek medical attention.

Side effects: anaphylaxis (life-threatening allergic reaction); anemia; appetite loss; chest congestion or tightness; chills; confusion; constipation; convulsions; diarrhea; difficulty urinating; dizziness; dry mouth, nose, or throat; earlier-than-expected menstrual period; exaggerated feeling of well-being; excessive perspiration; excitement; faintness; fatigue; fluttery or throbbing heartbeat; frequent urination; hallucinations; headache; hives; hysteria; inability to urinate; insomnia; irritability; lack of coordination; light sensitivity; low blood pressure; nausea; nervousness; rapid heartbeat; rash and swelling; restlessness; ringing in ears; sleepiness; stomach pain; stuffy nose; tingling or pins and needles; tremor; vertigo; vision problems; vomiting; weight gain; wheezing; yellow eyes and skin.

 No known less common or rare side effects.

Interactions

 Inform your doctor before combining Periactin with: sedatives such as Nembutal and Seconal, tranquilizers such as Librium and Valium. *Do not take with MAO inhibitors such as Nardil and Parnate.*

 Avoid alcohol while taking Periactin.

Special Cautions

 Should not be used during pregnancy or breastfeeding due to possible harm to the fetus or newborn.

 Seniors may develop dizziness or drowsiness, or low blood pressure.

 May cause hallucinations or convulsions in children.

 Do not take if sensitive to or allergic to this or similar medications.

Do not take if you have: angle-closure glaucoma, peptic ulcer, enlarged prostate, obstruction of neck and bladder, or obstruction of outlet of the stomach.

May cause drowsiness and impair your ability to drive a car or operate machinery. *Do not take part in any activity that requires alertness.*

Use with caution if you have: overactive thyroid, high blood pressure, heart disease, or circulatory problems.

Peridex

Generic name: Chlorhexidine gluconate

Peridex is an oral disinfectant. It is thought to eliminate bacteria which cause dental plaque.

℞ QUICK FACTS

Purpose

℞ Used to treat gingivitis (red and swollen gums) and to control gum bleeding caused by gingivitis.

Dosage

Should have a dental cleaning prior to Peridex treatment. When using Peridex, *do not dilute and do not eat or drink for several hours after using medication.*

. . . .

Usual adult dose: ½ fluid ounce, undiluted, to rinse with for 30 seconds in the morning and evening after brushing teeth. Spit out after rinsing and never swallow.

. . . .

Usual child dose: not generally prescribed for children.

. . . .

Missed dose: resume schedule after next brushing.

Side Effects

Overdose symptoms: (for accidental child overdose)— signs of alcohol intoxication (slurred speech, staggering, or sleepiness), upset stomach, nausea. If you suspect an overdose, immediately seek medical attention.

. . . .

More common side effects: change in taste; increase in plaque; staining of teeth, mouth, tooth fillings, dentures, or other mouth appliances.

 Less common side effects: irritation of the mouth, scaling of lining of the mouth.

Interactions

 No drug interactions reported.

 No known food/other substance interactions.

Special Cautions

 If pregnant or planning to become pregnant, inform your doctor immediately. Not known if Peridex appears in breast milk.

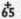 No special precautions apply to seniors.

 Follow doctor's instructions carefully for children 2 years and older.

 Do not use if sensitive to or allergic to Peridex unless directed by your doctor.

May stain front-tooth fillings, especially those with a rough surface. Is usually removed with a professional dental cleaning.

Not for treating periodontal disease.

May cause excess tartar buildup; have teeth cleaned every 6 months to avoid buildup.

Persantine

~~~~~~

Generic name: Dipyridamole

Other brand name: Pyridamole

Persantine is an anti-platelet agent and vasodilator. It prevents the aggregation of platelets and relieves chest pain by dilating heart blood vessels, thereby providing more oxygen to the heart.

℞ QUICK FACTS

Purpose

℞ Used to reduce blood clots in people who have had heart valve surgery, in combination with blood-thinning medications. Also used with aspirin to reduce damage from heart attack and prevent recurrence, to treat angina (crushing chest pain), and to prevent complications during heart bypass surgery.

Dosage

 Take on empty stomach with a full glass of water. May take with food or milk to avoid stomach upset. *Do not change brands without consulting your doctor.*

 Usual adult dose: 75 to 100 milligrams taken 4 times per day.

 Usual child dose: not generally prescribed for children under 12 years.

 Missed dose: take as soon as possible, unless within 4 hours of next dose. In that case, do not take missed dose; go back to regular schedule. *Do not double doses.*

Side Effects

 Overdose symptom: low blood pressure. If you suspect an overdose, immediately seek medical attention.

 More common side effects: abdominal distress, dizziness.

 Less common or rare side effects: angina (crushing chest pain), diarrhea, feeling flushed, headache, itching, liver problems, skin rash, vomiting.

Interactions

 Inform your doctor before combining Persantine with: blood thinners such as Coumadin, indomethacin (Indocin), ticlopidine (Ticlid), valproic acid (Depakene). *To avoid increased bleeding, take only the amount of aspirin prescribed by the same doctor prescribing Persantine. If you need medication for pain or fever, do not take extra aspirin without consulting the doctor who prescribed Persantine.*

 No known food/other substance interactions.

Special Cautions

 If pregnant or planning to become pregnant, inform your doctor immediately. Appears in breast milk; could affect a nursing infant.

 No special precautions apply to seniors.

 Not generally prescribed for children under 12 years.

 Use carefully if you have low blood pressure.

. . . .

Inform your doctor or dentist in the event of a medical emergency or surgery that you are taking Persantine.

Pertofrane

see NORPRAMIN

Phenaphen with Codeine

see TYLENOL WITH CODEINE

Phenazopyridine Hydrochloride

see PYRIDIUM

Phenelzine Sulfate

see NARDIL

Phenergan

Generic name: Promethazine hydrochloride

Phenergan is an antihistamine. Antihistamines block the effects of histamine, a body chemical that causes swelling and itching.

℞ QUICK FACTS

Purpose

℞ Used to relieve nasal stuffiness and inflammation, and red, inflamed eyes caused by hay fever and other allergies. Also used to treat itching, swelling, and redness from hives and other rashes, allergic reactions to blood transfusions. Prescribed with other medications to treat anaphylactic shock (severe allergic reaction). Also prescribed as a sedative for children and adults, to prevent and control nausea and vomiting before and after surgery, to prevent and treat motion sickness, and for pain after surgery.

Dosage

 Take exactly as prescribed.

 Usual adult dose: *for allergy*—oral dose of 25 milligrams taken before bedtime, or 12.5 milligrams before meals and before bed. *For motion sickness*—25 milligrams taken 2 times per day. First dose should be taken ½ to 1 hour before travel, and second dose 8 to 12 hours later. Then 25 milligrams in the morning and before evening meal. *For nausea and vomiting*—25 milligrams orally, or if cannot be tolerated, rectal suppository. Doctor may advise 12.5 to 25 milligrams every 4 to 6 hours if necessary. *For insomnia*—25 to 50 milligrams at bedtime.

. . . .

 Usual child dose: *for allergy*—a single 25 milligram dose at bedtime or 6.25 to 2.5 milligrams 3 times per day. *For motion sickness*—12.5 to 25 milligrams taken 2 times per day in tablet, syrup, or rectal suppository form. *For nausea and vomiting*—0.5 milligram per pound of body weight; age of child and severity of condition are taken into consideration. *For insomnia*—12.5 to 25 milligrams by tablet or rectal suppository at bedtime.

. . . .

Missed dose: *if taking on a regular schedule*—take as soon as possible, unless almost time for next dose. In that case, do not take missed dose; go back to regular schedule. *Do not double doses.*

Side Effects

 Overdose symptoms: difficulty breathing, dry mouth, fixed or dilated pupils, flushing, loss of consciousness, slowdown in brain activity, slowed heartbeat, stomach and intestinal problems, very low blood pressure. If you suspect an overdose, immediately seek medical attention.

 More common side effects: blurred vision, dizziness, dry mouth, increased or decreased blood pressure, nausea, rash, sedation, sleepiness, vomiting.

 Rare side effects: abnormal eye movements, blood disorders, confusion, disorientation, protruding tongue, sensitivity to light, stiff neck.

Interactions

 Inform your doctor before combining Phenergan with: certain antidepressants, including Elavil and Tofranil, narcotic pain relievers such as Demerol and Dilaudid, sedatives such as Halcion and Seconal, tranquilizers such as Xanax and Valium.

 Do not drink alcohol while taking Phenergan.

Special Cautions

 If pregnant or planning to become pregnant, inform your doctor immediately. May affect pregnancy test results. May appear in breast milk; could affect a nursing infant.

No special precautions apply to seniors.

 Follow doctor's instructions carefully for children 2 years and older. May cause drowsiness; supervise children carefully when bike-riding, roller-skating, or participating in other potentially hazardous activities.

 May cause drowsiness and impair your ability to drive a car or operate machinery. *Do not take part in any activity that requires alertness.* Doctor may reduce other medications you are currently taking if they also cause drowsiness.

Should not use if sensitive to or allergic to this or similar medications such as Thorazine, Mellaril, Stelazine, or Prolixin.

Phenergan may prompt seizures in people who already experience them.

Should not take if you have sleep apnea (periods of sleep when breathing stops).

Use with caution if you have: heart disease, high blood pressure or circulatory problems, liver problems, narrow-angle glaucoma, peptic ulcer or other abdominal obstructions, or urinary bladder obstruction due to enlarged prostate.

May raise blood sugar.

You may experience jaundice (yellow eyes and skin) during Phenergan therapy.

Inform your doctor if you experience any uncontrolled movements or unusual sensitivity to sunlight.

Phenergan with Codeine

‧‧

Generic ingredients: Promethazine hydrochloride with codeine phosphate

Other brand names: Pherazine with Codeine, Prometh with Codeine, Prothazine DC

Phenergan with Codeine is an antihistamine and cough suppressant. Antihistamines block the effects of histamine, a body chemical that causes swelling and itching. Cough suppressants act on the cough reflex center of the brain.

℞ QUICK FACTS

Purpose

℞ Used to relieve coughs and other symptoms of allergies and the common cold. Also helps control nausea and vomiting, relieve pain, and stop coughing.

Dosage

🄳 Take exactly as prescribed. Adhere to dosage level, never taking more than prescribed. If cough persists beyond 5 days, contact your doctor.

. . . .

💊 Usual adult dose: 1 teaspoonful (5 milliliters) every 4 to 6 hours, not to exceed 6 teaspoonfuls or 30 milliliters in 24 hours.

. . . .

🧸 Usual child dose: *for children 6 to 12 years*—½ to 1 teaspoonful (2.5 to 5 milliliters) every 4 to 6 hours, not to exceed 6 teaspoonfuls or 30 milliliters in 24 hours. *For children under 6 years*—¼ to ½ teaspoonful (1.25 to 2.5 milliliters) every 4 to 6 hours, not to exceed 9 milliliters for children weighing 40 pounds, 8 milliliters for 35 pounds, 7 milliliters for 30 pounds, and 6 milliliters for 25 pounds. Not generally prescribed for children under 2 years.

Missed dose: *if taking on a regular schedule*—take as soon as possible, unless almost time for next dose. In that case, do not take missed dose; go back to regular schedule. *Do not double doses.*

Side Effects

Overdose can be fatal. Overdose symptoms: bluish skin, cold or clammy skin, coma, convulsions, difficulty breathing, dilated pupils, dry mouth, extreme sleepiness, flushing, low blood pressure, muscle softness, nightmares, overexcitability, slow heartbeat, small pupils, stomach and intestinal problems, stupor, unconsciousness. If you suspect an overdose, immediately seek medical attention.

Side effects: blurred vision, constipation, convulsions, decreased amount of urine, depressed feeling, difficulty breathing, disorientation, dizziness, dizziness upon standing, dry mouth, exaggerated sense of well-being, fainting, faintness, fast or fluttery heartbeat, feeling of anxiety, restlessness, flushing, headache, hives, inability to urinate, increased or decreased blood pressure, itching, light-headedness, nausea, passing hallucinations, rapid heartbeat, rash, sedation, sleepiness, slow heartbeat, sweating, swelling due to fluid retention (including throat), vision changes, vomiting, weakness, yellowed skin or eyes.

Rare side effects: abnormal eye movements, blood disorders, confusion, protruding tongue, skin sensitivity to light, stiff neck.

Interactions

Inform your doctor before combining Phenergan with Codeine with: all antidepressants, including Nardil, Elavil, and Prozac; narcotic pain relievers such as Demerol and Dilaudid; sedatives such as Seconal, Halcion, and Dalmane; tranquilizers such as Xanax and Valium.

 Do not drink alcohol while taking Phenergan with Codeine.

Special Cautions

 If pregnant or planning to become pregnant, inform your doctor immediately. May affect pregnancy test results. May appear in breast milk; could affect a nursing infant.

 No special precautions apply to seniors.

 Follow doctor's instructions carefully for children 2 years and older. May cause drowsiness; supervise children carefully when bike-riding, roller-skating, or participating in other potentially hazardous activities. Use with extreme caution in young children.

 May cause drowsiness and impair your ability to drive a car or operate machinery. Do not take part in any activity that requires alertness. Doctor may reduce other medications you are currently taking if they also cause drowsiness.

Should not use if sensitive to or allergic to this or similar medications such as Thorazine, Mellaril, Stelazine, or Prolixin.

May cause or worsen constipation.

Use with caution if you have: a head injury, heart disease, high blood pressure or circulatory problems, liver or kidney problems, narrow-angle glaucoma, peptic ulcer or other abdominal obstructions, urinary bladder obstruction due to enlarged prostate, seizures, underactive thyroid, intestinal inflammation, Addison's disease, or recent stomach or intestinal or urinary tract surgery.

. . . .

Monitor use in very young, very elderly, or people in a weakened condition.

. . . .

Phenergan with Codeine may prompt seizures in people who already experience them.

. . . .

May raise blood sugar.

. . . .

Inform your doctor of any uncontrolled movements or if you experience unusual sensitivity to sunlight.

Phenindamine Tartrate with Chlorpheniramine Maleate and Phenylpropanolamine Hydrochloride

see NOLAMINE

Phenobarbital

Brand names: Barbita, Solfoton

Phenobarbital is a barbiturate and anticonvulsant. It acts as a depressant to the central nervous system.

℞ QUICK FACTS

Purpose

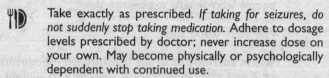

℞ Used to promote sleep and to treat certain types of epilepsy, including generalized or grand mal and partial seizures.

Dosage

🍴 Take exactly as prescribed. *If taking for seizures, do not suddenly stop taking medication.* Adhere to dosage levels prescribed by doctor; never increase dose on your own. May become physically or psychologically dependent with continued use.

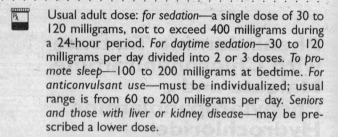

Usual adult dose: *for sedation*—a single dose of 30 to 120 milligrams, not to exceed 400 milligrams during a 24-hour period. *For daytime sedation*—30 to 120 milligrams per day divided into 2 or 3 doses. *To promote sleep*—100 to 200 milligrams at bedtime. *For anticonvulsant use*—must be individualized; usual range is from 60 to 200 milligrams per day. *Seniors and those with liver or kidney disease*—may be prescribed a lower dose.

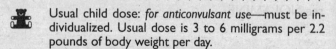

Usual child dose: *for anticonvulsant use*—must be individualized. Usual dose is 3 to 6 milligrams per 2.2 pounds of body weight per day.

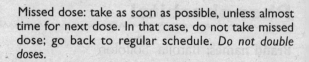

Missed dose: take as soon as possible, unless almost time for next dose. In that case, do not take missed dose; go back to regular schedule. *Do not double doses.*

Side Effects

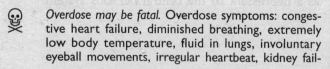

Overdose may be fatal. Overdose symptoms: congestive heart failure, diminished breathing, extremely low body temperature, fluid in lungs, involuntary eyeball movements, irregular heartbeat, kidney failure, lack of muscle coordination, low blood pressure, poor reflexes, skin reddening or bloody blisters, slowdown of central nervous system. If you suspect an overdose, immediately seek medical attention.

 Side effects: abnormal thinking; aggravation of existing emotional disturbances and phobias; agitation; anemia; angioedema (swelling of face around lips, tongue, and throat, swollen arms and legs, difficulty breathing); allergic reactions (localized swelling of the eyelids, cheeks, or lips, skin redness and inflammation); anxiety; confusion; constipation; decreased breathing; delirium; difficulty sleeping; dizziness; drowsiness; excitement; fainting; fever; hallucinations; headache; increased physical activity and muscle movement; irritability and hyperactivity in children; lack of muscle coordination; low blood pressure; muscle, nerve, or joint pain, especially in people with insomnia; nausea; nervousness; nightmares; psychiatric disturbances; rash; residual drowsiness; restlessness, excitement, and delirium when taken for pain; shallow breathing; sleepiness; slow heartbeat; slowdown of the nervous system; sluggishness; softening of bones; temporary cessation of breathing; vertigo; vomiting.

 No known less common or rare side effects.

Interactions

 Inform your doctor before combining phenobarbital with: all antidepressants, including Nardil, Elavil, and Prozac; narcotic pain relievers such as Demerol and Dilaudid; sedatives such as Seconal, Halcion, and Dalmane; tranquilizers such as Xanax and Valium.

 Do not drink alcohol while taking phenobarbital.

Special Cautions

 If pregnant or planning to become pregnant, inform your doctor immediately. Appears in breast milk; could affect a nursing infant.

 Seniors may be prescribed a lower dose. Can cause depression or confusion in seniors.

 Follow doctor's instructions carefully for children. May cause excitement in children.

 May cause drowsiness and impair your ability to drive a car or operate machinery. *Do not take part in any activity that requires alertness.*

Inform your doctor *before* taking phenobarbital if you have pain or are in constant pain.

Should not use if you have porphyria (metabolic disorder), liver disease, or lung disease that causes breathing problems, or if sensitive to or allergic to phenobarbital or other barbiturates.

If you have a history of depression or drug abuse, use with extreme caution.

Can cause depression or confusion in those with weakened conditions.

Use with caution if you have liver disease or adrenal gland problems.

Phenobarbital with Hyoscyamine Sulfate, Atropine Sulfate, and Scopolamine Hydrobromide

see DONNATAL

Phentermine Hydrochloride

see FASTIN

Phenylephrine Hydrochloride with Phenylpropanolamine Hydrochloride, Chlorpheniramine Maleate, Hyoscyamine Sulfate, Atropine Sulfate, and Scopolamine Hydrobromide

see RU-TUSS TABLETS

Phenylephrine Tannate with Chlorpheniramine Tannate and Pyrilamine Tannate

see RYNATAN

Phenytoin Sodium

see DILANTIN

Phospholine Iodine

Generic name: Echothiophate iodide

Phospholine Iodine is a miotic. It reduces fluid pressure in the eye by constricting the pupil and increasing the flow of fluid out of the eye.

℞ QUICK FACTS

Purpose

℞   Used to treat chronic open-angle glaucoma. Also used to treat secondary glaucoma, subacute or chronic angle-closure glaucoma either after or in the absence of surgery, and in children with accommodative esotropia (cross-eye).

Dosage

    Use exactly as directed by your doctor. If eye problems return after 1 or 2 years of treatment, your doctor may suggest surgery.

Usual adult dose: *for glaucoma*—0.03 percent solution used 2 times per day in the morning and at bedtime.

 Usual child dose: *for accommodative esotropia*—1 drop of 0.125 percent solution at bedtime for 2 or 3 weeks. May be reduced to 0.125 solution every other day or 0.06 percent solution every day.

 Missed dose: *for 1 dose every other day*—apply as soon as possible if it is the scheduled day. Otherwise, do not apply missed dose; go back to regular schedule. *For 1 dose per day*—apply as soon as possible unless it is the next day. Otherwise, do not apply missed dose, go back to regular schedule. *For 2 doses per day*—apply as soon as possible unless almost time for next dose. In that case, do not apply missed dose, go back to regular schedule. *Do not double doses.*

Side Effects

 Overdose symptoms: no specific information available. If you suspect an overdose, immediately seek medical attention.

 Side effects: ache above the eyes, blurred vision, burning or clouded eye lens, cyst formation, decreased pupil size, decreased visual sharpness, excess tears, eye pain, heart irregularities, increased eye pressure, inflamed iris, lid muscle twitching, nearsightedness, red eyes, stinging.

 No known less common or rare side effects.

Interactions

 Inform your doctor before taking Phospholine Iodine with Enlon, Mestinon, or Tensilon, which are used to treat myasthenia gravis (muscle weakness that affects muscles in the eyes, face, limbs, and throat).

No known food/other substance interactions.

Special Cautions

If pregnant or planning to become pregnant, inform your doctor immediately. No information available about the effects of Phospholine Iodine during pregnancy; should not be used if breastfeeding.

No special precautions apply to seniors.

Follow doctor's instructions carefully for children.

May cause vision problems; use caution if driving at night or when working in poor light.

Stop taking and immediately contact your doctor if you experience: breathing difficulties, diarrhea, inability to hold urine, muscle weakness, profuse sweating or salivation.

Doctor should perform regular check-ups if you are taking this medication for an extended period.

Pesticides such as Sevin and Trolene may increase side effects; use extra precautions if working with these chemicals—wear mask over mouth and nose, wash and change clothing frequently, and wash hands often.

Should not use if you have eye inflammation, angle-closure glaucoma or if sensitive to or allergic to this medication.

Use with caution if you have or ever had: bronchial asthma, detached retina, epilepsy, extreme low blood pressure, Parkinson's disease, peptic ulcer, recent heart attack, slow heartbeat, stomach or intestinal problems.

. . . .

Immediately contact your doctor if you notice heart problems.

Pilocar

Generic name: Pilocarpine hydrochloride

Other brand names: Adsorbocarpine, Akarpine, Isopto Carpine, Ocusert Pilo, Pilopine HS Gel

Pilocar is a miotic. It reduces fluid pressure in the eye by constricting the pupil and increasing the flow of fluid out of the eye.

℞ QUICK FACTS

Purpose

℞ Used to treat the pressure of open-angle glaucoma and to lower eye pressure prior to surgery for acute-angle closure glaucoma.

Dosage

 Take exactly as directed by your doctor, and be sure to take regularly. *Do not use if solution is discolored.*

 Usual dose: 1 or 2 drops up to 6 times per day. For severe attack, doctor will advise drops in the unaffected eye as well.

. . . .

 Usual child dose: not generally prescribed for children.

. . . .

Missed dose: apply as soon as possible, unless almost time for next dose. In that case, do not apply missed dose; go back to regular schedule. *Do not double doses.*

Side Effects

 Overdose symptoms: no specific information available. If you suspect an overdose, immediately seek medical attention.

 More common side effects: cloudy vision, detached retina, headache over eye, nearsightedness, reduced vision in poor light, spasms of eyelids, tearing eyes.

 Rare side effects: breathing difficulty, diarrhea, excessive salivation, fluid in lungs, high blood pressure, nausea, rapid heartbeat, sweating, vomiting.

Interactions

 No drug interactions reported.

 No known food/other substance interactions.

Special Cautions

 If pregnant or planning to become pregnant, inform your doctor immediately. May appear in breast milk; could affect a nursing infant.

 No special precautions apply to seniors.

 Not generally prescribed for children.

 May cause vision problems; use caution if driving at night or when working in poor light.

As there is no cure for glaucoma, you will most likely continue treatment for life.

. . . .
Should not use if sensitive to or allergic to this medication.
. . . .
Doctor will not prescribe if you should not have your pupils constricted.

Pilocarpine Hydrochloride

see PILOCAR

Pindolol

see VISKEN

Piroxicam

see FELDENE

Plaquenil

∿∿∿∿∿∿∿∿∿∿∿∿∿∿∿∿∿∿∿∿∿∿∿∿∿∿∿∿∿∿∿∿∿∿∿∿∿∿

Generic name: Hydroxychloroquine sulfate

Plaquenil is an anti-inflammatory/antimalarial agent.

℞ QUICK FACTS

Purpose

  Used to prevent and treat certain forms of malaria. Also used to treat symptoms of rheumatoid arthritis such as swelling, inflammation, stiffness, and joint pain, and for lupus erythematosus.

. . . .

Dosage

 Take exactly as prescribed, and complete the entire prescription.

 Usual adult dose: *for restraint or prevention of malaria*—400 milligrams taken once per day for 7 days. Preventive therapy should begin if possible 2 weeks before exposure. If not possible, doctor will prescribe 800 milligrams divided into 2 doses and taken 6 hours apart, continued for 8 weeks after leaving area where you may be exposed to malaria. *For acute malaria attack*—800 milligrams followed by 400 milligrams in 6 to 8 hours, and 400 milligrams on each of 2 consecutive days. Alternatively, doctor may prescribe a single dose of 800 milligrams. *For lupus*—400 milligrams once or twice per day, taken for several weeks or months depending on your response. Long-term therapy—200 to 400 milligrams per day. *For rheumatoid arthritis*—400 to 600 milligrams per day with food or milk. Reduced to 200 to 400 milligrams per day if condition improves within 4 to 12 weeks.

 Usual child dose: *for malaria*—dose based on the child's weight. Not prescribed to treat juvenile arthritis.

 Missed dose: *for 1 dose every 7 days*—take as soon as possible, then go back to regular schedule. *For 1 dose per day*—take as soon as possible, unless it is the next day. In that case, do not take missed dose, go back to regular schedule. *For 1 or more doses per day*—take as soon as possible, if within 1 hour of missed dose. Otherwise, do not take missed dose; go back to regular schedule. *Do not double doses.*

Side Effects

 Overdose symptoms can occur within 30 minutes. Overdose symptoms: convulsions, drowsiness, headache, heart problems and failure, inability to breathe, visual problems. If you suspect an overdose, immediately seek medical attention.

 Side effects of treatment for acute malarial attack: abdominal cramps, diarrhea, dizziness, lack or loss of appetite, mild headache, nausea, vomiting. Side effects of treatment for lupus and rheumatoid arthritis: abdominal cramps, abnormal eye pigmentation, anemia, bleaching of hair, blind spots, blood disorders, blurred vision, convulsions, decreased vision, diarrhea, difficulty focusing eyes, dizziness, emotional changes, excessive coloring of skin, eye muscle paralysis, "foggy" vision, halos around lights, headache, hearing loss, involuntary eyeball movement, irritability, itching, lack of muscle coordination, light flashes and streaks, light intolerance, loss of hair, loss or lack of appetite, muscle weakness, nausea, nervousness, nightmares, psoriasis, reading difficulties, ringing in ears, skin eruptions, skin inflammation and scaling, skin rash, vertigo, vomiting, weariness, weight loss.

 No known less common or rare side effects.

Interactions

 Inform your doctor before combining Plaquenil with any medication that may cause liver damage, aurothioglucose (Solganal), cimetidine (Tagamet), digoxin (Lanoxin).

 No known food/other substance interactions.

Special Cautions

 Avoid use during pregnancy except when your doctor judges the benefit outweighs the risks of taking this medication. May appear in breast milk; could affect a nursing infant.

 No special precautions apply to seniors.

 Follow doctor's instructions carefully for children. Should not use for long-term therapy with children.

 Do not take if you have psoriasis or porphyria (metabolic disorder); may increase severity of these conditions. Inform your doctor if you are taking medications that may cause dermatitis.

If sensitive to or allergic to this or similar medications such as Aralen or Chloroquin, should not take.

Notify your doctor if you experience any partial or complete loss of vision in small areas while taking this or similar medications; if so, should not take.

Doctor should perform eye exam at start of treatment and every 3 months for prolonged therapy. May experience progression of visual disturbances after Plaquenil therapy is completed.

Physical examinations to determine muscle weakness should be done on a periodic basis, as should blood cell counts.

Inform your doctor if you experience ringing in the ears or other ear problems.

Medication may be discontinued if no relief for rheumatoid arthritis has occurred within 6 months.

Use with caution if you are alcoholic and have liver or kidney problems.

Plendil

~~~~~~

Generic name: Felodipine

Plendil is a calcium channel blocker. It increases the amount of oxygen that reaches the heart muscle.

℞ QUICK FACTS

Purpose

℞   Used to treat high blood pressure.

Dosage

 Can take with or without food. Swallow tablet whole, never crush or chew. Continue taking if symptoms disappear; however, may take several weeks before you observe the full effects. If you miss a dose, or do not take regularly, blood pressure may increase.

 Usual adult dose: 5 milligrams once per day initially, then 5 to 10 milligrams, up to 20 milligrams once per day maximum for usual dose. *For seniors or those with liver problems*—maximum daily dose is 10 milligrams.

 Usual child dose: not generally prescribed for children.

 Missed dose: take as soon as possible, unless almost time for next dose. In that case, do not take missed dose; go back to regular schedule. *Do not double doses.*

Side Effects

 Overdose symptoms: severely low blood pressure, slow heartbeat. If you suspect an overdose, immediately seek medical attention.

 More common side effects: abdominal pain, back pain, chest pain, constipation, cough, diarrhea, dizziness, flushing, headache, indigestion, muscle cramps, nausea, pounding heartbeat, rash, runny nose, sore throat, swelling of legs and feet, tingling sensation, upper respiratory infection, weakness.

 Less common or rare side effects: anemia, angina pectoris (crushing chest pain), ankle pain, anxiety disorders, arm pain, arthritis, blurred vision, bronchitis, bruising, decreased sex drive, depression, difficulty sleeping, dry mouth, excessive nighttime urination, gas, generalized muscle pain, heart attack, hip pain, hives, impotence, inflammation of gums, inflammation of the nose, irregular heartbeat, irritability, itching, joint pain, knee pain, leg pain, low blood pressure, neck pain, nervousness, nosebleeds, painful or difficult urination, rapid heartbeat, respiratory infections, ringing in ears, shortness of breath, shoulder pain, sinus inflammation, sleepiness, sneezing, stomach and intestinal pain, tremor, unusual redness of the skin, urgent urination, vomiting, warm sensation.

Interactions

 Inform your doctor before combining Plendil with: beta-blockers such as Lopressor, Inderal, and Tenormin; cimetidine (Tagamet); digoxin (Lanoxin); epilepsy medications such as Tegretol and Dilantin; erythromycin (PCE, Eryc); phenobarbital; theophylline (Theo-Dur).

No known food/other substance interactions.

Special Cautions

 If pregnant or planning to become pregnant, inform your doctor immediately. Birth defects have appeared in animal studies. May appear in breast milk; could affect a nursing infant.

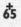 Seniors are prescribed lower doses, and should have blood pressure monitored while doctor is adjusting dosage.

 Not generally prescribed for children.

 If sensitive to or allergic to this or other calcium channel blockers, should not take.

May cause low blood pressure. Immediately notify your doctor if you experience light-headedness, heart racing, or chest pain.

Use with caution if you have congestive heart failure, especially if taking a beta-blocker such as Inderal or Tenormin.

May experience swelling of legs and feet in the first 2 to 3 weeks of starting medication.

To avoid swollen and sore gums, practice good dental hygiene.

In the case of liver disease, doctor will monitor blood pressure.

Polaramine

^^^

Generic name: Dexchlorpheniramine maleate

Other brand names: Dexchlor, Poladex, Polargen

Polaramine is an antihistamine. Antihistamines block the effects of histamine, a body chemical that causes swelling and itching.

℞ QUICK FACTS

Purpose

Used to treat allergy symptoms including: nasal stuffiness and inflammation, and eye irritation caused by hay fever and other allergies; itching, swelling, and redness from hives and other rashes; allergic reactions to blood transfusions; and in combination with other medications, anaphylactic shock (severe allergic reaction).

Dosage

Take exactly as prescribed.

. . . .

Usual adult dose: *Polaramine Repetabs Tablets*—one 4 or 6 milligram tablet at bedtime or every 8 to 10 hours during the day. *Polaramine Tablets*—1 tablet every 4 to 6 hours. *Polaramine Syrup*—1 teaspoon (2 milligrams) every 4 to 6 hours.

. . . .

Usual child dose: *Polaramine Repetabs Tablets*—children 12 years and over are prescribed adult dosage. *Children ages 6 to 11*—one 4 milligram tablet per day at bedtime. *Polaramine Tablets*—children 12 years and older are prescribed adult dose. *Children ages 6 to 11*—½ tablet every 4 to 6 hours. *Children 2 to 5 years*—¼ tablet every 4 to 6 hours. *Polaramine Syrup*—children 12 years and older are prescribed adult dose. *Children 6 to 11 years*—½ teaspoon (1

milligram) every 4 to 6 hours. *Children 2 to 5 years*—
¼ teaspoon (½ milligram) every 4 to 6 hours.

 Missed dose: *if taking on a regular schedule*—take as
soon as possible, unless almost time for next dose.
In that case, do not take missed dose; go back to
regular schedule. *Do not double doses.*

Side Effects

 Overdose symptoms: blurred vision, cardiovascular
collapse, convulsions, decreased alertness, difficulty
sleeping, dizziness, hallucinations, lack of muscle coordination, low blood pressure, ringing in ears, sedation, temporary failure to breathe, tremors. Symptoms in children: dry mouth, extremely high body
temperature, fixed or dilated pupils, flushing, stimulation, stomach and intestinal problems. If you suspect an overdose, immediately seek medical attention.

 More common side effects: mild to moderate drowsiness, thickening of mucus.

 Less common or rare side effects: anaphylactic
shock (severe allergic reaction); blurred vision; chest
congestion; chills; confusion; constipation; convulsions; diarrhea; difficulty sleeping; difficulty urinating;
disturbed coordination; dizziness; dry mouth, nose,
and throat; early menstruation; excessive perspiration; excitement (especially in children); extreme fatigue; exaggerated sense of well-being; fever; frequent urination; headache; hives; hysteria; irritability;
loss of appetite; low blood pressure; nausea; nervousness; nightmares; painful urination; pounding
heartbeat; premature heart contractions; rapid
heartbeat; rash; restlessness; ringing in ears; sedation; sensitivity to sun; sore throat; stomach upset
or pain; stuffy nose; sweating; tightness in chest; tingling or pins and needles; tiredness; tremor; unusual

bleeding or bruising; urinary retention; vertigo; vomiting; weakness; wheezing.

Interactions

 Inform your doctor before combining Polaramine with: antidepressants such as Elavil and Tofranil, blood thinners such as Coumadin, sedatives such as Nembutal and Seconal, tranquilizers such as Xanax and Valium. May hide effects of aspirin if taking aspirin in large doses. *Do not take Polaramine if you are taking MAO inhibitors such as Parnate and Nardil; may cause extremely low blood pressure.*

 Avoid alcohol during Polaramine therapy.

Special Cautions

 Should not be used during third trimester. If pregnant or planning to become pregnant, inform your doctor immediately. Appears in breast milk; could affect a nursing infant.

 May cause dizziness and low blood pressure in seniors.

 Follow doctor's instructions carefully for children. *Do not administer to premature infants or newborns.*

 Do not take if sensitive to or allergic to this or similar medications.

May cause drowsiness and impair your ability to drive a car or operate machinery. *Do not take part in any activity that requires alertness.*

Use with caution if you have: glaucoma, obstructive peptic ulcer or other stomach problems, symptoms of enlarged prostate, difficulty urinating, history of bronchial asthma, overactive thyroid, heart disease, circulatory problems, or high blood pressure.

Polymox

see AMOXIL

Polymyxin B Sulfate with Neomycin Sulfate and Hydrocortisone

see CORTISPORIN OPHTHALMIC SUSPENSION

Poly-Vi-Flor

Generic ingredients: Vitamins with fluoride

Other brand names: Florvite, Poly-Vitamins with Fluoride, Vi-Daylin/F

Poly-Vi-Flor is a multivitamin supplement containing fluoride. Vitamins are chemical substances that supplement nutritional deficiencies, and fluoride encourages remineralization and inhibits the cariogenic microbial process.

℞ QUICK FACTS

Purpose

℞ Used to provide fluoride to children 2 to 16 years and older when drinking water is deficient, and to build strong teeth and prevent cavities.

Dosage

 Do not give child more than prescribed dose, may discolor or cause pitting of teeth. Chew or crush tablet before swallowing.

 Usual adult dose: not generally prescribed for adults.

 Usual child dose: 1 tablet every day per doctor's advice.

 Missed dose: take as soon as possible, unless almost time for next dose. In that case, do not take missed dose; go back to regular schedule. *Do not double doses.*

Side Effects

 Overdose symptoms: no specific information available. If you suspect an overdose, immediately seek medical attention.

 More common side effects: none reported.

 Rare side effect: allergic rash.

Interactions

 If child is receiving fluoride from other medications or sources, should not take Poly-Vi-Flor.

 No known food/other substance interactions.

Special Cautions

 Not generally prescribed for pregnant or breastfeeding women.

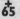 Not generally prescribed for seniors.

Follow doctor's instructions carefully for children.

 Before administering this medication to your child, check fluoride level of drinking water.

Contact your doctor if you notice white, brown, or black spots on your child's teeth.

Inform your doctor of any changes to drinking water or filtering systems.

This medication is not a substitute for brushing, flossing, and regular dental check-ups.

Ponstel

Generic name: Mefenamic acid

Ponstel is a nonsteroidal anti-inflammatory analgesic. It blocks the production of body chemicals called prostaglandins, which trigger pain.

℞ QUICK FACTS

Purpose

 Used to treat moderate pain (for not more than 7 days) and menstrual pain.

Dosage

 To avoid stomach upset, take with food, an antacid, or milk. Take exactly as prescribed.

 Usual adult dose: *for moderate pain*—500 milligrams followed by 250 milligrams every 6 hours if needed, for 1 week. *For menstrual pain*—500 milligrams followed by 250 milligrams every 6 hours for 2 to 3 days.

 Usual child dose: children 14 years and older are prescribed adult dose. Not generally prescribed for children under 14 years.

 Missed dose: *if taking on a regular schedule*—take as soon as possible, unless almost time for next dose. In that case, do not take missed dose; go back to regular schedule. *Do not double doses.*

Side Effects

 Overdose symptoms: no specific information available. If you suspect an overdose, immediately seek medical attention.

 More common side effects: abdominal pain, diarrhea, nausea, stomach and intestinal upset, vomiting.

 Less common or rare side effects: anemia, blurred vision, blood in urine, changes in liver function, constipation, difficult or painful urination, dizziness, drowsiness, ear pain, eye irritation, facial swelling due to fluid retention, fluttery or throbbing heartbeat, gas, headache, heartburn, hives, inability to sleep, increased need for insulin as a diabetic, kidney failure, labored breathing, loss of appetite, loss of color vision, nervousness, rash, red or purple skin spots, sweating, ulcers and internal bleeding.

Interactions

 Inform your doctor before combining Ponstel with: aspirin, blood thinners such as Coumadin, diuretics such as Lasix and HydroDIURIL, lithium (Lithonate), methotrexate.

No known food/other substance interactions.

Special Cautions

 Should not be used during latter stages of pregnancy, as it affects heart and blood vessels of fetus. If pregnant or planning to become pregnant, inform your doctor immediately. May appear in breast milk; could affect a nursing infant.

 No special precautions apply to seniors.

 Follow doctor's instructions carefully for children over 14 years.

 Do not take if you have stomach ulcerations or frequently recurring inflammation of stomach or intestines.

Do not take if sensitive to or allergic to Ponstel. Should not take if you have had asthma attacks, hay fever, or hives caused by aspirin or other nonsteroidal anti-inflammatory medications such as Motrin or Nuprin.

Stop taking and immediately contact your doctor if you experience rash, diarrhea, or other stomach problems.

Doctor should monitor for ulcers or internal bleeding if you take Ponstel regularly.

Should use with caution if you have kidney disease, heart failure, or liver disease.

May prolong bleeding time; if using a blood-thinning medication, use Ponstel with caution.

Potassium Chloride

see MICRO-K

Pravachol

~~~~~~

Generic name: Pravastatin sodium

Pravachol is an antihyperlipidemic (lipid-lowering) agent. It chemically interferes with the enzyme that synthesizes cholesterol, thereby decreasing the low-density lipoprotein (LDL) type of cholesterol associated with coronary artery disease and atherosclerosis.

℞ QUICK FACTS

Purpose

℞ Used to lower cholesterol in conjunction with a cholesterol-lowering diet for dangerously high cholesterol levels not controlled by diet alone.

Dosage

 Before starting Pravachol therapy, diet alone for 3 to 6 months should be tried to lower cholesterol. If cholesterol is still too high after 6 months, take medication exactly as prescribed. *Do not use Pravachol as a substitute for a cholesterol-lowering diet; it is a supplement to your diet.* Doctor may prescribe Questran or Colestid for greater cholesterol-lowering effect. Take Pravachol at least 1 hour before or 4 hours after taking the other medication. To get full effect of medication, must follow the diet and exercise program prescribed by your doctor.

Usual adult dose: 10 to 20 milligrams once per day at bedtime. Ongoing therapy—10 to 40 milligrams taken once per day at bedtime. *Seniors*—10 milligrams per day at bedtime. Ongoing therapy—up to 20 milligrams per day.

 Usual child dose: not generally prescribed.

 Missed dose: take as soon as possible, unless almost time for next dose. In that case, do not take missed dose; go back to regular schedule. *Do not double doses.*

Side Effects

 Overdose symptoms: no specific information available. If you suspect an overdose, immediately seek medical attention.

 Side effects: abdominal pain, allergic reaction, altered sense of taste, anxiety, appetite loss, breast swelling in men, chest pain, cold, constipation, cough, depression, diarrhea, difficulty sleeping, dizziness, eye movement difficulties, fatigue, flu, gas, hair loss, headache, heartburn, inflammation of nasal passages, jaundice (yellow skin and eyes), joint pain, lowered sex drive, memory loss, mild stomach or bowel discomfort, muscle aches or pain, nausea, nerve pain or twitching, numbness or tingling, penile erection problems, rash, sluggish facial muscles, tremor, urinary difficulties, vomiting.

 No known less common or rare side effects.

Interactions

 Inform your doctor before combining Pravachol with: cholestyramine (Questran), cimetidine (Tagamet), colestipol (Colestid), erythromycin (E.E.S. or Erythrocin), gemfibrozil (Lopid), immunosuppressive medications such as cyclosporine (Sandimmune), ketoconazole (Nizoral), niacin, warfarin (Coumadin).

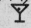 No known food/other substance interactions.

Special Cautions

 Must not take if pregnant; may cause birth defects. If pregnant or planning to become pregnant, inform your doctor immediately. Appears in breast milk; should not breastfeed, as the cholesterol-lowering effects of the medication may prove harmful to your baby.

 Seniors are prescribed a lower dose.

 Not generally prescribed for children.

 Do not take if sensitive to or allergic to Pravachol, or if you have liver disease.

Should not use if your high cholesterol is a result of: alcoholism, poorly controlled diabetes, underactive thyroid, or kidney or liver problem.

Doctor will perform blood tests regularly if you have had prior liver problems.

Immediately report any unexplained muscle pain, tenderness, or weakness, especially if accompanied by a fever. Doctor should check for muscle damage.

Pravastatin Sodium
see PRAVACHOL

Prazosin Hydrochloride

see MINIPRESS

Predate-S

see PEDIAPRED

Pred Forte

Generic name: Prednisolone acetate

Other brand names: Cortalone, Delta-Corf, Prelone

Pred Forte is an adrenocorticosteroid hormone. It works by regulating a variety of body processes, including fluid balance, temperature, and reaction to inflammation.

℞ QUICK FACTS

Purpose

℞ Used to treat redness, irritation, and swelling due to eye inflammation.

Dosage

 Use entire amount prescribed. *Do not share use of this prescription to avoid spreading infection.* Doctor may advise not wearing contacts as they may increase chance of infection. *Do not use longer than*

your doctor prescribes; overuse can cause eye damage.

 Usual adult dose: 1 to 2 drops under eyelid 2 to 4 times daily. During first 2 days of treatment, doctor may prescribe more frequent doses.

 Usual child dose: not generally prescribed for children.

 Missed dose: apply as soon as possible, unless almost time for next dose. In that case, do not apply missed dose; go back to regular schedule. *Do not double doses.*

Side Effects

 Overdose symptoms: no specific information available. However, if you suspect chronic overdose with Pred Forte, immediately seek medical attention. If accidentally swallowed, immediately seek medical attention.

 Side effects: cataract formation, increased pressure inside eyeball, perforation of eyeball, secondary infection with fungi or viruses.

 Occasionally ongoing use may cause side effects due to overload of steroid hormone, including "moon-faced" appearance, obese trunk, humped upper back, wasted limbs, and purple stretch marks on back. Will usually disappear once medication is stopped; however, medication must be stopped gradually.

Interactions

 Inform your doctor before combining Pred Forte with other forms of prednisolone acetate.

No, known food/other substance interactions.

Special Cautions

 If pregnant or planning to become pregnant, inform your doctor immediately. Not known if Pred Forte appears in breast milk.

 No special precautions apply to seniors.

 Not generally prescribed for children.

 Do not use if you have an untreated, pus-forming eye infection.

Do not take if sensitive to or allergic to this medication. Contains sodium bisulfite, which can cause life-threatening asthmatic reactions, especially in people with asthma.

Should not use if you have herpes or other eye viruses, tuberculosis of the eye, or a fungal disease of the eye.

Doctor should closely monitor Pred Forte use, as there is a risk of developing cataracts.

If the cornea of the eye has persistent ulceration, may be a secondary infection requiring medical evaluation.

Eye pressure should be checked on a regular basis to avoid vision loss.

Prednisolone Acetate

see PRED FORTE

Prednisolone Sodium Phosphate

see PEDIAPRED

Prednisone

see DELTASONE

Premarin

~~~~~~

Generic name: Conjugated estrogens

Other brand names: Estracon, Progens Tabs

Premarin is an estrogen replacement/antineoplastic/anti-osteoporotic. It mimics the action of naturally produced estrogen, inhibits the growth of hormone-sensitive tissue in some cancers, enhances calcium and phosphate retention, and limits bone decalcification.

℞ QUICK FACTS

Purpose

℞ Used to reduce symptoms of menopause. Also used for teenagers who do not mature at usual rate, to relieve symptoms of certain cancers, and to relieve dry, itchy external genitals and vaginal irritation. Prescribed along with diet, calcium supplements, and exercise to prevent osteoporosis.

Dosage

🍴D Take exactly as prescribed. *Do not share prescription.*

Usual adult dose: *for menopause symptoms*—0.3 to 1.25 milligrams per day. *For vaginitis*—0.3 to 1.25 milligrams or more per day. *For low estrogen levels due to reduced ovary function*—2.5 to 7.5 milligrams per day, in divided doses for 20 days, followed by a rest period of 10 days. *For ovary removal or failure*—1.25 milligrams per day, 3 weeks on and 1 week off Premarin. *For osteoporosis*—0.625 milligram per day, 3 weeks on and 1 week off. *For breast cancer (women and men)*—10 milligrams taken 3 times per day for at least 3 months. *For relief of symptoms of advanced androgen-dependent prostate cancer*—1.25 to 2.5 milligrams taken 3 times per day. *Vaginal cream—for atrophic vaginitis or severe itching*—2 to 4 grams (½ applicator) per day inserted into vagina or lowest dose possible, used for 3 weeks and off for 1 week. Women with uterus intact should be monitored for endometrial cancer.

 Usual child dose: follow doctor's individualized dose.

 Missed dose: take as soon as possible, unless almost time for next dose. In that case, do not take missed dose; go back to regular schedule. *Do not double doses.*

Side Effects

 Overdose symptoms: no specific information available. If you suspect an overdose, immediately seek medical attention.

 Side effects: abdominal cramps, abnormal vaginal bleeding, bloating, breast swelling and tenderness, depression, dizziness, enlargement of benign tumors in uterus, fluid retention, gallbladder disease, hair loss from scalp, increased body hair, intolerance to contact lenses, migraine headache, nausea, vomiting, sex-drive changes, skin darkening (especially on the face), skin rash or redness, swelling of wrists and ankles, vaginal yeast infection, weight gain or loss, yellow eyes and skin.

 No known less common or rare side effects.

Interactions

 Inform your doctor before combining Premarin with: barbiturates such as phenobarbital; blood thinners such as Coumadin; epilepsy medications such as Dilantin; major tranquilizers such as Thorazine; oral diabetic medications such as Micronase; rifampin (Rifadin); thyroid preparations such as Synthroid; tricyclic antidepressants such as Elavil and Tofranil; vitamin C.

 No known food/other substance interactions.

Special Cautions

 If pregnant or planning to become pregnant, inform your doctor immediately, may harm fetus.

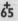 No special precautions apply to seniors.

 Follow doctor's individualized instructions for children.

 Do not take if you have had an allergic or bad reaction to this medication, or undiagnosed vaginal bleeding.

Notify your doctor immediately if you experience: abdominal pain, tenderness, or swelling; unusual vaginal bleeding; coughing up blood; pain in chest or calves; severe headache; dizziness or faintness; sudden shortness of breath; vision changes; yellowing of skin.

Should not take Premarin if you have breast cancer or other estrogen-dependent cancer unless your doctor makes an exception.

· ·

Women taking this medication after menopause at higher risk for gallbladder disease.

· ·

Risk of blood clots increased with Premarin therapy.

Prilosec

~~~~~~

Generic name: Omeprazole

Prilosec is a gastric acid secretion inhibitor. It inhibits the production of gastric acid.

℞ QUICK FACTS

Purpose

℞ Used to treat active duodenal ulcer, gastroesophageal reflux disease (GERD—backflow of acid stomach contents), and severe erosive esophagitis on a short-term (4 to 8 weeks) basis. Also used to treat Zollinger-Ellison syndrome (too much stomach acid secretion), multiple endocrine adenomas (benign tumors), and systemic mastocytosis (cancerous cells), on a long-term basis.

Dosage

 Take before meals for best results. May take with an antacid. Swallow capsules whole; not to be crushed or chewed. May take several days to see results; must adhere to dosage schedule.

· ·

 Usual adult dose: *for short-term treatment of active duodenal ulcer*—20 milligrams once per day. *For severe erosive esophagitis or GERD*—20 milligrams per day for 4 to 8 weeks. *For pathological hypersecretory conditions*—60 milligrams once per day. If taking more than 80 milligrams per day, doctor will divide into smaller doses.

Usual child dose: not generally prescribed for children.

Missed dose: take as soon as possible, unless almost time for next dose. In that case, do not take missed dose; go back to regular schedule. *Do not double doses.*

Side Effects

Overdose symptoms: no specific information available. If you suspect an overdose, immediately seek medical attention.

More common side effects: abdominal pain, diarrhea, headache, nausea, vomiting.

Less common or rare side effects: abdominal swelling, abnormal dreams, aggression, anemia, anxiety, apathy, back pain, breast development in males, blood in urine, changes in liver function, chest pain, confusion, constipation, cough, depression, difficulty sleeping, discolored feces, dizziness, dry mouth, dry skin, fatigue, fever, fluid retention and swelling, fluttery heartbeat, frequent urination, gas, general feeling of illness, hair loss, hallucinations, hepatitis, high blood pressure, hives, irritable colon, itching, joint and leg pain, loss of appetite, low blood sugar, muscle cramps and pain, nervousness, nosebleeds, pain, pain in testicles, rapid heartbeat, rash, ringing in ears, skin inflammation, sleepiness, slow heartbeat, taste distortion, tingling or pins and needles, throat pain, tremors, upper respiratory infection, urinary tract infection, vertigo, weakness, weight gain, yellow eyes and skin.

Interactions

 Inform your doctor before combining Prilosec with: ampicillin-containing medications such as Spectrobid, cyclosporine (Sandimmune), diazepam (Valium), disulfiram (Antabuse), iron (Feosol), ketoconazole (Nizoral), phenytoin (Dilantin), warfarin (Coumadin).

 Avoid excessive amounts of caffeine during Prilosec therapy.

Special Cautions

 If pregnant or planning to become pregnant, inform your doctor immediately. May appear in breast milk; could affect a nursing infant.

 No special precautions apply to seniors.

 Not generally prescribed for children.

 Not for long-term use after ulcer has healed. Safety of prolonged use has yet to be established.

If sensitive to or allergic to this medication, should not take.

Primidone

see MYSOLINE

Principen

see OMNIPEN

Prinivil

see ZESTRIL

Prinzide

see ZESTORETIC

Probucol

see LORELCO

Procainamide Hydrochloride

see PROCAN SR

Procan SR

Generic name: Procainamide hydrochloride

Other brand names: Promine, Pronestyl-SR

Procan SR is an anti-arrhythmic. It corrects irregular heartbeats by altering nerve impulses within the heart to achieve a more normal rhythm.

℞ QUICK FACTS

Purpose

 Used to treat severe irregular heartbeats (arrhythmias), either tachycardia (too fast) or bradycardia (too slow).

Dosage

 Take prescribed amount only; never increase dosage. Swallow tablet whole; should not chew or crush. Adhere to schedule; skipping or missing doses or changing intervals may cause condition to worsen and may be dangerous.

 Usual adult dose: doses and intervals are determined based on your doctor's assessment of your heart disease, age, and kidney functioning. *Younger people with normal kidney function*—total daily dose of 50 milligrams per 2.2 pounds of body weight, divided into smaller doses and taken every 6 hours. *People over age 50 or those with reduced kidney, liver, or heart function*—prescribed lower doses with longer intervals between doses.

 Usual child dose: not generally prescribed for children.

 Missed dose: take as soon as possible, if within 4 hours of scheduled dose. Otherwise, do not take missed dose, go back to regular schedule. *Do not double doses.*

Side Effects

☠ Overdose symptoms: changes in heart function and heartbeat. If you suspect an overdose, immediately seek medical attention.

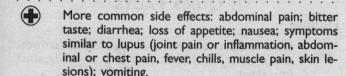 More common side effects: abdominal pain; bitter taste; diarrhea; loss of appetite; nausea; symptoms similar to lupus (joint pain or inflammation, abdominal or chest pain, fever, chills, muscle pain, skin lesions); vomiting.

Less common side effects: depression, dizziness, fluid retention, flushing, giddiness, hallucinations, hives, itching, rash, weakness. Rare side effects: anemia, changes in blood counts, low blood pressure.

Interactions

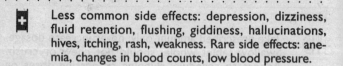 Inform your doctor before combining Procan SR with: anti-arrhythmic medications such as quinidine (Quinidex), propranolol (Inderal), and mexiletine (Mexitil); lidocaine; medications that ease muscle spasms such as benztropine (Cogentin) and trihexyphenidyl (Artane); neuromuscular blocking agents such as succinylcholine (Anectine).

No known food/other substance interactions.

Special Cautions

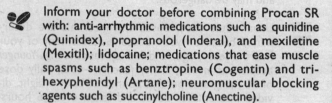 If pregnant or planning to become pregnant, inform your doctor immediately. Appears in breast milk, could affect a nursing infant.

65 People over age 50 are prescribed lower doses.

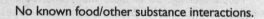 Not generally prescribed for children.

STOP Within first 3 months of therapy can cause serious blood disorders. Doctor will order blood count weekly for the first 12 weeks of therapy and then careful monitoring.

Immediately contact your doctor if you experience: joint or muscle pain, dark urine, yellowing skin or eyes, muscular weakness, chest or abdominal pain, appetite loss, diarrhea, hallucinations, dizziness, depression, wheezing, cough, easy bruising or bleeding, tremors, palpitations, rash, soreness or ulcers in mouth, sore throat, fever, or chills.

Doctor should not prescribe if you have lupus erythematosus or heartbeat irregularity known as "torsade de pointes."

Doctor will closely monitor you if you have had: kidney or liver disease, or myasthenia gravis (disease causing muscle weakness, especially in face and neck).

Should not take if you have complete or incomplete heart block without a pacemaker, or if you have had an allergic reaction to procaine or similar local anesthetics, or aspirin.

Use with caution if you have ever had congestive heart failure or other heart disease.

Procardia

Generic name: Nifedipine

Other brand names: Adalat, Procardia XL

Procardia is a calcium channel blocker. It increases the amount of oxygen that reaches the heart muscle.

℞ Quick Facts

Purpose

 Used to treat angina (crushing chest pain). Also used to treat high blood pressure.

Dosage

 Continue to take exactly as prescribed even if symptoms subside. Must take on a regular basis in order for medication to be effective, and may take several weeks before you get the full benefit of Procardia. Take at the same time each day. May take with food; *do not chew or crush tablets. Do not substitute brands.*

 Usual adult dose: *Procardia*—one 10 milligram capsule taken 3 times per day. Range may be from 10 to 20 milligrams taken 3 times per day, up to 120 to 180 milligrams per day maximum. *Procardia XL*—one 30 or 60 milligram tablet taken once per day.

 Usual child dose: not generally prescribed for children.

 Missed dose: take as soon as possible, unless almost time for next dose. In that case, do not take missed dose; go back to regular schedule. *Do not double doses.*

Side Effects

 Overdose symptoms: dizziness, extremely low blood pressure, flushing, fluttering heartbeat, loss of consciousness, nausea, nervousness, swelling due to fluid retention, vomiting. If you suspect an overdose, immediately seek medical attention.

 More common side effects: constipation; cough; dizziness; fatigue; fluid retention (ankle or leg swelling); giddiness; headache; heartburn; heat sensation;

light-headedness; low blood pressure; mood changes; muscle cramps; nasal congestion; nausea; sore throat; swelling of arms, legs, hands, feet; tremors; wheezing.

Less common side effects: abdominal pain, blurred vision, chest congestion, chills, cramps, diarrhea, difficult or labored breathing, difficulty in balance, difficulty sleeping, drowsiness, dry cough, dry mouth, excessive sweating, fever, flushing, fluttering heartbeat, gas, general chest pain, hives, impotence, indigestion, itching, jitteriness, joint pain, leg cramps, muscle and bone inflammation, nervousness, pain, production of large amounts of pale urine, rash, sexual difficulties, shakiness, shortness of breath, skin inflammation, sleep disturbances, sleepiness, stiff joints, tingling or pins and needles, weakness. Rare side effects: abnormal or terrifying dreams, anemia, anxiety, arthritis, back pain, belching, blood in urine, breast pain, breathing disorders, dark stools containing blood, decreased sex drive, depression, distorted taste, dulled sense of touch, excessive urination at night, facial swelling, fainting, fever, gout, gum irritation, hair loss, hepatitis, hives, hot flashes, increased angina, increased sweating, inflammation of sinuses, irregular heartbeat, migraine, muscle incoordination, muscle pain, muscle tension, nosebleeds, painful or difficult urination, paranoia, rapid heartbeat, reddish or purplish spots under the skin, ringing in ears, swelling around the eyes, tearing eyes, temporary blindness, upper respiratory tract infection, vague feeling of illness, vertigo, vision changes, vomiting, weight gain.

Interactions

Inform your doctor before combining Procardia with: cimetidine (Tagamet); digitalis (Lanoxin); other heart and blood pressure medications such as propranolol (Inderal) and metoprolol (Lopressor).

No known food/other substance interactions.

Special Cautions

 If pregnant or planning to become pregnant, inform your doctor immediately. Not known if Procardia appears in breast milk.

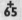 No special precautions apply to seniors.

 Not generally prescribed for children.

 There may be an increased risk of heart attack or death with Procardia.

Should not use if sensitive to or allergic to Procardia or other calcium channel blockers such as Adalat and Calan.

At beginning of therapy and when dose is increased, may experience low blood pressure, making you feel light-headed or faint. May also occur if you are taking beta-blockers such as Tenormin or Inderal; doctor should monitor blood pressure.

Small risk of increased angina at the beginning of therapy and when dose is increased; contact your doctor if this occurs.

Shell from Procardia XL tablets may appear in your stool; this is normal.

If doctor stops beta-blocker therapy, should be gradually stopped. If you have tight aortic stenosis (narrowing of aortic valve that obstructs blood flow from the heart to the body) and were taking a beta-blocker, doctor will monitor your condition.

. . . .

Use with caution if you have stomach or intestinal narrowing.

. . . .

Inform your doctor or dentist in the event of a medical emergency or prior to surgery or dental treatment that you are taking Procardia.

. . . .

To avoid moderate swelling of the arms, hands, legs, and feet, doctor may prescribe a diuretic.

Prochlorperazine

see COMPAZINE

Progestin

see ORAL CONTRACEPTIVES

Promethazine Hydrochloride

see PHENERGAN

Promethazine Hydrochloride with Codeine Phosphate

see PHENERGAN WITH CODEINE

Pronestyl-SR
see PROCAN SR

Propafenone
see RYTHMOL

Propine
∧∧

Generic name: Dipivefrin hydrochloride

Propine is an antiglaucoma agent. It decreases eye fluid production and enhances outflow. It is a "prodrug," a drug that is not active by itself but is converted in the body to an active form.

℞ QUICK FACTS

Purpose

 Used to treat chronic open-angle glaucoma.

Dosage

 Use exactly as prescribed, and use regularly. Will most likely continue treatment for life, as there is no cure for glaucoma. Wash hands before and after use, and do not touch the applicator to your eye or any other surface.

- -

 Usual adult dose: I drop in eye(s) every 12 hours. May take ½ hour for medication to work, will experience maximum results within I hour.

- -

Usual child dose: not generally prescribed for children.

 Missed dose: take as soon as possible, unless almost time for next dose. In that case, do not take missed dose; go back to regular schedule. *Do not double doses.*

Side Effects

 Overdose symptoms: no specific information available. If you suspect an overdose, immediately seek medical attention.

 More common side effects: burning and stinging, red eyes.

 Less common or rare side effects: allergic reactions, change in heart rhythm, conjunctivitis, extreme dilation of pupils, increased heart rate or blood pressure, increased sensitivity to light.

Interactions

 No significant drug interactions reported.

 No known food/other substance interactions.

Special Cautions

 If pregnant or planning to become pregnant, inform your doctor immediately. May appear in breast milk; could affect a nursing infant.

 No special precautions apply to seniors.

 Not generally prescribed for children.

Do not use if you have narrow-angle glaucoma unless directed by your doctor.

May blur vision or cause other problems for a short while. *Do not drive, operate machinery or participate in any other hazardous activity.*

If sensitive to or allergic to Propine should not use.

Propoxyphene Napsylate with Acetaminophen

see DARVOCET-N

Propranolol Hydrochloride

see INDERAL

Propulsid

Generic name: Cisapride

Propulsid is a gastrointestinal stimulant. It stimulates the production of acetylcholine in the gastrointestinal tract and thus restores the ability of the stomach and intestines to move food through the gastrointestinal tract.

℞ Quick Facts

Purpose

 Used to treat nighttime heartburn, which is a result of gastroesophageal reflux disease (GERD), a condition in which there is a backflow of the acid contents of the stomach.

Dosage

 Take 15 minutes prior to meals and at bedtime. Continue to take as prescribed, even if symptoms disappear.

 Usual adult dose: 10 milligrams taken 4 times per day. Doctor may increase dosage up to 20 milligrams taken 4 times per day.

 Usual child dose: not generally prescribed for children.

 Missed dose: take as soon as possible, unless almost time for next dose. In that case, do not take missed dose, go back to regular schedule. *Do not double doses.*

Side Effects

 Overdose symptoms: frequent urination or bowel movements, gas, gurgling and rumbling in stomach, retching. If you suspect an overdose, immediately seek medical attention.

 More common side effects: abdominal pain, bloating or gas, constipation, diarrhea, headache, inflamed nasal passages and sinuses, nausea, pain, upper respiratory and viral infections.

 Less common side effects: abnormal vision, anxiety, back pain, chest pain, coughing, depression, dehydration, dizziness, fever, fatigue, frequent urination, indigestion, insomnia, itching, inflammation of the vagina, joint pain, muscle pain, nervousness, rash, sore throat, urinary tract infection, vomiting. Rare side effects: dry mouth, fluid retention and swelling,

migraines, rapid heartbeat, sleepiness, throbbing
heartbeat, tremor.

Interactions

Inform your doctor before combining Propulsid
with: antispasmodics such as dicyclomine (Bentyl)
and benztropine (Cogentin); cimetidine (Tagamet);
ranitidine (Zantac); tranquilizers such as Librium,
Valium, and Xanax; warfarin (Coumadin). If taking
warfarin, doctor should perform a blood test 1
week after starting Propulsid and after Propulsid
therapy is completed.

May increase the effects of alcohol.

Special Cautions

If pregnant or planning to become pregnant, inform
your doctor immediately. Appears in breast milk;
could affect a nursing infant.

No special precautions apply to seniors.

Not generally prescribed for children.

If you suffer from blockage or bleeding of the intestines or stomach, or if sensitive to or allergic to
this medication, should not take.

Proscar

Generic name: Finasteride

Proscar is an androgen synthesis inhibitor. It inhibits
steroid 5∝-reductase, an enzyme responsible for forming androgen 5∝-dihydrotestosterone (DHT) in adult
males. DHT influences development of the prostate gland.

℞ QUICK FACTS

Purpose

℞ Used to shrink an enlarged prostate. Also prescribed for baldness and as a preventive measure against prostate cancer.

Dosage

May take with or without food. Read patient information package that comes with prescription each time prescription is renewed.

Usual adult dose: *for men only*—one 5 milligram tablet per day.

Usual child dose: not prescribed for children.

Missed dose: take as soon as possible, unless almost time for next dose. In that case, do not take missed dose; go back to regular schedule. *Do not double doses.*

Side Effects

Overdose symptoms: no specific information available. If you suspect an overdose, immediately seek medical attention.

Side effects: decreased amount of semen in ejaculation, decreased sex drive, impotence.

No known less common or rare side effects.

Interactions

No significant drug interactions reported.

No known food/other substance interactions.

Special Cautions

 Not prescribed for women. If accidentally taken by a pregnant woman carrying a male fetus, may cause abnormal development of genital organs. Men taking Proscar should use a condom if having intercourse with a pregnant woman; semen may contain small amounts of Proscar. Pregnant women should be careful not to touch a crushed Proscar tablet.

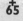 No special precautions apply to senior men.

 Not prescribed for children.

 Do not take if sensitive to or allergic to Proscar.

Before prescribing Proscar doctor should rule out infection, bladder obstruction, prostate cancer, and bladder disorders.

Differing responses to this medication may occur: early relief from urinary problems, no relief for 6 months to a year, no relief after a year's time.

Doctor should periodically monitor for prostate cancer; Proscar is not a treatment for prostate cancer.

ProSom

Generic name: Estazolam

ProSom is a benzodiazepine sedative. It selectively reduces the activity of certain brain chemicals.

℞ QUICK FACTS

Purpose

 Used to treat insomnia on a short-term basis. Insomnia may include: difficulty falling asleep, frequently waking up during the night, or waking too early in the morning.

Dosage

 Take exactly as prescribed, usually at bedtime. *Do not suddenly stop taking ProSom if you have a history of seizures; follow doctor's instructions for gradually tapering off medication. Also if you have no history of seizures, gradually taper off medication per doctor's instructions.*

 Usual adult dose: 1 milligram at bedtime; some may require 2 milligrams. *For seniors, physically run-down individuals, those with kidney or liver problems, or breathing problems*—0.5 to 1 milligram (½ to 1 tablet).

 Usual child dose: not generally prescribed for children.

 Missed dose: only take at bedtime as needed. Not necessary to make up missed doses.

Side Effects

 Overdose symptoms: confusion, depressed breathing, drowsiness and eventually coma, lack of coordination, slurred speech. If you suspect an overdose, immediately seek medical attention.

 More common side effects: abnormal coordination, cold symptoms, decreased movement or activity, dizziness, general feeling of illness, hangover, headache, leg and foot pain, nausea, nervousness, sleepiness, weakness.

 Less common or rare side effects: abnormal pain, abnormal dreaming, abnormal thinking, abnormal vision, acne, agitation, allergic reaction, altered taste, anxiety, apathy, arm and hand pain, arthritis, asthma, back pain, black stools, body pain, chest pain, chills, confusion, constant involuntary eye movement, constipation, cough, decreased appetite, decreased hearing, decreased reflexes, depression, difficult or labored breathing, double vision, dry mouth, dry skin, ear pain, emotional changeability, fainting, fever, flushing, frequent urination, gas, hallucinations, hostility, inability to hold urine, inability to urinate, increased appetite, indigestion, inflamed sinuses, itching, lack of coordination, little or no urine flow, loss of memory, menstrual cramps, muscle stiffness, nasal inflammation, neck pain, nighttime urination, nosebleed, numbness or tingling around mouth, purple or reddish skin spots, rapid and/or heavy breathing, rash, ringing in ears, seizure, sleep problems, sore throat, stupor, swollen breast, thirst, throbbing or fluttering heartbeat, tingling or pins and needles, tremor, twitch, urgency to urinate, vaginal discharge or itching, vomiting, weight gain or loss.

Interactions

 Inform your doctor before combining ProSom with: anticonvulsants such as Dilantin, Tegretol, and Depakene; antihistamines such as Benadryl and Chlor-Trimeton; antipsychotics such as Haldol and Mellaril; barbiturates such as phenobarbital; MAO inhibitors such as Nardil and Parnate; narcotics such as Percodan and Tylox; tranquilizers such as Valium and Xanax; or any other medication that slows the central nervous system.

Do not drink alcohol during ProSom therapy; may make you comatose or dangerously slow your breathing.

Special Cautions

 Do not take if pregnant; may cause birth defects. If taking ProSom or a similar medication just before birth, you may deliver a baby that has poor muscle tone and experiences withdrawal symptoms. If pregnant or planning to become pregnant, inform your doctor immediately. Is believed to appear in breast milk; could affect a nursing infant.

 Seniors should use with caution, may require lower dose.

 Not generally prescribed for children.

 Do not take if sensitive to or allergic to ProSom or other Valium-type medications.

May cause drowsiness and impair your ability to drive a car or operate machinery. *Do not take part in any activity that requires alertness.*

Due to potential addictiveness of ProSom, should be prescribed for short-term therapy. Even after short-term therapy, may experience withdrawal symptoms after discontinuing medication. Withdrawal symptoms may include: mild and temporary insomnia; irritability; and, less frequently, abdominal and muscle cramps, convulsions, sweating, tremors, and vomiting.

Proventil

Generic name: Albuterol sulfate

Other brand names: Proventil Syrup/Inhaler/ Repetabs; Ventolin Syrup/Inhalation Aerosol/Tablets; Volmax Extended Release Tablets

Proventil is a bronchodilator. It acts on the muscles of the bronchi (breathing tubes) to relieve bronchospasms, thereby allowing air to move freely to and from the lungs.

℞ QUICK FACTS

Purpose

℞ Used to relieve wheezing and shortness of breath associated with asthma, bronchitis, and emphysema. Also used to prevent bronchial spasm due to exercise.

Dosage

 Follow your doctor's instructions carefully. To avoid stomach irritation, take tablets and oral syrup with food, unless your doctor directs otherwise. Proventil inhaler should not be used with other aerosol bronchodilators. *Do not exceed your doctor's recommended dose; can be dangerous and may worsen asthma symptoms. Do not change brands without consulting your doctor.*

 Usual adult dose: *inhalation aerosol—Ventolin and Proventil for sudden or severe bronchial spasm, or prevention of asthma symptoms—*2 inhalations every 4 to 6 hours. *For exercise-induced bronchial spasm—*2 inhalations 15 minutes prior to exercise. *Tablets—*2 or 4 milligrams taken 3 to 4 times per day. *Syrup—*1 or 2 teaspoonfuls 3 or 4 times per day. *Ventolin Rotocaps for inhalation—*contents of one 200-microgram capsule inhaled every 4 to 6 hours using Rotahaler inhalation device. *Inhalation solution—*2.5 milligrams taken 3 to 4 times per day by nebulization. (Dilute 0.5 milliliter of the solution for inhalation with

2.5 milliliters of sterile normal saline solution.) *Ventolin nebules inhalation solution*—2.5 milligrams taken 3 or 4 times per day by nebulization. *Proventil Repetabs and Volmax extended release tablets*—8 milligrams every 12 hours. *Seniors*—2 milligrams taken 3 or 4 times per day for tablet or syrup form. If prescribed dose does not relieve or worsens symptoms, immediately contact your doctor.

 Usual child dose: *inhalation aerosol*—Proventil and Volmax are not prescribed for children under age 12; for children 12 years and older, adult dose is prescribed. Ventolin is not prescribed for children under age 4; for children 4 years and older, adult dose is prescribed. *Tablets*—2 milligrams taken 3 or 4 times per day for children 6 to 12 years. *Syrup*—1 teaspoonful taken 3 to 4 times per day for children 6 to 14 years. For children 2 to 6 years—0.1 milligram per 2.2 pounds of body weight, up to 4 milligrams taken 3 times per day. If prescribed dose does not relieve or worsens symptoms, immediately contact your doctor.

 Missed dose: take forgotten dose as soon as possible; take remaining doses for that day at equally spaced intervals. *Do not double doses.*

Side Effects

 Overdose symptoms: high blood pressure, low potassium level, radiating chest pain, rapid heartbeat, seizures. If you suspect an overdose, immediately seek medical attention.

 More common side effects: aggression, anxiety, cough, diarrhea, dizziness, excitement, general bodily discomfort, headache, heartburn, increased appetite, increased blood pressure, indigestion, irritability, labored breathing, light-headedness, muscle cramps, nausea, nervousness, nightmares, nosebleed, overactivity, palpitations, rapid heartbeat, rash, ringing in the ears, shakiness, sleeplessness, stomachache, stuffy nose, throat irritation, tooth discoloration, tremors, vomiting, wheezing, worsening bronchospasm.

 Less common side effects: chest pain (sometimes crushing) or discomfort, difficulty urinating, drowsiness, dry mouth and throat, flushing, high blood pressure, muscle spasm, restlessness, sweating, unusual taste, vertigo, weakness. Rare side effects from inhaler: hoarseness, increased breathing or wheezing, skin rash or hives, unusual and unexpected swelling of mouth and throat.

Interactions

 Inform your doctor before combining Proventil with: antidepressants such as Elavil and Nardil; beta-blockers (heart and blood pressure medications such as Inderal, Tenormin, and Sectral); medications similar to Proventil such as Alupent, Brethaire, Isuprel, and epinephrine.

 No known food/other substance interactions.

Special Cautions

 If pregnant or planning to become pregnant, inform your doctor immediately. Not known whether Proventil appears in breast milk.

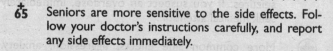 Seniors are more sensitive to the side effects. Follow your doctor's instructions carefully, and report any side effects immediately.

 Proventil and Volmax are not generally prescribed for children under the age of 12; Ventolin is not generally prescribed for children under the age of 4.

If sensitive to or allergic to this medication or similar medications, should not take.

Notify your doctor before using Proventil if you have: cardiovascular or convulsive disorder, high blood pressure, abnormal heartbeat, overactive thyroid gland, diabetes, epilepsy, enlarged prostate, or glaucoma.

Provera

Generic name: Medroxyprogesterone acetate

Other brand names: Amen, Curretab, Cycrin, Depo-Provera

Provera is a progestin and antineoplastic. It suppresses ovulation, causes thickening of cervical mucus, and induces sloughing of the lining of the uterus, and inhibits the growth of progestin-sensitive endometrial or renal cancer tissue.

℞ Quick Facts

Purpose

 Used when menstrual periods have ceased or a female hormone imbalance is causing the uterus to bleed abnormally. Depo-Provera is used as a contraceptive injection, and to treat endometrial cancer. Also prescribed for endometriosis, menopause symptoms, sexually aggressive behavior in men, and sleep apnea (temporary breathing failure while sleeping).

Dosage

 Take with or between meals. *Do not change brands unless directed by your doctor.*

 Usual adult dose: *to restore menstrual periods*—5 to 10 milligrams daily for 5 to 10 days. Should experience bleeding for 3 to 7 days after stopping Provera. *For abnormal uterine bleeding due to hormonal imbalance*—5 to 10 milligrams starting on the 16th or 21st day of your menstrual cycle, for 5 to 10 days. Should experience bleeding for 3 to 7 days after stopping Provera.

 Usual child dose: not generally prescribed for children.

 Missed dose: take as soon as possible, unless almost time for next dose. In that case, do not take missed dose; go back to regular schedule. *Do not double doses.*

Side Effects

 Overdose symptoms: no specific information available. If you suspect an overdose, immediately seek medical attention.

 Side effects: acne; anaphylaxis (life-threatening allergic reaction); blood clot in a vein, lungs, or brain; breakthrough bleeding between menstrual periods; breast tenderness or sudden or excessive flow of milk; cervical erosion or changes in secretions; depression; excessive growth of hair; fever; fluid retention; hair loss; headache; hives; insomnia; itching; lack of menstruation; menstrual flow changes; spotting; nausea; rash; skin discoloration; sleepiness; weight gain or loss; yellowed eyes and skin.

No known less common or rare side effects.

Interactions

 Inform your doctor before combining Provera with Aminoglutethimide (Cytadren).

 No known food/other substance interactions.

Special Cautions

 Should not take during first 4 months of pregnancy; may cause birth defects. If pregnant or planning to become pregnant, inform your doctor immediately. Provera is no longer used to prevent miscarriage. *Do not use Provera as a pregnancy test.* Appears in breast milk; could affect a nursing infant.

 No special precautions apply to seniors.

 Not generally prescribed for children.

 Do not take if sensitive to or allergic to Provera.

Do not take if you have: cancer of the breast or genital organs, liver disease or a liver condition, a dead fetus in the uterus, undiagnosed bleeding from the vagina, history of or current blood clots.

Before starting Provera, doctor will perform a complete physical exam, including your breasts, and pelvic organs (Pap test).

May cause some fluid retention; inform your doctor of any condition you have that is aggravated by fluid retention, such as epilepsy, migraine, asthma, or heart or kidney problems.

. . . .

May mask onset of menopause—regular menstrual bleeding may continue.

. . . .

If you have a history of depression, Provera may cause depression. Doctor will stop Provera if you become depressed.

. . . .

If you are diabetic, doctor should closely monitor your reaction to Provera.

. . . .

May increase risk of blood clots. Notify your doctor immediately if you experience: pain with swelling, warmth, and redness in leg vein; coughing or shortness of breath; vision problems (loss of some or all of vision or seeing double); migraine; or weakness or numbness in an arm or leg.

Prozac
∿∿

Generic name: Fluoxetine hydrochloride

Prozac is a cyclic antidepressant. It increases the concentration of certain chemicals necessary for nerve transmission in the brain.

℞ QUICK FACTS

Purpose

   Used to treat major depression—continuing depression that interferes with daily functioning, such as changes in appetite, sleep habits, and mind or body coordination, decreased sex drive, increased fatigue, feelings of guilt or worthlessness, difficulty concentrating, slowed thinking, suicidal thoughts. Also used to treat obesity, eating disorders, and obsessive-compulsive disorders.

. . . .

Dosage

 Take exactly as prescribed, and at the same time each day.

 Usual adult dose: 20 milligrams per day, taken in the morning. Doses over 20 milligrams should be divided into 2 doses. Total maximum dose is 80 milligrams per day. *For individuals with kidney or liver disease*—may have dose adjusted by doctor. *Seniors*—dose is individualized.

 Usual child dose: not generally prescribed for children.

 Missed dose: take as soon as possible, unless several hours have passed. In that case, do not take missed dose; go back to regular schedule. *Do not double doses.*

Side Effects

 Overdose symptoms: agitation, nausea, restlessness, vomiting. If you suspect an overdose, immediately seek medical attention.

 More common side effects: abnormal dreams, agitation, anxiety, bronchitis, chills, diarrhea, dizziness, drowsiness and fatigue, hay fever, inability to fall or stay asleep, increased appetite, lack or loss of appetite, light-headedness, nausea, nervousness, sweating, tremors, weakness, weight loss, yawning.

 Less common side effects: abnormal ejaculation, abnormal gait, abnormal stoppage of menstrual flow, acne, amnesia, apathy, arthritis, asthma, belching, bone pain, breast cysts, breast pain, brief loss of consciousness, bursitis, chills and fever, conjunctivitis (pink eye), convulsions, dark or tarry stool, difficulty swallowing, dilation of pupils, dimness of vision, dry skin, ear pain, eye pain, exaggerated feeling of well-being, excessive bleeding, facial swelling due to fluid retention, fluid retention, hair loss, hallucinations, hangover effect, hiccups, high or low blood pressure, hives, hostility, impotence, increased sex drive, inflammation of the esophagus, inflammation of the gums, inflammation of the stomach lining, inflammation of the tongue, inflammation of the vagina, intolerance of light, involuntary movement, irrational ideas, irregular heartbeat, jaw or neck pain, lack of muscle coordination, low blood pressure upon standing, low blood sugar, migraine, mouth inflammation, neck pain and rigidity, nosebleed, ovarian disorders, paranoid reaction, pelvic pain, pneumonia, rapid breathing, rapid heartbeat, ringing in ears, severe chest pain, skin inflammation, skin rash, thirst, twitching, uncoordinated movements, urinary disorders, vague feeling of bodily discomfort, vertigo, weight gain. Rare side effects: antisocial behavior, blood in urine, bloody diarrhea, bone disease, breast enlargement, cataracts, colitis, coma, deafness, decreased reflexes, dehydration, double vision, drooping of eyelids, duodenal ulcer, enlarged abdomen, enlargement of liver, enlargement or increased activity of thyroid gland, excess growth of coarse hair on face and chest, excess uterine or vaginal bleeding, extreme muscle tension, eye bleeding, female milk production, fluid accumulation and swelling in the head, fluid buildup in larynx and lungs, gallstones, glaucoma, gout, heart attack, hepatitis, high blood sugar, hysteria, inability to control bowel movements, increased salivation, inflammation of eyes and eyelids, inflammation of gallbladder, inflammation of small intestine, inflammation of tissue below the skin, kidney disorders, lung inflammation, menstrual disorders, miscarriage, mouth sores, muscle inflammation or bleeding, muscle spasms, painful sexual intercourse for women, psoriasis, rashes, reddish or purplish skin spots, reduction of body temperature, rheumatoid arthritis, seborrhea, shingles, skin discoloration, skin inflammation and disorders, slowing of heart rate, slurred speech, spitting blood, stomach ulcer, stupor, suicidal thoughts, taste loss, temporary cessation of breathing, tingling sensation around mouth, tongue discoloration and swelling, urinary tract disorders, vomiting blood, yellow eyes and skin.

Interactions

 Do not take Prozac if you are using a MAO inhibitor such as Nardil and Parnate, may cause fatal reaction. Inform your doctor before combining Prozac with: carbamazepine (Tegretol), diazepam (Valium), digitalis (Lanoxin), flecainide (Tambocor), lithium (Eskalith), medications that act on the central nervous system such as Xanax and Valium, other antidepressants (Elavil), tryptophan, vinblastine (Velban), warfarin (Coumadin). **Also notify your doctor of any other prescription or nonprescription medications you are taking.**

 Do not drink alcohol while taking Prozac.

Special Cautions

 If pregnant or planning to become pregnant, inform your doctor immediately. May appear in breast milk; could affect a nursing infant.

 Dose is individualized for seniors.

 Not generally prescribed for children.

 Do not take if you have recently had a heart attack, have kidney or liver disease, or diabetes.

May cause drowsiness and impair your ability to drive a car or operate machinery. *Do not take part in any activity that requires alertness.*

If sensitive to or allergic to this or similar medications, should not take. Immediately stop taking Prozac if you experience skin rash or hives.

Use with caution if you have a history of seizures.

Inform your doctor if you experience dizziness or actually faint when standing from sitting or lying down.

Psorcon

Generic name: Diflorasone diacetate

Other brand names: Florone, Maxiflor

Psorcon is an anti-inflammatory and topical corticosteroid. It stimulates the synthesis of enzymes required to decrease the inflammatory response.

℞ QUICK FACTS

Purpose

Used to treat the inflammatory and itching symptoms of skin disorders that respond to topical application of steroids.

Dosage

Use exactly as prescribed, on skin only. Keep away from the eyes. Never use large amounts over large areas or cover with airtight dressings unless directed by your doctor. *Use only for disorder for which it was prescribed.*

Usual adult dose: thin film of ointment to affected area 1 to 3 times per day. Doctor may recommend airtight bandages for psoriasis or stubborn skin conditions; if infection occurs, discontinue bandages.

 Usual child dose: limited to least amount that is effective. Long-term treatment may affect growth and development in children. Avoid covering treated area with waterproof diapers or plastic pants.

 Missed dose: apply as soon as possible, unless several hours have passed. In that case, do not apply missed dose; go back to regular schedule.

Side Effects

 Overdose symptoms: unlikely, though long-term or prolonged use can produce side effects throughout the body such as: weight gain, reddening and rounding of face and neck, growth of excess body and facial hair, high blood pressure, emotional disturbances, loss of energy due to high blood sugar, and increase in frequency of urination. If you suspect an overdose, immediately seek medical attention.

 Side effects: burning, dryness, eruptions resembling acne, excessive discoloration of the skin, excessive growth of hair, inflammation of hair follicles, inflammation around the mouth, irritation, itching, prickly heat, secondary infection, severe inflammation of the skin, softening of the skin, stretch marks, stretching or thinning of the skin.

 No known less common or rare side effects.

Interactions

 No drug interactions reported.

 No known food/other substance interactions.

Special Cautions

 If pregnant or planning to become pregnant, inform your doctor immediately. Not known whether Psorcon appears in breast milk.

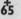 No special precautions apply to seniors.

 Follow doctor's instructions carefully for children.

 If sensitive to or allergic to this medication or similar medications (antifungals, steroids), you should not use. Inform your doctor if any irritation or allergic reaction occurs.

Pyridamole

see PERSANTINE

Pyridium

Generic name: Phenazopyridine hydrochloride

Other brand names: Azo-Standard, Baridium, Di-Azo, Diridone, Phenazodine, Pyridiate, Urodine

Pyridium is a urinary analgesic. Analgesics reduce pain.

℞ QUICK FACTS

Purpose

 Used to treat the pain, burning, urgency, frequency, and irritation caused by infection, trauma, catheters, or various surgical procedures in the lower urinary tract.

Dosage

 Take after meals, and exactly as prescribed by your doctor.

 Usual adult dose: two 100-milligram tablets or one 100-milligram tablet taken 3 times per day after meals. Should not take for more than 2 days if you are also taking an antibiotic.

 Usual child dose: not generally prescribed for children.

 Missed dose: take as soon as possible, unless several hours have passed. In that case, do not take missed dose; go back to regular schedule. *Do not double doses.*

Side Effects

 Overdose symptoms: changes in kidney, liver, and blood functioning. If you suspect an overdose, immediately seek medical attention.

 Side effects: abdominal upset; headache; itching; rash; severe allergic reaction (rash, difficulty breathing, fever, rapid heartbeat, convulsions).

 No known less common or rare side effects.

Interactions

 No drug interactions reported.

 No known food/other substance interactions.

Special Cautions

 If pregnant or planning to become pregnant, inform your doctor immediately. Not known whether Pyridium appears in breast milk.

 No special precautions apply to seniors.

 Follow doctor's instructions carefully for children.

 Urine will turn orange to red in color, and may stain fabric. May also stain contact lenses.

Avoid if sensitive to or allergic to Pyridium, or if you have kidney disease.

Quazepam

see DORAL

Questran

Generic name: Cholestyramine

Other brand name: Questran Light

Questran is an antihyperlipidemic (lipid-lowering) agent. It chemically interferes with the enzyme that synthesizes cholesterol, thereby decreasing the low-density lipoprotein (LDL) type of cholesterol associated with coronary artery disease and atherosclerosis.

℞ QUICK FACTS

Purpose

℞ Used to lower cholesterol levels in people with primary hypercholesterolemia (too much low-density lipoprotein [LDL] cholesterol). Also prescribed for hyperglyceridemia (excess fat is stored in the body). Also used for itching associated with gallbladder obstruction.

Dosage

 Is a supplement to, not a substitute for, the diet and exercise program prescribed by your doctor; to achieve full benefit of medication, must adhere to diet and exercise.

 Usual adult dose: *powder*—initially—1 single-dose packet or 1 level scoopful taken 1 to 2 times per day. Maintenance dose—2 to 4 packets or scoopfuls per day divided into 2 doses. Doctor may suggest taking in smaller doses. *Tablet*—4 grams taken 1 to 2 times per day to start. Maintenance dose—8 to 16 grams per day divided into 2 doses, up to 24 grams per day total.

 Usual child dose: follow doctor's instructions, is prescribed in limited circumstances.

 Missed dose: take as soon as possible, unless almost time for next dose. In that case, do not take missed dose; go back to regular schedule. *Do not double doses.*

Side Effects

 Overdose symptoms: no reported cases; however, potential overdose symptoms would be obstruction of the stomach and intestines. If you suspect an overdose, immediately seek medical attention.

 Most common side effect: constipation.

 Less common or rare side effects: abdominal discomfort, anemia, anxiety, arthritis, asthma, backache, belching, black stools, bleeding around teeth, blood in urine, brittle bones, burnt odor to urine, dental cavities, diarrhea, difficulty swallowing, dizziness, drowsiness, fainting, fatigue, fluid retention, gas, headache, heartburn, hiccups, hives, increased sex drive, increased tendency to bleed due to vitamin K deficiency, indigestion, inflammation of the eye, inflammation of the pancreas, irritation around the anal area, irritation of the skin and tongue, joint pain, lack or loss of appetite, muscle pain, nausea, night blindness due to vitamin A deficiency, painful or difficult urination, rash, rectal bleeding and/or pain, ringing in ears, shortness of breath, sour taste, swollen glands, tingling sensation, ulcer attack, vertigo, vitamin D deficiency, vomiting, weight gain or loss, wheezing.

Interactions

 Inform your doctor before combining Questran with: chlorothiazide (Diuril), digitalis (Lanoxin), oral diabetes medications (DiaBeta or Diabinese), penicillin G (Pentids), phenobarbital, phenylbutazone (Butazolidin), propranolol (Inderal), tetracycline (Achromycin V), thyroid medication (Synthroid), warfarin (Coumadin). Doctor may advise taking other medications 1 hour before or 4 to 6 hours after taking Questran. May experience exaggerated effects of digitalis if you stop Questran.

 Questran may interfere with the digestion and absorption of fats, including fat-soluble vitamins such as A, D, and K.

Special Cautions

 If pregnant or planning to become pregnant, inform your doctor immediately. May appear in breast milk; could affect a nursing infant.

 No special precautions apply to seniors.

 Is prescribed in limited circumstances for children.

 Do not take if being treated for gallbladder obstruction.

Inform your doctor *before* taking Questran if you have phenylketonuria, a genetic disorder; as well as any disease that contributes to increased blood cholesterol such as hypothyroidism (reduced thyroid function), diabetes, nephrotic syndrome (kidney and blood vessel disorder), dysproteinemia, or obstructive liver disease.

. . . .

If sensitive to or allergic to, should not take.

. . . .

Contact your doctor if cholesterol levels are not reduced within the first month of therapy.

. . . .

May induce or worsen constipation and aggravate hemorrhoids; contact your doctor if either occurs.

. . . .

In younger and smaller individuals, extended use may change acidity in bloodstream. Doctor should monitor these individuals on a regular basis.

Quinapril Hydrochloride

see ACCUPRIL

Quinidex Extentabs

Generic name: Quinidine sulfate

Other brand names: Cin-Quin, Novaquinidin, Quinora

Quinidex is an anti-arrhythmic. It alters nerve impulses within the heart to regulate heartbeat.

℞ QUICK FACTS

Purpose

℞ Used to correct irregular heart rhythms and to slow an abnormally fast heartbeat.

. . . .

Dosage

 Adhere to regular dosage schedule, taking only the prescribed amount, not increasing or decreasing dose. Swallow tablets whole, not crushed or chewed. May take with water, milk, or other liquid.

 Usual adult dose: 1 or 2 tablets every 8 to 12 hours.

 Usual child dose: not generally prescribed for children.

 Missed dose: take as soon as possible, if within 2 hours of next dose. Otherwise, do not take missed dose; go back to regular schedule. *Do not double doses.*

Side Effects

 Overdose symptoms: abnormal heart rhythms, changes in heart function, coma, decreased breathing, decreased production of urine, fluid in the lungs, low blood pressure, seizures. If you suspect an overdose, immediately seek medical attention.

 Most common side effects: abdominal pain, diarrhea, hepatitis, inflammation of esophagus (gullet), loss of appetite, nausea, vomiting.

 Less common or rare side effects: allergic reaction (swelling of face, lips, tongue, throat, arms and legs, sore throat, fever and chills, difficulty swallowing, chest pain); anemia; apprehension; asthma attack; blind spots; blood clots; blurred vision; changes in skin pigmentation; confusion; delirium; depression; dilated pupils; disturbed color perception; double vision; eczema; excitement; fainting; fever; fluid retention; flushing; headache; hearing changes; hepatitis; hives; inability to breathe; intense itching; intolerance to light; irregular heartbeats; joint pain; lack of coordination; low blood pressure; lupus erythematosus; mental decline; muscle pain; night blindness; psoriasis; rash; reddish or purplish spots below the skin; skin eruptions and scaling; skin sensitivity to light; vertigo; vision changes. Another possible side effect is cinchonism—a condition with symptoms such as ringing in ears, loss of hearing, dizziness, light-headedness, headache, nausea, disturbed vision.

Interactions

 Digoxin (Lanoxin) concentrations may increase or double when taken with Quinidex. Inform your doctor before combining Quinidex with: amiodarone (Cordarone); antacids with magnesium such as Maalox and Mylanta; antidepressants such as Elavil and Tofranil; antispasmodics such as Bentyl; aspirin; blood thinners such as Coumadin; cimetidine (Tagamet); diuretics such as Diamox and Daranide; decamethonium; disopyramide (Norpace); ketoconazole (Nizoral); major tranquilizers such as Stelazine and Thorazine; nifedipine (Procardia); phenobarbital; phenytoin (Dilantin); physostigmine (Antilirium); ranitidine (Zantac); reserpine (Diupres); rifampin (Rifadin); sodium bicarbonate; sucralfate (Carafate); thiazide diuretics such as Dyazide and HydroDIURIL; verapamil (Calan).

 No known food/other substance interactions.

Special Cautions

 If pregnant or planning to become pregnant, inform your doctor immediately. Appears in breast milk, could affect a nursing infant.

 No special precautions apply to seniors.

 Not generally prescribed for children.

Do not confuse with quinine, which is prescribed for nighttime leg cramps and malaria.

Should not take if you have certain heartbeat irregularities such as heart block; or if you have myasthenia gravis (abnormal muscle weakness); or if sensitive to or allergic to Quinidine or cinchona derivatives. In rare cases there have been severe allergic reactions.

Use with caution if you have: poorly controlled heart disease or circulatory problems, partial heart block, kidney or liver disease.

Immediately contact your doctor if you faint.

If you develop an unexplained fever contact your doctor; may be a sign of liver damage.

Quinidine Sulfate
see QUINIDEX EXTENTABS

Do not confuse with quinine, which is prescribed for nighttime leg cramps and malaria.

Should not take if you have certain heartbeat irregularities such as heart block, or if you have myasthenia gravis (abnormal muscle weakness), or if sensitive to or allergic to Quinidine or cinchona derivatives. In rare cases there have been severe allergic reactions.

Use with caution if you have poorly controlled heart disease or circulatory problems, partial heart block, kidney or liver disease.

Immediately contact your doctor if you faint.

If you develop an unexplained fever, contact your doctor; may be a sign of liver damage.

Quinidine Sulfate
see QUINIDEX EXTENTABS

~~~~~~

Ramipril

see ALTACE

Ranitidine Hydrochloride

see ZANTAC

Reglan

~~~~~~

Generic name: Metoclopramide hydrochloride

Other brand names: Clopra, Maxolon, Octamide, Reclomide

Reglan is a dopamine antagonist and anti-emetic. It acts on the brain's vomiting center to control or prevent nausea and vomiting, and it stimulates stomach and intestinal movement.

℞ QUICK FACTS

Purpose

℞ Used to treat diabetic gastroparesis, a condition in which the stomach does not contract. Also used to treat heartburn in the case of gastroesophageal reflux disease (GERD—backflow of stomach contents into esophagus). Also prescribed to prevent nausea and vomiting as a result of cancer chemotherapy and surgery.

Dosage

 Take 30 minutes prior to meals. Therapy lasts for 4 to 12 weeks; beyond 12 weeks is not recommended. If you suffer from diabetic "lazy stomach" (gastric stasis) on a recurring basis, doctor may advise taking Reglan as it reoccurs.

 Usual adult dose: *for GERD*—10 to 15 milligrams taken up to 4 times per day, 30 minutes prior to meals and at bedtime. *For intermittent symptoms*—single dose of 20 milligrams per day. *For gastric stasis*—10 milligrams 30 minutes prior to meals and at bedtime for 2 to 8 weeks. *Seniors*—5 milligrams per dose for GERD.

 Usual child dose: not generally prescribed for children.

 Missed dose: take as soon as possible, unless almost time for next dose. In that case, do not take missed dose; go back to regular schedule. *Do not double doses.*

Side Effects

 Overdose symptoms: disorientation, drowsiness, involuntary movements. If you suspect an overdose, immediately seek medical attention.

 Most common side effects: drowsiness, fatigue, lassitude, restlessness.

 Less common or rare side effects: breast development in males, confusion, continual discharge of milk from breasts, depression, diarrhea, dizziness, fluid retention, frequent urination, hallucinations, headache, high or low blood pressure, high fever, hives, impotence, inability to hold urine, insomnia, menstrual irregularities, nausea, rapid or slow heartbeat, rash, rigid muscles, slow movement, swollen tongue or throat, tremor, vision problems, wheezing, yellowed eyes and skin. May also cause Parkinson-like symptoms, including slow movements, rigidity, tremor, or a mask-like facial appearance. May cause tardive dyskinesia, with symptoms such as jerky or writhing involuntary movements, particularly of the tongue, face, mouth, or jaw; involuntary movements of the arms and legs; grimacing; tongue-thrusting; locking of jaw; rigid backward arching of the body; and loud or labored breathing. Also can cause intense restlessness, with symptoms such as anxiety, agitation, foot-tapping, pacing, inability to sit still, jitteriness, and insomnia.

Interactions

 Inform your doctor before combining Reglan with: acetaminophen (Tylenol); antispasmodics such as Bentyl and Pro-Banthine; cimetidine (Tagamet); digoxin (Lanoxin); insulin; MAO inhibitors such as Nardil and Parnate; levodopa (Dopar or Sinemet); narcotic painkillers such as Percocet and Demerol; sleeping pills such as Dalmane, Halcion, and Restoril; tetracycline (Achromycin or Sumycin); tranquilizers such as Valium and Xanax. Insulin dosage schedule for diabetics may be adjusted during Reglan therapy.

 Do not drink alcohol during Reglan therapy.

Special Cautions

 If pregnant or planning to become pregnant, inform your doctor immediately. Appears in breast milk; could affect a nursing infant.

 Seniors are prescribed lower doses.

Not generally prescribed for children.

 Do not take if you have: sensitivity to or allergic reaction to Reglan; pheochromocytoma (nonmalignant tumor causing hypertension); epilepsy; or a medication that may cause side effects such as jerks, tremors, grimaces, other writhing movements.

May cause drowsiness and impair your ability to drive a car or operate machinery. *Do not take part in any activity that requires alertness.*

If you suffer from Parkinson's disease, either avoid Reglan or use very cautiously.

May cause mild to severe depression; inform your doctor if you have a history of depression.

Avoid if you have obstruction, perforation, or hemorrhage of the stomach or small bowel that might be aggravated by increased stomach and small-bowel movement.

Use with caution if you have high blood pressure.

Relafen

Generic name: Nabumetone

Relafen is a nonsteroidal anti-inflammatory (NSAID). It works by blocking the production of prostaglandins, which may trigger pain.

℞ QUICK FACTS

Purpose

 Used to treat the inflammation, swelling, stiffness, and joint pain associated with rheumatoid arthritis and osteoarthritis.

Dosage

 May take with or without food; take exactly as prescribed.

 Usual adult dose: 1,000 milligrams as a single dose. May be increased up to 2,000 milligrams per day, taken once or 2 times per day. Doctor will prescribe lowest effective dose for chronic pain.

 Usual child dose: not generally prescribed for children.

 Missed dose: take as soon as possible, unless almost time for next dose. In that case, do not take missed dose; go back to regular schedule. *Do not double doses.*

Side Effects

 Overdose symptoms: no specific information available. If you suspect an overdose, immediately seek medical attention.

 More common side effects: abdominal pain, constipation, diarrhea, dizziness, fluid retention, gas, headache, indigestion, itching, nausea, rash, ringing in ears.

 Less common side effects: dry mouth; fatigue; inability to fall or stay asleep; increased sweating; inflammation of the mouth; inflammation of the stomach; nervousness; sleepiness; vomiting. Rare side effects:

agitation; anxiety; confusion; dark, tarry, or bloody stools; depression; difficult or labored breathing; difficulty swallowing; fluid retention; general feeling of illness; hives; increase or loss of appetite; large blisters; pins and needles; pneumonia or lung inflammation; sensitivity to light; severe allergic reactions; skin peeling; stomach and intestinal inflammation and/or bleeding; tremors; ulcers; vaginal bleeding; vertigo; vision changes; weakness; weight gain; yellow eyes or skin.

Interactions

 Inform your doctor before combining Relafen with: blood thinners such as coumadin; diuretics such as HydroDIURIL or Lasix; lithium (Lithonate); methotrexate.

 No known food/other substance interactions.

Special Cautions

 If pregnant or planning to become pregnant, inform your doctor immediately. May appear in breast milk; could affect a nursing infant.

 No special precautions apply to seniors.

 Not generally prescribed for children.

 Do not take if sensitive to or allergic to this medication or if you have experienced allergic reactions, asthma attacks, hives, or other allergic reactions with Relafen, aspirin, or other similar medications.

Be aware that ulcers or internal bleeding can occur with or without warning.

Use with caution if you have liver or kidney disease.

May cause fluid retention and swelling; use with caution if you have high blood pressure or congestive heart failure.

Increased sensitivity to light may occur during Relafen therapy.

Restoril

Generic name: Temazepam

Other brand name: Razepam

Restoril is a benzodiazepine sedative/hypnotic. It is thought to work as a depressant to the central nervous system.

℞ QUICK FACTS

Purpose

℞ Used to treat insomnia—difficulty falling asleep, waking up frequently during the night, waking up early in the morning.

Dosage

🄳 Take exactly as prescribed; must not increase dosage unless directed by your doctor.

  Usual adult dose: 15 milligrams at bedtime, may range from 7.5 to 30 milligrams depending on your needs. *Seniors*—7.5 milligrams or lowest effective dose.

Usual child dose: not generally prescribed for children.

 Missed dose: take on an as-needed basis only.

Side Effects

 Overdose symptoms: coma, confusion, diminished reflexes, loss of coordination, low blood pressure, labored or difficult breathing, seizures, sleepiness, slurred speech. If you suspect an overdose, immediately seek medical attention.

 More common side effects: dizziness, drowsiness, fatigue, headache, nausea, nervousness, sluggishness.

 Less common or rare side effects: abdominal discomfort, abnormal sweating, agitation, anxiety, backache, blurred vision, burning eyes, confusion, constant involuntary movement of the eyeball, depression, diarrhea, difficult or labored breathing, dry mouth, exaggerated feeling of well-being, fluttery or throbbing heartbeat, hallucinations, hangover, increased dreaming, lack of coordination, loss of appetite, loss of equilibrium, loss of memory, nightmares, overstimulation, restlessness, tremors, vertigo, vomiting, weakness. Side effects from rapid decrease in or sudden withdrawal from Restoril: abdominal and muscle cramps, convulsions, feeling of discomfort, inability to fall asleep or stay asleep, sweating, tremors, vomiting.

Interactions

 Inform your doctor before combining Restoril with: antidepressants such as Elavil, Nardil, Parnate, and Tofranil; antihistamines such as Benadryl; barbiturates such as phenobarbital and Seconal; major tranquilizers such as Mellaril and Thorazine; narcotic pain relievers such as Percocet and Demerol; oral contraceptives; tranquilizers such as Valium and Xanax.

 Do not take with alcohol during Restoril therapy; the effects of alcohol may be intensified.

Special Cautions

 Do not take if pregnant or planning to become pregnant; use of drug increases number of birth defects. May appear in breast milk; could affect a nursing infant.

 Seniors are prescribed lower doses to avoid oversedation, dizziness, confusion, and lack of muscle coordination.

 Not generally prescribed for children.

 May impair your ability to drive a car or operate machinery. *Do not take part in any activity that requires alertness.*

Tell your doctor *before* starting Restoril if you have a history of depression, kidney or liver problems, or chronic lung disease.

Inform your doctor if you need this medication beyond 7 to 10 days.

Prolonged use may cause a tolerance to Restoril. May also cause physical dependence.

May experience trouble sleeping for 1 or 2 nights after stopping Restoril.

Retin-A

~~~~~~

Generic name: Tretinoin

Other brand names: Retinoic Acid, Vitamin A Acid

Retin-A is an acne preparation. It works by increasing the regenerating skin cells.

℞ QUICK FACTS

Purpose

℞   Used to treat acne.

Dosage

 Take exactly as prescribed. Avoid eyes, mouth, angles of the nose, and mucous membranes.

 Usual adult dose: apply once per day at bedtime, covering affected area lightly. Avoid oversaturating area. Should observe results in 2 to 3 weeks, and 6 weeks before major results. May experience slight stinging or warmth upon application.

 Usual child dose: not generally prescribed for children.

 Missed dose: resume schedule next day.

Side Effects

 Overdose symptoms: redness, peeling, or discomfort. If you suspect an overdose, immediately notify your doctor.

⊕ More common side effects: excessively red, puffy, blistered, or crusted skin.

Less common side effects: darkening or lack of color of the skin.

Interactions

 Inform your doctor before combining Retin-A with: preparations containing sulfur; resorcinol (used in ointments to treat acne); salicylic acid. Doctor may advise "resting" skin before using any of these skin preparations.

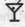 No known food/other substance interactions.

Special Cautions

 If pregnant or planning to become pregnant, inform your doctor immediately. Not known if Retin-A appears in breast milk.

 No special precautions apply to seniors.

 Not generally prescribed for children.

 Use with extreme caution if you have eczema.

Use caution during Retin-A therapy when using: other topical medications; medicated or abrasive soaps and cleaners; drying soaps and cosmetics; products with high amounts of alcohol, astringents, spices, or lime.

Immediately notify your doctor if you experience sensitivity reaction or irritation.

Acne may worsen initially after starting Retin-A therapy, inform your doctor if this occurs.

Keep away from heat and flames; this medication is flammable.

. . . .

Avoid excessive exposure to sunlight and sunlamps when using Retin-A.

Retrovir

ᴧᴧ

Generic name: Zidovudine

Other brand name: AZT

Retrovir is an antiviral. It inhibits the progression of the HIV virus, thus slowing the progression of AIDS.

℞ QUICK FACTS

Purpose

℞ Used to slow the progress of the human immunodeficiency virus (HIV) in adults, which can lead to acquired immune deficiency syndrome (AIDS). Also prescribed to treat HIV positive children over 3 months. Symptoms include: significant weight loss, fever, diarrhea, infections, and nervous system problems.

Dosage

 Take exactly as prescribed. *Do not share Retrovir, and do not increase prescribed dose.*

. . . .

 Usual adult dose: *capsules and syrup—With HIV symptoms, including AIDS—*initially 200 milligrams (two 100-milligram capsules or 4 teaspoons of syrup) taken every 4 hours around the clock. After 1 month doctor may reduce dose to 100 milligrams taken every 4 hours around the clock. *Without HIV symptoms—*100 milligrams taken every 4 hours while awake.

. . . .

Usual child dose: *3 months to 12 years*—individually determined based on weight, not to exceed 200 milligrams every 6 hours. Not prescribed for children under 3 months.

 Missed dose: take as soon as possible, unless almost time for next dose. In that case, do not take missed dose; go back to regular schedule. *Do not double doses.*

Side Effects

 Overdose symptoms: nausea, vomiting. If you suspect an overdose, immediately seek medical attention.

 More common side effects: change in sense of taste, constipation, diarrhea, difficult or labored breathing, dizziness, fever, general feeling of illness, inability to fall or stay asleep, indigestion, loss of appetite, muscle pain, nausea, rash, severe headache, sleepiness, stomach and intestinal pain, sweating, tingling or pins and needles, vomiting, weakness.

 Less common or rare side effects: acne, anxiety, back pain, belching, bleeding from rectum, bleeding gums, body odor, changeable emotions, chest pain, chills, confusion, cough, decreased mental sharpness, depression, difficulty swallowing, dimness of vision, excess sensitivity to pain, fainting, fatigue, flu-like symptoms, frequent urination, gas, hearing loss, hives, hoarseness, increase in urine volume, inflammation of the sinuses or nose, itching, joint pain, light intolerance, mouth sores, muscle spasm, nervousness, nosebleed, painful or difficult urination, sore throat, swelling of the lip, swelling of the tongue, tremor, twitching, vertigo.

Interactions

 Inform your doctor before combining Retrovir with: acetaminophen (Tylenol); amphotericin B (Fungizone); doxorubicin (Adriamycin, a cancer medication); aspirin; dapsone; flucytosine (Ancobon); indomethacin (Indocin); interferon (Intron A or Roferon); pentamidine (NebuPent or Pentam); phenytoin (Dilantin); probenecid (Benemid); vinblastine (Velban); vincristine (Oncovin). Combining Retrovir with phenytoin may cause seizures.

 No known food/other substance interactions.

Special Cautions

 If pregnant or planning to become pregnant, inform your doctor immediately. Has been shown to protect fetus from contracting HIV. May appear in breast milk; could affect a nursing infant.

 No special precautions apply to seniors.

 Follow doctor's instructions carefully for children.

 Inform your doctor *before* taking Retrovir if you have a kidney or liver disorder.

If you have bone marrow disease, use Retrovir with extreme caution.

Retrovir use may lead to blood diseases such as: granulocytopenia (sharp decrease in white blood cells called granulocytes) and anemia severe enough to require blood transfusions.

May develop opportunistic infections—unusual infections that develop when the immune system is compromised. Doctor should do frequent blood counts.

. . . .

Side effects are more frequent and severe in individuals whose infection is more advanced.

. . . .

May be difficult to distinguish side effects from symptoms of HIV or infections caused by HIV.

. . . .

Should not take if you have had a life-threatening reaction to Retrovir. Inform your doctor if you develop any sensitivity reaction such as a rash.

. . . .

Long-term safety and effectiveness are unknown.

. . . .

Retrovir has not been shown to reduce the risk of transmitting HIV through sexual contact or blood contamination.

Rheumatrex

see METHOTREXATE

Ridaura

Generic name: Auranofin

Ridaura, a gold preparation, is an anti-arthritic. It is thought to reduce inflammation by altering the immune system.

℞ QUICK FACTS

Purpose

℞ Used to treat rheumatoid arthritis in individuals who get no relief with use of nonsteroidal anti-inflammatory medications such as Anaprox, Dolobid, Indocin, and Motrin. Most effective in early stages of active joint inflammation.

Dosage

 Take orally, as prescribed by your doctor. Most other gold preparations are injected. Ridaura therapy is usually combined with a non-medication treatment plan. May take 3 to 6 months to see results.

 Usual adult dose: 6 milligrams per day in a single dose or divided into 2 smaller doses. After 6 months—doctor may increase dose to 9 milligrams per day divided into 3 smaller doses.

 Usual child dose: not generally prescribed for children.

 Missed dose: if taking 1 dose per day—take as soon as possible, unless it is the next day. In that case, do not take missed dose; go back to regular schedule. If taking 2 or more doses per day—take as soon as possible, unless almost time for next dose. In that case, do not take missed dose; go back to regular schedule. *Do not double doses.*

Side Effects

 Overdose symptoms: no specific information available. If you suspect an overdose, immediately seek medical attention.

 More common side effects: loose stools or diarrhea in approximately 50% who take Ridaura. Also may cause abdominal pain and gas; blood-cell abnormalities resulting in bleeding; bronchitis; bruising; conjunctivitis (pink eye); fever; gold dermatitis (skin inflammation); indigestion; itching; loss of appetite; metallic taste; nausea; rash; sores in mouth; vomiting.

 Less common or rare side effects: altered sense of taste, anemia, black or bloody stools, blood in urine, constipation, difficulty swallowing, fluid retention and swelling, hair loss, hives, inflammation of tongue or gums, intestinal inflammation with ulcers, stomach or intestinal bleeding, yellowed eyes and skin.

Interactions

 Inform your doctor before combining Ridaura with: penicillamine (Cuprimine), phenytoin (Dilantin).

 No known food/other substance interactions.

Special Cautions

 Ridaura may cause birth defects. If pregnant or planning to become pregnant, inform your doctor immediately. Injected gold appears in breast milk; could affect a nursing infant.

 No special precautions apply to seniors.

 Not generally prescribed for children.

 Do not take if you have had any of the following reactions to taking gold medications: anaphylaxis (life-threatening allergic reaction); blood or bone marrow disorder; fibrosis (scar tissue) in the lungs; serious bowel inflammation; skin peeling.

Immediately inform your doctor if you experience bruising easily; or small, red or purplish skin discolorations appear.

Doctor will monitor you closely during Ridaura therapy if you have: inflammatory bowel disease, kidney or liver disease, skin rash.

Practice good oral hygiene during Ridaura therapy.

Ongoing blood and urine tests will be performed to check for unwanted effects.

Risperdal

Generic name: Risperidone

Risperdal is an antipsychotic. It is thought to work by blocking certain chemicals involved in nerve transmission in the brain.

℞ QUICK FACTS

Purpose

 Used to treat symptoms of severe mental illness, including schizophrenia.

Dosage

 Do not change dosage unless directed by your doctor; may cause unwanted side effects.

 Usual adult dose: 1 milligram taken 2 times per day, increased to 2 milligrams on day 2, and 3 milligrams on day 3. Doctor may increase dosage at weekly intervals. Most people experience maximal effect in the range of 4 to 6 milligrams per day. *For individuals*

with liver or kidney disease—dose is cut in half, with increases by the ½ tablet. *Seniors*—half of usual dose.

 Usual child dose: not generally prescribed for children.

 Missed dose: take as soon as possible, unless almost time for next dose. In that case, do not take missed dose; go back to regular schedule. *Do not double doses.*

Side Effects

 Overdose symptoms: drowsiness, low blood pressure, rapid heartbeat, sedation. If you suspect an overdose, immediately seek medical attention.

 More common side effects: abdominal pain, abnormal walk, agitation, aggression, anxiety, chest pain, constipation, coughing, decreased activity, diarrhea, difficulty with orgasm, diminished sexual desire, dizziness, dry skin, erection and ejaculation problems, excessive menstrual bleeding, fever, headache, inability to sleep, increased dreaming, increased duration of sleep, indigestion, involuntary movements, joint pain, lack of coordination, nasal inflammation, nausea, overactivity, rapid heartbeat, rash, reduced salivation, respiratory infection, sleepiness, sore throat, tremor, underactive reflexes, urination problems, vomiting, weight gain.

 Less common side effects: abnormal vision, back pain, dandruff, difficult or labored breathing, increased saliva, sinus inflammation, toothache.

Interactions

 Inform your doctor before combining Risperdal with: blood pressure medications such as Aldomet,

Procardia, and Vasotec; bromocriptine mesylate (Parlodel); carbamazepine (Tegretol); clozapine (Clozaril); levodopa (Sinemet or Dopar); quinidine (Quinidex). Medications such as Valium, Percocet, Demerol, and Haldol may slow central nervous system and cause other serious side effects. Inform your doctor before taking any other medication.

 Alcohol use during Risperdal therapy may cause drowsiness.

Special Cautions

 If pregnant or planning to become pregnant, inform your doctor immediately. Not known if Risperdal appears in breast milk.

 Seniors are prescribed lower doses. Senior women at a higher risk for developing tardive dyskinesia, a condition with symptoms such as involuntary muscle spasms and facial and body twitches.

 Not generally prescribed for children.

 May cause neuroleptic malignant syndrome (NMS), a potentially fatal disorder with symptoms such as: muscle stiffness, fast heartbeat or irregular pulse, increased sweating, high fever, high or low blood pressure.

May impair your ability to drive a car or operate machinery. *Do not take part in any activity that requires alertness.*

Inform your doctor of any involuntary movement; Risperdal increases risk for tardive dyskinesia, a condition with symptoms such as involuntary muscle spasms and facial and body twitches.

If sensitive to or allergic to this or other major tranquilizers, should not take.

. . . .

Use with caution if you have: kidney, liver, or heart diseases; seizures; breast cancer; thyroid disorders; or any other diseases affecting metabolism; or if you have exposure to intense heat.

. . . .

Symptoms of overdose may be masked, as well as symptoms of intestinal obstruction, brain tumor, and Reye's syndrome.

. . . .

May experience dizziness when standing, rapid heartbeat, or fainting at beginning of Risperdal therapy.

Risperidone
see RISPERDAL

Ritalin

Generic name: Methylphenidate hydrochloride

Other brand name: Ritalin-SR

Ritalin is a central nervous system stimulant. It simultaneously increases mental alertness and decreases fatigue.

℞ QUICK FACTS

Purpose

 Used to treat attention deficit disorder (ADD) in children, with such symptoms as: continual problems with moderate to severe distractibility, short attention span, hyperactivity, emotional changeability, and impulsiveness. Also used to treat narcolepsy in adults.

Dosage

 Take exactly as prescribed. Should take 30 to 45 minutes prior to meals. If Ritalin causes sleep problems, give last dose to child before 6 PM. Never chew or crush tablets; swallow whole. Treatment program should include psychological, educational, and social elements.

 Usual adult dose: *tablets*—20 to 30 milligrams per day taken in 2 or 3 doses. *SR tablets*—work for 8 hours, may be substituted for tablets if dosage is comparable.

 Usual child dose: *tablets*—5 milligrams taken 2 times per day before breakfast and lunch; increased by doctor 5 to 10 milligrams per week, up to 60 milligrams. *SR tablets*—check with doctor to see if they can be substituted for tablets. If no benefits are observed in 1 month, doctor may discontinue Ritalin. Not prescribed for children under 6 years.

 Missed dose: give to child as soon as possible. Give remainder of doses at regularly spaced intervals for the day. *Do not double doses.*

Side Effects

 Overdose symptoms: agitation, confusion, convulsions possibly followed by coma, delirium, drying of mucous membranes, enlarging of pupil of the eye, exaggerated elation, extremely high body temperature, flushing, hallucinations, headache, high blood pressure, irregular or rapid heartbeat, muscle twitching, sweating, tremors, vomiting. If you suspect an overdose, immediately seek medical attention.

 More common side effects: inability to fall or stay asleep; nervousness—doctor's reducing dose usually prevents these side effects. Other more common side effects (in children): loss of appetite, abdominal pain, weight loss with long-term therapy, inability to fall or stay asleep, abnormally fast heartbeat.

 Less common or rare side effects: abdominal pain, abnormal heartbeat, abnormal muscular movements, blood pressure changes, chest pain, dizziness, drowsiness, fever, headache, hives, jerking, joint pain, loss of appetite, nausea, palpitations, pulse changes, rapid heartbeat, reddish or purplish skin spots, skin reddening, skin inflammation with peeling, skin rash, Tourette's syndrome, weight loss during long-term treatment.

Interactions

 Inform your doctor before combining Ritalin with: anticonvulsants such as phenobarbital, Dilantin, and Mysoline; antidepressants such as Tofranil, Anafranil, and Norpramin; blood thinners such as Coumadin; EpiPen; guanethidine (Ismelin); MAO inhibitors such as Nardil and Parnate; phenylbutazone (Butazolidin).

 No known food/other substance interactions.

Special Cautions

 If pregnant or planning to become pregnant, inform your doctor immediately. Not known if Ritalin appears in breast milk.

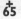 No special precautions apply to seniors.

Not prescribed for children under 6 years. Long-term use may suppress growth.

 Doctor will perform complete history *before* prescribing Ritalin.

May develop addiction or tolerance to this medication; changes to dose should be regulated by your doctor.

Should not take if you have: anxiety; agitation; glaucoma; seizure disorder; tension; tics; or a family history of Tourette's syndrome; or if you are sensitive to or allergic to Ritalin.

Not used to treat stress or psychiatric disorders in children, or normal fatigue or treatment of severe depression.

If you have high blood pressure, should be monitored during Ritalin therapy.

May experience visual disturbances.

Robaxin

Generic name: Methocarbamol

Other brand names: Marbaxin, Robamol

Robaxin is a skeletal muscle relaxant agent. It is thought to work by acting as a central nervous system depressant.

℞ QUICK FACTS

Purpose

℞ Used to treat severe muscular aches, sprains, and strains. May also be prescribed to control the neuromuscular manifestations of tetanus.

Dosage

🍴 Take exactly as prescribed, no more or less than prescribed dose. Should be part of a recovery program that includes physical therapy and rest.

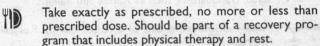 Usual adult dose: *Robaxin*—3 tablets taken 4 times per day. Long-term therapy dose is 2 tablets taken 4 times per day. *Robaxin-750*—2 tablets taken 4 times per day. Long-term therapy dose is 1 tablet taken every 4 hours or 2 tablets taken 3 times per day.

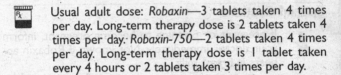 Usual child dose: not generally prescribed for children under 12 years.

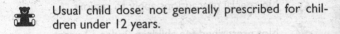 Missed dose: take as soon as possible, unless an hour has passed. In that case, do not take missed dose; go back to regular schedule. *Do not double doses.*

Side Effects

☠ Overdose symptoms: no specific information available. If you suspect an overdose, immediately seek medical attention.

➕ Side effects: blurred vision, conjunctivitis (pink eye), dizziness, drowsiness, fever, headache, hives, itching, light-headedness, nasal congestion, nausea, rash.

No known less common or rare side effects.

Interactions

 Inform your doctor before combining Robaxin with: narcotic pain relievers such as Percocet and Tylenol with Codeine; sleep aids such as Halcion and Seconal; tranquilizers such as Xanax and Valium.

 Use caution/avoid use of alcohol during Robaxin therapy.

Special Cautions

 If pregnant or planning to become pregnant, inform your doctor immediately. Not known if Robaxin appears in breast milk.

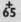 No special precautions apply to seniors.

 Not prescribed for children under 12 years.

 May impair your ability to drive a car or operate machinery. *Do not take part in any activity that requires alertness.*

Is not for use in place of physical therapy or rest.

Use caution not to rush the healing process during Robaxin therapy, as the injury may temporarily feel better.

Should not take if sensitive to or allergic to Robaxin or similar medications.

May experience brown, green, or black urine during Robaxin therapy.

Rocaltrol

~~~~~~

Generic name: Calcitriol

Rocaltrol is a vitamin D synthetic. It replaces the lack of active vitamin D that is produced by the kidneys.

℞ QUICK FACTS

Purpose

℞ Used to treat hypocalcemia (very low blood calcium levels) and bone damage in people on dialysis, and those with hypoparathyroidism (decreased functioning of the parathyroid glands).

Dosage

 Take plenty of fluids to avoid dehydration during Rocaltrol therapy.

. . . .

 Usual adult dose: *for people on dialysis*—0.25 microgram per day, doctor may increase. *For hypoparathyroidism*—0.25 microgram per day, taken in the morning. Doctor may increase dose. Usual range for adults is 0.5 to 2 micrograms per day.

. . . .

 Usual child dose: *for hypoparathyroidism*—0.25 microgram per day, taken in the morning, initially. Doctor may prescribe between 0.25 to 0.75 microgram per day for children 1 to 5 years, and 0.5 to 2 micrograms per day for most children 6 years and older.

. . . .

 Missed dose: *if taking 1 dose every other day and you remember the same day*—take as soon as possible, then go back to regular schedule. *If taking 1 dose every other day and you remember the next day*—take as soon as possible, skip a day, then go back to regular schedule. *If taking 1 dose every day*—take as soon as possible, unless it is the next day. In that case, do not take missed dose; go back to regular schedule. *Do not double doses.*

Side Effects

 Overdose symptoms: coma, confusion, extreme drowsiness. If you suspect an overdose, immediately seek medical attention.

 More common side effects: *initial side effects*—bone pain, constipation, dry mouth, extreme sleepiness, headache, metallic taste, muscle pain, nausea, vomiting, weakness. *Later side effects*—abnormal thirst, decreased sex drive, elevated cholesterol levels, excessive urination, inflamed eyes, irregular heartbeat, itchy skin, kidney problems, light intolerance, loss of appetite, nighttime urination, runny nose, very high body temperature, weight loss, yellowing skin.

 Rare side effects: mental disturbances, red patches on arms and hands with irregular or circular shapes.

Interactions

 Inform your doctor before combining Rocaltrol with: cholestyramine (Questran), digitalis (Lanoxin).

 Check with your doctor before taking antacids such as Maalox (if you are on dialysis), calcium supplements, and vitamin D with Rocaltrol.

Special Cautions

 If pregnant or planning to become pregnant, inform your doctor immediately. May appear in breast milk; could affect a nursing infant.

$\overset{+}{65}$ No special precautions apply to seniors.

Follow doctor's instructions carefully for children.

 Doctor may recommend a special diet or calcium supplements during Rocaltrol therapy. Inform your doctor if you are already taking medications with calcium or a calcium supplement.

Should not use if you have high blood levels of calcium or vitamin D poisoning.

Rogaine, Topical

Generic name: Minoxidil

Rogaine is a hair growth stimulant in its lotion form. It is thought to improve the blood supply to the hair follicles, thus stimulating growth.

℞ QUICK FACTS

Purpose

 Used to treat baldness in men and thinning hair in women.

Dosage

 Use exactly as prescribed. *Do not increase dose; causes side effects and does not speed up hair growth process.* Apply to dry scalp only, and keep on scalp for at least 4 hours. Wash your hands thoroughly after application. For external use only.

 Usual adult dose: 1 milliliter of Rogaine Topical to affected scalp area 2 times per day, not to exceed 2 milliliters per day. May take up to 4 months to observe results. If you have hair growth, continue dosage for additional or continued growth.

Usual child dose: not generally prescribed for children.

 Missed dose: no need to make up dose; go back to regular schedule with next dose. *Do not increase the amount you apply after a missed dose or for any other reason.*

Side Effects

 Overdose symptoms: no specific information available. If you suspect an overdose, immediately seek medical attention.

 Side effects: aches and pains, arthritis symptoms, anxiety, back pain, blood disorders, bone fractures, bronchitis, changes in blood pressure, changes in pulse rate, chest pain, conjunctivitis (pink eye), depression, diarrhea, dizziness, dry skin or flaking scalp, ear infections, eczema, exhaustion, facial swelling, faintness, fluid retention, genital infections and irritation, growth of excess body hair, headache, hives, increased hair loss, itching, light-headedness, menstrual and breast changes, nausea, pounding heartbeat, runny nose, sexual dysfunction, skin redness, sinus inflammation, skin irritation and other allergic reactions, vision changes, vomiting, weight gain.

 No known less common or rare side effects.

Interactions

 No drug interactions reported.

 No known food/other substance interactions.

Special Cautions

 May cause birth defects. If pregnant or planning to become pregnant, inform your doctor immediately.

May appear in breast milk; could affect a nursing infant.

 No special precautions apply to seniors.

 Not generally prescribed for children.

 If sensitive to or allergic to, should not use.

Scalp should be free of infections or other irritations before using Rogaine Topical, as they may increase absorption of Rogaine Topical, thus increasing the risk of side effects.

People with high blood pressure or taking blood pressure medication may be at risk for adverse effects.

Doctor should monitor progress after 1 month and every 6 months thereafter.

Avoid using Rogaine Topical with other topical medications that increase skin absorption or contain petroleum jelly.

Rondec

Generic ingredients: Carbinoxamine maleate with pseudoephedrine hydrochloride

Other brand names: Carbiset Tablets, Carbodec Syrup, Carbodec Tablets

Rondec is an antihistamine and decongestant combination. It works by blocking the effects of histamine, a body chemical that narrows air passages, reducing swelling and itching, and drying secretions.

℞ QUICK FACTS

Purpose

Used to treat nasal inflammation and runny nose, hay fever, and other allergies.

Dosage

Take exactly as prescribed.

Usual adult dose: *tablet or syrup form*—1 tablet or 1 teaspoonful (5 milliliters) taken 4 times per day. *Rondec-TR tablet*—1 tablet taken 2 times per day. *For mild cases or sensitivity*—may be prescribed lower doses.

Usual child dose: *tablet or syrup form*—children 6 years and older use adult dosage. Children 18 months to 6 years—½ teaspoonful (2.5 milliliters) taken 4 times per day. *Rondec-TR tablet*—children 12 years and older use adult dosage, not recommended for children under 12 years. *For mild cases or sensitivity*—may be prescribed lower doses.

Missed dose: take as soon as possible, unless almost time for next dose. In that case, do not take missed dose, go back to regular schedule. *Do not double doses.*

Side Effects

Overdose symptoms: no specific information about Rondec. Overdose symptoms for antihistamine and pseudoephedrine overdose: abdominal cramps, coma, convulsions, diarrhea, difficulty sleeping, difficulty urinating, dizziness, drowsiness, dry mouth, excitement, fever, flushing, fluttery heartbeat, headache, high blood pressure followed by low blood pressure, irregular heartbeat, irritability, loss of appetite, metallic taste, nausea, restlessness, talkativeness, tremor, vomiting. In children—may cause death. Other symptoms: coma, convulsions, excitement, fever, fixed and dilated pupils, flushed face, hallucinations, lack of muscle coordination, tremors. If you suspect an overdose, immediately seek medical attention.

 Side effects: convulsions, diarrhea, difficulty breathing, dizziness, double vision, dry mouth, excitability in children (rare), hallucinations, headache, heartburn, increased blood pressure, increased heart rate, increased production of urine, insomnia, loss of appetite, nausea, nervousness, painful or difficult urination, pallor, sedation, stimulation, tremors, vomiting, weakness.

 No known less common or rare side effects.

Interactions

 Inform your doctor before combining Rondec with: beta-blockers such as Tenormin and Inderal; depression medications such as Elavil and Nardil; high blood pressure medications such as Aldomet, Diupres, and Inversine; MAO inhibitors such as Nardil and Parnate; sedatives such as Halcion and Restoril; tranquilizers such as Xanax and Valium.

 Do not drink alcohol during Rondec therapy.

Special Cautions

 If pregnant or planning to become pregnant, inform your doctor immediately. Not known if Rondec appears in breast milk.

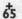 Use with caution if over age 60.

 Follow doctor's instructions carefully for children.

Do not take Rondec if you are taking MAO inhibitors or if sensitive to or allergic to Rondec.

May cause drowsiness and impair your ability to drive a car or operate machinery. Do not take part in any activity that requires alertness.

Avoid Rondec if you have: asthma attack, narrow-angle glaucoma, difficulty urinating, peptic ulcer, severe high blood pressure, coronary artery disease.

Use with caution if you have overactive thyroid, diabetes, or enlarged prostate.

Rowasa

Generic name: Mesalamine

Other brand names: Asacol, Pentasa

Rowasa is an anti-inflammatory. It works specifically to reduce inflammation of the bowel.

℞ QUICK FACTS

Purpose

℞ Used to treat mild to moderate ulcerative colitis (inflammation of the large intestine and rectum). Also used to treat inflammation of the lower colon and rectum.

Dosage

 Take suspension enema, suppositories, capsule, or tablet exactly as prescribed. *Do not crush or chew capsule or tablet; swallow whole.*

Usual adult dose: *suspension enema*—1 rectal enema (60 milliliters) per day at bedtime and retained for 8 hours. Treatment lasts 3 to 6 weeks. *Rowasa suppositories*—1 rectal suppository (500 milligrams) taken 2 times per day. Should retain for 1 to 3 hours or longer. Treatment lasts 3 to 6 weeks. *Pentasa capsules*—4 capsules taken 4 times per day. *Asacol tablets*—2 tablets taken 3 times per day for 6 weeks.

Usual child dose: not generally prescribed for children.

Missed dose: take as soon as possible, unless almost time for next dose. In that case, do not take missed dose; go back to regular schedule. *Do not double doses.*

Side Effects

Overdose symptoms: no serious overdose effects reported for Rowasa. Overdose symptoms of Pentasa or Asacol: confusion, diarrhea, drowsiness, headache, hyperventilation, ringing in ears, sweating, vomiting. If you suspect an overdose, immediately seek medical attention.

More common side effects: *Rowasa suspension enema*—flu-like symptoms, gas, headache, nausea, stomach pain or cramps. *Rowasa suppositories*—diarrhea, dizziness, gas, headache, stomach pain. *Pentasa and Asacol*—diarrhea, headache, nausea.

Less common side effects: *Rowasa suspension enema*—back pain, bloating, diarrhea, dizziness, fever, hemorrhoids, itching, leg or joint pain, pain on insertion of enema tip, rash, rectal pain, sore throat, tiredness, weakness. *Rowasa suppositories*—acne, cold symptoms, fever, inflammation of the colon, nausea, rash, rectal pain, swelling, weakness. Rare side effects: *Pentasa and Asacol*—abdominal pain; abdominal swelling; acne; belching; blood in urine; bloody diarrhea; breast pain; bruising; conjunctivitis (pink eye); constipation; depression; difficulty sleeping; difficulty swallowing; dizziness; dry skin; duodenal ulcer; eczema; fever; fluid retention; general feeling of illness; hair loss; hives; inflammation of pancreas; itching; joint pain; Kawasaki-like syndrome (rash, swollen glands, fever, mouth inflammation, strawberry tongue); lack or loss of appetite; leg cramps; menstrual irregularities; mouth sores and infections; muscle pain; nail problems; palpitations; rash; rectal bleeding; sensitivity to light; skin eruptions; sleepiness; stomach and intestinal bleeding; stool changes; sweating; thirst; tingling or pins and needles; ulcer of the esophagus; uncontrollable bowel movements; urinary frequency; weakness; worsening of ulcerative colitis; vomiting. Rare side effects: *Rowasa suspension*—constipation, hair loss, insomnia, swelling of arms or legs, urinary burning.

Interactions

 Inform your doctor before combining Rowasa with sulfasalazine (Azulfidine).

 No known food/other substance interactions.

Special Cautions

 If pregnant or planning to become pregnant, inform your doctor immediately. Appears in breast milk; could affect a nursing infant.

 No special precautions apply to seniors.

 Not generally prescribed for children.

 Stop taking medicine and contact your doctor immediately if you experience: bloody diarrhea, cramping, fever, rash, severe headache, sudden, severe stomach pain.

. . . .

Should not use if sensitive to or allergic to this medication, salicylates (aspirin), or sulfites. Stop using and contact your doctor if you develop rash or fever. Severe asthma attack due to sulfites in suspension enema may result (rarely) in death.

. . . .

If you have a history of kidney disease or are using other anti-inflammatory medications such as Dipentum, doctor should monitor kidney function.

. . . .

In rare cases, pericarditis (inflammation of membrane surrounding heart) has occurred with Rowasa use.

. . . .

May aggravate colitis.

. . . .

Suspension enema may stain clothes and fabrics.

Roxanol

see MS CONTIN

Ru-Tuss Tablets

Generic ingredients: Phenylephrine hydrochloride with phenylpropanolamine hydrochloride, chlorpheniramine maleate, Hyoscyamine sulfate, atropine sulfate, and scopolamine hydrobromide

Other brand names: Allerest, Condrin-LA, Conex D.A., Contac 12-hour, Dehist, Demazin, Drize, Dura-Vent/A, Genamin, Myminic, Oragest T.D.,

Ornade, Resaid S.R., Rhinolar-Ex 12, Triaminic, Trind, Triphenyl

Ru-Tuss is an antihistamine and decongestant combination. It works by blocking the effects of histamine, a body chemical that narrows air passages, reducing swelling and itching, and drying secretions.

℞ QUICK FACTS

Purpose

 Used to treat runny or stuffy nose, nasal drip, itching, watery eyes, and scratchy or itchy throat caused by allergies, colds, and other irritations of the sinus, nose, and upper respiratory tract.

Dosage

 Take exactly as prescribed. Swallow tablets whole; do not crush or chew.

 Usual adult dose: 1 tablet in the morning and 1 tablet in the evening.

 Usual child dose: not generally prescribed for children under 12 years.

Missed dose: take as soon as possible, unless almost time for next dose. In that case, do not take missed dose; go back to regular schedule. *Do not double doses.*

Side Effects

 Antihistamine overdose may result in convulsions and death in children. Overdose symptoms: coma, delirium, fever, rapid breathing, respiratory failure, stupor. If you suspect an overdose, immediately seek medical attention.

Side effects: allergic reactions (rash or hives), blood disorders, blurred vision, constipation, diarrhea, dilated pupils, dizziness, drowsiness, dry mouth, dry nose and other mucous membranes, exhaustion, faintness, frequent urination, giddiness, increased chest congestion, insomnia, itching, lack of coordination, loss of appetite, low blood pressure or high blood pressure, nausea, nervousness, painful or difficult urination, pounding heartbeat, rapid heartbeat, ringing in the ears, stomach upset, tightness in the chest, vision changes, vomiting.

 No known less common or rare side effects.

Interactions

 Do not take Ru-Tuss while taking antidepressants such as Nardil and Parnate. Inform your doctor before combining Ru-Tuss Tablets with sleep medications such as Halcion and Dalmane, or tranquilizers such as Xanax and Valium.

 Do not drink alcohol when taking Ru-Tuss.

Special Cautions

 If pregnant or planning to become pregnant, inform your doctor immediately; pregnant women should not use.

 No special precautions apply to seniors.

 Not generally prescribed for children under 12 years.

 May cause drowsiness and impair your ability to drive a car or operate machinery. *Do not take part in any activity that requires alertness.*

. . . . . .

Avoid if you are sensitive to or allergic to antihistamines or the ingredients in Ru-Tuss, or if you have glaucoma or bronchial asthma.

. . . . . .

Use with caution if you have bladder obstruction, high blood pressure, cardiovascular disease, or an overactive thyroid.

Rynatan

Generic ingredients: Phenylephrine tannate with chlorpheniramine tannate and pyrilamine tannate

Other brand names: Decotan Tablets, R-Tannamine, R-Tannate, Tanoral, Triotann, Tri-Tannate

Rynatan is an antihistamine and decongestant combination. It works by blocking the effects of histamine, a body chemical that narrows air passages, thus reducing swelling and itching and drying secretions.

℞ QUICK FACTS

Purpose

℞ Used to treat runny nose and nasal congestion caused by the common cold, inflamed sinuses, hay fever, and other respiratory conditions.

Dosage

 Take exactly as prescribed.

. . . . . .

 Usual adult dose: 1 or 2 tablets every 12 hours.

. . . . . .

 Usual child dose: *pediatric suspension for ages 6 and over*—1 to 2 teaspoonfuls (5 to 10 milliliters) every

12 hours; *for ages 2 to 5*—½ to 1 teaspoonful (2.5 to 5 milliliters) every 12 hours; *for children under 2 years*—doctor will determine dosage.

 Missed dose: take as soon as possible, unless almost time for next dose. In that case, do not take missed dose; go back to regular schedule. *Do not double doses.*

Side Effects

 Antihistamine overdose may result in convulsions and death in children. Overdose symptoms: slowing of central nervous system, depression, and overstimulation (restlessness to convulsions). If you suspect an overdose, immediately seek medical attention.

 Side effects: drowsiness; dry nose, mouth, and throat; extreme calm; stomach and intestinal problems.

 No known less common or rare side effects.

Interactions

 Inform your doctor before combining Rynatan with: MAO inhibitors such as Nardil; sedatives such as Halcion and Dalmane; tranquilizers such as Xanax and Valium.

 Do not drink alcohol when taking Rynatan.

Special Cautions

 If pregnant or planning to become pregnant, inform your doctor immediately. Should not take if breastfeeding.

 No special precautions apply to seniors.

Follow doctor's instructions carefully for children. Not to be given to newborns.

 May cause drowsiness and impair your ability to drive a car or operate machinery. *Do not take part in any activity that requires alertness.*

Avoid use if sensitive to or allergic to Rynatan or other antihistamines and decongestants.

Use with caution if you have: high blood pressure, heart disease, circulatory problems, overactive thyroid gland, narrow-angle glaucoma, or enlarged prostate gland.

Rythmol

Generic name: Propafenone

Rythmol is an anti-arrhythmic. It alters nerve impulses within the heart to regulate heartbeat.

℞ QUICK FACTS

Purpose

 Used to correct heartbeat irregularities, including ventricular arrhythmias.

Dosage

 May take with or without food. Take exactly as prescribed, maintaining a constant level in the blood.

 Usual adult dose: 150 milligrams every 8 hours, up to 900 milligrams per day maximum. Treatment usually begins in the hospital.

Usual child dose: not generally prescribed for children.

 Missed dose: take as soon as possible, unless almost time for next dose or more than 4 hours past missed dose. Otherwise, do not take missed dose; go back to regular schedule. *Do not double doses.*

Side Effects

 Overdose symptoms: convulsions (rarely), heartbeat irregularities, sleepiness. Symptoms are worse in the first 3 hours of taking medication. If you suspect an overdose, immediately seek medical attention.

 More common side effects: constipation, dizziness, heartbeat abnormalities, nausea, unusual taste in the mouth, vomiting.

 Other side effects: abdominal pain or cramps; anemia; angina (crushing chest pain); anxiety; blood disorders; blurred vision; breathing difficulties; bruising; cardiac arrest; coma; confusion; congestive heart failure; depression; diarrhea; dreaming abnormalities; drowsiness; dry mouth; eye irritation; fainting or near fainting; fatigue; fever; flushing; gas; hair loss; headache; heart palpitations; heartbeat abnormalities (rapid, irregular, slow); hot flashes; impotence; increased blood sugar; indigestion; inflamed esophagus, stomach, or intestines; insomnia; itching; joint pain; kidney disease; kidney failure; lack of coordination; liver dysfunction; loss of appetite; loss of balance; low blood pressure; memory loss; muscle cramps; muscle weakness; numbness; pain; psychosis; rash; red or purple skin spots; ringing in the ears; seizures; speech abnormalities; sweating; swelling due to fluid retention; tingling or pins and needles; tremor; unusual smell sensations; vertigo; vision abnormalities; weakness.

Interactions

 Inform your doctor before combining Rythmol with: beta-blockers such as Inderal and Lopressor; cimetidine (Tagamet); digitalis (Lanoxin); local anesthetics such as Novocaine; quinidine (Cardioquin); warfarin (Coumadin).

 No known food/other substance interactions.

Special Cautions

 May cause birth defects. If pregnant or planning to become pregnant, inform your doctor immediately. Should not take if breastfeeding.

 No special precautions apply to seniors.

 Not generally prescribed for children.

 Do not take if sensitive to or allergic to Rythmol.

Doctor will not prescribe Rythmol if you have: abnormally slow heartbeat; certain heartbeat irregularities such as atrioventricular block or "sick sinus" syndrome not corrected by a pacemaker; cardiogenic shock; chronic bronchitis or emphysema; congestive heart failure; mineral (electrolyte) imbalance; severe low blood pressure.

If you have a pacemaker, doctor must monitor settings or reprogram during Rythmol therapy.

May interfere with blood cell manufacturing. Immediately contact your doctor if you experience fever, chills, or sore throat, especially during first 3 months of therapy.

· · · · · · · · · · · · · · · · · · · ·
May cause or worsen heartbeat irregularities. Doctor should perform electrocardiogram (EKG) before and during treatment.
· · · · · · · · · · · · · · · · · · · ·
At risk for a lupus-like illness with symptoms such as rashes and arthritic symptoms. Doctor may stop Rythmol if your blood contains ANA (antinuclear antibodies).

Sandimmune

Generic name: Cyclosporine

Sandimmune is an immunosuppressant. It prevents the body from rejecting foreign material.

℞ QUICK FACTS

Purpose

℞ Used after organ transplant surgery to prevent rejection of transplanted organ by suppressing the body's immune system. Also used to treat organ rejection in people treated with Imuran, another immunosuppressant. Also prescribed to treat alopecia areata (localized hair loss), aplastic anemia (red and white blood cell deficiency), Crohn's disease (chronic inflammation of the digestive tract), nephropathy (kidney disease), psoriasis, and dermatomyositis (inflammation of skin and muscles, causing weakness and rash). Used also for bone marrow, pancreas, and lung procedures.

Dosage

 Sandimmune is always prescribed with prednisone or another steroid. Take exactly as prescribed, at the same time each day. May take with or without food, but be consistent. May mix liquid form with room-temperature milk, chocolate milk, or orange juice, but use the same liquid each day. Use glass container, not plastic for mixing liquid, and drink as soon as you prepare it. Rinse glass with more liquid and drink to get full dose. Maintain good oral hygiene during Sandimmune therapy. *Do not rinse or wash pipette used to transfer Sandimmune liquid unless absolutely necessary. In that case, dry thoroughly before using again.*

 Usual adult dose: dose is determined to suit individual needs. 15 milligrams every 4 to 12 hours before the transplant and for 1 to 2 weeks after the transplant is the usual dose range. May be prescribed a maintenance dose of 5 to 10 milligrams per 2.2 pounds of body weight.

 Usual child dose: determined to suit child's needs on an individualized basis.

 Missed dose: take as soon as possible if less than 12 hours have passed. Otherwise, do not take missed dose; go back to regular schedule. *Do not double doses.*

Side Effects

 Overdose symptoms: no specific information available; however, liver and kidney problems may result from overdose. If you suspect an overdose, immediately seek medical attention.

 Most common side effects: excessive growth of gums, high blood pressure, hirsutism (excessive hairiness), kidney damage, tremor. Other common side effects: abdominal discomfort, acne, anemia, blood clots, breast development in males, convulsions, cramps, diarrhea, flushing, headache, liver damage, nausea and vomiting, numbness or tingling, sinus inflammation.

 Less common side effects: allergic reactions, anemia, appetite loss, brittle fingernails, confusion, fever, fluid retention, hearing loss, hiccups, high blood sugar, inflamed eyes, muscle pain, peptic ulcer, ringing in the ears, stomach inflammation. Rare side effects: anxiety, blood in the urine, chest pain, constipation, depression, hair breaking, heart attack, itching, joint pain, mouth sores, night sweats, sluggishness, stomach and upper intestinal bleeding, swallowing difficulty, visual disturbance, weakness, weight loss.

Interactions

Do not use oral contraceptives with Sandimmune unless directed by your doctor. Avoid vaccines during Sandimmune therapy. Inform your doctor before combining Sandimmune with: amphotericin B (Fungizone I.V.), bromocriptine (Parlodel), calcium blockers such as Calan and Cardizem, carbamazepine (Tegretol), cimetidine (Tagamet), danazol (Danocrine), diclofenac (Voltaren), digoxin (Lanoxin or Lanoxicaps), erythromycin (E.E.S. or Erythrocin), fluconazole (Diflucan), gentamicin (Garamycin), itraconazole (Sporanox), ketoconazole (Nizoral), lovastatin (Mevacor), melphalan (Alkeran), methylprednisolone (Medrol or Solu-Medrol), metoclopramide (Reglan), phenobarbital, phenytoin (Dilantin), potassium-sparing diuretics such as Midamor and Aldactone, prednisolone (Hydeltra), ranitidine (Zantac), rifampin (Rifadin or Rimactane), tobramycin (Nebcin), trimethoprim with sulfamethoxazole (Bactrim or Septra), vancomycin (Vancocin).

No known food/other substance interactions.

Special Cautions

If pregnant or planning to become pregnant, inform your doctor immediately. Appears in breast milk; could affect a nursing infant.

No special precautions apply to seniors.

Follow doctor's instructions carefully for children.

Doctor will monitor levels of Sandimmune to prevent toxicity due to overdosing or organ rejection due to underdosing.

Oral Sandimmune therapy may last indefinitely after surgery.

At increased risk for infection and malignancies, including skin cancer and lymph system cancer.

High doses of Sandimmune may result in liver and kidney damage. Doctor may allow your body to reject a transplanted organ rather than give high doses of Sandimmune.

Risk of convulsions is increased if taking large doses of Methylprednisolone (Medrol or Solu-Medrol).

Sectral

Generic name: Acebutolol hydrochloride

Sectral is a beta-adrenergic blocking agent (beta-blocker). Beta-blockers decrease the workload of the heart and help regulate the heartbeat.

℞ QUICK FACTS

Purpose

 Used to treat high blood pressure, angina (crushing chest pain), and abnormal heart rhythms.

Dosage

 Take with or without food as directed by your doctor. Take exactly as prescribed, even if symptoms disappear. Must be taken regularly for Sectral to be effective.

 Usual adult dose: *for hypertension*—400 milligrams per day in a single dose or 2 doses of 200 milligrams each in the case of mild to moderate hypertension. Maximum daily dose is 800 milligrams. *For severe hypertension*—may be prescribed up to 1,200 milligrams per day divided into 2 doses. *For irregular heartbeat*—400 milligrams per day divided into 2 doses, initially. Doctor may increase to 600 to 1,200 milligrams per day. *Seniors*—dose based on individual needs; not prescribed more than 800 milligrams per day.

 Usual child dose: not generally prescribed for children.

 Missed dose: take dose *unless within 4 hours of next dose. Otherwise, do not take the missed dose; go back to your regular schedule. Do not double doses.*

Side Effects

 Overdose symptoms: changes in heartbeat (unusually slow, unusually fast, or irregular), severe dizziness or fainting; difficulty breathing; bluish-colored fingernails or palms; seizures. If you suspect an overdose, immediately seek medical attention.

 More common side effects: abnormal vision, chest pain, constipation, cough, decreased sexual ability, depression, diarrhea, dizziness, fatigue, frequent urination, gas, headache, indigestion, joint pain, nasal inflammation, nausea, shortness of breath or difficulty breathing, strange dreams, swelling due to fluid retention, trouble sleeping, weakness.

 Less common side effects: abdominal pain, anxiety, back pain, burning eyes, cold hands and feet, conjunctivitis, dark urine, excessive urination at night, eye pain, fever, heart failure, impotence, low blood pressure, muscle pain, nervousness, painful or difficult urination, rash, slow heartbeat, throat inflammation, vomiting, wheezing.

Interactions

 Inform your doctor before combining Sectral with: albuterol (the airway-opening drug Ventolin); certain blood pressure medicines such as reserpine (Diupres); certain over-the-counter remedies and nasal drops such as Afrin, Neo-Synephrine, and Sudafed; nonsteroidal anti-inflammatory drugs such as Motrin and Voltaren; oral diabetes drugs such as Micronase.

 No known food/other substance interactions.

Special Cautions

 If pregnant or plan to become pregnant, inform your doctor immediately. Appears in breast milk; could affect a nursing infant.

 Dosage level may be adjusted to meet particular needs.

 Not generally prescribed for children.

 If you experience difficulty breathing, or develop hives or large areas of swelling, immediately seek medical attention. You may be having a serious allergic reaction.

Use caution if you have had congestive heart failure, very slow heart rate, or heart block.

Sectral should not be stopped suddenly, can cause increased chest pain and heart attack.

People with asthma, seasonal allergies, other bronchial conditions, coronary artery disease, or kidney or liver disease should use caution.

If you are diabetic, immediately inform your doctor. Sectral may cover the symptoms of low blood sugar or alter blood sugar levels.

Notify your doctor or dentist in a medical emergency or before surgery.

Seldane

Generic name: Terfenadine

Other brand name: Seldane-D

Seldane is an antihistamine. Antihistamines block the effects of histamine, a body chemical that causes swelling and itching.

℞ QUICK FACTS

Purpose

℞ Used to treat sneezing, runny nose, stuffiness, itching, and tearing eyes from hay fever.

Dosage

  Take only when needed. Swallow tablets whole, not to be crushed or chewed. *Do not increase dose unless under the direction of your doctor.*

Usual adult dose: *Seldane*—1 tablet (60 milligrams) taken 2 times per day. *Seldane-D*—1 tablet taken 2 times per day.

 Usual child dose: not generally prescribed for children under 12 years.

 Missed dose: *if taking Seldane regularly*—take as soon as possible, unless almost time for next dose. In that case, do not take missed dose; go back to regular schedule. *Do not double doses.*

Side Effects

 Overdose symptoms: changes in heartbeat, confusion, fainting, headache, irregular heartbeat, nausea, seizures. If you suspect an overdose, immediately seek medical attention.

 More common side effects: *Seldane*—drowsiness, fatigue, headache, stomach and intestinal problems. *Seldane-D*—drowsiness; dry mouth, nose, and throat; headache; insomnia; loss of appetite; nausea; nervousness.

 Less common or rare side effects: *Seldane*—confusion, cough, depression, dizziness, dry mouth, dry nose, dry throat, excessive or spontaneous milk flow, fainting, frequent urination, hair thinning or loss, hepatitis, hives, increased appetite, irregular heartbeat, insomnia, itching, low blood pressure, menstrual disorders and pain, nightmares, nosebleeds, palpitations, rapid heartbeat, seizures, sensitivity to light, severe allergic reaction, sore throat, sweating, tingling or pins and needles, tremor, vision changes, weakness, wheezing. *Seldane-D*—blurred vision, change in bowel habits, change in taste, confusion, cough, depression, disorientation, dizziness, excessive or spontaneous flow of milk, fatigue, flareup of psoriasis, frequent urination, hair loss, hepatitis, hives, increased appetite, increased energy, increased physical activity, irregular heartbeat, irritability, itching, menstrual disorders, muscle twitches, nightmares, nosebleeds, palpitations, rapid heartbeat, rash, restlessness, seizures, sensitivity to light, severe allergic reaction, sore throat, stomach and intestinal upset, sweating, tingling or pins and needles, tremors, upper respiratory infection, vision problems, vomiting, weakness, wheezing.

Interactions

 Do not take Seldane with: clarithromycin (Biaxin), erythromycin (PCE or E-Mycin), itraconazole (Sporanox), ketoconazole (Nizoral), troleandomycin (Tao Capsules). Inform your doctor before combining Seldane with: amiodarone (Cordarone), astemizole (Hismanal), bepridil (Vascor), disopyramide (Norpace), probucol (Lorelco), procainamide (Pronestyl or Procan), quinidine (Quinaglute or Quinidex). Seldane-D may interact with: MAO inhibitors (Nardil or Parnate), mecamylamine (Inversine), methyldopa, reserpine (Diupres).

 No known food/other substance interactions.

Special Cautions

 If pregnant or plan to become pregnant, inform your doctor immediately. *Do not take if breastfeeding.*

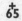 No special precautions apply to seniors.

 Not generally prescribed for children.

 Do not take if sensitive to or allergic to this medication, or if you have liver disease.

Avoid Seldane if you have severe high blood pressure or heart disease.

Causes much less drowsiness than other antihistamines.

Use with caution if you have diabetes, glaucoma, or enlarged prostate.

Seldane-D
see SELDANE

Selegiline Hydrochloride
see ELDEPRYL

Septra

Generic ingredients: Trimethoprim with sulfamethoxazole

Other brand names: Bactrim, Bactrim DS, Bactrim Pediatric, Cotrim, Cotrim DS, Cotrim Pediatric, Co-Trimoxazole, Septra DS, SMZ-TMP, Sulfatrim DS, Uroplus, Uroplus DS

Septra is a sulfa antibiotic. It prevents the proliferation of nutrients needed to grow infecting bacteria.

℞ QUICK FACTS

Purpose

℞ Used to treat urinary tract infections; severe middle ear infections in children; chronic bronchitis in adults that has developed into a serious condition; intestinal inflammation from severe bacterial infection; pneumonia in patients with suppressed immune system (pneumocystis carinii pneumonia); and for traveler's diarrhea.

Dosage

 Drink plenty of fluids during Septra therapy to avoid sediment in urine and stone formation. Take exactly as prescribed; works best to keep a constant amount in the system. Should take doses at evenly spaced intervals. Use measuring spoon dispensed by pharmacy if taking suspension form.

 Usual adult dose: *for urinary tract infections and intestinal inflammation*—1 Septra DS tablet or 2 Septra tablets, or 4 teaspoonfuls (20 milliliters) of pediatric suspension every 12 hours for 10 to 14 days. Intestinal inflammation therapy is 5 days. *For worsening chronic bronchitis*—1 Septra DS tablet or 2 Septra tablets, or 4 teaspoonfuls (20 milliliters) of pediatric suspension every 12 hours for 14 days. *For pneumocystis carinii pneumonia*—20 milligrams of trimethoprim and 100 milligrams of sulfamethoxazole per 2.2 pounds of body weight per 24 hour period, divided into equal doses taken every 6 hours. Therapy lasts 14 days. *For traveler's diarrhea*—1 Septra DS tablet, or 2 Septra tablets, or 4 teaspoonfuls (20 milliliters) of pediatric suspension every 12 hours for 5 days. *Seniors*—consult with doctor before starting Septra, especially if you have impaired kidney or liver function or are taking other medications.

Usual child dose: *for urinary tract or middle ear infections*—Children 22 pounds—1 teaspoonful (5 milliliters); children 44 pounds—2 teaspoonfuls (10 milliliters) or 1 tablet; children 66 pounds—3 teaspoonfuls (15 milliliters) or 1½ tablets; children 88 pounds—4 teaspoonfuls (20 milliliters) or 2 tablets or 1 DS tablet. Dosage is for children 2 months and older, given every 12 hours for 10 days. *For intestinal inflammation*—same as for urinary tract and middle ear infections, but taken for 5 days. *For pneumocystis carinii pneumonia*—Children 18 pounds—1 teaspoonful (5 milliliters); children 35 pounds—2 teaspoonfuls (10 milliliters) or 1 tablet; children 53 pounds—3 teaspoonfuls (15 milliliters) or 1½ tablets; children 70 pounds—4 teaspoonfuls (20 milliliters) or 2 tablets or 1 DS tablet.

 Missed dose: take as soon as possible, unless almost time for next dose. In that case, do not take missed dose; go back to regular schedule. *Do not double doses.*

Side Effects

 Overdose symptoms: blood or sediment in the urine, colic, confusion, dizziness, drowsiness, fever, headache, lack or loss of appetite, mental depression, nausea, unconsciousness, vomiting, yellowed eyes and skin. If you suspect an overdose, immediately seek medical attention.

 More common side effects: hives, lack or loss of appetite, nausea, skin rash, vomiting.

 Less common or rare side effects: abdominal pain, allergic reactions, anemia, chills, convulsions, depression, diarrhea, eye irritation, fatigue, fever, hallucinations, headache, hepatitis, inability to fall or stay asleep, inability to urinate, increased urination, inflammation of heart muscle, inflammation of mouth and/or tongue, itching, joint pain, kidney failure, lack of feeling or concern, lack of muscle coordination, loss of appetite, low blood sugar, meningitis (inflammation of brain or spinal cord), muscle ache, nausea, nervousness, red or raised rash, redness and swelling of the tongue, ringing in the ears, scaling of dead skin due to inflammation, sensitivity to light, severe skin welts or swelling, skin eruptions, skin peeling, vertigo, weakness, yellowing of eyes and skin.

Interactions

 Inform your doctor before combining Septra with: amantadine (Symmetrel), blood thinners such as Coumadin, diuretics (in seniors) such as HydroDIURIL, methotrexate (Rheumatrex), oral diabetes medications such as Micronase.

 No known food/other substance interactions.

Special Cautions

 If pregnant or plan to become pregnant, inform your doctor immediately. Appears in breast milk; could affect a nursing infant.

 Seniors should consult with doctor before starting Septra, especially if you have impaired kidney or liver function or are taking other medications.

 Follow doctor's instructions carefully for children.

 Do not take if you have megaloblastic anemia, a blood disorder from a lack of folic acid, unless directed by your doctor.

Rare and sometimes fatal reactions have occurred when taking Septra. Immediately contact your doctor if you experience: skin rash, sore throat, fever, joint pain, cough, shortness of breath, abnormal skin paleness, reddish or purplish skin spots, or yellowing of skin or eyes.

· · · · · · · · · · · · · · · · · ·

At risk for Stevens-Johnson syndrome (severe eruptions around mouth, anus, or eyes); progressive disintegration of outer skin layer; sudden and severe liver damage; severe blood disorder (agranulocytosis); lack of red and white blood cells due to bone marrow disorder.

· · · · · · · · · · · · · · · · · ·

Doctor should perform blood counts frequently.

· · · · · · · · · · · · · · · · · ·

Avoid if sensitive to or allergic to Septra or other sulfa medications.

· · · · · · · · · · · · · · · · · ·

Not for use to prevent middle ear infections, or for prolonged use with this infection. Also not for use with streptococcal pharyngitis (inflammation of the pharynx due to streptococcus bacteria).

· · · · · · · · · · · · · · · · · ·

Inform your doctor if you have folic acid deficiency; are a chronic alcoholic; are taking anticonvulsants; have been diagnosed as having malabsorption syndrome, poor nutritional state, severe allergies, or bronchial asthma.

· · · · · · · · · · · · · · · · · ·

At risk for more side effects if you have acquired immune deficiency syndrome (AIDS).

Ser-Ap-Es

∿∿∿∿∿∿∿∿∿∿∿∿∿∿∿∿∿∿∿∿∿∿∿∿∿∿∿∿∿∿∿∿∿∿∿

Generic ingredients: Serpasil (reserpine) with Apresoline (hydralazine hydrochloride) and Esidrix (hydrochlorothiazide)

Ser-Ap-Es is an antihypertensive. It improves blood flow throughout the body and helps the body eliminate urine, which lowers blood pressure.

℞ QUICK FACTS

Purpose

℞   Used to treat high blood pressure. It combines the blood pressure medications Serpasil and Apresoline with Esidrix, a thiazide diuretic.

Dosage

Take exactly as prescribed, even if symptoms disappear. Must keep to schedule, missing doses may worsen high blood pressure. May take several weeks to see effects of medication.

Usual adult dose: no more than 0.25 milligram per day (2½ tablets). Dosage is determined on individual needs.

Usual child dose: not generally prescribed for children.

Missed dose: take as soon as possible, unless almost time for next dose. In that case, do not take missed dose; go back to regular schedule. *Do not double doses.*

Side Effects

Overdose symptoms: coma, confusion, constricted pupils, calf muscle cramps, decreased amounts of urine, diarrhea, dizziness, drowsiness, fatigue, flushing, headache, heart attack, inability to urinate, increased amounts of urine, increased salivation, irregular heartbeat, low blood pressure, low body temperature, nausea, rapid heartbeat, severe fluid loss, shock, slow heartbeat, slowed breathing, thirst, tingling or pins and needles, vomiting, weakness. If you suspect an overdose, immediately seek medical attention.

Side effects: angina (crushing chest pain); anemia; anxiety; blockage in intestines; blood disorders; blurred vision; breast development in males; breast engorgement; change in potassium levels; chills; conjunctivitis (pink eye); constipation; cramping (stomach and intestinal); deafness; decreased sex drive; depression; diarrhea; difficult or labored breathing; difficult or painful urination; disorientation; dizziness; dizziness when standing up; drowsiness; dry mouth; enlarged spleen; eye disorders; fainting; fever; fluid in the lungs; fluid retention; flushing; glaucoma; headache; hepatitis; high blood sugar; hives; impotence; inflammation of lungs; inflammation of pancreas; inflammation of salivary glands; irregular heartbeat; irritation of stomach; itching; joint pain; loss of appetite; low blood pressure; muscle aches; muscle cramps; muscle spasm; nasal congestion; nausea; nervousness; nightmares; nosebleeds; numbness; parkinsonism syndrome (tremors, muscle weakness, shuffling walk, stooped posture, drooling); pounding heartbeat; rapid heartbeat; rash; red or purple skin discoloration; respiratory distress; restlessness; skin peeling; skin sensitivity to light; slow heartbeat; sugar in the urine; teary eyes; tingling or pins and needles; tremors; vertigo; vision changes; vomiting; weakness; weight gain; yellow eyes and skin.

No known less common or rare side effects.

Interactions

Inform your doctor before combining Ser-Ap-Es with: ACTH (adrenal hormone); amphetamines such as Dexedrine; antidepressant MAO inhibitors such as Nardil and Parnate; central nervous system medications such as Cylert and Desoxyn; digitalis (Lanoxin); elavil; insulin; lithium (Eskalith); nonsteroidal anti-inflammatory medications such as Motrin; norepinephrine (Levophed); other high blood pressure medications such as Aldomet and Vasotec; quinidine (Quinidex); steroids such as Deltasone; sympathetic nervous system stimulants such as epinephrine, ephedrine, isoproterenol, metaraminol, tyramine, and phenylephrine.

 No known food/other substance interactions.

Special Cautions

 If pregnant or plan to become pregnant, inform your doctor immediately. Appears in breast milk; could affect a nursing infant.

 No special precautions apply to seniors.

 Not generally prescribed for children.

 Do not take if sensitive to or allergic to this medication or sulfa medications. If you have a history of allergies or bronchial asthma, at higher risk for allergic reaction.

Avoid Ser-Ap-Es if being treated for depression.

Should not take if you have: an active peptic ulcer; ulcerative colitis (chronic inflammation of the large intestine and rectum); coronary artery disease; rheumatic heart disease; or if unable to urinate or are receiving electroshock therapy.

Notify your doctor or dentist prior to a medical emergency or surgery that you are taking Ser-Ap-Es.

Doctor may prescribe a potassium supplement or advise you to eat foods high in potassium (bananas and orange juice), as diuretics may cause your body to lose potassium.

. . . .

May cause depression that can last several months after Ser-Ap-Es therapy. Immediately contact your doctor if you experience: despondency, waking early in the morning, loss of appetite, impotence, loss of self-esteem.

. . . .

Use cautiously if you have gallstones.

. . . .

May activate or aggravate symptoms of lupus erythematosus.

. . . .

Doctor will monitor you if you have coronary artery, kidney, or liver disease.

. . . .

May mask symptoms of low blood sugar or alter blood sugar levels. Inform your doctor if you are diabetic.

. . . .

On rare occasion abnormal amounts of uric acid in the blood may occur, leading to an attack of gout.

Serax

Generic name: Oxazepam

Serax is a benzodiazepine tranquilizer. It reduces the activity of certain chemicals in the brain.

℞ QUICK FACTS

Purpose

℞ Used to treat anxiety disorders. Very effective for anxiety, tension, agitation, and irritability in seniors. Also used to treat acute alcohol withdrawal.

. . . .

Dosage

 Take exactly as prescribed.

 Usual adult dose: *for mild to moderate anxiety with tension, irritability, agitation*—10 to 15 milligrams taken 3 or 4 times per day. *For severe anxiety, depression with anxiety, alcohol withdrawal*—15 to 30 milligrams taken 3 or 4 times per day. *Seniors*—10 milligrams taken 3 times per day. Doctor may increase up to 15 milligrams taken 3 or 4 times per day.

 Usual child dose: doctor will determine dosage on an individual basis for children 6 to 12 years. Not prescribed for children under 6 years.

 Missed dose: take as soon as possible, if within an hour of scheduled time. Otherwise, do not take missed dose; go back to regular schedule. *Do not double doses.*

Side Effects

 Overdose symptoms: no specific information available. If you suspect an overdose, immediately seek medical attention.

 Most common side effect: drowsiness.

 Less common or rare side effects: blood disorders, change in sex drive, dizziness, excitement, fainting, headache, hives, liver problems, loss or lack of muscle control, nausea, skin rashes, sluggishness or unresponsiveness, slurred speech, swelling due to fluid retention, tremors, vertigo, yellowed eyes and skin. Side effects due to sudden withdrawal from Serax: abdominal and muscle cramps, convulsions, depressed mood, inability to fall or stay asleep, sweating, tremors, vomiting.

Interactions

 Inform your doctor before combining Serax with: antihistamines such as Benadryl, narcotic painkillers such as Percocet and Demerol, sedatives such as Seconal and Halcion, tranquilizers such as Valium and Xanax.

 Avoid alcohol during Serax therapy. Serax intensifies the effects of alcohol.

Special Cautions

 Do not take if pregnant or planning to become pregnant. Serax increases the risk of birth defects. May appear in breast milk; could affect a nursing infant.

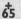 Seniors are generally prescribed lower doses.

 Follow doctor's instructions carefully for children 6 to 12 years. Not generally prescribed for children under 6 years.

 May cause drowsiness and impair your ability to drive a car or operate machinery. *Do not take part in any activity that requires alertness.*

Inform your doctor *before* starting Serax if you have any heart problems; may cause drop in blood pressure.

Before taking Serax, inform your doctor of any aspirin allergies or other allergies. May be at increased risk for allergic reaction to coloring agent used in 15-milligram tablet.

May be addictive and lose effectiveness over the long term. May also develop a tolerance to Serax. Doctor will gradually reduce dose at the end of therapy to avoid withdrawal symptoms.

Avoid if sensitive to or allergic to Serax or other tranquilizers such as Valium.

Not used to treat everyday tension or anxiety.

Should not use if you are under treatment for mental disorders more serious than anxiety.

Serpasil with Apresoline and Esidrix

see SER-AP-ES

Sertan

see MYSOLINE

Sertraline

see ZOLOFT

Silvadene Cream 1%

Generic name: Silver sulfadiazine

Other brand names: SSD AF, SSD Cream, Thermazene

Silvadene Cream 1% is a topical antibacterial. It inhibits the growth of bacteria by affecting the biochemicals or nutrients necessary for bacteria to sustain life.

℞ QUICK FACTS

Purpose

℞ Used to treat and prevent infections in people with 2nd and 3rd degree burns. Also used to treat several bacteria, including yeast.

Dosage

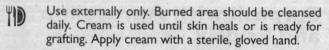 Use externally only. Burned area should be cleansed daily. Cream is used until skin heals or is ready for grafting. Apply cream with a sterile, gloved hand.

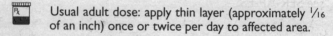 Usual adult dose: apply thin layer (approximately $\frac{1}{16}$ of an inch) once or twice per day to affected area.

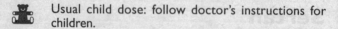 Usual child dose: follow doctor's instructions for children.

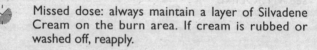 Missed dose: always maintain a layer of Silvadene Cream on the burn area. If cream is rubbed or washed off, reapply.

Side Effects

☠ Overdose symptoms: no specific information available. If you suspect an overdose, immediately seek medical attention.

✚ Side effects: areas of dead skin, burning sensation, rash, red or raised rash on body, skin discoloration.

✚ No known less common or rare side effects.

Interactions

 Inform your doctor before combining use of Silvadene Cream 1% with: topical enzymes such as Panafil and Santyl that contain collagenase, papain, or sutilains; or cimetidine (Tagamet).

 No known food/other substance interactions.

Special Cautions

 If pregnant or plan to become pregnant, inform your doctor immediately. *Do not use at the end of pregnancy.* Other sulfa medications appear in breast milk, affecting nursing infants.

 No special precautions apply to seniors.

 Follow doctor's instructions carefully for children. *Do not use on premature infants or newborns under 2 months.*

 Avoid if sensitive to or allergic to other sulfa medications such as Septra.

If burn wounds are extensive, Silvadene may be absorbed into bloodstream, which may lead to side effects throughout the body.

Silver Sulfadiazine

see SILVADENE CREAM 1%

Simvastatin

see ZOCOR

Sinemet CR

Generic ingredients: Carbidopa with levodopa

Sinemet CR is an antiparkinsonism agent. It corrects the chemical imbalance, thereby relieving symptoms of Parkinson's disease. Levodopa treats the Parkinson's symptoms, and carbidopa prevents vitamin B_6 from destroying the levodopa.

℞ QUICK FACTS

Purpose

℞ Used to treat the symptoms of Parkinson's disease—muscle stiffness, tremor, and weakness. Also used to treat similar symptoms caused by encephalitis (brain fever), carbon monoxide poisoning, or manganese poisoning.

Dosage

 Take after meals, swallowing tablets whole; do not chew or crush tablets. Important to take dose at the same time each day; most effective with a constant level in the blood. Only doctor should change dose or add other Parkinson's disease products to the therapy program. *Do not abruptly discontinue medication; may result in muscle rigidity, high temperature, and mental changes.*

 Usual adult dose: *for mild to moderate symptoms*—1 tablet taken 2 times per day. Initially, doses should be every 4 to 8 hours, then adjusted to each patient's needs. Long-term dose is 2 to 8 tablets per day taken in divided doses every 4 to 8 hours while awake.

Usual child dose: not generally prescribed for children.

 Missed dose: take as soon as possible, unless almost time for next dose. In that case, do not take missed dose; go back to regular schedule. *Do not double doses.*

Side Effects

 Overdose symptoms: muscle twitches, inability to open the eyes. If you suspect an overdose, immediately seek medical attention.

 More common side effects: confusion, hallucinations, nausea, uncontrollable jerking or twitching.

 Less common or rare side effects: abdominal or stomach pain, abnormal dreams, agitation, anemia, anxiety, back pain, bitter taste, bizarre breathing patterns, bleeding from stomach, blurred vision, burning sensation on tongue, chest pain, clumsiness in walking, common cold, constipation, convulsions, cough, dark sweat, dark urine, delusions, depression, diarrhea, disorientation, dizziness, dizziness upon standing, dream abnormalities, drooling, drowsiness, dry mouth, euphoria, eyelid twitching, faintness, falling, fatigue, fever, flatulence, fluid retention, flushing, hair loss, headache, heart attack, heart palpitations, heartburn, hiccups, high or low blood pressure, hoarseness, hot flashes, increased hand tremor, insomnia or other sleep disorders, irregular heartbeat, leg pain, locked jaw, loss of appetite, malignant melanoma, memory problems, mental changes, muscle cramps, muscle twitching, nervousness, numbness, "on-off" phenomena, paralysis of certain muscles and unwanted movement of others, paranoia, persistent erection, phlebitis (vein swelling), rash, shortness of breath, shoulder pain, slowed physical movements, sore throat, speech impairment, stomach ulcer, suicidal tendencies, swallowing difficulties, sweating, teeth-grinding, tingling or pins and needles, upper respiratory infection, upset stomach, urinary frequency, urinary incontinence, urinary retention, urinary tract infections, weakness, weight loss or gain, writhing or flailing movements, vomiting.

Interactions

Inform your doctor before combining Sinemet CR with: antacids such as Di-Gel and Maalox, anticonvulsants such as Dilantin, antiparkinson medications such as Artane and Cogentin, antihypertensives such as Aldomet and Clonidine, iron products such as Feosol, isoniazid (Nydrazid), major tranquilizers such as Haldol and Thorazine, MAO inhibitors such as Nardil and Parnate, methionine medications such as Odor-Scrip and Pedameth, metoclopramide (Reglan), papaverine (Pavabid), pyridoxine (Vitamin B₆), tranquilizers such as Valium and Xanax, tricyclic antidepressants such as Elavil and Tofranil. Must discontinue MAO inhibitors at least 2 weeks prior to starting Sinemet CR therapy.

No known food/other substance interactions.

Special Cautions

If pregnant or plan to become pregnant, inform your doctor immediately. Not known if Sinemet CR appears in breast milk.

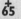

No special precautions apply to seniors.

Not generally prescribed for children.

Do not take if sensitive to or allergic to Sinemet CR.

Doctor should not prescribe if you have an undiagnosed mole or history of melanoma.

Inform your doctor *before* starting Sinemet CR therapy if you have: bronchial asthma, cardiovascular or lung disease, endocrine (gland) disorder, history of heart attack or heartbeat irregularity, history of active peptic ulcer, kidney or liver disorder, wide-angle glaucoma.

Sinemet is a regular, noncontrolled form of Sinemet CR. If taking regular Sinemet, may need higher dose of Sinemet CR to get same kind of relief, and may take longer to start working than the first morning dose of regular Sinemet.

Doctor should monitor blood, liver, heart, and kidney during long-term Sinemet CR therapy.

If taking levodopa alone, discontinue it for at least 8 hours before starting Sinemet CR.

Carbidopa ingredient in Sinemet CR will not eliminate levodopa side effects. May produce levodopa side effects, since it helps levodopa reach the brain. Doctor may reduce dose if you experience involuntary movement side effects.

May cause depression; inform your doctor if you have any mental or emotional problems.

Sinequan

Generic name: Doxepin hydrochloride

Other brand name: Adapin

Sinequan is a tricyclic antidepressant. It is thought to relieve depression by increasing the concentration of chemicals necessary for nerve transmissions in the brain.

℞ QUICK FACTS

Purpose

℞ Used to treat depression and anxiety. It relieves tension, improves sleep, elevates mood, increases energy, and eases feelings of fear, guilt, apprehension, and worry. Effective when depression is psychological, associated with alcoholism, or a result of another disease or psychotic depressive disorders.

Dosage

 Take exactly as prescribed. May take several weeks to observe effects of medication.

 Usual adult dose: *mild to moderate illness*—75 milligrams per day. Range may be from 25 to 150 milligrams per day, depending on an individual's needs. 150-milligram capsule for long-term therapy only, and not as a starting dose. *More severe illness*—may be prescribed up to 300 milligrams per day. *Seniors*—dosage is carefully adjusted by your doctor.

 Usual child dose: not generally prescribed for children under 12 years.

 Missed dose: *if taking several doses per day*—take as soon as possible; then take remaining doses for the day at evenly spaced intervals. If almost time for next dose, do not take missed dose; go back to regular schedule. *If taking single dose at bedtime*—if it is the next morning, skip missed dose and return to regular schedule. *Do not double doses.*

Side Effects

Overdose symptoms: blurred vision, coma, convulsions, decreased intestinal movement, dilated pupils, drowsiness, excessive mouth dryness, high or low body temperature, irregular or rapid heartbeat, low or high blood pressure, overactive reflexes, severe breathing problems, stupor, urinary problems. If you suspect an overdose, immediately seek medical attention.

Most common side effect: drowsiness.

Less common or rare side effects: blurred vision, breast development in males, bruises, buzzing or ringing in ears, changes in sex drive, chills, confusion, constipation, diarrhea, difficulty urinating, disorientation, dizziness, dry mouth, enlarged breasts, fatigue, fluid retention, flushing, fragmented or incomplete movements, hair loss, hallucinations, headache, high fever, high or low blood sugar, inappropriate breast milk secretion, indigestion, inflammation of mouth, itching and skin rash, lack of muscle control, loss of appetite, loss of coordination, low blood pressure, nausea, nervousness, numbness, poor bladder control, rapid heartbeat, red or brownish skin spots, seizures, sensitivity to light, severe muscle stiffness, sore throat, sweating, swelling of testicles, taste disturbances, tingling sensation, tremors, vomiting, weakness, weight gain, yellow eyes and skin.

Interactions

Do not take MAO inhibitors such as Nardil and Parnate with Sinequan; may result in death. Inform your doctor before combining Sinequan with: amphetamines such as Dexedrine; antihistamines such as Benadryl and Tavist; baclofen (Lioresal); benztropine (Cogentin); carbamazepine (Tegretol); central nervous system depressants such as Darvon and

Xanax; cimetidine (Tagamet); clonidine (Catapres); epinephrine (EpiPen); fluoxetine (Prozac); guanethidine (Ismelin); quinidine (Quinidex); tolazamide (Tolinase). Also inform your doctor of any nonprescription medications you are taking.

 Do not drink alcohol during Sinequan therapy.

Special Cautions

 If pregnant or plan to become pregnant, inform your doctor immediately. May appear in breast milk; could affect a nursing infant.

 Seniors should use with caution.

 Not generally prescribed for children under 12 years.

 Do not take if you have glaucoma or difficulty urinating unless directed by your doctor.

May cause drowsiness and impair your ability to drive a car or operate machinery. *Do not take part in any activity that requires alertness.*

Avoid if sensitive to or allergic to this medication or similar antidepressants.

May decrease seizure threshold.

Inform your doctor or dentist in medical emergency or before surgery that you are taking Sinequan.

Sodium Fluoride

see LURIDE

Sodium Sulamyd

Generic name: Sulfacetamide sodium

Other brand names: AK-Sulf Forte, AK-Sulf Ointment, Bleph-10, Cetamide, Isopto Cetamide, Sodium Sulamyd 10%, Sodium Sulamyd 30%, Sulamyd, Sulf-10, Sulfair 15, Sulten-10

Sodium Sulamyd is a sulfa antibiotic. It inhibits the growth of bacteria by affecting the biochemicals or nutrients necessary for bacteria to sustain life.

℞ Quick Facts

Purpose

℞ Used to treat eye inflammations, corneal ulcer, and other eye infections. Used with oral sulfa medications to treat trachoma.

Dosage

🍽 Use exactly as prescribed, comes in eyedrop and ointment form. Doctor may advise using both forms at the same time.

  Usual adult dose: *ophthalmic solution 30%*—For inflamed eyes or corneal ulcer—1 drop inside lower eyelid every 2 hours. For trachoma—2 drops every 2 hours. *Ophthalmic solution 10%*—1 or 2 drops inside lower eyelid every 2 or 3 hours during the day and less at night. *Ophthalmic ointment 10%*—apply small amount 4 times per day and at bedtime.

  Usual child dose: follow doctor's instructions carefully.

Missed dose: apply as soon as possible, unless almost time for next dose. In that case, do not apply missed dose; go back to regular schedule.

Side Effects

 Overdose symptoms: no specific information available. If you suspect an overdose, immediately seek medical attention.

 Most common side effect: eye irritation causing stinging and burning. If prolonged irritation, doctor may discontinue.

 Rare side effect: severe blistering skin rash.

Interactions

 Avoid using medications containing silver.

 No known food/other substance interactions.

Special Cautions

 If pregnant or plan to become pregnant, inform your doctor immediately. Not known if Sodium Sulamyd appears in breast milk.

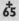 No special precautions apply to seniors.

 Follow doctor's instructions carefully for children.

 Do not use if sensitive to or allergic to this or other sulfa medications. If you have taken other sulfa medications in the past, may have developed a hidden allergy to sulfa drugs. Monitor for symptoms such as rash, itching, or other allergy signs. If you develop allergy, stop taking medication and contact your doctor.

May develop fungus infection not treatable with this medication. Inform your doctor if you have a pus-producing eye infection.

Eye ointment may delay healing of cornea.

Solfoton

see PHENOBARBITAL

Soma

Generic name: Carisoprodol

Other brand names: Sodol, Soprodol

Soma is a muscle relaxant. It is thought to act as a central nervous system depressant; the sedative effect indirectly relaxes skeletal muscles.

℞ QUICK FACTS

Purpose

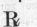

Used to treat acute, painful muscle strains and spasms. Is part of a program of physical therapy, exercise, and rest.

Dosage

Take exactly as prescribed. Suddenly stopping Soma may cause withdrawal symptoms such as: abdominal cramps, chilliness, headache, insomnia, and nausea.

Usual adult dose: one 350-milligram tablet taken 3 times per day and at bedtime.

Usual child dose: not generally prescribed for children under 12 years.

 Missed dose: take as soon as possible if only an hour has passed. Otherwise, do not take missed dose; go back to regular schedule. *Do not double doses.*

Side Effects

 Overdose may be fatal. Overdose symptoms: coma, shock, stupor. If you suspect an overdose, immediately seek medical attention.

 Side effects: agitation, depression, dizziness, drowsiness, facial flushing, fainting, headache, hiccups, inability to fall or stay asleep, irritability, light-headedness upon standing, loss of coordination, nausea, rapid heart rate, stomach upset, tremors, vertigo, vomiting.

 No known less common or rare side effects.

Interactions

 Inform your doctor before combining Soma with: antidepressants such as Elavil, Tofranil, and Nardil; major tranquilizers such as Haldol, Stelazine, and Thorazine; sedatives such as Nembutal and Halcion; tranquilizers such as Librium, Valium, and Xanax.

 Use caution if you drink alcohol during Soma therapy; may intensify the effects of alcohol.

Special Cautions

 If pregnant or plan to become pregnant, inform your doctor immediately. Appears in breast milk; could affect a nursing infant.

No special precautions apply to seniors.

 Not generally prescribed for children under 12.

 Do not increase physical activity over what doctor recommends. Soma may temporarily relieve symptoms, making it seem feasible to increase activity.

Do not take if you have porphyria (blood disorder).

May impair mental and physical ability to drive a car or operate machinery. *Do not take part in any activity that requires alertness.*

Inform your doctor *before* taking Soma if you have a history of drug dependence.

Avoid if sensitive to or allergic to Soma or similar medications such as meprobamate (Miltown).

First dose of Soma may produce (in rare cases): agitation, confusion, disorientation, dizziness, double vision, enlargement of pupils, extreme weakness, exaggerated feeling of well-being, lack of coordination, speech problems, temporary loss of vision, temporary paralysis of arms and legs. Symptoms usually last a few hours. Immediately contact your doctor if you experience any of these symptoms.

Allergic reactions may occur between 1st and 4th doses in patients taking Soma for the first time: itching, red skin welts, skin rash. More severe allergic reactions: asthmatic attacks, dizziness, fever, low blood pressure, shock, stinging of eyes, swelling due to fluid retention, weakness.

Use cautiously if you have liver or kidney problems.

Spectazole Cream

Generic name: Econazole nitrate

Spectazole Cream is an antifungal. It destroys and prevents the growth of fungi.

℞ QUICK FACTS

Purpose

℞ Used to treat ringworm (tinea), athlete's foot (tinea pedis), jock itch (tinea cruris), fungal infection of the entire body (tinea corporis), and skin infection causing yellow or brown-colored skin eruptions (tinea versicolor). Also prescribed for yeast infections of the skin caused by candida fungus.

Dosage

 Take exactly as prescribed. Use entire medication, even if symptoms disappear before medication is finished. *Do not apply near the eyes.*

 Usual adult dose: *for athlete's foot, jock itch, tinea corporis, tinea versicolor*—cover affected area with cream once per day. Athlete's foot is treated for 1 month, jock itch and tinea corporis are treated for 2 weeks, and tinea versicolor is usually treated for 2 weeks. *For yeast infections*—apply cream to affected area 2 times per day for 2 weeks.

 Usual child dose: follow doctor's instructions carefully.

 Missed dose: apply as soon as possible, unless almost time for next dose. In that case, do not apply missed dose; go back to regular schedule.

Side Effects

 Overdose symptoms: no specific information available. If you suspect an overdose, immediately seek medical attention.

 More common side effects: burning, itching, skin redness, stinging.

 Less common or rare side effect: itchy rash.

Interactions

 No drug interactions reported.

 No food/other substance interactions reported.

Special Cautions

 If pregnant or plan to become pregnant, inform your doctor immediately. Only use in first trimester if essential to your health. May appear in breast milk; could affect a nursing infant.

 No special precautions apply to seniors.

 Follow doctor's instructions carefully for children.

 Avoid use if sensitive to or allergic to Spectazole.

Stop using and contact your doctor if you develop an allergy.

Spironolactone
see ALDACTONE

Spironolactone with Hydrochlorothiazide

see ALDACTAZIDE

Sporanox

Generic name: Itraconazole

Sporanox is an antifungal. It destroys and prevents the growth of fungi.

℞ QUICK FACTS

Purpose

℞ Used to treat two types of fungal infections—blastomycosis (rare infection caused by inhaling a fungus found in wood and soil, and affecting lungs, bones, and skin); and histoplasmosis (infection caused by inhaling fungal spores, and affecting lungs, heart, and blood). Also used to treat fungal infections in people with weak immune systems such as AIDS patients.

Dosage

 Take exactly as prescribed, with food. Finish entire prescription, otherwise infection may return.

 Usual adult dose: two 100-milligram capsules taken with food once per day. Doctor may increase by 100 milligrams at a time up to 400 milligrams per day if no improvement or if infection spreads. Doses over 200 milligrams per day are divided into smaller doses. Therapy lasts a minimum of 3 months or until infection has disappeared.

Usual child dose: not generally prescribed for children.

 Missed dose: take as soon as possible, unless almost time for next dose. In that case, do not take missed dose; go back to regular schedule. *Do not double doses.*

Side Effects

 Overdose symptoms: no specific information available. If you suspect an overdose, immediately seek medical attention.

 More common side effects: diarrhea, fatigue, fever, headache, high blood pressure, nausea, rash, swelling due to water retention, vomiting.

 Less common side effects: abdominal pain, decreased sex drive, dizziness, feeling of general discomfort, itching, loss of appetite, reproductive disorders such as male impotence, extreme sleepiness. Rare side effects: depression, gas, male breast development, male breast pain, ringing in ears, sleeplessness.

Interactions

 Serious heart problems and death have occurred in rare cases when taking Seldane or Hismanal with Sporanox. Inform your doctor before combining Sporanox with: antiulcer medications such as Tagamet and Zantac; astemizole (Hismanal); blood thinners such as Coumadin; carbamazepine (Tegretol); cyclosporine (Sandimmune); digoxin (Lanoxin); isoniazid (INH); oral diabetes medications such as DiaBeta, Diabinese, Glucotrol, and Micronase; phenytoin (Dilantin); rifampin (Rifadin or Rimactane); terfenadine (Seldane).

No known food/other substance interactions.

Special Cautions

 If pregnant or plan to become pregnant, inform your doctor immediately. Appears in breast milk; could affect a nursing infant.

 No special precautions apply to seniors.

 Not generally prescribed for children.

 Avoid if sensitive to or allergic to Sporanox or similar antifungal medications.

Doctor should monitor you if you have liver disease. Immediately contact your doctor if you develop symptoms such as: unusual fatigue, loss of appetite, nausea, vomiting, jaundice, dark urine, or pale stool.

SSD Cream

see SILVADENE CREAM 1%

Stelazine

Generic name: Trifluoperazine hydrochloride

Stelazine is a phenothiazine tranquilizer. It is thought to work by blocking chemicals involved in nerve transmission in the brain.

℞ QUICK FACTS

Purpose

℞ Used to treat severe mental disturbances and anxiety that does not respond to normal tranquilizers.

Dosage

If using liquid concentrate, must dilute. May use carbonated beverage, coffee, fruit juice, milk, tea, tomato juice, or water, or puddings, soups, and other semisolid foods. *Do not take with alcohol.*

Usual adult dose: *for nonpsychotic anxiety*—2 to 4 milligrams per day, divided into 2 equal doses. *Do not take more than 6 milligrams per day or take medication for more than 12 weeks. For psychotic disorders*—4 to 10 milligrams per day, divided into 2 equal doses, up to 40 milligrams per day. *Seniors*—prescribed lower doses.

Usual child dose: *for psychotic conditions*—1 milligram per day as a single dose or divided into 2 doses. Doctor will prescribe up to 15 milligrams per day. Dose is determined based on weight and severity of illness. Children must be closely monitored or hospitalized during Stelazine therapy. Not prescribed for children under 6 years.

Missed dose: *if taking 1 dose per day*—take as soon as possible, then go back to regular schedule. If you remember the next day, do not take missed dose; go back to regular schedule. *If taking more than 1 dose per day*—take as soon as possible if within an hour of scheduled time. Otherwise, do not take missed dose; go back to regular schedule. *Do not double doses.*

Side Effects

Overdose symptoms: agitation, coma, convulsions, difficulty breathing, difficulty swallowing, dry mouth, extreme sleepiness, fever, intestinal blockage, irregular heart rate, low blood pressure, restlessness. If you suspect an overdose, immediately seek medical attention.

Side effects: abnormal milk secretion; abnormal sugar in urine; abnormalities in movement and posture; agitation; allergic reactions; anemia; asthma; blood disorders; blurred vision; body rigidly arched backward; breast development in males; chewing movements; constipation; constricted pupils; difficulty swallowing; dilated pupils; dizziness; drooling; drowsiness; dry mouth; ejaculation problems; exaggerated or excessive reflexes; excessive or spontaneous milk flow; eye problems causing fixed gaze; eye spasms; fatigue; fever or high fever; flu-like symptoms; fluid accumulation and swelling (including the brain); fragmented movements; headache; heart attack; high or low blood sugar; hives; impotence; inability to urinate; increase in appetite and weight; infections; insomnia; intestinal blockage; involuntary movements of tongue, face, mouth, jaw, arms, and legs; irregular blood pressure, pulse, and heartbeat; irregular or no menstrual periods; jitteriness; lightheadedness; liver damage; lockjaw; loss of appetite; low blood pressure; mask-like face; muscle stiffness and rigidity; nasal congestion; nausea; persistent; painful erections; pill-rolling movement; protruding tongue; puckering of mouth; puffing of cheeks; purple or red skin spots; rapid heartbeat; restlessness; rigid arms, feet, head, and muscles; seizures; sensitivity to light; shuffling walk; skin inflammation and peeling; skin itching, pigmentation, reddening, or rash; spasms in jaw, face, tongue, neck, hands, feet, back, and mouth; sweating; swelling of throat; totally unresponsive state; tremors; twisted neck; weakness; yellowing of skin and eyes.

 No known less common or rare side effects.

Interactions

 Inform your doctor before combining Stelazine with: anticonvulsants such as Dilantin; atropine (Donnatal); blood thinners such as Coumadin; guanethidine (Ismelin); propranolol (Inderal); thiazide diuretics such as Dyazide. Extreme drowsiness occurs if combining Stelazine with: tranquilizers such as Valium, narcotic painkillers such as Percocet, antihistamines such as Benadryl, and barbiturates such as phenobarbital.

 Avoid using alcohol; causes extreme drowsiness.

Special Cautions

 If pregnant or plan to become pregnant, inform your doctor immediately. Appears in breast milk; could affect a nursing infant.

 Seniors are susceptible to low blood pressure and tardive dyskinesia (involuntary muscle spasms and twitches in the face and body). Senior women have higher risk for tardive dyskinesia.

 Follow doctor's instructions carefully for children over 6 years. Not prescribed for children under 6 years.

 May impair ability to drive a car or operate machinery. *Do not take part in any activity that requires alertness.*

Immediately contact your doctor if you experience fever; sore throat, mouth, or gums; or flu-like symptoms.

Follow doctor's instructions for gradually tapering off medication when therapy ends.

At risk for tardive dyskinesia (potentially permanent involuntary muscle spasms and twitches in the face and body). Ask your doctor about your particular risk.

Avoid if you have liver damage or an abnormal bone marrow or blood condition.

At risk for neuroleptic malignant syndrome—high body temperature, rigid muscles, irregular pulse or blood pressure, rapid or abnormal heartbeat, and excessive perspiration.

Use with caution if you have or ever had: brain tumor, breast cancer, intestinal blockage, glaucoma, heart or liver disease, or seizures; or if exposed to pesticides or extreme heat.

May mask overdose symptoms of other medications, and may cause difficulty in doctor diagnosing intestinal obstruction, brain tumor, and Reye's syndrome.

Inform your doctor of any allergic reaction to other major tranquilizers.

May cause allergic reaction if you have asthma.

Contact your doctor if you experience vision problems.

Stimate

see DDAVP

Stuartnatal Plus

Generic ingredients: Supplemental vitamins and minerals

Other brand names: Materna, Natalins

Stuartnatal Plus is a nutritional supplement. It supplies missing nutrients to a pregnant woman.

℞ QUICK FACTS

Purpose

℞ Used to provide a supply of critical nutrients during pregnancy and after childbirth. Also used to improve nutritional status before a pregnancy. Contains iron, calcium, zinc, and folic acid.

Dosage

 Take exactly as prescribed.

 Usual adult dose: 1 tablet per day.

 Usual child dose: not generally prescribed for children.

 Missed dose: take as soon as possible, then return to regular schedule.

Side Effects

 Overdose symptoms: no specific information available. If you suspect an overdose, immediately seek medical attention.

 No known more common side effects.

 No known less common or rare side effects.

Interactions

 No drug interactions reported.

 No known food/other substance interactions.

Special Cautions

 No cautions for pregnancy or breastfeeding.

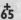 No special precautions apply to seniors.

 Not generally prescribed for children.

 Take on a regular basis.

Sucralfate
see CARAFATE

Sulfacetamide Sodium
see SODIUM SULAMYD

Sulfasalazine

see AZULFIDINE

Sulfisoxazole

see GANTRISIN

Sulindac

see CLINORIL

Sumatriptan Succinate

see IMITREX INJECTION

Sumycin

see ACHROMYCIN V CAPSULES

Suprax

Generic name: Cefixime

Suprax is a cephalosporin antibiotic. It interferes with
the production of certain biochemicals necessary for
bacteria to sustain life.

℞ Quick Facts

Purpose

℞ Used to treat bacterial infections of the chest, ears, urinary tract, and throat, and for uncomplicated gonorrhea.

Dosage

 Can take with or without food. Take with food if you have stomach upset. Food does slow down absorption rate. Use specially marked measuring spoon from pharmacy if taking liquid form. Shake liquid well before using. Finish entire prescription; otherwise infection may reappear.

. . . .

 Usual adult dose: *for infections other than gonorrhea*— 400 milligrams per day as a single dose or a 200-milligram tablet taken every 12 hours. May be prescribed lower dose if you have kidney disease. *For uncomplicated gonorrhea*—a single 400-milligram dose. *Seniors*—prescribed lower doses.

. . . .

 Usual child dose: 8 milligrams per 2.2 pounds of body weight per day. May give as a single dose or in 2 half doses every 12 hours, per doctor's instructions. Children over 110 pounds or over 12 years are prescribed adult dose. Suspension form is prescribed for middle ear infection because it is generally more effective than the tablet form. Not prescribed for children under 6 months.

. . . .

 Missed dose: *if taking 1 dose per day*—take as soon as possible. Wait 10 to 12 hours before taking next dose, then go back to regular schedule. If you remember the next day, do not take missed dose; go back to regular schedule. *If taking 2 doses per day*— take as soon as possible, and take next dose in 5 to

6 hours. Then go back to regular schedule. *If taking 3 doses per day*—take as soon as possible, and take next dose in 2 to 4 hours. Then go back to regular schedule. *Do not double doses.*

Side Effects

 Overdose symptoms: blood in urine, diarrhea, nausea, upper abdominal pain, vomiting. If you suspect an overdose, immediately seek medical attention.

 More common side effects: abdominal pain, gas, indigestion, loose stools, mild diarrhea, nausea, vomiting.

 Less common side effects: colitis, dizziness, fever, headaches, hives, itching, skin rashes, vaginitis. Rare side effects: bleeding, decrease in urine output, seizures, severe abdominal or stomach cramps, severe diarrhea (sometimes with blood), shock, skin redness.

Interactions

 No drug interactions reported.

 No known food/other substance interactions.

Special Cautions

 If pregnant or plan to become pregnant, inform your doctor immediately. May appear in breast milk; could affect a nursing infant.

65 Seniors are prescribed lower doses to accommodate decreasing kidney function.

 Follow doctor's instructions carefully for children.

Inform your doctor before taking Suprax if allergic to any form of penicillin or cephalosporin antibiotics; at risk for extremely severe allergic reaction.

Suprax may cause false urine-sugar test results. If diabetic, inform your doctor that you are taking Suprax before being tested. *Do not change diet or diabetes medication dosage unless directed by your doctor.*

Doctor may test to verify that Suprax is effective against your particular infection. *Do not share medication with others who have infections.*

Tell your doctor *before* starting Suprax therapy if you have a history of stomach or intestinal disease such as colitis, or kidney disorder.

Immediately contact your doctor if you experience allergic symptoms.

Notify your doctor right away if your symptoms either do not improve or worsen.

If you experience nausea, vomiting, or severe diarrhea, talk with your doctor before taking diarrhea medication. Some such as Lomotil and paregoric may worsen or prolong diarrhea.

At risk for secondary infection if used when not directed by your doctor.

Surmontil

Generic name: Trimipramine maleate

Surmontil is a tricyclic antidepressant. It is thought to relieve depression by increasing the concentration of chemicals necessary for nerve transmissions in the brain.

℞ QUICK FACTS

Purpose

℞ Used to treat depression.

Dosage

 May take in a single dose at bedtime or in smaller doses throughout the day. Continue taking medication as prescribed, even if there is no immediate effect. May take up to 4 weeks to observe results. If Surmontil is stopped suddenly, may experience nausea, headache, and general feeling of illness; follow doctor's instructions on stopping medication.

 Usual adult dose: 75 milligrams per day divided into smaller doses. Doctor may increase up to 150 milligrams per day divided into smaller doses. Single dose is recommended for long-term therapy; doses range from 50 to 150 milligrams per day. *Seniors and adolescents*—50 milligrams per day, up to 100 milligrams per day, according to doctor's instructions.

 Usual child dose: not generally prescribed for children.

 Missed dose: take as soon as possible, unless almost time for next dose. In that case, do not take missed dose; go back to regular schedule. *If taking 1 dose per day at bedtime*—do not take missed dose in the morning; may cause disturbing side effects during the day. Go back to regular schedule. *Do not double doses.*

Side Effects

Surmontil overdose can be fatal. Overdose symptoms: agitation, coma, convulsions, difficulty breathing, dilated pupils, discolored bluish skin, drowsiness, heart failure, high fever, involuntary movement, irregular heart rate, lack of coordination, low blood pressure, muscle rigidity, rapid heartbeat, restlessness, shock, stupor, sweating, vomiting. If you suspect an overdose, immediately seek medical attention.

Side effects: abdominal cramps, agitation, anxiety, black tongue, blocked intestine, blood disorders, blurred vision, breast development in males, confusion (especially in seniors), constipation, delusions, diarrhea, difficulty urinating, dilated pupils, disorientation, dizziness, drowsiness, dry mouth, excessive or spontaneous milk flow, fatigue, fever, flushing, fluttery or throbbing heartbeat, frequent urination, hair loss, hallucinations, headache, heart attack, high blood pressure, high blood sugar, hives, impotence, increased or decreased sex drive, inflammation of the mouth, insomnia, irregular heart rate, lack of coordination, loss of appetite, low blood pressure, low blood sugar, nausea, nightmares, numbness, peculiar taste in mouth, purple or reddish-brown skin spots, rapid heartbeat, restlessness, ringing in the ears, seizures, sensitivity to light, skin itching, skin rash, sore throat, stomach upset, stroke, sweating, swelling of breasts, swelling of face and tongue, swelling of testicles, swollen glands, tingling or pins and needles, tremors, visual problems, vomiting, weakness, weight gain or loss, yellowing of skin and eyes.

No known less common or rare side effects.

Interactions

 Do not start Surmontil for 2 weeks after taking MAO *inhibitors such as Nardil and Parnate; may cause death.* Inform your doctor before taking Surmontil with: antispasmodics such as Cogentin, cimetidine (Tagamet), guanethidine (Ismelin), local anesthetics, local decongestants such as Dristan Nasal Spray, oral nasal decongestants such as Sudafed, stimulants such as EpiPen, thyroid medications such as Synthroid.

 Alcohol may cause extreme drowsiness and potentially serious side effects.

Special Cautions

 Not known if Surmontil affects pregnancy or appears in breast milk. If pregnant or plan to become pregnant, inform your doctor immediately.

 Seniors are prescribed lower doses.

 Not generally prescribed for children.

 May impair ability to drive a car or operate machinery. *Do not take part in any activity that requires alertness.*

Avoid if you are recovering from a recent heart attack, or if sensitive to or allergic to this or similar medications such as Tofranil.

Use with caution if you have glaucoma, heart disease, liver disease, thyroid disease; are taking thyroid medication; or have problems urinating.

Synalgos-DC

Generic ingredients: Dihydrocodeine bitartrate with aspirin and caffeine

Synalgos-DC is a narcotic analgesic. It relieves pain and gives a feeling of well-being.

℞ QUICK FACTS

Purpose

℞   Used to treat moderate to moderately severe pain.

Dosage

    Take exactly as prescribed. *Do not increase dose unless directed by your doctor.*

. . . .

    Usual adult dose: 2 capsules taken every 4 hours as needed. *Seniors*—dose adjusted to accommodate condition of health.

. . . .

    Usual child dose: not generally prescribed for children under 12 years.

. . . .

    Missed dose: *if taking on a regular schedule*—take as soon as possible, unless almost time for next dose. In that case, do not take missed dose; go back to regular schedule. *Do not double doses.*

Side Effects

    Overdose symptoms: no specific information available. If you suspect an overdose, immediately seek medical attention.

. . . .

    Side effects: constipation, dizziness, drowsiness, itching, light-headedness, nausea, sedation, skin reactions, vomiting.

. . . .

No known less common or rare side effects.

Interactions

 Inform your doctor before combining Synalgos-DC with: narcotic pain relievers such as Percocet and Demerol, sedatives such as Halcion and Seconal, tranquilizers such as Valium and Xanax. Taking Coumadin may cause internal bleeding. Taking antigout medications such as Benemid may alter the effects of Synalgos-DC.

 Avoid alcohol or reduce intake during Synalgos-DC therapy; it slows brain activity and intensifies the effects of alcohol.

Special Cautions

 If pregnant or plan to become pregnant, inform your doctor immediately. May appear in breast milk; could affect a nursing infant.

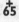 Dose is determined according to senior's physical condition.

 Not generally prescribed for children under 12 years.

 May cause drowsiness and impair ability to drive a car or operate machinery. *Do not take part in any activity that requires alertness.*

May be habit-forming if taken for a prolonged period; tell your doctor *before* starting Synalgos-DC if you have been addicted to drugs.

Inform your doctor *before* taking Synalgos-DC if you have stomach ulcer or blood-clotting disorder.

Avoid if sensitive to or allergic to this medication, other narcotic pain relievers, or aspirin.

Synthroid

Generic name: Levothyroxine

Other brand names: Levothroid, Levoxine

Synthroid is a synthetic thyroid hormone. It works exactly as the natural thyroid hormone produced in the body, regulating specific body functions.

℞ QUICK FACTS

Purpose

℞ Used to treat any of the following conditions: thyroid hormone deficiency; at risk for or have developed a goiter; as a suppression test to determine if the thyroid is producing too much hormone; if you have had radiation therapy to treat or prevent thyroid gland cancer.

Dosage

 Take exactly as prescribed, not increasing or decreasing dose. Take dose at same time each day. If unable to swallow tablet, may mix into a spoonful of liquid or sprinkle over a small amount of food such as applesauce, and take right away. May take indefinitely if thyroid is not producing enough hormone. Doctor will monitor level of hormone through blood tests.

 Usual adult dose: tailored to meet individual needs. *Seniors, people with angina (crushing chest pain)*—prescribed lower doses.

Usual child dose: tailored to meet individual needs.

 Missed dose: take as soon as possible, unless almost time for next dose. In that case, do not take missed dose; go back to regular schedule. *Do not double doses.*

Side Effects

 Overdose symptoms: abdominal cramps, chest pain, diarrhea, excessive sweating, fever, headaches, heat intolerance, irregular heartbeat, nervousness, palpitations, rapid heartbeat, tremors, trouble sleeping, weight loss. If you suspect an overdose, immediately seek medical attention.

 Side effects: other than overdose symptoms, side effects are rare. Children may lose hair, but this is rare. Excessive or rapid increase in dose may lead to overstimulation of thyroid gland. Overstimulation symptoms: abdominal cramps, changes in appetite, chest pain, diarrhea, fever, headache, heat intolerance, increased heart rate, irregular heartbeat, irritability, nausea, nervousness, palpitations, sleeplessness, sweating, tremors, weight loss.

 No known less common or rare side effects.

Interactions

 Inform your doctor before combining Synthroid with: antacids such as Mylanta; antidiabetic medications such as Diabinese and Glucotrol; blood thinners such as Coumadin; cholestyramine medications such as Questran; colestipol (Colestid); epinephrine (EpiPen); estrogen or contraceptive pills such as Ortho-Novum and Premarin; insulin; lovastatin (Mevacor); phenytoin (Dilantin); tricyclic antidepressants such as Elavil and Tofranil. Blood test results may be altered if you are taking: androgens, corticosteroids such as Decadron and prednisone, estrogens such as Premarin, iodine-containing medications, oral contraceptives containing estrogen, or salicylate-containing medications such as aspirin.

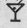 No known food/other substance interactions.

Special Cautions

 May take during pregnancy or breastfeeding if taking due to thyroid hormone deficiency.

 Seniors are prescribed lower dose.

 Follow doctor's instructions carefully for children.

 Not for use as a weight-loss medication. Overdose may cause life-threatening side effects, especially if taking with an appetite suppressant.

Doctor should not prescribe if: sensitive to or allergic to Synthroid; thyroid gland is overproducing thyroid hormone; or if adrenal glands are underproducing corticosteroid hormone.

If you have diabetes mellitus or diabetes insipidus, or if your body produces too little adrenal corticosteroid hormone, Synthroid will worsen your symptoms. Dosages for medications of these disorders will be adjusted during Synthroid therapy.

Tacrine Hydrochloride

see COGNEX

Tagamet

Generic name: Cimetidine

Tagamet is an anti-ulcer/gastric acid secretion inhibitor. It blocks the effects of histamine in the stomach, which reduces stomach acid secretion.

℞ QUICK FACTS

Purpose

℞ Used to treat stomach and intestinal ulcers and related conditions, including: active duodenal (upper intestinal) ulcers; active benign stomach ulcers; erosive gastroesophageal reflux disease (backflow of stomach acid contents); prevention of upper abdominal bleeding in the critically ill; and excess acid conditions such as Zollinger-Ellison syndrome (peptic ulcer with too much acid). Also used for maintenance therapy for duodenal ulcer; to treat acne; stress-induced ulcers; herpes virus infections (including shingles); abnormal hair growth in women; and overactivity of parathyroid gland.

Dosage

  Take with or without food. May take several days to feel effects of Tagamet; continue taking medication even if there seems to be no reduction of symptoms. Avoid excessive amounts of caffeine; *do not take antacids within 1 to 2 hours of taking Tagamet.*

Usual adult dose: *for active duodenal ulcer*—800 milligrams taken once per day at bedtime; or 300 milligrams taken 4 times per day with meals and at bedtime; 400 milligrams taken twice per day in the morning and bedtime. Most therapy lasts 4 weeks. *For active benign gastric ulcer*—800 milligrams taken once per day at bedtime or 300 milligrams taken 4 times per day with meals and at bedtime. *For erosive gastroesophageal reflux disease*—total of 1,600 milligrams per day divided into 2 doses of 800 milligrams or 400 milligrams taken 4 times per day for 12 weeks. *For pathological hypersecretory condition*—300 milligrams taken 4 times per day with meals and at bedtime. Doctor may prescribe up to 2,400 milligrams per day. *Seniors*—may be prescribed lower dose depending on individual needs.

Usual child dose: not generally prescribed for children under 16 years. However, doctor may use in limited cases. Doses range from 20 to 40 milligrams per 2.2 pounds of body weight.

Missed dose: take as soon as possible, unless almost time for next dose. In that case, do not take missed dose; go back to regular schedule. *Do not double doses.*

Side Effects

Overdose symptoms: respiratory failure, increased heartbeat, exaggerated side effects, or unresponsiveness. If you suspect an overdose, immediately seek medical attention.

More common side effects: breast development in men, headache.

 Less common side effects: agitation, anxiety, confusion, depression, disorientation, hallucinations may occur in the severely ill being treated for over 1 month—these are temporary. Rare side effects: allergic reactions, anemia, blood disorders, diarrhea, dizziness, fever, hair loss, impotence, inability to urinate, joint pain, kidney disorders, liver disorders, mild rash, muscle pain, pancreas inflammation, rapid heartbeat, skin inflammation or peeling, sleepiness, slow heartbeat.

Interactions

 Inform your doctor before combining Tagamet with: anti-arrhythmic heart medications such as Cordarone, Tonocard, Quinidex, and Procan; antidiabetic medications such as Micronase and Glucotrol; antifungal medications such as Diflucan and Nizoral; aspirin; Augmentin; benzodiazepine tranquilizers such as Valium and Librium; beta-blockers such as Inderal and Lopressor; calcium blockers such as Cardizem, Calan, and Procardia; chlorpromazine (Thorazine); cisapride (Propulsid); cyclosporine (Sandimmune); digoxin (Lanoxin); narcotic pain relievers such as Demerol and Morphine; metoclopramide (Reglan); metronidazole (Flagyl); nicotine (Nicoderm); paroxetine (Paxil); pentoxifylline (Trental); phenytoin (Dilantin); quinine (Quinamm); sucralfate (Carafate); theophylline (Theo-Dur); warfarin (Coumadin).

 Avoid alcohol during Tagamet therapy; intensifies the effects of alcohol. Smoking cigarettes during Tagamet therapy may slow healing process.

Special Cautions

 If pregnant or planning to become pregnant, inform your doctor immediately. Appears in breast milk; could affect a nursing infant.

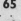 Seniors are generally prescribed lower doses.

 In limited cases is prescribed for children under 16 years.

 Do not take if allergic to Tagamet.

Ulcers can be completely healed with short-term treatment of Tagamet. Recurrence rate may be slightly higher with Tagamet than other forms of therapy; however, Tagamet is usually prescribed for the severe cases.

Tell your doctor if you are being treated for a kidney or liver disorder.

Individuals over age 50, or with kidney disease, or those who are critically ill, may experience mental confusion during Tagamet therapy. This is a temporary condition.

Talwin Compound

Generic ingredients: Pentazocine hydrochloride with aspirin

Talwin Compound is a narcotic analgesic. It relieves pain and gives a feeling of well-being.

℞ QUICK FACTS

Purpose

 Used to treat moderate pain.

Dosage

 Take exactly as prescribed; *do not increase dose unless directed by your doctor.* Abruptly stopping medication may result in withdrawal symptoms.

 Usual adult dose: 2 caplets taken 3 or 4 times per day.

 Usual child dose: not generally prescribed for children under 12 years.

 Missed dose: *if taking on a regular schedule*—take as soon as possible, unless almost time for next dose. In that case, do not take missed dose; go back to regular schedule. *Do not double doses.*

Side Effects

 Overdose may cause inability to breathe, leading to death. Overdose symptoms: coma, confusion, convulsions, diarrhea, dizziness, gasping, headache, heavy perspiration, nausea, rapid breathing, rapid heart rate, ringing in the ears, thirst, vomiting. If you suspect an overdose, immediately seek medical attention.

 More common side effects: confusion, disorientation, dizziness, feelings of elation, hallucinations, headache, light-headedness, nausea, sedation, sweating, vomiting.

 Less common side effects: blurred vision, constipation, depression, difficulty focusing, disturbed dreams, fainting, flushing, inability to fall or stay asleep, lowered blood pressure, rapid heart rate, rash, weakness. Rare side effects: abdominal distress, chills, diarrhea, excitement, facial swelling, fluid retention, hives, inability to urinate, irritability, lack or loss of appetite, ringing in the ears, skin peeling, tingling sensation, tremors, troubled or slowed breathing.

Interactions

 Inform your doctor before combining Talwin Compound with: benzodiazepines such as Valium and Xanax, MAO inhibitors such as Nardil, other analgesics such as Demerol, sleep aids such as Dalmane and Halcion. These medications may lead to overdose symptoms. Blood thinners such as Coumadin may cause bleeding. Use of narcotics, including methadone, may cause withdrawal symptoms.

Limit use of alcohol when taking Talwin Compound; the effects of alcohol are intensified.

Special Cautions

 If pregnant or planning to become pregnant, inform your doctor immediately. Not known if Talwin Compound appears in breast milk.

 No special precautions apply to seniors.

 Not generally prescribed for children under 12 years.

 Do not share Talwin Compound with others.

 May cause drowsiness and impair your ability to drive a car or operate machinery. *Do not take part in any activity that requires alertness.*

Before taking Talwin Compound, inform your doctor if you have kidney or liver disorder; experience seizures; have severe bronchial asthma or respiratory problems.

· ·

Use extremely cautiously if you have head injury. May cause breathing trouble and pressure on the skull, and may mask or hide pain from a head injury.

· ·

Use with caution if you have had a heart attack or are nauseated or vomiting.

· ·

May cause physical and psychological dependence. Inform your doctor of any drug addiction problems.

· ·

Avoid if sensitive to or allergic to pentazocine or salicylates (aspirin), or similar medications.

· ·

Due to risk of Reye's syndrome, should not give Talwin Compound to children and teenagers who have chicken pox or the flu.

· ·

Tell your doctor if you have an ulcer. Talwin Compound may irritate stomach lining and cause bleeding.

Tambocor

^^^

Generic name: Flecainide acetate

Tambocor is an anti-arrhythmic. It alters nerve impulses within the heart to regulate heartbeat.

℞ QUICK FACTS

Purpose

Used to treat certain heart rhythm irregularities, such as paroxysmal atrial fibrillation (sudden attack or worsening of irregular heartbeat in which upper chamber of the heart beats irregularly and very rapidly); and paroxysmal supraventricular tachycardia (sudden attack or worsening of abnormally fast but regular heart rate occurring intermittently).

Dosage

 Usually Tambocor therapy is started in the hospital. Once you are out of the hospital, you must follow your doctor's instructions carefully or you are at risk for serious heartbeat disturbances.

 Usual adult dose: 50 to 100 milligrams taken every 12 hours. Doctor may increase dose every 4 days by 50 milligrams every 12 hours until condition is stabilized. If you have alkaline urine as a result of being a vegetarian or have a kidney disorder, you may need a lower dosage, as Tambocor will be processed and eliminated at a slower pace in the body.

 Usual child dose: not generally prescribed for children.

 Missed dose—take as soon as possible, if within 6 hours of next dose. Otherwise, do not take missed dose; go back to regular schedule. *Do not double doses.*

Side Effects

 Moderate overdose can be fatal. Overdose symptoms: slowed or rapid heartbeat, other cardiac problems, fainting, low blood pressure, nausea, vomiting, convulsions, and heart failure. If you suspect an overdose, immediately seek medical attention.

 Side effects: congestive heart failure, heart block, heart attack, new or worsened heartbeat abnormalities. Other side effects: abdominal pain; angina (crushing chest pain); anxiety; apathy; appetite loss;

chest pain; confusion; constipation; convulsions; decreased sex drive; depression; diarrhea; difficult or labored breathing; dizziness; dry mouth; edema (fluid accumulation in tissues); exaggerated feeling of well-being; excessive urine; eye pain or irritation; faintness; fainting; fatigue; fever; flushing; gas; hair loss; headache; heart palpitations; high or low blood pressure; hives; impotence; inability to urinate; indigestion; insomnia; intolerance of light; involuntary eye movements; itching; joint pain; lack of coordination; loss of sense of identity; lung inflammation or other conditions; malaise (feeling ill); memory loss; morbid dreams; muscle pain; nausea; numbness or tingling; paralysis; rash; reduced sensitivity to touch; ringing in the ears; skin inflammation and peeling; sleepiness; speech problems; stupor; sweating; swollen lips, tongue, or mouth; taste changes; tremor; twitching; vertigo; vision problems (blurred vision, difficulty focusing, double vision, spots before eyes); vomiting; weakness; wheezing.

No known less common or rare side effects.

Interactions

Inform your doctor before combining Tambocor with: amiodarone (Cordarone); beta-blockers such as Inderal, Tenormin, and Sectral; carbamazepine (Tegretol); cimetidine (Tagamet); diltiazem (Cardizem); disopyramide (Norpace); nifedipine (Procardia); phenobarbital; phenytoin (Dilantin); verapamil (Calan or Isoptin).

No known food/other substance interactions.

Special Cautions

If pregnant or planning to become pregnant, inform your doctor immediately. Appears in breast milk; could affect a nursing infant.

 **65** No special precautions apply to seniors.

 Not generally prescribed for children.

 STOP Doctor should carefully explain risks of taking Tambocor *before* prescribing. Can cause or worsen heartbeat irregularities and heart failure.

A high or low level of potassium should be stabilized *before* starting Tambocor.

At increased risk for severe cardiac side effects if you have a history of congestive heart failure or a weak heart.

If you wear a pacemaker, it may need to be adjusted; doctor will closely monitor.

In the case of liver disease, doctor will monitor your blood. Tambocor can build up in your body.

Doctor will closely monitor if you have kidney failure.

Tamoxifen Citrate

see NOLVADEX

Tavist

Generic name: Clemastine fumarate

Other brand names: Tavist-1, Tavist-D

Tavist is an antihistamine. Antihistamines block the effects of histamine, a body chemical that causes swelling and itching.

℞ QUICK FACTS

Purpose

 Used to treat hay fever symptoms including sneezing, runny nose, itching, and watery eyes. Also used to treat mild allergic skin reactions such as hives and swelling; to reduce itching and swelling; and to dry up eye, nose, and throat secretions.

Dosage

 Take exactly as prescribed.

 Usual adult dose: *Tavist tablets*—1 tablet taken 3 times per day, not to exceed 3 tablets per day. *Tavist-1 tablets*—1 tablet taken 2 times per day, not to exceed 6 tablets per day. *Tavist syrup—For hay fever*—2 teaspoonfuls taken 2 times per day, not to exceed 12 teaspoonfuls per day. *For hives and swelling*—4 teaspoonfuls taken 2 times per day, not to exceed 12 teaspoonfuls per day.

 Usual child dose: *for hay fever*—1 teaspoon taken 2 times per day, not to exceed 6 teaspoonfuls per day. *For hives and swelling*—2 teaspoonfuls taken 2 times per day, not to exceed 6 teaspoonfuls per day. Not prescribed for children under 12 years.

 Missed dose: *if taking on a regular schedule*—take as soon as possible, unless almost time for next dose. In that case, do not take missed dose; go back to regular schedule. *Do not double doses.*

Side Effects

Overdose symptoms: coma, convulsions, drowsiness, dry mouth, fever, fixed or dilated pupils, flushing, stimulation (especially in children), stomach and intestinal problems. Overdose symptoms in children: bluish color to the skin; convulsions; excitement; hallucinations; high body temperature; slow, twisting movements of hand and arms; tremors; twitching; uncoordinated movements. If you suspect an overdose, immediately seek medical attention.

More common side effects: disturbed coordination, dizziness, drowsiness, extreme calm, sleepiness, upset stomach.

Less common or rare side effects: acute inflammation of the inner ear; anemia; blurred vision; chills; confusion; constipation; convulsions; diarrhea; difficulty sleeping; difficulty urinating; double vision; dry mouth, nose, and throat; early menstruation; exaggerated sense of well-being; excessive perspiration; excitement; fatigue; frequent urination; headache; hives; hysteria; inability to urinate; increased chest congestion; irregular heartbeat; irritability; loss of appetite; low blood pressure; nausea; nerve inflammation; nervousness; palpitations; rapid heartbeat; rash; restlessness; ringing in the ears; sensitivity to light; severe allergic reaction (anaphylactic shock); stuffy nose; tightness of chest; tingling or pins and needles; tremor; vertigo; vomiting; wheezing.

Interactions

Avoid Tavist if you are taking a MAO inhibitor such as Nardil or Parnate. Inform your doctor before combining Tavist with: sedatives such as Nembutal and Seconal, tranquilizers such as Xanax and Valium.

Do not drink alcohol while taking Tavist, it increases the effects of alcohol.

Special Cautions

 If pregnant or planning to become pregnant, inform your doctor immediately. Avoid Tavist if breastfeeding.

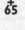 Seniors at higher risk for experiencing dizziness, sedation, or low blood pressure.

 Not generally prescribed for children under 12.

 Do not take if sensitive to or allergic to this or antihistamines with similar compounds.

May cause drowsiness and impair your ability to drive a car or operate machinery. *Do not take part in any activity that requires alertness.*

Use with extreme caution if you have narrow-angle glaucoma, peptic ulcer, intestinal blockage, bladder obstruction, or enlarged prostate.

Use with caution if you have history of bronchial asthma, heart disease, circulatory problems, overactive thyroid, or high blood pressure.

Tegretol

Generic name: Carbamazepine

Other brand name: Epitol, Atretol

Tegretol is an anticonvulsant. It acts as a depressant to the central nervous system.

℞ QUICK FACTS

Purpose

Used to treat seizure disorders, including certain types of epilepsy. Also used to treat trigeminal neuralgia (severe jaw pain), and pain in the tongue and throat. Also prescribed for alcohol withdrawal, cocaine addiction, emotional disorders such as depression and abnormally aggressive behavior, migraine headaches, and "restless legs."

Dosage

Always take with meals. Shake suspension well before using. *Do not suddenly stop if taking for seizures; may cause severe brain damage or death.*

. . . .

Usual adult dose: *for seizures*—one 200-milligram tablet taken 2 times per day or 1 teaspoonful taken 4 times per day. Doctor may increase at weekly intervals by adding 200-milligram or 2-teaspoonful doses up to 3 or 4 times per day. Dose should not exceed 1,200 milligrams per day. Usual maintenance dose ranges from 800 to 1,200 milligrams per day. *For trigeminal neuralgia*—one 100-milligram tablet taken 2 times per day or ½ teaspoonful 4 times on day 1. Doctor may increase by increments of 100 milligrams every 12 hours or 2 teaspoonfuls 4 times per day. Maximum daily dose—1,200 milligrams. Maintenance dose—400 to 800 milligrams per day.

. . . .

Usual child dose: *for seizures—children 6 to 12 years*—one 100-milligram tablet taken 2 times per day or ½ teaspoonful taken 4 times per day. Doctor may increase at weekly intervals by adding 100 milligrams or 1 teaspoonful 3 or 4 times per day. Maximum dose is 1,000 milligrams per day divided into 3 or 4 doses. Maintenance dose—400 to 800 milligrams per day. *For children over 12 years—same as adult dose.* Not generally prescribed for children under 6 years.

 Missed dose: take as soon as possible, unless almost time for next dose. In that case, do not take missed dose; go back to regular schedule. Call your doctor if you miss more than 1 dose in a day. *Do not double doses.*

Side Effects

 Overdose symptoms: coma, convulsions, dizziness, drowsiness, inability to urinate, involuntary rapid eye movements, irregular or reduced breathing, lack or absence of urine, lack of coordination, low or high blood pressure, muscle twitching, nausea, pupil dilation, rapid heartbeat, restlessness, severe muscle spasm, shock, tremors, unconsciousness, vomiting, writhing movements. Most signs of overdose occur within 1 to 3 hours. If you suspect an overdose, immediately seek medical attention.

 More common side effects: dizziness, drowsiness, nausea, unsteadiness, vomiting.

 Other side effects: abdominal pain, abnormal heartbeat and rhythm, abnormal involuntary movements, abnormal sensitivity to sound, aching joints and muscles, agitation, anemia, blood clots, blurred vision, chills, confusion, congestive heart failure, constipation, depression, diarrhea, double vision, dry mouth and throat, fainting and collapse, fatigue, fever, fluid retention, frequent urination, hair loss, hallucinations, headache, hepatitis, hives, impotence, inability to urinate, inflammation of the mouth and tongue, inflamed eyes, involuntary movements of the eyeball, itching, kidney failure, labored breathing, leg cramps, liver disorders, loss of appetite, loss of coordination, low blood pressure, pneumonia, reddened skin, reddish or purplish skin spots, reduced urine volume, ringing in ears, sensitivity to light, skin inflammation and scaling, skin peeling, skin rashes, skin pigmentation changes, speech difficulties, stomach problems, sweating, talkativeness, tingling sensation, worsening of high blood pressure, yellow skin and eyes.

Interactions

 Inform your doctor before combining Tegretol with antiseizure medications such as phenytoin (Dilantin) or primidone (Mysoline); may reduce effectiveness of Tegretol. Other anticonvulsants may change thyroid gland function. Haldol and Depakene may be reduced if taken with Tegretol. erythromycin, cimetidine (Tagamet), Darvon, Rifamate, or calcium channel blockers such as Calan raise the amount of Tegretol in the bloodstream to dangerous levels. Lithium may cause serious nervous system side effects. Oral contraceptives combined with Tegretol may result in blood spotting and reduction in contraceptive's effectiveness. Theo-Dur, Vibramycin, Dilantin, and Coumadin activity may be significantly affected.

 No known food/other substance interactions.

Special Cautions

 Birth defects have been reported with Tegretol use. If pregnant or planning to become pregnant, inform your doctor immediately. Appears in breast milk; could affect a nursing infant.

 Doctor will monitor level of Tegretol in your blood to determine the correct dosage. Seniors may experience agitation or confusion with Tegretol.

 Follow doctor's instructions carefully. Not generally prescribed for children under 6 years.

In rare cases may cause severe, fatal skin reactions. Immediately contact your doctor if you experience skin problems.

May cause drowsiness and impair your ability to drive a car or operate machinery. *Do not take part in any activity that requires alertness.*

Talk with your doctor before starting Tegretol if you have: history of heart, liver or kidney damage, adverse blood reaction to any medication, glaucoma, or allergic reactions to other medications.

Immediately inform your doctor if you experience: fever, sore throat, ulcers in the mouth, easy bruising, or red or purple skin spots. May be symptoms of a blood disorder caused by Tegretol.

Avoid if you have: history of bone marrow depression (reduced function), sensitivity to Tegretol, sensitivity to tricyclic antidepressants such as Elavil, or if taking a MAO inhibitor such as Nardil or Parnate. Wait at least 2 weeks before starting Tegretol if you have taken MAO inhibitors.

Not prescribed for minor aches and pains.

Temazepam
see RESTORIL

Temovate

Generic name: Clobetasol propionate

Temovate is a topical adrenocorticoid/anti-inflammatory. It interferes with the natural body mechanisms that produce rash, itching, or inflammation.

℞ QUICK FACTS

Purpose

℞ Used to treat itching and inflammation of moderate to severe scalp conditions. Scalp application is for short-term treatment; cream and ointment are for short-term treatment of skin conditions on the body.

Dosage

 Take exactly as prescribed. Keep away from eyes.

 Usual adult dose: *cream or ointment*—gently rub thin layer into affected area 2 times per day, in the morning and evening. Treatment should not exceed 2 weeks. Area should not be covered, avoid using more than 50 grams (1 large tube). *Scalp application*—apply to affected scalp area 2 times per day, in the morning and night. Treatment should not exceed 2 weeks. Area should not be covered, avoid using more than 50 grams (1 large tube).

 Usual child dose: *for children 12 years and older*—same as adult dose. Not prescribed for children under 12 years.

 Missed dose: apply as soon as possible, unless almost time for next dose. In that case, do not apply missed dose, go back to regular schedule.

Side Effects

 Overdose symptoms: increase in blood sugar, Cushing's syndrome (moon-shaped face, emotional disturbances, high blood pressure, weight gain, and body and facial hair growth in women). If you suspect an overdose, immediately seek medical attention.

 More common side effects: *Temovate cream*—localized stinging or burning. *Temovate ointment*—burning sensation, irritation, itching. *Temovate scalp application*—burning and/or stinging sensation, scalp pustules, tingling.

 Less common side effects: *Temovate cream*—cracks and grooves in skin, itching. *Temovate ointment*—cracking of skin, finger numbness, inflammation of hair follicles, localized red spots that become pale or white with pressure, stinging, unusual skin redness. *Temovate scalp application*—eye irritation, hair loss, headache, itching, skin inflammation, tenderness, tightness of scalp. Rare side effects of all forms of Temovate: acne, additional infections, allergic contact skin reactions, dryness, excessive hair growth, prickly heat, skin softening.

Interactions

 No drug interactions reported.

No known food/other substance interactions.

Special Cautions

 Strong corticosteroids such as Temovate cause birth defects in animals. Temovate may also be absorbed into the skin. If pregnant or planning to become pregnant, inform your doctor immediately. Not known if Temovate appears in breast milk.

65 No special precautions apply to seniors.

Not generally prescribed for children under 12.

To avoid absorption into bloodstream: never use large amounts over large areas of the body, *and do not cover with airtight bandages unless specifically directed by your doctor.*

Should not use if sensitive to or allergic to this or other corticosteroids, or any of the ingredients in corticosteroids. If scalp infection is present, avoid using Temovate Scalp Application.

Not to be used for other than condition for which Temovate was prescribed.

Inform your doctor of any localized side effects.

Tenex

Generic name: Guanfacine hydrochloride

Tenex is an antihypertensive. It works to reduce blood pressure by reducing nerve impulses to the heart and arteries.

℞ QUICK FACTS

Purpose

 Used to treat high blood pressure. May be prescribed alone or with other high blood pressure medications such as thiazide diuretics.

Dosage

 May take several weeks to observe full effects of medication. Take Tenex regularly for it to be effective; continue to take even if you feel well. Causes drowsiness, so take at bedtime. *Do not stop taking abruptly.*

Usual adult dose: 1 milligram per day taken at bed-time. Doctor may increase after 3 to 4 weeks up to 2 milligrams per day. Doctor will adjust doses if you have kidney damage and are also taking phenytoin (Dilantin).

 Usual child dose: not generally prescribed for children under 12 years.

 Missed dose: take as soon as possible, unless almost time for next dose. In that case, do not take missed dose; go back to regular schedule. *Do not double doses.*

Side Effects

 Overdose symptoms: drowsiness, lethargy, slowed heartbeat, very low blood pressure. If you suspect an overdose, immediately seek medical attention.

 More common side effects: constipation, dizziness, dry mouth, fatigue, headache, impotence, sleepiness, weakness.

 Less common or rare side effects: abdominal pain, amnesia, breathing difficulties, chest pain, confusion, conjunctivitis (pinkeye), decreased sex drive, depression, diarrhea, difficulty swallowing, fainting, heart palpitations, indigestion, insomnia, itching, leg cramps, malaise (vague feeling of illness), nausea, numbness or tingling skin, purplish skin spots, rash and peeling, runny nose, skin inflammation, slow heartbeat, upset stomach, urinary incontinence, vision disturbance.

Interactions

 Inform your doctor before combining Tenex with: barbiturates such as Amytal, Seconal, and Tuinal; benzodiazepines such as Tranxene, Valium, and

Xanax; phenothiazines such as Mellaril, Stelazine, and Thorazine; phenytoin (Dilantin).

 No known food/other substance interactions.

Special Cautions

 Should not be taken if pregnant. If pregnant or planning to become pregnant, inform your doctor immediately. Not known if Tenex appears in breast milk.

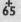 No special precautions apply to seniors.

 Not generally prescribed for children under 12.

 May cause drowsiness and dizziness and impair your ability to drive a car or operate machinery. *Do not take part in any activity that requires alertness.*

Doctor should closely monitor during Tenex therapy if you have: chronic kidney or liver failure, heart disease, history of stroke, recent heart attack.

If you stop taking abruptly, may cause nervousness, rapid pulse, anxiety, heartbeat irregularities, and rebound high blood pressure—higher blood pressure than before treatment began. Rebound high blood pressure usually occurs 2 to 4 days after the end of therapy, and will disappear over 2 to 4 days.

Tenoretic

Generic name: Atenolol with chlorthalidone

Tenoretic is a beta-adrenergic blocking agent (beta-blocker) and diuretic combination. Beta-blockers decrease the workload of the heart and help to regulate heartbeat. Diuretics lower blood pressure by helping the body produce and eliminate more urine.

℞ QUICK FACTS

Purpose

℞ Used to treat high blood pressure. Combines a beta-blocker, which decreases the force and rate of heart contractions; and a diuretic, which makes the body produce and eliminate more urine, thereby lowering blood pressure. Can be used alone or with other high blood pressure medications.

Dosage

 May take with or without food, per doctor's instructions. Take exactly as prescribed, even if symptoms disappear. Try not to miss dose; condition may worsen if not taken regularly. Should not be stopped suddenly, for this can increase chest pain; dosage must be reduced gradually.

 Usual adult dose: starting dose—one Tenoretic-50 tablet taken 1 time per day. Doctor may increase up to one Tenoretic-100 tablet taken 1 time per day. Dose is tailored to meet individual needs, and may be combined with other high blood pressure medications. *For kidney disorder*—dose will be adjusted accordingly.

 Usual child dose: not generally prescribed for children.

 Missed dose: take as soon as possible, *unless within 8 hours of next dose. In that case, do not take missed dose; go back to regular dose. Do not double doses.*

Side Effects

 Overdose symptoms: no specific information available for Tenoretic. Symptoms of atenolol overdose: bronchospasm, congestive heart failure, low blood pressure, low blood sugar, slow heartbeat, sluggishness, wheezing. Symptoms of chlorthalidone component overdose: dizziness, nausea, weakness. If you suspect an overdose, immediately seek medical attention.

 More common side effects: dizziness, fatigue, nausea, slow heartbeat.

 Less common side effects: blood disorders, constipation, cramping, decreased sexual activity, depression, diarrhea, difficult or labored breathing, dizziness when getting up, drowsiness, excessive thirst, hair loss, headache, high blood sugar, hives, impotence, light-headedness, loss of appetite, low potassium leading to symptoms like dry mouth, muscle pain or cramps, muscle spasm, Peyronie's disease (deformity of the penis), psoriasis-like rash, rash, reddish or purplish spots on the skin, restlessness, skin sensitivity to light, sluggishness or unresponsiveness, stomach irritation, sugar in the urine, tingling or pins and needles, tiredness, vertigo, visual disturbances, vomiting, weak or irregular heartbeat, weakness, worsening of psoriasis, yellow eyes and skin.

Interactions

 Inform your doctor before combining Tenoretic with: blood pressure medicines containing reserpine; clonidine (Catapres); epinephrine (EpiPen); insulin; lithium (Eskalith); nasal decongestants; other blood pressure drugs.

No known food/other substance interactions.

Special Cautions

 If pregnant or planning to become pregnant, inform your doctor immediately. May cause harm to a developing fetus. Appears in breast milk; could affect a nursing infant.

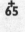 Seniors with reduced kidney function may be prescribed a lower dosage.

 Not generally prescribed for children.

 Do not take if you have: heart block (conduction disorder); heart failure; inability to urinate; inadequate blood supply to the circulatory system (cardiogenic shock); sensitivity for allergic reaction to atenolol or chlorthalidone or similar drugs, or other sulfur drugs; slow heartbeat.

May cause drowsiness and impair your ability to drive a car or operate machinery. *Do not take part in any activity that requires alertness.*

Can cause heartbeat to become too slow.

Use with caution with: asthma, coronary artery disease, kidney disease, history of severe congestive heart failure, seasonal allergies, or other bronchial conditions.

May mask the symptoms of low blood sugar or alter blood sugar levels.

Notify your doctor or dentist in a medical emergency or before surgery.

Tenormin

∿∿∿∿∿∿∿∿∿∿∿∿∿∿∿∿∿∿∿∿∿∿∿∿∿∿∿∿∿∿∿∿∿

Generic name: Atenolol

Tenormin is a beta-adrenergic blocking agent (beta-blocker). Beta-blockers decrease the workload of the heart and help regulate the heartbeat.

℞ QUICK FACTS

Purpose

Used in the treatment of high blood pressure, angina (chest pain) and heart attack. Also prescribed for alcohol withdrawal, prevention of migraine, and anxiety.

Dosage

May take with or without food, per doctor's instructions. Take exactly as prescribed, even if symptoms disappear. If taking once a day, try not to miss dose; condition may worsen if not taken regularly. Should not be stopped suddenly, can increase chest pain; dosage must be reduced gradually.

. . . .

Usual adult dose: 50 milligrams per day in 1 dose, taken alone or with a diuretic. Will see full effect in 1 to 2 weeks. Doctor may increase up to 100 milligrams per day maximum. *Angina*—50 milligrams per day in 1 dose, taken alone or with a diuretic. Will see full effect in 1 week. Doctor may increase up to 100 milligrams per day maximum, and is individualized. *For heart attack*—dose is individualized. *Seniors*—dose is individualized.

. . . .

Usual child dose: not generally prescribed for children.

. . . .

Missed dose: take as soon as possible, *unless within 8 hours of next dose. In that case, do not take missed dose; go back to regular dose. Do not double doses.*

Side Effects

 Overdose symptoms: bronchospasm, changes in breathing, congestive heart failure, low blood pressure, low blood sugar, slow heartbeat, sluggishness, wheezing. If you suspect an overdose, immediately seek medical attention.

 More common side effects: dizziness, fatigue, nausea, slow heartbeat.

 Less common or rare side effects: depression, diarrhea, difficult or labored breathing, dizziness upon standing up, drowsiness, headache, heart failure, impotence, light-headedness, low blood pressure, penile deformity, psoriasis-like rash, red or purple spots on the skin, rapid heartbeat, slow heartbeat, sluggishness, temporary hair loss, tiredness, vertigo, wheezing, worsening of psoriasis.

Interactions

 Inform your doctor before taking Tenormin with: ampicillin (Omnipen), calcium-containing antacids such as Tums, calcium-blocking blood pressure drugs such as Calan and Cardizem, certain blood pressure drugs such as reserpine (Diupres), epinephrine (Epipen), insulin, oral diabetes drugs such as Micronase, quinidine (Quindex).

 No known food/other substance interactions.

Special Cautions

 If pregnant or planning to become pregnant, inform your doctor immediately. May cause harm to a developing fetus. Appears in breast milk; could affect a nursing infant.

 Dose is individualized for seniors.

 Not generally prescribed for children.

STOP *Do not take if you have: heart failure, inadequate blood supply to the circulatory system (cardiogenic shock), heart block (conduction disorder), severely slow heartbeat.*

With high blood pressure, must be taken regularly to be effective.

Can cause heartbeat to become too slow.

Use with caution if you have: asthma, coronary artery disease, kidney disease, history of severe congestive heart failure, seasonal allergies or other bronchial conditions.

May mask the symptoms of low blood sugar or alter blood sugar levels.

Notify your doctor or dentist in a medical emergency or before surgery.

Tenuate

Generic name: Diethylpropion hydrochloride

Other brand names: Tenuate Dospan, Tepanil, Tepanil Ten-tab

Tenuate is a non-amphetamine appetite suppressant. It relieves hunger by altering nerve impulses to the appetite control center of the brain.

℞ QUICK FACTS

Purpose

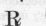 Used on a short-term basis as part of a weight reduction plan that includes behavior modification. Comes in immediate and controlled release forms.

Dosage

 Take exactly as prescribed. May be habit-forming. *Do not crush or chew tablets; swallow them whole.*

 Usual adult dose: *immediate-release*—one 25-milligram tablet taken 3 times per day, 1 hour before meals. To avoid night hunger, take 1 tablet in the middle of the evening. *Tenuate Dospan controlled-release*—one 75-milligram tablet taken once per day, in midmorning.

 Usual child dose: not generally prescribed for children under 12 years.

 Missed dose: *immediate-release*—go back to regular schedule at the next meal. *Tenuate Dospan controlled-release*—take as soon as possible, unless it is the next day. In that case, do not take missed dose; go back to regular schedule. *Do not double doses.*

Side Effects

 Overdose symptoms: abdominal cramps, assaultiveness, confusion, depression, diarrhea, elevated blood pressure, fatigue, hallucinations, irregular heartbeat, lowered blood pressure, nausea, overactive reflexes, panic state, rapid breathing, restlessness, tremors, vomiting. If you suspect an overdose, immediately seek medical attention.

 Side effects: abdominal discomfort, abnormal redness of the skin, anxiety, blood pressure elevation, blurred vision, breast development in males, bruising, changes in sex drive, chest pain, constipation, depression, diarrhea, difficulty with voluntary movements, dizziness, drowsiness, dryness of the mouth, feelings of discomfort, feelings of elation, feeling of illness, hair loss, headache, hives, impotence, inability to fall or stay asleep, increased heart rate, increased seizures in epileptics, increased sweating, increased volume of diluted urine, irregular heartbeat, jitteriness, menstrual upset, muscle pain, nausea, nervousness, overstimulation, painful urination, palpitations, pupil dilation, rash, restlessness, shortness of breath or labored breathing, stomach and intestinal disturbances, tremors, unpleasant taste, vomiting.

 No known less common or rare side effects.

Interactions

 Inform your doctor before combining Tenuate with: blood pressure medications such as Ismelin; insulin; phenothiazine medications such as the major tranquilizer Thorazine.

 Do not drink alcohol during Tenuate therapy.

Special Cautions

 If pregnant or planning to become pregnant, inform your doctor immediately. Appears in breast milk; could affect a nursing infant.

65 No special precautions apply to seniors.

Not generally prescribed for children under 12.

 Do not take if you have: severe hardening of the arteries, overactive thyroid, glaucoma, severe high blood pressure, agitation, history of drug abuse, or have taken a MAO inhibitor within the last 14 days.

May impair your ability to drive a car or operate machinery. *Do not take part in any activity that requires alertness.*

Tenuate loses effectiveness after a few weeks; stop medication rather than increase dosage.

Avoid if sensitive to or allergic to this or other appetite suppressants.

Use with caution if you have heart disease.

At risk for increase in convulsions if you have epilepsy.

Inform your doctor if you start to rely on Tenuate to maintain a state of well-being; can cause psychological dependence.

Tepanil
see TENUATE

Terazol 3

Generic name: Terconazole

Other brand name: Terazol 7

Terazol 3 is an antifungal. It destroys and prevents the growth of fungi.

℞ QUICK FACTS

Purpose

℞   Used to treat candidiasis, a yeast-like infection of the vulva and vagina.

Dosage

 Apply as prescribed by your doctor. Comes in cream and suppository form. Wear cotton underwear during Terazol therapy. Dry genital area thoroughly after a shower, bath, or swim. Change from damp or wet clothing as soon as possible. *Do not use tampons, as they absorb the medication. Do not douche unless specifically directed by your doctor.* Scratching may cause more irritation and cause infection to spread. Use full course of treatment even if symptoms disappear; otherwise infection can return. Continue using during your menstrual period.

 Usual adult dose: *vaginal cream*—1 full applicator (5 grams) inserted vaginally once per day at bedtime for 3 consecutive days. *Vaginal suppositories*—1 suppository inserted vaginally once per day at bedtime for 3 consecutive days. Terazol-7 is usually prescribed for 7 consecutive days.

 Usual child dose: not generally prescribed for children.

 Missed dose: take as soon as possible, unless almost time for next dose. In that case, do not take missed dose; go back to regular schedule. *Do not double doses.*

Side Effects

 Overdose symptoms: no reported overdose symptoms. However, if you suspect an overdose, immediately seek medical attention.

 More common side effects: body pain, burning, genital pain, headache, menstrual pain.

 Less common side effects: abdominal pain, chills, fever, itching.

Interactions

 No drug interactions reported.

 No known food/other substance interactions.

Special Cautions

 Should not use during first 3 months of pregnancy (first trimester) since the drug is absorbed from the vagina. Not known if Terazol 3 appears in breast milk.

 No special precautions apply to seniors.

 Not generally prescribed for children.

 Avoid if sensitive to or allergic to Terazol 3.

Contact your doctor if you develop: irritation, allergic reaction, fever, chills, or flu-like symptoms.

Either use nonlatex condoms or avoid sexual intercourse to prevent reinfection.

Can interact with latex products (diaphragms, some condoms) and compromise their effectiveness.

Terazosin Hydrochloride

see HYTRIN

Terbutaline Sulfate

see BRETHINE

Terconazole

see TERAZOL 3

Terfenadine

see SELDANE

Tessalon

Generic name: Benzonatate

Tessalon is a non-narcotic antitussive agent. It works by acting on the brain to suppress the cough reflex.

℞ QUICK FACTS

Purpose

℞   Used to relieve a cough.

Dosage

 Swallow capsule whole, should not be chewed. *Chewing capsule may temporarily numb mouth and throat, causing choking or severe allergic reaction.*

 Usual adult dose: one 100-milligram perle taken 3 times per day, as needed, up to 600 milligrams or 6 perles per day.

 Usual child dose: for children over 10—same as adults.

 Missed dose: take as soon as possible, unless almost time for next dose. In that case, do not take missed dose; go back to regular schedule. *Do not double doses.*

Side Effects

 Overdose symptoms: mouth and throat numbness if capsules are chewed or dissolved; restlessness; tremors; convulsions. If you suspect an overdose, immediately seek medical attention.

 Side effects: allergic reactions, burning sensation in the eyes, constipation, dizziness, extreme calm, headache, itching, mental confusion, nausea, numbness in chest, skin eruptions, stuffy nose, upset stomach, vague "chilly" feeling, visual hallucinations.

 No known less common or rare side effects.

Interactions

 Inform your doctor before combining Tessalon with other prescription medications. On rare occasions bizarre behavior, confusion, and visual hallucinations have occurred.

No known food/other substance interactions.

Special Cautions

 If pregnant or planning to become pregnant, inform your doctor immediately. Not known if Tessalon appears in breast milk.

 No special precautions apply to seniors.

 Not generally prescribed for children under 10 years. Follow doctor's instructions carefully for children ages 10 and older.

 Avoid if sensitive to or allergic to this or similar medications, such as local anesthetics.

Tetracycline Hydrochloride
see ACHROMYCIN V CAPSULES

Tetracyn
see ACHROMYCIN V CAPSULES

Thalitone
see HYGROTON

Theo-Dur

Generic name: Theophylline

Other brand names: *Sustained-action—*
Aerolate Capsules, Constant-T, Elixophyllin SR,
Quibron-T/SR, Respbid, Slo-bid Gyrocaps,
Slo-Phyllin Gyrocaps, Susaire, Theobid Duracaps,
Theobid Jr. Duracaps, Theoclear L.A., Theocron,
Theo-Dur Sprinkle, Theolair-SR, Theophylline S.R.,
Theo-Sav, Theospan-SR, Theo-24, Theovent,
T-Phyl, Uniphyl. *Extended-release—*Accubron,
Aquaphyllin, Asmalix, Bronkodyl, Elixomin,
Elixophyllin, Lanophyllin, Quibron-T, Slo-Phyllin,
Theoclear, Theolair, Theostat

Theo-Dur is a xanthine bronchodilator. It works by relaxing the smooth muscle of the bronchial airways, thereby opening air passages to the lungs.

℞ QUICK FACTS

Purpose

℞ Used to prevent or relieve asthma, chronic bronchitis, and emphysema. Active ingredient is theophylline, a chemical cousin of caffeine.

Dosage

 Take exactly as prescribed. Comes in extended-
release and sustained-action forms. Swallow extended-release form whole; never crush or swallow;
and may take with or without food. Must take sustained-action (Theo-Dur Sprinkle) 1 hour before or
2 hours after a meal. May swallow capsule whole or
empty contents onto a spoonful of soft (not hot)
food, not crushing or chewing contents. Follow with

glass of cool water or juice. Only doctor or pharmacist should change brands.

Usual adult dose: *extended-release*—initially 1 Theo-Dur 200-milligram tablet every 12 hours. Doctor will gradually increase up to 900 milligrams per day. *Theo-Dur Sprinkle*—no more than 200 milligrams every 12 hours. Doctor may increase up to 900 milligrams per day. Dose may be divided into 3 doses.

Usual child dose: *extended-release*—*55 to 76 pounds*—500 milligrams. *Extended-release*—*77 through 154 pounds*—600 milligrams. *Theo-Dur Sprinkle*—*children ages 6 to 8*—24 milligrams per 2.2 pounds of body weight. *Theo-Dur Sprinkle*—*children ages 9 to 11*—20 milligrams per 2.2 pounds of body weight. *Theo-Dur Sprinkle*—*children ages 12 to 15*—18 milligrams per 2.2 pounds of body weight. For children under 55 pounds—liquid preparation recommended before switching to tablet or sprinkle form.

Missed dose: take as soon as possible, unless almost time for next dose. In that case, do not take missed dose, go back to regular schedule. *Do not double doses.*

Side Effects

Overdose symptoms: flu shot or influenza may cause usual dose to act like an overdose. Most of side effects are caused by slight overdose. Mild overdose symptoms: nausea and restlessness. *Larger overdose may cause serious heartbeat irregularities, convulsions, or death.* If you suspect an overdose, immediately seek medical attention.

Most common side effects: restlessness, nausea. Other side effects: convulsions, diarrhea, disturbances of heart rhythm, excitability, flushing, frequent urination, hair loss, headache, heart palpitations, high blood sugar, irritability, low blood pressure, muscle twitching, nausea, rapid breathing, rapid heartbeat, rash, restlessness, sleeplessness, stomach pain, vomiting, vomiting blood. May also cause or worsen heartbeat abnormalities. Contact your doctor if you notice significant change in your heart rate or rhythm.

 No known less common or rare side effects.

Interactions

 Inform your doctor before combining Theo-Dur with: allopurinol (Lopurin or Zyloprim); cimetidine (Tagamet); ciprofloxacin (Cipro); ephedrine in medications (Primatene, Tedral, or Rynatuss); erythromycin (E.E.S., ERYC, or Erythrocin); lithium carbonate (Eskalith or Lithobid); oral contraceptives; phenytoin (Dilantin); propranolol (Inderal); rifampin (Rifadin, Rifamate, or Rimactane); troleandomycin (Tao).

 Avoid large amounts of caffeine-containing beverages.

Special Cautions

 If pregnant or planning to become pregnant, inform your doctor immediately. Appears in breast milk, causing irritability and other harm to nursing baby.

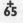 Seniors should use with precaution, especially males over 55 with chronic lung disease.

 Follow doctor's instructions carefully for children over 10 years.

 Do not take if sensitive to or allergic to Theo-Dur, or if you have an active peptic ulcer.

If epileptic, make sure your antiseizure medication is the correct dose before taking Theo-Dur.

Use cautiously if you have or had: sustained a high fever, heart disease or liver failure, high blood pressure, low blood oxygen, alcoholism, or history of stomach ulcers.

Theophylline
see THEO-DUR

Thermazene
see SILVADENE CREAM 1%

Thioridazine Hydrochloride
see MELLARIL

Thiothixene
see NAVANE

Thorazine

Generic name: Chlorpromazine

Other brand names: Ormazine, Promapar, Promaz, Sonazine, Thor-Prom

Thorazine is an antipsychotic/anti-emetic. It calms certain areas of the brain while enabling the rest of the brain to function normally.

℞ QUICK FACTS

Purpose

℞ Used to reduce symptoms of psychotic disorders such as schizophrenia; to treat severe behavior disorders in children (hyperactivity and combativeness) on a short-term basis; and to treat the hyperenergetic phase of manic-depressive illness. Also used for nausea and vomiting, and to relieve restlessness and apprehension prior to surgery. Also prescribed to treat tetanus; uncontrollable hiccups; and attacks of severe abdominal pain with psychiatric disturbances; cramps in the arms and legs; and muscle weakness (porphyria).

Dosage

 If using liquid concentrate, dilute with carbonated drink, coffee, fruit juice, milk, tea, tomato juice, water, puddings, or soups. Take immediately after preparing. *Do not take antacids such as Gelusil at the same time; should have 1 or 2 hours between taking the two. Do not discontinue unless directed by your doctor, or you may experience serious withdrawal symptoms.*

 Usual adult dose: *psychotic disorders*—30 to 75 milligrams per day, divided into 3 or 4 equal doses. Doctor may increase by 20 to 50 milligrams at semi-weekly intervals. *For nausea and vomiting*—10 to 25 milligrams in tablet form taken every 4 to 6 hours as needed. Doctor may also prescribe one 100-milligram suppository every 6 to 8 hours. *For uncontrollable hiccups*—75 to 200 milligrams per day divided into 3 or 4 equal doses. *For porphyria*—75 to 200

·

milligrams per day divided into 3 or 4 equal doses.
Seniors—generally prescribed lower doses due to risk
of low blood pressure and tardive dyskinesia.

 Usual child dose: *for severe behavior problems, nausea,
and vomiting*—based on child's weight. Oral dose—
¼ milligram for each 1 pound of weight, taken every
4 to 6 hours as needed. Rectal dose—½ milligram
per 1 pound of body weight, taken every 6 to 8
hours as needed. Not generally prescribed for children under 6 months.

 Missed dose: *if taking 1 dose per day*—take as soon
as possible, unless almost time for next dose. In that
case, do not take missed dose; go back to regular
schedule. *If taking more than 1 dose per day*—take as
soon as possible, unless within 1 hour of next dose.
In that case, do not take missed dose; go back to
regular schedule. *Do not double doses.*

Side Effects

 Thorazine overdose may be fatal. Overdose symptoms:
agitation, coma, convulsions, difficulty breathing, difficulty swallowing, dry mouth, extreme sleepiness,
fever, intestinal blockage, irregular heart rate, low
blood pressure, restlessness. Overdose symptoms
may be hidden, as Thorazine prevents vomiting. If
you suspect an overdose, immediately seek medical
attention.

 Side effects: abnormal milk secretion; abnormalities
in movement and posture; agitation; anemia; asthma;
blood disorders; breast development in males; chewing movements; constipation; difficulty breathing;
difficulty swallowing; dizziness; drooling; drowsiness;
dry mouth; ejaculation problems; eye problems
causing fixed gaze; fainting; fever; flu-like symptoms;
fluid accumulation and swelling; headache; heart attack; high or low blood sugar; hives; impotence; in-

ability to urinate; inability to move or talk; increase
of appetite; infections; insomnia; intestinal blockage;
involuntary movement of arms and legs, tongue,
face, mouth, or jaw; irregular blood pressure, pulse,
and heartbeat; irregular or no menstrual periods; jitteriness; light-headedness; lockjaw; mask-like face;
muscle stiffness and rigidity; narrow or dilated
pupils; nasal congestion; nausea; pain and stiffness in
the neck; persistent or painful erections; pill-rolling
motion; protruding tongue; puckering of the mouth;
puffing of the cheeks; rapid heartbeat; red or purple skin spots; rigid arms, feet, head, and muscles
(including the back); seizures; sensitivity to light; severe allergic reactions; shuffling walk; skin inflammation and peeling; sore throat; spasms in jaw, face,
tongue, neck, mouth, and feet; sweating; swelling of
breasts in women; swelling of the throat; tremors;
twitching in the body, neck, shoulders, and face;
twisted neck; visual problems; weight gain; yellowed
skin and eyes.

No known less common or rare side effects.

Interactions

Inform your doctor before combining Thorazine
with: anesthetics; anticonvulsants such as Dilantin;
antispasmodics such as Cogentin; atropine (Donnatal); barbiturates such as phenobarbital; blood
thinners such as Coumadin; Captopril (Capoten);
cimetidine (Tagamet); diuretics such as Dyazide;
epinephrine (EpiPen); guanethidine (Ismelin); lithium
(Lithonate); MAO inhibitors such as Nardil and Parnate; narcotics such as Percocet; propranolol (Inderal). Demerol and other narcotics may cause extreme drowsiness.

Avoid alcohol use during Thorazine therapy.

Special Cautions

 If pregnant or planning to become pregnant, inform your doctor immediately. Appears in breast milk; could affect a nursing infant.

 Seniors are prescribed lower doses due to increased risk for low blood pressure and tardive dyskinesia, a condition marked by involuntary muscle spasms and twitches in the face and body. Senior women are particularly at risk.

 Follow doctor's instructions carefully for children.

 At risk for neuroleptic malignant syndrome, which may be fatal. Symptoms: extremely high body temperature, rigid muscles, mental changes, irregular pulse or blood pressure, rapid heartbeat, sweating, and changes in heart rhythm.

May impair your ability to drive a car or operate machinery. *Do not take part in any activity that requires alertness.*

Ask your doctor about the risk of tardive dyskinesia, a condition marked by involuntary muscle movements.

Avoid if allergic to any major tranquilizers containing phenothiazine.

Use with caution if you have or had: asthma; brain tumor; breast cancer; intestinal blockage; emphysema; glaucoma; heart, kidney, or liver disease; respiratory infections; seizures; abnormal bone marrow or blood condition; exposure to pesticides; exposure to extreme heat.

May mask symptoms of brain tumor, intestinal blockage, and Reye's syndrome.

Thorazine can suppress cough reflex, making it difficult to vomit.

Sunlight sensitivity may be increased.

Side effects may worsen over time with prolonged therapy.

Thyroid Hormone

see ARMOUR THYROID

Thyroid Strong

see ARMOUR THYROID

Tigan

Generic name: Trimethobenzamide hydrochloride

Other brand names: Tebamide Suppositories, Tegamide, T-Gen, Ticon, Tiject-20, Trimazide

Tigan is an anti-emetic. It is thought to act by inhibiting impulses to the vomiting center in the brain.

℞ QUICK FACTS

Purpose

℞   Used to control nausea and vomiting.

Dosage

 Take exactly as prescribed. If using suppository and it is too soft, can chill in refrigerator for approximately 30 minutes or run cold water over suppository while still in the wrapper. Insert suppository well up into rectum.

 Usual adult dose: *capsules*—one 250-milligram capsule taken 3 or 4 times per day. *Suppositories*—1 suppository (200 milligrams) inserted rectally 3 or 4 times per day.

 Usual child dose: *capsules*—for children weighing 30 to 90 pounds—one or two 100-milligram capsules taken 3 or 4 times per day. *Suppositories*—for children weighing under 30 pounds—½ suppository (100 milligrams) inserted rectally 3 or 4 times per day. For children weighing 30 to 90 pounds—½ to one 200-milligram suppository inserted rectally 3 or 4 times per day. *Pediatric suppositories*—for children weighing under 30 pounds—1 suppository (100 milligrams) inserted rectally 3 or 4 times per day. For children weighing 30 to 90 pounds—1 or 2 suppositories (100 to 200 milligrams) rectally 3 or 4 times per day.

 Missed dose: take as soon as possible, unless almost time for next dose. In that case, do not take missed dose; go back to regular schedule. *Do not double doses.*

Side Effects

 Overdose symptoms: no specific information available. If you suspect an overdose, immediately seek medical attention.

Side effects: allergic-type skin reactions, blurred vision, coma, convulsions, depression, diarrhea, disorientation, dizziness, drowsiness, headache, muscle cramps, severe muscle spasm, tremors, yellowed eyes and skin.

 No known less common or rare side effects.

Interactions

 Inform your doctor before combining Tigan with: central nervous system medications such as phenothiazines (tranquilizers and anti-emetics); barbiturates such as phenobarbital; medications derived from belladonna such as Donnatal; if you are dehydrated; or have a severe disease with fever, inflammation of the stomach, intestines, or brain.

 Avoid using alcohol with Tigan.

Special Cautions

 If pregnant or planning to become pregnant, inform your doctor immediately. Not known if Tigan appears in breast milk.

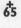 Seniors should use with caution if you have severe illness with high fever, brain inflammation, stomach or intestinal inflammation, or dehydration.

 Follow doctor's instructions carefully for children. Not for use to treat simple vomiting in children; used for prolonged vomiting due to a known disease. Use with caution if you have severe illness with high fever, brain inflammation, stomach or intestinal inflammation, or dehydration. May be link to Reye's syndrome if used to treat viral illnesses in children. *Do not use suppositories in premature or newborn infants.*

Do not take if sensitive to. Do not use suppositories if allergic to benzocaine or other local anesthetics.

May impair your ability to drive a car or operate machinery. *Do not take part in any activity that requires alertness.*

If you have a weakened condition, use with caution if you have severe illness with high fever, brain inflammation, stomach or intestinal inflammation, or dehydration.

Antinausea effects may mask conditions such as appendicitis or overdose of other medications.

Tilade

Generic name: Nedocromil sodium

Tilade is an anti-asthmatic. It works by stimulating the synthesis of enzymes needed to decrease the inflammatory response.

℞ QUICK FACTS

Purpose

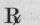 Used to control asthma symptoms in people who have mild to moderate bronchial asthma.

Dosage

 Must inhale properly and regularly to be effective, even if there are no symptoms. Follow doctor's instructions carefully. Tilade Inhaler is not to be used with other mouthpieces. Tilade does not stop an

asthma attack; continue to take during an attack
with a bronchodilator to relieve the acute attack.

 Usual adult dose: 2 inhalations 4 times per day at
regular intervals. If this dosage level is effective, doctor will try reducing after a while.

 Usual child dose: children 12 years and older are
prescribed adult doses. Not generally prescribed for
children under 12 years.

 Missed dose: take as soon as possible, unless almost
time for next dose. In that case, do not take missed
dose; go back to regular schedule. *Do not double
doses.*

Side Effects

 Overdose symptoms: no specific information available. If you suspect an overdose, immediately seek
medical attention.

 More common side effects: chest pain, coughing, headache, nausea, inflamed nose, sore throat, unpleasant
taste, upper respiratory tract infection, wheezing.

 Less common side effects: abdominal pain, bronchitis, diarrhea, difficult or labored breathing, difficulty
speaking, dizziness, dry mouth, fatigue, increased
sputum, indigestion, viral infection, vomiting.

Interactions

 No drug interactions reported.

 No known food/other substance interactions.

Special Cautions

 If pregnant or planning to become pregnant, inform your doctor immediately. May appear in breast milk; could affect a nursing infant.

- -

 No special precautions apply to seniors.

- -

 Not generally prescribed for children under 12 years.

- -

 Immediately discontinue if you experience coughing and wheezing.

- -

Avoid if sensitive to or allergic to Tilade or any of its ingredients.

Timolol Maleate

see TIMOPTIC

Timoptic
∧∧

Generic name: Timolol maleate

Other brand names: Blocadren Oral, Timoptic Ocudose, Timoptic-XE

Timoptic is an anti-glaucoma ophthalmic solution/topical beta-blocker. It reduces eye pressure by decreasing eye fluid production and increasing the fluid outflow from the eye.

℞ QUICK FACTS

Purpose

℞ Used to treat glaucoma.

Dosage

 Use exactly as prescribed. If using Ocudose, use immediately after opening individual unit and throw out leftover solution. If using Timoptic-XE, shake *only 1 time* before each use. If using other eye medications, apply at least 10 minutes before applying Timoptic-XE. *Do not allow tip of dispenser to actually touch the eye.*

 Usual adult dose: *Timoptic*—1 drop of 0.25% solution in the affected eye 2 times per day. Doctor may switch to 0.5% solution if you do not respond to the initial dose. *Timoptic-XE*—1 drop of 0.25% or 0.5% solution in the affected eye once per day.

 Usual child dose: not generally prescribed for children.

 Missed dose: *if using once per day*—apply as soon as possible, unless it is the next day. In that case, do not take missed dose; go back to regular schedule. *If using more than once per day*—apply as soon as possible, unless almost time for next dose. In that case, do not take missed dose; go back to regular schedule. *Do not double doses.*

Side Effects

 Overdose symptoms: no specific information about Timoptic. However, beta-blocker overdose symptoms: extremely slow heart rate, low blood pressure, severe heart failure, wheezing. If you suspect an overdose, immediately seek medical attention.

Side effects: allergic reactions, anxiety, chest pain, confusion, conjunctivitis (pink eye), cough, depression, diarrhea, difficult or labored breathing, disorientation, dizziness, double vision, drooping eyelid, dry mouth, eye discharge, eye irritation and inflammation, eye itching and tearing, fainting, fatigue, fluid in the lungs, hair loss, hallucinations, headache, heart failure, high blood pressure, hives, impotence, inability to breathe, increase in signs or symptoms of myasthenia gravis (severe muscle weakness), indigestion, inflammation of the eyelid, irregular heartbeat, loss of appetite, low blood pressure, nausea, nervousness, pain, rash, sensation of a foreign body in the eye, sleepiness, slow heartbeat, stroke, stuffy nose, throbbing or fluttering heartbeat, tingling or pins and needles, upper respiratory infection, visual disturbances, weakness, wheezing, worsened angina (crushing chest pain).

 No known less common or rare side effects.

Interactions

 Inform your doctor before combining Timoptic with: epinephrine (EpiPen), catecholamine-depleting medications such as blood pressure medications containing reserpine (Serpasil), calcium antagonists such as Cardizem and Isoptin, digitalis (Lanoxin). Avoid using with other topical beta-blockers; use with caution if taking oral beta-blockers such as Inderal and Tenormin.

 No known food/other substance interactions.

Special Cautions

 If pregnant or planning to become pregnant, inform your doctor immediately. Appears in breast milk; could affect a nursing infant.

Seniors may have some sensitivity and should immediately report eye infection to your doctor.

 Not generally prescribed for children.

STOP *Do not use if you have: bronchial asthma, history of bronchial asthma, or other serious breathing conditions such as emphysema; slow heartbeat, heart block, active heart failure, or inadequate blood supply to the circulatory system; or if sensitive or allergic to Timoptic.*

May mask symptoms of overactive thyroid.

Antiglaucoma effect decreases if using medication for a prolonged period.

Medication is absorbed into the body and may affect other parts of the body.

Use with caution if you have poor cerebral circulation or history of heart failure.

Let your doctor know of any allergies.

May mask symptoms of low blood sugar; diabetics should inform their doctor of their condition.

Tell your doctor or dentist in medical emergency or before surgery that you are taking Timoptic.

Tobramycin

see TOBREX

Tobrex

‹‹

Generic name: Tobramycin

Tobrex is an aminoglycoside ophthalmic antibiotic. It prevents the growth and multiplication of infecting bacteria.

℞ QUICK FACTS

Purpose

℞ Used to treat bacterial infections of the eye.

Dosage

 Apply eye drops and ointment exactly as prescribed. Use Tobrex for entire time prescribed, even if symptoms disappear.

- -

 Usual adult dose: *solution*—1 or 2 drops into affected eye every 4 hours for mild to moderate infection. 2 drops every hour until improvement for severe infection. Gradually reduce dose before stopping. *Ointment*—½ inch ribbon into affected eye 2 or 3 times per day for mild to moderate infection. ½ inch ribbon into affected eye every 3 or 4 hours until improvement for severe infection. Gradually reduce dose before stopping.

- -

 Usual child dose: individually tailored by doctor.

 Missed dose: apply as soon as possible, unless it is the next day. In that case, do not take missed dose; go back to regular schedule.

Side Effects

☠ Overdose symptoms: corneal redness and inflammation, excessive eye tearing, lid itching and swelling. If you suspect an overdose, immediately seek medical attention.

 Side effects: abnormal redness of eye tissue, allergic reactions, lid itching, lid swelling.

 No known less common or rare side effects.

Interactions

 Inform your doctor before combining Tobrex with other prescription eye antibiotics.

 No known food/other substance interactions.

Special Cautions

 If pregnant or planning to become pregnant, inform your doctor immediately. May appear in breast milk; could affect a nursing infant.

 No special precautions apply to seniors.

 Follow doctor's instructions carefully for children.

 Avoid if sensitive to or allergic to Tobrex or any of its ingredients. If you experience allergic reaction, stop using and immediately contact your doctor.

May cause a secondary infection not treatable by Tobrex.

Ophthalmic ointments can slow healing of corneal wounds.

Tocainide Hydrochloride
see TONOCARD

Tofranil

∧∧

Generic name: Imipramine hydrochloride

Other brand names: Janimine, SK-Pramine, Tofranil-PM, Typramine

Tofranil is a tricyclic antidepressant. It is thought to relieve depression by increasing the concentration of the chemicals necessary for nerve transmission to the brain.

℞ QUICK FACTS

Purpose

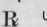 Used to treat depression.

Dosage

 May take with or without food. Follow doctor's instructions for stopping Tofranil. *Do not stop medication if there is no immediate effect, can take 4 to 6 weeks to see improvement.*

· ·

 Usual adult dose: 75 milligrams per day, up to 150 and to a maximum of 200 milligrams per day. *Seniors and adolescents*—30 to 40 milligrams per day, up to a maximum of 100 milligrams per day.

· ·

 Usual child dose: *is only used for bedwetting as a short-term therapy.* Dose is no more than 2.5 milligrams per each 2.2 pounds of body weight, and usually begins at 25 milligrams per day. Give dose to child 1 hour before bedtime. After 1 week, doctor may increase dose to 50 milligrams per day (children 6–11 years) or 75 milligrams per day (children ages 12 and up), taken in 1 dose at bedtime or divided into 2 doses, taken at mid-afternoon and bedtime.

· ·

Missed dose: *if taking one dose per day at bedtime—do not take dose in the morning and contact your doctor. If taking more than 1 dose per day—take as soon as possible, unless almost time for next dose. In that case, do not take missed dose; go back to regular schedule. Do not double doses.*

Side Effects

Overdose may cause death. Overdose symptoms: agitation, bluish skin, coma, convulsions, difficulty breathing, dilated pupils, drowsiness, heart failure, high fever, involuntary writhing or jerky movements, irregular or rapid heartbeat, lack of coordination, low blood pressure, overactive reflexes, restlessness, rigid muscles, shock, stupor, sweating, vomiting. If you suspect an overdose, immediately seek medical attention.

Side effects: abdominal cramps, agitation, anxiety, blackening of tongue, bleeding sore, blood disorders, blurred vision, breast development in males, confusion, congestive heart failure, constipation or diarrhea, cough, delusions, dilated pupils, disorientation, dizziness, drowsiness, dry mouth, episodes of elation or irritability, excessive or spontaneous milk flow, fatigue, fever, flushing, frequent urination or difficulty or delay in urinating, hair loss, hallucinations, headache, heart attack, heart failure, high blood pressure, high or low blood sugar, high pressure of fluid in eyes, hives, impotence, increased or decreased sex drive, inflammation of the mouth, insomnia, intestinal blockage, irregular heartbeat, lack of coordination, light-headedness, loss of appetite, nausea, nightmares, numbness in hands and feet, odd taste in mouth, palpitations, purple or reddish-brown skin spots, rapid heartbeat, restlessness, ringing in the ears, seizures, sensitivity to light, skin itching and rash, sore throat, stomach upset, stroke, sweating, swelling due to fluid retention (especially face and tongue), swelling of breasts, swelling of testicles, swollen glands, tendency to fall, tingling or pins and needles, tremors, visual problems, vomiting, weakness, weight gain or loss, yellowed skin and eyes. Most common side effect in children treated for bedwetting: nervousness, sleep disorders, stomach and intestinal problems, tiredness. Other side effects in children: anxiety, collapse, constipation, convulsions, emotional instability, fainting.

 No known less common or rare side effects.

Interactions

 Fatal reactions have occurred when Tofranil is taken with MAO inhibitors such as Nardil and Parnate. Do not take Tofranil for 2 weeks after taking a MAO inhibitor. Inform your doctor before combining Tofranil with: albuterol (Proventil or Ventolin); anticholinergics such as Cogentin; antihypertensives such as Wytensin; barbiturates such as Nembutal and Seconal; carbamazepine (Tegretol); central nervous system depressants such as Xanax and Valium; cimetidine (Tagamet); clonidine (Catapres); decongestants such as Sudafed; epinephrine (EpiPen); fluoxetine (Prozac); guanethidine (Ismelin); methylphenidate (Ritalin); norepinephrine; phenytoin (Dilantin); thyroid medications. May experience extreme drowsiness if taking Tofranil with narcotic painkillers such as Percocet or sleeping medications such as Valium.

 Extreme drowsiness or other serious side effects may occur if using alcohol with Tofranil.

Special Cautions

 If pregnant or planning to become pregnant, inform your doctor immediately. May appear in breast milk; could affect a nursing infant.

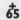 Seniors are prescribed lower doses.

 Children are at higher risk for overdose due to increased sensitivity. Follow doctor's instructions carefully for children. Not generally prescribed for children under 6 years.

 May impair your ability to drive a car or operate machinery. *Do not take part in any activity that requires alertness.*

Avoid use if recovering from a heart attack.

Use with caution if you have or ever had: narrow-angle glaucoma; difficulty urinating; heart, liver, kidney, or thyroid disease; seizures; or if taking thyroid medication.

Inform your doctor if a sore throat or fever develops when taking Tofranil.

May cause sensitivity to sunlight.

Doctor will discontinue Tofranil if you are having elective surgery.

Tolbutamide

see ORINASE

Tolectin

Generic name: Tolmetin sodium

Other brand names: Tolectin DS, Tolectin 200, Tolectin 600

Tolectin is a nonsteroidal anti-inflammatory drug. It works by blocking the production of prostaglandins, which may trigger pain.

℞ QUICK FACTS

Purpose

℞ Used to treat the inflammation, swelling, stiffness, and joint pain associated with rheumatoid arthritis and osteoarthritis. Used for acute episodes and long-term treatment. Also used to treat juvenile rheumatoid arthritis.

Dosage

 Take with food if you experience stomach irritation. Lying down for 20 to 30 minutes after taking medication may alleviate upset stomach.

 Usual adult dose: 1,200 milligrams divided into 3 doses of 400 milligrams each, taken in the morning, afternoon, and at bedtime. Doctor may adjust dose after 1 to 2 weeks. Dosage range—600 to 1,800 milligrams per day divided into 3 doses.

 Usual child dose: 20 milligrams per 2.2 pounds of body weight per day, divided into 3 or 4 smaller doses. Dosage range—15 to 30 milligrams per 2.2 pounds of body weight per day. Not generally prescribed for children under 2 years.

 Missed dose: take as soon as possible, unless almost time for next dose. In that case, do not take missed dose; go back to regular schedule. *Do not double doses.*

Side Effects

 Overdose symptoms: no specific information available. If you suspect an overdose, immediately seek medical attention.

 More common side effects: abdominal pain, change in weight, diarrhea, dizziness, gas, headache, heartburn, high blood pressure, indigestion, nausea, stomach and intestinal upset, swelling due to fluid retention, vomiting, weakness.

 Less common or rare side effects: anemia, blood in urine, chest pain, congestive heart failure, constipation, depression, drowsiness, fever, hepatitis, hives, inflammation of the mouth or tongue, kidney failure, painful urination, peptic ulcer, purple or reddish skin spots, ringing in the ears, severe allergic reactions, skin irritation, stomach inflammation, stomach or intestinal bleeding, urinary tract infection, visual disturbances, yellow eyes and skin.

Interactions

 Inform your doctor before combining Tolectin with: aspirin, blood thinners such as Coumadin, carteolol (Cartrol), diuretics such as Lasix, glyburide (Micronase), lithium (Lithonate), methotrexate.

 No known food/other substance interactions.

Special Cautions

 If pregnant or planning to become pregnant, inform your doctor immediately. Appears in breast milk; could affect a nursing infant.

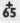 Seniors are susceptible to kidney problems while taking Tolectin.

Follow doctor's instructions carefully for children.

 May cause drowsiness and impair your ability to drive a car or operate machinery. *Do not take part in any activity that requires alertness.*

Ulcers or internal bleeding may occur suddenly; doctor should do frequent check-ups if you take Tolectin regularly.

Use with caution if you have heart disease or high blood pressure, Tolectin can increase water retention.

Avoid if sensitive to or allergic to other NSAIDs or if you have had asthma, hives, or nasal inflammation caused by aspirin or other NSAIDs.

May cause kidney problems if you have heart failure or liver disease, or take diuretics.

If you develop symptoms of liver problems such as yellow skin and eyes, notify your doctor. Doctor will discontinue Tolectin.

Contact your doctor if you experience visual disturbances.

Tolmetin Sodium

see TOLECTIN

Tonocard

Generic name: Tocainide hydrochloride

Tonocard is an anti-arrhythmic. It suppresses irregular heartbeats and helps to achieve a normal rhythm.

℞ QUICK FACTS

Purpose

℞ Used to treat arrhythmias: severe irregular heartbeats that are slower than normal (bradycardia) or faster than normal (tachycardia). Effective in treating ventricular arrhythmias.

Dosage

 Take on a regular schedule for Tonocard to be effective. If not taken regularly, may worsen symptoms.

 Usual adult dose: 400 milligrams every 8 hours. Dose range—1,200 to 1,800 milligrams per day divided into 3 doses. *For individuals with reduced kidney or liver function*—dose is lowered. *Seniors*—prescribed Tonocard with caution.

 Usual child dose: not generally prescribed for children.

 Missed dose: take as soon as possible, unless more than 2 hours after scheduled dose time have passed. In that case, do not take missed dose, go back to regular schedule. *Do not double doses.*

Side Effects

 Overdose symptoms: no specific information available; however, likely signs of overdose would appear in the central nervous system, followed by stomach and intestinal disorders, leading to convulsions and heart and lung slowing or stopping. If you suspect an overdose, immediately seek medical attention.

More common side effects: confusion or disorientation, dizziness or vertigo, diarrhea, excessive sweating, hallucinations, increased irregular heartbeat, lack of coordination, loss of appetite, nausea, nervousness, rash, tingling or pins and needles, tremor, vision disturbances, vomiting.

 Less common side effects: arthritis, anxiety, chest pain, congestive heart failure, drowsiness, exhaustion, fatigue, headache, hearing loss, hot or cold feelings, involuntary eyeball movement, joint pain, low blood pressure, muscle pain, pounding heartbeat, rapid heartbeat, ringing in ears, sleepiness, slow heartbeat, sluggishness, unsteadiness, walking disturbances. Rare side effects: abdominal pain, agitation, allergic reactions, anemia, angina (crushing chest pain), blood clots in lungs, blood disorders, changes in blood counts, changes in heart function, chills, cinchonism (sensitivity reaction), cold hands and feet, coma, constipation, decreased mental ability, decreased urination, depression, difficulty breathing, difficulty speaking, difficulty sleeping, difficulty swallowing, disturbed behavior, disturbed dreams, dizziness on standing, double vision, dry mouth, earache, enlarged heart, fainting, fever, fluid in lungs, fluid retention, flushing, general bodily discomfort, hair loss, heart attack, hepatitis, hiccups, high blood pressure, hives, increased urination, lung disorders, memory loss, muscle cramps, muscle twitching or spasm, myasthenia gravis, neck pain or pain extending from the neck, pallor, pneumonia, seizures, skin peeling, slurred speech, smell disturbance, stomach upset, taste disturbance, thirst, weakness, yawning, yellow eyes and skin.

Interactions

 Inform your doctor before combining Tonocard with: the anesthetic lidocaine (Xylocaine), blood pressure medications such as metoprolol (Lopressor), other anti-arrhythmics such as Quinidex, Procan, and Mexitil.

 No known food/other substance interactions.

Special Cautions

 Animal studies have shown increase in stillbirths and spontaneous abortions. If pregnant or planning to become pregnant, inform your doctor immediately. May appear in breast milk; could affect a nursing infant.

 Seniors are prescribed Tonocard with caution.

 Not generally prescribed for children.

 Do not take if you have heart block and you do not have a pacemaker, or if sensitive to or allergic to Tonocard or local anesthetics.

In first 3 months at increased risk for serious blood and lung disorders. Inform your doctor immediately if you experience: painful or difficult breathing, wheezing, cough, easy bruising or bleeding, tremors, palpitations, rash, soreness or ulcers in the mouth or throat, fever, and chills.

May worsen congestive heart failure.

Inform your doctor or dentist in a medical emergency or before surgery that you are taking Tonocard.

Topicort

Generic name: Desoximetasone

Other brand name: Topicort LP

Topicort is a topical adrenocorticoid/anti-inflammatory. It interferes with the natural body mechanisms that produce rash, itching, or inflammation.

℞ QUICK FACTS

Purpose

℞ Used to treat inflammation and itching caused by many skin conditions.

Dosage

 Use only on skin; keep away from eyes. Never cover affected area unless directed by your doctor. Use sparingly and not for prolonged periods of time. *Do not cover affected areas unless directed by your doctor or use for other than prescribed condition.*

. . . .

 Usual adult dose: apply thin layer to affected area 2 times per day.

. . . .

 Usual child dose: use as little as possible; follow doctor's dosage instructions carefully.

. . . .

 Missed dose: apply only as needed, in the smallest amount required.

Side Effects

 Overdose symptoms: Cushing's syndrome (moon-shaped face, emotional disturbances, high blood pressure, weight gain, and in women, baldness or growth of body or facial hair) or diabetes. If you suspect an overdose, immediately seek medical attention.

. . . .

 Side effects: acne-like pimples, blistering, burning of the skin, dryness, excessive growth of hair, inflammation of hair follicles, irritation, itching, loss of skin pigmentation, prickly heat, secondary infection, skin inflammation around the mouth, rash, redness, stretch marks on the skin, thinning of the skin.

 No known less common or rare side effects.

Interactions

 No drug interactions reported.

 No known food/other substance interactions.

Special Cautions

 If pregnant or planning to become pregnant, inform your doctor immediately. Not known if Topicort appears in breast milk.

 No special precautions apply to seniors.

 Follow doctor's instructions carefully for children. If using for genital rash in infants, use caution not to use tight diapers or plastic pants; air must be able to circulate. Long-term use may interfere with a child's growth and development.

 Do not use if sensitive to or allergic to Topicort.

Toprol XL

see LOPRESSOR

Toradol

Generic name: Ketorolac tromethamine

Other brand name: Acular Eye Drops

Toradol is a nonsteroidal anti-inflammatory drug. It works by blocking the production of prostaglandins, which may trigger pain.

℞ QUICK FACTS

Purpose

℞ Used for short-term therapy to relieve pain.

Dosage

 Works faster if taken on an empty stomach; however, may take with an antacid to relieve stomach upset. Take with a full glass of water, and *do not lie down for 20 minutes after taking to prevent upper digestive tract irritation.*

 Usual adult dose: 10 milligrams taken as needed, every 4 to 6 hours, up to a maximum of 40 milligrams per day.

 Usual child dose: not generally prescribed for children.

 Missed dose: *if taking on a regular schedule*—take as soon as possible, unless almost time for next dose. In that case, do not take missed dose; go back to regular schedule. *Do not double doses.*

Side Effects

 Overdose symptoms: no specific information available. If you suspect an overdose, immediately seek medical attention.

 More common side effects: diarrhea, dizziness, drowsiness, headache, indigestion, itching, nausea, stomach and intestinal pain, swelling due to fluid retention.

Less common side effects: abdominal fullness, constipation, gas, high blood pressure, inflammation of the mouth, rash, red or purple skin spots, sweating, vomiting. Rare side effects: abnormal dreams, allergic reactions, anemia, asthma, belching, black stools, blood in urine, convulsions, decreased amount of urine, difficult or labored breathing, exaggerated feeling of well-being, fainting, fever, fluid in the lungs, flushing, gastritis (inflammation of stomach lining), hallucinations, hives, increased appetite, kidney failure, kidney inflammation, loss of appetite, low blood pressure, nosebleeds, pallor, peptic ulcer, skin inflammation and flaking, Stevens-Johnson syndrome (skin peeling), stomach and intestinal bleeding, swelling of the throat or tongue, throbbing heartbeat, tremors, vertigo, weight gain.

Interactions

 Inform your doctor before combining Toradol with: aspirin, blood thinners such as Coumadin, diuretics such as Lasix and Dyazide, lithium (Lithonate), methotrexate, probenecid (Benemid).

 No known food/other substance interactions.

Special Cautions

 If pregnant or planning to become pregnant, inform your doctor immediately. Appears in breast milk; could affect a nursing infant.

 Seniors should use with caution.

 Not generally prescribed for children.

 Do not take if you are allergic to Toradol, or if you have had allergic reactions to aspirin or medications similar to

Toradol such as nasal polyps; swelling of the face, limbs, and throat; hives; wheezing; or light-headedness.

Ulcers or internal bleeding can occur suddenly; doctor should perform frequent check-ups if you take Toradol regularly.

Use with caution if you have kidney or liver disease, may cause liver inflammation; if you have high blood pressure or heart disease, Toradol can increase water retention.

Trandate

see NORMODYNE

Tranxene

Generic name: Clorazepate dipotassium

Other brand names: Tranxene-SD, Tranxene-SD Half Strength

Tranxene is a benzodiazepine tranquilizer. It reduces the activity of certain chemicals in the brain.

℞ QUICK FACTS

Purpose

℞ Used to treat anxiety disorders and for short-term relief of anxiety.

Dosage

🍽️D. Take exactly as prescribed. Follow doctor's instructions for stopping medication; otherwise may experience withdrawal. Never change dose unless directed by your doctor.

Usual adult dose: *for anxiety*—Tranxene—30 milligrams divided into several smaller doses. Doses range from 15 to 60 milligrams. Can also take in a single dose at bedtime, starting at 15 milligrams, and adjusted by your doctor. *Tranxene-SD*—one 22.5 milligram tablet every 24 hours. Not for initial dosing. *Tranxene-SD Half Strength*—one 11.25 milligram tablet every 24 hours. Not for initial dosing. *For anxiety associated with depression*—prescribed lower dose. *For acute alcohol withdrawal*—30 milligrams per day to start, increased by doctor to 90 milligrams per day after 2 days; then dose is reduced, and continually reduced gradually. Should be used under strict supervision by your doctor for alcohol withdrawal. *When used with anti-epileptic medications*—7.5 milligrams taken 3 times per day. Doctor may increase by 7.5 milligrams per week to a maximum of 90 milligrams per day. *Seniors*—7.5 to 15 milligrams per day for anxiety.

Usual child dose: *when used with anti-epileptic medications*—children over 12 years—7.5 milligrams taken 3 times per day. Doctor may increase by 7.5 milligrams per week to a maximum of 90 milligrams per day. For children 9 to 12 years—7.5 milligrams taken 3 times per day. Doctor may increase by 7.5 milligrams per week to a maximum of 60 milligrams per day.

Missed dose: take as soon as possible, if within one hour of missed dose. Otherwise, do not take missed dose; go back to regular schedule. *Do not double doses.*

Side Effects

 Overdose symptoms: coma, low blood pressure, sedation. If you suspect an overdose, immediately seek medical attention.

 Most common side effect: drowsiness.

 Less common or rare side effects: blurred vision, depression, difficulty sleeping or falling asleep, dizziness, dry mouth, double vision, fatigue, genital and urinary tract disorders, headache, irritability, lack of muscle coordination, mental confusion, nervousness, tremors, skin rashes, slurred speech, stomach and intestinal disorders, tremor. Side effects due to abruptly stopping Tranxene: diarrhea, difficulty sleeping or falling asleep, hallucinations, impaired memory, irritability, muscle aches, nervousness, tremors.

Interactions

 Inform your doctor before combining Tranxene with: barbiturates such as Nembutal and Seconal, MAO inhibitors such as Nardil and Parnate, major tranquilizers such as Mellaril and Thorazine, narcotic pain relievers such as Demerol and Percodan.

 Do not drink alcohol during Tranxene therapy.

Special Cautions

 Increased risk of birth defects with benzodiazepine tranquilizers; avoid use during pregnancy. May appear in breast milk; could affect a nursing infant.

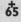 Seniors are prescribed lower doses, at risk for becoming unsteady or oversedated.

 Follow doctor's instructions carefully for children over 12 years.

Do not take if you have narrow-angle glaucoma.

May cause drowsiness and impair your ability to drive a car or operate machinery. *Do not take part in any activity that requires alertness.*

Avoid if sensitive to or allergic to Tranxene.

Not prescribed for anxiety or tension related to everyday stress, or for serious conditions such as depression or severe psychological disorders.

Trazodone Hydrochloride

see DESYREL

Trental

Generic name: Pentoxifylline

Trental is a blood-viscosity reducer. It reduces blood thickness and increases the ability of red blood cells to modify their shape.

℞ QUICK FACTS

Purpose

 Used to allow blood to flow more freely, thereby relieving painful leg cramps (intermittent claudication). Also used to treat dementia; strokes; circulatory and nerve disorders caused by diabetes; and Raynaud's syndrome (blood vessel disorder in which exposure to cold causes white fingers and toes). Also prescribed to treat impotence and increase sperm motility in infertile men.

Dosage

 Swallow tablet whole; *do not break, crush, or chew.* Take exactly as prescribed.

 Usual adult dose: one 400-milligram controlled-release tablet taken 3 times per day with meals. Effects are seen within 2 to 4 weeks; therapy usually does not last for more than 8 weeks. If you experience side effects related to the stomach or central nervous system, doctor will reduce dose, or stop medication if side effects persist.

 Usual child dose: not generally prescribed for children.

 Missed dose: take as soon as possible, unless almost time for next dose. In that case, do not take missed dose; go back to regular schedule. *Do not double doses.*

Side Effects

 Overdose symptoms usually appear within 4 to 5 hours and may last 12 hours. Overdose symptoms: agitation, convulsions, fever, flushing, loss of consciousness, low blood pressure, sleepiness. If you suspect an overdose, immediately seek medical attention.

 Side effects: abdominal discomfort; allergic reaction (swelling of face, lips, tongue, throat, arms, legs, sore throat, fever and chills, difficulty swallowing, chest pain); anxiety; bad taste in the mouth; blind spot in vision; blurred vision; brittle fingernails; chest pain (sometimes crushing); confusion; conjunctivitis (pink eye); constipation; depression; difficult or labored breathing; dizziness; dry mouth or thirst; earache;

excessive salivation; flu-like symptoms; fluid retention; general feeling of bodily discomfort; headache; hives; indigestion; inflammation of the gallbladder; irregular heartbeat; itching; laryngitis; loss of appetite; low blood pressure; nosebleeds; rash; seizures; sore throat or swollen neck glands; stuffy nose; tremor; vomiting; weight change.

 No known less common or rare side effects.

Interactions

 Inform your doctor before combining Trental with: blood thinners such as Coumadin, clot inhibitors such as Persantine, ulcer medications such as Tagamet.

 No known food/other substance interactions.

Special Cautions

 If pregnant or planning to become pregnant, inform your doctor immediately. Appears in breast milk; could affect a nursing infant.

 No special precautions apply to seniors.

 Not generally prescribed for children.

 Do not take if you have recently had a stroke or bleeding in the retina of the eye, or if sensitive to or allergic to Trental, caffeine, theophylline, or theobromine.

Doctor should periodically test your blood if you are taking a blood thinner, have recently had surgery, have a peptic ulcer or other disorder that involves bleeding.

Trental is not a substitute for physical therapy or surgery.

. . . .

On occasion, cases of crushing chest pain, low blood pressure, and irregular heartbeat have been experienced by people with heart disease and brain disorders.

Tretinoin
see RETIN-A

Triamcinolone Acetonide
(for adults only)
see NASACORT

Triamcinolone Acetonide
(for adults and children)
see AZMACORT

Triamterene with Hydrochlorothiazide
see MAXZIDE

Triavil

Generic ingredients: Amitriptyline hydrochloride with perphenazine

Other brand name: Etrafon

Triavil is a tricyclic antidepressant and tranquilizer combination. Tricyclic antidepressants are thought to relieve depression by increasing the concentration of the chemicals necessary for nerve transmission to the brain, and tranquilizers reduce the activity of certain chemicals in the brain.

℞ QUICK FACTS

Purpose

℞ Used to treat anxiety, agitation, and depression. Also used to treat people with schizophrenia who are depressed and people with insomnia, fatigue, loss of interest, loss of appetite, or a slowing of physical and mental reactions.

Dosage

 May take with or without food. Follow doctor's instructions for stopping Triavil to avoid withdrawal symptoms.

 Usual adult dose: no more than 4 tablets of Triavil 4-50 or 8 tablets of any other strength per day. May take several days to weeks to see improvement. *For nonpsychotic anxiety and depression*—1 tablet of Triavil 2-25 or 4-25 taken 3 or 4 times per day, or 1 tablet of Triavil 4-50 taken twice per day. *For anxiety in people with schizophrenia*—2 tablets of Triavil 4-25 taken 3 times per day. Doctor may advise taking another Triavil 4-25 tablet at bedtime if needed. *For ongoing use*—1 tablet of Triavil 2-25 or 4-25 taken 2 to 4 times per day, or 1 tablet of Triavil 4-50 taken twice per day. *Seniors and adolescents*—1 tablet of Triavil 4-10 taken 3 or 4 times per day.

Usual child dose: not generally prescribed for children.

 Missed dose: take as soon as possible, unless within 2 hours of next dose. In that case, do not take missed dose, go back to regular schedule. *Do not double doses.*

Side Effects

 Triavil overdose may be fatal. Overdose symptoms: abnormalities of posture and movements, agitation, coma, convulsions, dilated pupils, drowsiness, extremely low body temperature, eye movement problems, high fever, heart failure, overactive reflexes, rapid or irregular heartbeat, rigid muscles, stupor, very low blood pressure, vomiting. If you suspect an overdose, immediately seek medical attention.

 Side effects: abnormal milk secretions; abnormalities of movements and posture; anxiety; asthma; black tongue; blood disorders; blurred vision; bodily rigidity, arched backward; breast development in males; change in pulse rate; chewing movements; coma; confusion; constipation; convulsions; delusions; diarrhea; difficulty breathing; difficulty concentrating; difficulty swallowing; dilated pupils; disorientation; dizziness; drowsiness; dry mouth; eating abnormal amounts of food; ejaculation failure; episodes of elation or irritability; excessive or spontaneous flow of milk; excitement; exhaustion; eye problems; eye spasms; eyes in a fixed position; fatigue; fever; fluid accumulation and swelling (throat and brain, face and tongue, arms and legs); frequent urination; hair loss; hallucinations; headache; heart attacks; hepatitis; high blood pressure; high fever; high or low blood pressure; hives; impotence; inability to stop moving; inability to urinate; increased or decreased sex drive; inflammation of the mouth; insomnia; intestinal blockage; intolerance to light; involuntary jerky movements of the tongue, face, mouth, lips, jaw, body, or arms and legs; irregular blood pressure, pulse, and heartbeat; irregular menstrual periods; lack of coordination; light-headedness upon standing; liver problems; lockjaw; loss or increase of appetite; low blood pressure; muscle stiffness; nasal congestion; nausea; nightmares; odd taste in mouth; overactive reflexes; pain and stiffness around neck; palpitations; protruding tongue; puckering of the mouth; puffing of the cheeks; purple or reddish-brown spots on skin; rapid heartbeat; restlessness; rigid arms and feet, head, and muscles; ringing in the ears; salivation; sedation; seizures; sensitivity to light; severe allergic reactions; skin rash or inflammation; scaling; spasms in the hands and feet; speech problems; stomach upset; stroke; sweating; swelling of breasts; swelling of testicles; swollen glands; tingling or pins and needles and numbness in hands and feet; tremors; twisted neck; twitching in the body, neck, shoulders, and face; uncontrollable and involuntary urination; urinary problems; visual problems; vomiting; weakness; weight gain or loss; writhing movements; yellowed skin and eyes.

 No known less common or rare side effects.

Interactions

 Inform your doctor before combining Triavil with: airway-opening medications such as Proventil; anticonvulsants such as Dilantin; antidepressant MAO inhibitors such as Nardil and Parnate; antihistamines such as Benadryl; antispasmodics such as Bentyl; atropine (Donnatal); barbiturates such as phenobarbital; blood thinners such as Coumadin; cimetidine (Tagamet); disulfiram (Antabuse); epinephrine (EpiPen); ethchlorvynol (Placidyl); fluoxetine (Prozac); furazolidone (Furoxone); guanethidine (Ismelin); major tranquilizers such as Haldol; narcotic analgesics such as Percocet; thyroid medications such as Synthroid. Narcotics, painkillers, and sleep medications may cause extreme drowsiness if used with Triavil.

 Alcohol taken with Triavil can cause extreme drowsiness and other serious side effects.

Special Cautions

 If pregnant or planning to become pregnant, inform your doctor immediately. May cause false-positive pregnancy test results. Not recommended for nursing mothers.

 Seniors are prescribed a lower dose. Senior women at increased risk for tardive dyskinesia—involuntary muscle spasms and twitches in the face and body.

 Not generally prescribed for children. Adolescents should follow doctor's instructions carefully.

 May cause drowsiness and impair your ability to drive a car or operate machinery. *Do not take part in any activity that requires alertness.*

Inform your doctor before starting Triavil if you have or had: glaucoma; difficulty urinating; breast cancer; seizures; heart, liver, or thyroid disease; or if exposed to pesticides or extreme heat.

May mask symptoms of brain tumor, intestinal blockage, overdose of other medications.

At risk for tardive dyskinesia, condition marked by involuntary muscle spasms and twitches in the face and body.

Avoid if allergic to any of the ingredients of Triavil.

Should not use if you have recently had a heart attack or have an abnormal bone marrow condition.

Stop taking Triavil and inform your doctor if you develop a fever.

Triazolam

see HALCION

Tridesilon

Generic name: Desonide

Other brand name: DesOwen

Tridesilon is a topical adrenocorticoid/anti-inflammatory. It interferes with the natural body mechanisms that produce rash, itching, or inflammation.

℞ QUICK FACTS

Purpose

℞ Used to treat the itching and inflammation of a variety of skin disorders.

Dosage

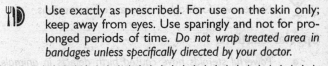 Use exactly as prescribed. For use on the skin only; keep away from eyes. Use sparingly and not for prolonged periods of time. *Do not wrap treated area in bandages unless specifically directed by your doctor.*

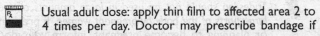 Usual adult dose: apply thin film to affected area 2 to 4 times per day. Doctor may prescribe bandage if

using for psoriasis or other conditions that do not respond well to medication.

 Usual child dose: same as adult dose.

 Missed dose: apply as soon as possible, unless almost time for next dose. In that case, do not take missed dose; go back to regular schedule. *Do not double doses.*

Side Effects

 Overdose symptoms: increase in blood sugar and Cushing's syndrome (moon-shaped face, emotional disturbances, high blood pressure, weight gain, and in women, baldness or growth of body or facial hair) or diabetes. If you suspect an overdose, immediately seek medical attention.

 Side effects: acne, additional infections, allergic reactions of the skin, burning of the skin, dryness, excessive growth of hair, irritation, itching, loss of skin pigmentation, prickly heat, rash, skin inflammation around the mouth, skin softening, stretch marks. Side effects in children: delayed weight gain, headaches, slowed growth.

 No known less common or rare side effects.

Interactions

 No drug interactions reported.

 No known food/other substance interactions.

Special Cautions

 Powerful steroids have caused birth defects in animals. Tridesilon should not be used in large amounts or over large parts of the body by pregnant women. If pregnant or planning to become pregnant, inform your doc-

tor immediately. Not known if Tridesilon appears in breast milk.

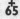 No special precautions apply to seniors.

 Follow doctor's instructions carefully for children. Avoid covering treated area with plastic pants or waterproof diapers.

 Avoid if sensitive to or allergic to Tridesilon.

Inform your doctor if an irritation develops.

Trifluoperazine Hydrochloride

see STELAZINE

Trihexyphenidyl Hydrochloride

see ARTANE

Trilisate

Generic name: Choline magnesium trisalicylate

Other brand name: Tricosal

Trilisate is a non-narcotic analgesic anti-inflammatory. It reduces pain and inflammation.

℞ Quick Facts

Purpose

 Used to treat symptoms of rheumatoid arthritis, osteoarthritis, and other forms of arthritis on a long-term basis. Also prescribed for acute painful shoulder; mild to moderate pain in general; fever; and juvenile rheumatoid arthritis.

Dosage

 Take exactly as prescribed. Comes in tablet or liquid form. May take 2 to 3 weeks to observe the effects of this medication.

 Usual adult dose: *for rheumatoid arthritis, osteoarthritis, more severe arthritis, and acute painful shoulder—*1,500 milligrams taken 2 times per day or 3,000 milligrams taken once per day. *For mild to moderate pain or fever—*2,000 to 3,000 milligrams per day divided into 2 equal doses. *Seniors—*2,250 milligrams per day divided into 3 doses of 750 milligrams. Liquid is prescribed for those who cannot swallow tablets.

 Usual child dose: *for inflammation or pain—*children weighing 81 pounds or less—50 milligrams per 2.2 pounds of body weight taken 2 times per day. Children weighing over 81 pounds—2,250 milligrams per day divided into 2 doses. Liquid is prescribed for those who cannot swallow tablets.

 Missed dose: *if taking on a regular basis—*take as soon as possible, unless almost time for next dose. In that case, do not take missed dose; go back to regular schedule. *Do not double doses.*

Side Effects

Overdose symptoms: confusion, diarrhea, dizziness, drowsiness, headache, hearing impairment, rapid breathing, ringing in ears, sweating, vomiting. If you

suspect an overdose, immediately seek medical attention.

 More common side effects: constipation, diarrhea, heartburn, indigestion, nausea, ringing in the ears, stomach pain and upset, vomiting.

 Less common side effects: dizziness, drowsiness, headache, hearing impairment, light-headedness, sluggishness. Rare side effects: asthma, blood in stool, bruising, confusion, distorted sense of taste, hallucinations, hearing loss, hepatitis, hives, inflammation of upper gastric tract, itching, loss of appetite, nosebleed, rash, skin eruptions or discoloration, stomach or intestinal ulcers, swelling due to fluid accumulation, weight gain.

Interactions

 Inform your doctor before combining Trilsate with: antacids such as Gaviscon or Maalox; antigout medications; blood thinners such as Coumadin; Diamox; diabetes medications such as insulin, Micronase, and Tolinase; methotrexate; other salicylates such as aspirin; phenytoin (Dilantin); steroids such as prednisone; valproic acid (Depakene).

 No known food/other substance interactions.

Special Cautions

 If pregnant or planning to become pregnant, inform your doctor immediately. Appears in breast milk; could affect a nursing infant.

 Seniors are prescribed a lower dose.

 Follow doctor's instructions carefully for children. Should not be used by children or teenagers who have chicken pox or flu symptoms—increases risk of Reye's syndrome (rare neurological disorder).

 Inform your doctor *before* starting Trilisate if you have asthma and are allergic to aspirin. Avoid if sensitive to or allergic to Trilisate.

Use with caution if you have: severe or recurring kidney or liver disorder, gastritis (inflammation of stomach lining), or stomach or intestinal disorder.

Trimethobenzamide Hydrochloride
see TIGAN

Trimethoprim with Sulfamethoxazole
see SEPTRA

Trimipramine Maleate
see SURMONTIL

Trimox
see AMOXIL

Trinalin Repetabs

Generic name: Azatadine with pseudoephedrine

Trinalin Repetabs is an antihistamine and decongestant combination. Antihistamines block the action of histamine, a chemical the body produces during an allergic reaction. Decongestants reduce nasal congestion, making it easier to breathe.

℞ QUICK FACTS

Purpose

 Used to treat nasal stuffiness and middle ear congestion caused by hay fever and ongoing nasal inflammation.

Dosage

 Take exactly as prescribed; *do not exceed dosage.*

Usual adult dose: 1 tablet taken 2 times per day.

 Usual child dose: for children ages 12 and over—1 tablet taken 2 times per day. Not generally prescribed for children under 12 years.

 Missed dose: *if taking on a regular schedule*—take as soon as possible, unless almost time for next dose. In that case, do not take missed dose; go back to regular schedule. *Do not double doses.*

Side Effects

 Overdose may be fatal. Overdose symptoms: anxiety, bluish color caused by lack of oxygen, blurred vision, chest pain, coma, convulsions, decreased mental alertness, delusions, difficulty sleeping, difficulty urinating, dizziness, excitement, extreme calm (sedation), exaggerated sense of well-being, fluttery heartbeat, giddiness, hallucinations, headache, high blood pressure or low blood pressure, irregular heartbeat, lack of muscle coordination, muscle tenseness, muscle weakness, nausea, perspiration, rapid heartbeat, restlessness, ringing in the ears, temporary interruption of breathing, thirst, tremors, vomiting. Overdose symptoms more common in children: dry mouth, fixed or dilated pupils, flushing, overstimulation, stomach and intestinal problems, very high body temperature. If you suspect an overdose, immediately seek medical attention.

Side effects: abdominal cramps; acute inflammation of the inner ear; anemia; anxiety; blood disorders; blurred vision; chest pain; chills; confusion; constipation; convulsions; diarrhea; difficulty breathing; dilated pupils; disturbed coordination; dizziness; dry mouth, nose, and throat; early menstruation; exaggerated feeling of well-being; excessive perspiration; excitement; extreme calm (sedation); fatigue; fear; fluttery heartbeat; frequent urination; hallucinations; headache; high blood pressure; hives; hysteria; increased chest congestion; increased sensitivity to light; insomnia; irregular heartbeat; irritability; loss of appetite; low blood pressure; nausea; nervousness; painful or difficult urination; pale skin; rapid heartbeat; rash; restlessness; ringing in the ears; severe allergic reaction; sleepiness; stuffy nose; tension; tightness in the chest; tingling or pins and needles; tremor; upset stomach; urinary retention; vertigo; vomiting; weakness; wheezing.

No known less common or rare side effects.

Interactions

Inform your doctor before combining Trinalin Repetabs with: antacids such as Maalox; barbiturates such as Phenobarbital; beta-blocking blood pressure drugs such as Tenormin and Inderal; blood thinners such as Coumadin; Digitalis (Lanoxin); drugs for depression such as Prozac and Elavil; high blood pressure drugs such as Aldomet and Inversine; Kaolin (Kaopectate); MAO-inhibitor drugs (antidepressants such as Nardil or Parnate); sedatives such as Nembutal and Seconal; tranquilizers such as Xanax and Valium.

 Alcohol may increase the effects of this medication; *do not drink alcohol when taking medication.*

Special Cautions

 Antihistamines can cause severe reactions in babies when used in last 3 months of pregnancy. If pregnant or planning to become pregnant, inform your doctor immediately. May appear in breast milk; could affect a nursing infant so avoid if breastfeeding.

 May cause dizziness, extreme calm (sedation), and low blood pressure in seniors. *Also more likely to cause side effects such as confusion, convulsions, hallucinations, and death in seniors.*

 Not prescribed for children under 12 years.

 May cause drowsiness and impair your ability to drive a car or operate machinery. *Do not take part in any activity that requires alertness.*

Should not take if you have: difficulty urinating; overactive thyroid; narrow-angle glaucoma; sensitivity to azatadine or pseudoephedrine; severe heart disease; severe high blood pressure; or if you take MAO inhibitors (antidepressants).

Use with caution if you have: bladder obstruction due to enlarged prostate or other bladder problems, diabetes, heart disease, high blood pressure, history of bronchial asthma, increased eye pressure, peptic ulcer or other upper intestinal obstruction.

Can be habit-forming at high doses.

Tripelennamine Hydrochloride
see PBZ-SR

T-Stat
see ERYTHROMYCIN, TOPICAL

Tussionex

Generic ingredients: Hydrocodone polistirex with chlorpheniramine polistirex

Tussionex is a cough suppressant and antihistamine combination. It works by acting on the brain to suppress the cough reflex and blocks the action of histamine, a chemical the body produces during an allergic reaction.

℞ QUICK FACTS

Purpose

℞ Used to relieve coughs and upper respiratory colds and allergies.

Dosage

 Take exactly as prescribed, not diluted with other liquids or medications. Shake well before using.

 Usual adult dose: *1 teaspoonful (5 milliliters) every 12 hours; do not exceed more than 2 teaspoonfuls in 24 hours.*

 Usual child dose: *for children ages 6 to 12—½ teaspoonful every 12 hours; do not exceed more than 1 teaspoonful in 24 hours. For children over 12 years—follow doctor's instructions. Not generally prescribed for children under 6 years.*

 Missed dose: *if taking on a regular schedule—take as soon as possible, unless almost time for next dose. In that case, do not take missed dose; go back to regular schedule. Do not double doses.*

Side Effects

 Overdose symptoms: blue skin color due to lack of oxygen, cardiac arrest, cold and clammy skin, decreased or difficult breathing, extreme sleepiness leading to stupor or coma, low blood pressure, muscle flabbiness, slow heartbeat, temporary cessation of breathing. If you suspect an overdose, immediately seek medical attention.

 Side effects: anxiety, constipation, decreased mental and physical performance, difficulty breathing, difficulty urinating, dizziness, drowsiness, dry throat, emotional dependence, exaggerated feeling of depression, exaggerated sense of well-being, extreme calm, fear, itching, mental clouding, mood changes, nausea, rash, restlessness, sluggishness, tightness in chest, vomiting.

No known less common or rare side effects.

Interactions

 Inform your doctor before combining Tussionex with: antidepressant MAO inhibitors such as Nardil and Parnate; antihistamines such as Benadryl; antispasmodic medications such as Bentyl and Cogentin; anxiety medications such as Xanax and Valium; depression medications such as Elavil and Prozac; major tranquilizers such as Thorazine and Compazine; narcotics such as Percocet and Demerol.

 Do not drink alcohol when taking this medication.

Special Cautions

 If pregnant or planning to become pregnant, inform your doctor immediately. May appear in breast milk; could affect a nursing infant. There may be a risk of physical dependence in infants born to mothers taking narcotics such as Tussionex.

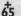 Seniors should use with caution.

 Follow doctor's instructions carefully for children.

 Do not take if sensitive to or allergic to any ingredients in Tussionex.

May cause drowsiness and impair your ability to drive a car or operate machinery. *Do not take part in any activity that requires alertness.*

May cause tolerance and dependence if used for several weeks, as it contains a mild narcotic.

Use with caution if you have lung disease or breathing disorder, may produce slowed or irregular breathing. Also use with caution if you have: narrow-angle glaucoma, asthma, enlarged prostate, urinary difficulties, intestinal disorder, liver or kidney disease, underactive thyroid gland, Addison's disease (disorder of adrenal glands), or if you have recently had a head injury.

. . . .

Can mask a severe abdominal condition or cause internal blockage.

Tussi-Organidin DM

Generic ingredients: Organidin (iodinated glycerol) with dextromethorphan hydrobromide

Other brand names: Iophen DM, IoTuss-DM, Par-Glycerol DM, Tussi-R-Gen, DM, Tusso-DM

Tussi-Organidin DM is a cough suppressant/expectorant combination. It works by acting on the brain to suppress the cough reflex and increases the amount of mucus produced, thereby changing a nonproductive cough into a productive one.

℞ QUICK FACTS

Purpose

℞   Used to relieve dry, irritating coughs associated with bronchitis and bronchial asthma.

Dosage

    Take exactly as prescribed. May take 3 to 4 weeks to see results, or doctor may discontinue after 4 weeks if no result.

Usual adult dose: 1 to 2 teaspoonfuls taken every 4 hours.

 Usual child dose: ½ to 1 teaspoonful taken every 4 hours.

 Missed dose: take as soon as possible, unless almost time for next dose. In that case, do not take missed dose; go back to regular schedule. *Do not double doses.*

Side Effects

 Overdose symptoms: no serious symptoms reported. However, if you suspect an overdose, immediately seek medical attention.

 No known common side effects.

 Rare side effects: allergic reaction to iodides; drowsiness; rash; stomach and intestinal irritation or disturbances.

Interactions

 Inform your doctor before combining Tussi-Organidin DM with: antidepressant MAO inhibitors such as Nardil and Parnate, antithyroid medications such as propylthiouracil and methimazole (Tapazole), lithium (Lithonate or Cibalith-S Syrup).

 No known food/other substance interactions.

Special Cautions

 May cause damage to the thyroid in a developing fetus. Stop taking immediately and inform your doctor if pregnant or planning to become pregnant. May appear in breast milk; could affect a nursing infant.

Seniors should use with caution.

 Follow doctor's instructions carefully for children. Use cautiously in children with cystic fibrosis; they are at risk for enlarged thyroid. May cause episodes of adolescent acne. *Not for newborn infants.*

 Do not take if sensitive to or allergic to any ingredients in Tussi-Organidin DM. Stop using if you experience rash or allergic reaction.

Use very cautiously (or not at all) if you have thyroid disease.

Skin inflammations may occur with long-term use.

Tylenol

Generic name: Acetaminophen

Other brand names: Aspirin Free Anacin, Bromo Seltzer, Datril, Liquiprin, Panadol

Tylenol is an antipyretic (fever-reducing) and analgesic combination. It works to relieve pain in people who cannot take aspirin.

℞ QUICK FACTS

Purpose

 Used to relieve simple headaches and muscle aches; the minor aches and pains of bursitis, arthritis, rheumatism, neuralgia (nerve inflammation), sprains, overexertion, and menstrual cramps; and the discomfort of fever due to colds and the flu.

Dosage

 Take medication only as needed. Follow instructions on the label.

 Usual adult dose: *Regular Strength*—1 to 2 tablets taken 3 or 4 times per day. *Extra Strength Tylenol Headache Plus*—2 caplets every 6 hours, not to exceed 8 caplets in any 24-hour period.

 Usual child dose: *for children 12 years and older*—prescribed adult doses. *For children 6 to 12 years—Regular Strength*—½ to 1 tablet taken 3 or 4 times per day. *Children's Tylenol*—give every 4 hours, but not more than 5 doses per day. *Chewable Tablets*—4 tablets (children 6 to 8 years), 5 tablets (children 9 to 10 years), 6 tablets (children 11 to 12 years). *Elixir and Suspension Liquid*—2 teaspoonfuls (children 6 to 8 years), 2½ teaspoonfuls (children 9 to 10 years), 3 teaspoonfuls (children 11 to 12 years). Use special measuring cup provided. *For children under 6 years—Regular Strength*—give only on the advice of your doctor. *Children's Tylenol*—give every 4 hours, but no more than 5 doses per day. *Chewable Tablets*—2 tablets (children 2 to 3 years), 3 tablets (children 4 to 5 years). *Elixir and Suspension Liquid*—½ teaspoonful (children 4 to 11 months), ¾ teaspoonful (children 12 to 23 months), 1 teaspoonful (children 2 to 3 years), 1½ teaspoonfuls (children 4 to 5 years). Use special measuring cup provided. *Infant's Tylenol Drops and Suspension Drops*—0.4 milliliter (children 0 to 3 months), 0.8 milliliter (children 4 to 11 months), 1.2 milliliters (children 12 to 23 months), 1.6 milliliters (children 2 to 3 years), 2.4 milliliters (children 4 to 5 years). *Do not give Tylenol Headache Plus to children under 12 years.*

 Missed dose: take only as needed.

Side Effects

 Overdose symptoms: nausea, vomiting, appetite loss, excessive perspiration, confusion, drowsiness or exhaustion, abdominal tenderness, low blood pressure, abnormal heart rhythms, yellowing of the skin and eyes, and liver and kidney failure. If you suspect an overdose, immediately seek medical attention.

 No known common side effects.

 Rare side effects: allergic reaction with symptoms such as rash, hives, swelling, or difficulty breathing.

Interactions

 Inform your doctor before combining Tylenol with: cholestyramine (Questran), isoniazid (Nydrazid), nonsteroidal anti-inflammatory drugs such as Dolobid and Motrin, oral contraceptives, phenytoin (Dilantin), warfarin (Coumadin), zidovudine (Retrovir).

 Alcohol increases the chances for liver toxicity. Avoid alcohol if Tylenol is regularly taken in large doses.

Special Cautions

 If pregnant or planning to become pregnant, or if you are breastfeeding, inform your doctor immediately.

 No special precautions apply to seniors.

 Follow doctor's instructions carefully for children.

 Do not use for more than 10 days to relieve pain, or for more than 3 days to reduce fever unless specifically instructed by your doctor.

Stop using and contact your doctor if you develop a sensitivity reaction or allergic reaction.

Use with caution if you have kidney or liver disease or viral infections of the liver.

Tylenol with Codeine

Generic name: Acetaminophen with codeine

Other brand names: Aceta with Codeine, Capital with Codeine, Phenaphen with Codeine, Ty-tabs

Tylenol with Codeine is an antipyretic (fever-reducing) and narcotic analgesic combination. It relieves pain and gives the patient a feeling of well-being.

℞ QUICK FACTS

Purpose

℞ Used to treat mild to moderately severe pain.

Dosage

 Take with meals or milk to avoid upset stomach, unless doctor advises otherwise. More effective if taken at onset of pain than when pain is intense. Take only per your doctor's instructions.

 Usual adult dose: *to relieve pain*—15 to 60 milligrams of codeine and 300 to 1,000 miligrams of acetaminophen taken every 4 hours as needed. Maximum dose per day—360 milligrams of codeine and 4,000 milligrams of acetaminophen. Doctor may also prescribe elixir form; usual dose is 1 tablespoonful taken every 4 hours as needed. *Seniors*—prescribed with caution.

Usual child dose: *children 12 years and over*—prescribed adult doses. *Children 3 to 6 years*—1 teaspoonful taken 3 or 4 times per day. *Children 7 to 12 years*—2 teaspoonfuls taken 3 or 4 times per day.

 Missed dose: *if taking on a regular schedule*—take as soon as possible, unless almost time for next dose. In that case, do not take missed dose; go back to regular schedule. *Do not take double doses.*

Side Effects

 Severe overdosage of Tylenol with Codeine can cause death. Overdose symptoms: bluish skin; cold and clammy skin; coma due to low blood sugar; decreased, irregular, or stopped breathing; extreme sleepiness progressing to stupor or coma; general bodily discomfort; heart attack; kidney failure; liver failure; low blood pressure; muscle weakness; nausea; slow heartbeat; vomiting. If you suspect an overdose, immediately seek medical attention.

 More common side effects: dizziness, light-headedness, nausea, sedation, shortness of breath, vomiting.

 Less common side effects: abdominal pain, allergic reactions, constipation, depressed feeling, exaggerated feeling of well-being, itchy skin. Rare side effects: decreased breathing at higher doses.

Interactions

 Inform your doctor before combining Tylenol with Codeine with: antipsychotic drugs such as Clozaril and Thorazine; anticholinergic drugs such as Cogentin; general anesthetics; MAO inhibitors such as Nardil; other narcotic painkillers such as Darvon; tranquilizers such as Xanax and Valium; tricyclic antidepressants such as Elavil and Tofranil.

Alcohol may increase sedative effects; *do not drink alcohol when taking this medication.*

Special Cautions

 If pregnant or planning to become pregnant, inform your doctor immediately. Used regularly in large doses during pregnancy can result in fetal addiction. At higher doses may cause breathing difficulty in mother and newborn.

 Seniors should use with caution.

 Follow doctor's instructions carefully for children 3 years and older. Not generally prescribed for children under 3 years.

 Contains sulfites, which may cause serious, even life-threatening allergic reaction. People with asthma at higher risk.

May cause drowsiness and impair your ability to drive a car or operate machinery. *Do not take part in any activity that requires alertness.*

Should not take if sensitive to or allergic to Tylenol or codeine.

If taken for prolonged periods, may cause physical and psychological addiction. Those with prior addiction problems are more at risk for Tylenol with Codeine addiction.

Tell your doctor if you have or currently experience the following: asthma; difficulty urinating; enlarged prostate; head injury; liver, kidney, thyroid, or adrenal disease; problems with drug or alcohol addiction; stomach problems such as an ulcer.

Ultracef

see DURICEF

Ultrase

see PANCREASE

Urised

Generic ingredients: Methenamine with methylene blue, phenyl salicylate, benzoic acid, atropine sulfate, and hyoscyamine

Other brand names: Atrosept, Dolsed, Hexalol, Prosed/DS, TracTabs 2X, U-Tract, UAA, Uridon Modified, Urimed, Urinary Antiseptic No. 2, Uriseptic, Uritab, Uritin, Uro-Ves

Urised is an analgesic, antispasmodic, and antiseptic combination. It works to relieve pain, slow bowel action, and reduce stomach acid.

℞ QUICK FACTS

Purpose

℞   Used to treat lower urinary tract discomfort resulting from inflammation or diagnostic procedures. Also used to treat cystitis (inflammation of bladder and ureters); urethritis (inflammation of urethra); trigonitis (inflammation of mucous membrane of the bladder).

Dosage

 Take exactly as prescribed. Drink plenty of fluids to assist medication to work better and relieve discomfort. *Do not exceed dose prescribed by your doctor.*

 Usual adult dose: 2 tablets taken 4 times per day.

 Usual child dose: *for children 6 years and older*—doctor will individualize dose. Not generally prescribed for children under 6 years.

 Missed dose: take as soon as possible, unless almost time for next dose. In that case, do not take missed dose; go back to regular schedule. *Do not double doses.*

Side Effects

 Overdose symptoms: abdominal pain; bladder and abdominal irritation; bloody diarrhea; bloody urine; burning pain in throat and mouth; circulatory collapse; coma; dilated pupils; dizziness; dry nose, mouth, and throat; elevated blood pressure; extremely high body temperature; headache; hot, dry, flushed skin; painful and frequent urination; pallor (paleness); pounding heartbeat; rapid heartbeat; respiratory failure; ringing in ears; sweating; vomiting; weakness; white sores in mouth. If you suspect an overdose, immediately seek medical attention.

 Side effects from long-term use: acute urinary retention (in men with enlarged prostate), blurry vision, difficulty urinating, dizziness, dry mouth, flushing, rapid pulse, skin rash.

No known less common or rare side effects.

Interactions

 Inform your doctor before combining Urised with: Acetazolamide (Diamox); potassium supplements such as Slow-K; sodium bicarbonate antacids such as Alka-Seltzer; sulfa medications such as Gantrisin, Gantanol, Bactrim, and Septra.

 Limit use of foods that produce alkaline urine, such as sodium bicarbonate, antacids, and orange juice.

Special Cautions

 If pregnant or planning to become pregnant, inform your doctor immediately. May appear in breast milk; could affect a nursing infant.

 No special precautions apply to seniors.

 Follow doctor's instructions carefully for children.

 Avoid if you have: glaucoma, bladder blockage, cardiospasm, or a disorder that obstructs the passage of food through the stomach.

Should not take if sensitive to or allergic to Urised or similar medications.

Use with caution if you have heart disease.

Doctor may test urine for acidity with phenapthazine paper. Vitamin C may be recommended if urine is not acidic enough.

May turn urine blue or blue-green, and may discolor stools.

Urispas

Generic name: Flavoxate hydrochloride

Urispas is a urinary tract spasmolytic. It relieves smooth muscle spasm primarily in the urinary tract.

℞ QUICK FACTS

Purpose

 Used to prevent urinary tract spasms and relieve painful or difficult urination; urinary urgency; excessive nighttime urination; pubic area pain; frequency of urination; and inability to hold urine caused by urinary tract infections. Is usually taken in combination with antibiotics.

Dosage

 Take exactly as prescribed.

 Usual adult dose: one or two 100-milligram tablets taken 3 or 4 times per day. Doctor may reduce dose as symptoms improve.

 Usual child dose: not generally prescribed for children under 12 years.

Missed dose: take as soon as possible, unless almost time for next dose. In that case, do not take missed dose; go back to regular schedule. *Do not double doses.*

Side Effects

 Overdose symptoms: convulsions; decreased ability to sweat (warm and/or red skin, dry mouth, increased body temperature); hallucinations; increased heart rate and blood pressure; mental confusion. If you suspect an overdose, immediately seek medical attention.

 Side effects: allergic skin reactions including hives, blurred vision and vision changes, drowsiness, dry mouth, fluttery heartbeat, headache, high body temperature, mental confusion (especially seniors), nausea, nervousness, painful or difficult urination, rapid heartbeat, vertigo, vomiting.

 No known less common or rare side effects.

Interactions

 No drug interactions reported.

 No known food/other substance interactions.

Special Cautions

 If pregnant or planning to become pregnant, inform your doctor immediately. May appear in breast milk; could affect a nursing infant.

 Seniors at higher risk for mental confusion.

 Not generally prescribed for children under 12 years.

 May blur vision and cause drowsiness, impairing your ability to drive a car or operate machinery. *Do not take part in any activity that requires alertness.*

Avoid Urispas if you have: stomach or intestinal blockage, muscle relaxation problems (especially the sphincter muscle), abdominal bleeding, or urinary tract blockage.

Use with caution if you have glaucoma.

Ursodiol

see ACTIGALL

Valium

Generic name: Diazepam

Other brand names: Valrelease, Vazepam

Valium is an anti-anxiety agent, skeletal muscle relaxant, amnesic agent, anticonvulsant, and sedative, as well as a benzodiazepine agent. It is thought to relieve anxiety by depressing the central nervous system. It also reduces the activity of certain chemicals in the brain.

℞ QUICK FACTS

Purpose

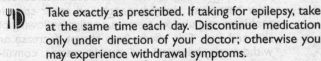

Used to treat anxiety disorders and for short-term relief of the symptoms of anxiety. Also used to treat symptoms of alcohol withdrawal; to relax muscles; to relieve uncontrolled muscle movements caused by cerebral palsy and lower-body paralysis; to control involuntary movement of the hands (athetosis); to relax tight, aching muscles; and in combination with other medication to treat convulsive disorders.

Dosage

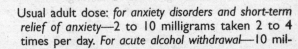

Take exactly as prescribed. If taking for epilepsy, take at the same time each day. Discontinue medication only under direction of your doctor; otherwise you may experience withdrawal symptoms.

Usual adult dose: *for anxiety disorders and short-term relief of anxiety*—2 to 10 milligrams taken 2 to 4 times per day. *For acute alcohol withdrawal*—10 milligrams taken 3 or 4 times in the first 24 hours, then 5 milligrams taken 3 or 4 times per day as needed. *For muscle spasm*—2 to 10 milligrams taken 3 or 4 times per day. *For convulsive disorders*—2 to 10 milligrams taken 2 to 4 times per day. *Seniors*—2 to 2.5 milligrams taken 1 or 2 times per day. Doctor may increase if needed.

 Usual child dose: *for children 6 months and older*—1 to 2.5 milligrams taken 3 or 4 times per day. Doctor may increase if needed.

 Missed dose: take as soon as possible, unless almost time for next dose. In that case, do not take missed dose; go back to regular schedule. *Do not double doses.*

Side Effects

 Overdose symptoms: coma, confusion, diminished reflexes, sleepiness. If you suspect an overdose, immediately seek medical attention.

 More common side effects: drowsiness, fatigue, lightheadedness, loss of muscle coordination.

 Less common side effects: anxiety, blurred vision, changes in salivation, changes in sex drive, confusion, constipation, depression, difficulty urinating, dizziness, double vision, hallucinations, headache, inability to hold urine, low blood pressure, nausea, overstimulation, rage, seizures, skin rash, sleep disturbances, slow heartbeat, slurred speech and other speech problems, stimulation, tremors, vertigo, yellowing of skin and eyes. Side effects from abrupt decrease or withdrawal: abdominal and muscle cramps, convulsions, sweating, tremors, vomiting.

Interactions

 Inform your doctor before combining Valium with: anticonvulsants such as Dilantin, antidepressants such as Elavil and Prozac, barbiturates such as phenobarbital, cimetidine (Tagamet), digoxin (Lanoxin), disulfiram (Antabuse), fluoxetine (Prozac), isoniazid (Nydrazid), levodopa (Larodopa or Sinemet), major tranquilizers such as Mellaril and Thorazine, MAO inhibitors such as Nardil, narcotics such as Percocet, omeprazole (Prilosec), oral contraceptives, propoxyphene (Darvon), ranitidine (Zantac), rifampin (Rifadin).

Do not drink alcohol during Valium therapy.

Special Cautions

 Do not take if pregnant or planning to become pregnant. Valium increases risk of birth defects.

 Seniors are prescribed lower doses to avoid oversedation or incoordination.

 Follow doctor's instructions carefully for children over 6 months of age.

 Do not take if you have glaucoma.

May cause drowsiness and impair your ability to drive a car or operate machinery. *Do not take part in any activity that requires alertness.*

Can be addictive or habit-forming.

Avoid if sensitive to or allergic to Valium.

. . . .
Valium is not for anxiety or tension related to everyday stress or for mental disorders more serious than anxiety.
. . . .
Use with caution if you have kidney or liver problems.

Valproic Acid

see DEPAKENE

Valrelease

see VALIUM

Vancenase

see BECLOVENT INHALATION AEROSOL

Vaseretic

Generic ingredients: Enalapril maleate with hydrochlorothiazide

Vaseretic is an angiotensin-converting enzyme (ACE) inhibitor and thiazide diuretic combination. It blocks the production of chemicals responsible for constricting blood vessels and helps your body eliminate fluids, thereby lowering blood pressure.

℞ QUICK FACTS

Purpose

℞ Used to treat high blood pressure.

Dosage

 Take exactly as prescribed, and on a regular basis for it to be effective. May take several weeks to observe effects. Once symptoms disappear, continue to take.

 Usual adult dose: once blood pressure has stabilized—1 or 2 tablets taken once per day. Maximum dose is 2 tablets per day. Doctor should discontinue diuretics before prescribing Vaseretic.

 Usual child dose: not generally prescribed for children.

 Missed dose: take as soon as possible, unless almost time for next dose. In that case, do not take missed dose; go back to regular schedule. *Do not double doses.*

Side Effects

 Overdose symptoms: dehydration, low blood pressure. If you suspect an overdose, immediately seek medical attention.

 More common side effects: cough, diarrhea, dizziness, drop in blood pressure upon standing, fatigue, headache, impotence, low potassium levels, muscle cramps, nausea, rash, tingling or pins and needles, weakness.

 Less common or rare side effects: abdominal pain; abnormal skin sensations such as numbness, prickling, or burning; back pain; black stools; blood clots in lungs; blurred vision; bronchitis; chest pain; confusion; decrease in sex drive; depression; disturbances in heart rhythm; dry eyes; dry mouth; excessive sweating; fainting; fluid in the lungs; flushing; gas; gout; heart attack; hepatitis; hives; hoarseness; inability to sleep; indigestion; inflammation of mouth and tongue; inflammation of the pancreas; itching; joint pain; kidney failure; loss of appetite; loss of coordination; loss of hair; low blood pressure; nervousness; rapid heartbeat; restlessness; ringing in ears; runny nose; sensitivity to light; shortness of breath; sleepiness; sore throat; stroke; tearing; urinary tract infections; vomiting; yellow eyes and skin.

Interactions

Inform your doctor before combining Vaseretic with: barbiturates; certain other antihypertensives; corticosteroids such as prednisone; digitalis (Lanoxin); insulin; lithium; narcotic painkillers; nonsteroidal anti-inflammatory medications such as Naprosyn and Motrin; norepinephrine; oral antidiabetic medications such as Micronase; potassium supplements; potassium-containing salt substitutes; potassium-sparing diuretics such as Midamor.

Do not drink alcohol while taking Vaseretic.

Special Cautions

May cause birth defects, premature birth, or death to newborns. If pregnant or planning to become pregnant, inform your doctor immediately. Appears in breast milk; could affect a nursing infant.

No special precautions apply to seniors.

Not generally prescribed for children.

Should not take if you have history of angioedema (swelling of face, extremities, and throat) or inability to urinate. *If swelling of these areas or of the eyes, lips, or tongue occurs, immediately seek medical help; may be an emergency situation.*

May cause drowsiness and impair your ability to drive a car or operate machinery. *Do not take part in any activity that requires alertness.*

Avoid if sensitive to or allergic to this or similar medications or other sulfa medications.

Inform your doctor immediately if you experience chest pain, sore throat, or fever.

Doctor will monitor kidney function during Vaseretic therapy.

Use with caution if you have liver disease or lupus erythematosus, and congestive heart failure—which may cause low blood pressure.

Excessive fluid loss may cause low blood pressure. Excessive sweating, dehydration, severe diarrhea, or vomiting may cause fluid loss.

Avoid excessive sunlight.

If you have diabetes, your doctor will monitor your blood sugar levels.

VasoClear

see NAPHCON-A

Vasotec

∿∿∿∿∿∿∿∿∿∿∿∿∿∿∿∿∿∿∿∿∿∿∿∿∿∿∿∿∿∿∿∿∿∿∿∿∿∿

Generic name: Enalapril maleate

Vasotec is an angiotensin-converting enzyme (ACE) inhibitor. It blocks the production of chemicals responsible for constricting blood vessels.

℞ QUICK FACTS

Purpose

℞   Used to treat high blood pressure.

Dosage

 Take exactly as prescribed, and on a regular basis for
it to be effective. May take several weeks to observe
effects. Once symptoms disappear, continue to take.
May take with or without food. *Do not use salt substitutes with potassium unless directed by your doctor.*

 Usual adult dose: *for hypertension (in people not taking
a diuretic)*—5 milligrams taken once per day to start.
Ongoing dose—10 to 40 milligrams per day as a single dose or divided into smaller doses. *For hypertension (in people who are taking a diuretic)*—2.5 milligrams to start. Doctor may suggest stopping
diuretic 2 to 3 days before taking Vasotec. Regular
dose is carefully prescribed. *For kidney disorder*—doctor will adjust dose according to severity of kidney
disease. *For heart failure*—2.5 milligrams taken 1 or 2
times per day to start. Doctor may prescribe using
with digitalis and diuretics if you have heart disease.
Regular dose is 5 to 20 milligrams per day taken as a
single dose or 2 doses. Maximum dose per day is 40
milligrams taken as a single dose or in 2 doses.

Usual child dose: not generally prescribed for children.

 Missed dose: take as soon as possible, unless almost time for next dose. In that case, do not take missed dose; go back to regular schedule. *Do not double doses.*

Side Effects

 Overdose symptoms: sudden drop in blood pressure. If you suspect an overdose, immediately seek medical attention.

 Side effects: abdominal pain; abnormal skin sensations such as numbness or prickling; anaphylactic shock (severe allergic reactions); angina (crushing chest pain); angioedema (swelling of the face, lips, tongue, throat, arms, legs, and difficulty swallowing); asthma; blood abnormalities; blood clot in lung and tissue loss; blurred vision; breast enlargement in males; bronchitis; confusion; conjunctivitis (pink eye); constipation; cough; dark or tarry stools containing blood; decreased urination; depression; diarrhea; difficulty breathing; difficulty sleeping; digestive difficulty and stomach discomfort; dizziness; dry eyes; dry mouth; excessive perspiration; fainting; fatigue; flank pain; fluid in lungs; flushing; hair loss; headache; heart palpitations; heart rhythm disturbances; hepatitis; herpes zoster; hives; impotence; inflammation of mouth and tongue; itching; lack of muscle coordination; loss of appetite; loss of sense of smell; low blood pressure; muscle cramps; nausea; nervousness; pneumonia; pounding heartbeat; rapid or slow heartbeat; rash; red skin (like sunburn); ringing in ears; runny nose; sensitivity to light; sleepiness; sore throat and hoarseness; stroke; taste alteration; tearing; tingling, pins and needles or burning sensation; upper respiratory infection; upset stomach; urinary tract infection; vertigo; vomiting; weakness; wheezing.

- -

 No known less common or rare side effects.

Interactions

 Inform your doctor before combining Vasotec with: diuretics such as Lasix or HydroDIURIL, potassium-sparing diuretics such as aldactazide, potassium supplements such as K-Lyte or K-Tab, potassium-containing salt substitutes, lithium. Serious blood disorders have occurred when using Captopril, another ACE inhibitor, with Vasotec.

- -

 No known food/other substance interactions.

Special Cautions

 May cause birth defects, premature birth, or death to newborns. If pregnant or planning to become pregnant, inform your doctor immediately. Appears in breast milk; could affect a nursing infant.

- -

 No special precautions apply to seniors.

- -

 Not generally prescribed for children.

- -

 Should not take if you have history of angioedema (swelling of face, extremities, and throat) or inability to urinate. *If swelling of these areas or of the eyes, lips, or tongue occurs, immediately seek medical help; may be an emergency situation.*

- -

May cause drowsiness and impair your ability to drive a car or operate machinery. *Do not take part in any activity that requires alertness.*

Avoid if sensitive to or allergic to this or similar medications.

Very low blood pressure may develop if taking high doses of diuretics with Vasotec. At increased risk if you have heart disease, kidney disease, potassium imbalance, or salt imbalance.

Inform your doctor immediately if you experience chest pain, sore throat, or fever.

Excessive fluid loss may cause low blood pressure. Excessive sweating, dehydration, severe diarrhea, or vomiting may cause fluid loss.

Venlafaxine Hydrochloride
see EFFEXOR

Ventolin
see PROVENTIL

Verapamil Hydrochloride
see CALAN

Vicodin

Generic ingredients: Hydrocodone bitartrate with acetaminophen

Other brand names: Amacodone, Anexsia,
Anodynos-DHC, Bancap HC, Co-Gesic, Dolacet,
Duradyne DHC, Hydrocet, Hydrogesic, Hy-Phen,
Margesic-H, Lorcet, Lortab, Norcet, Stagesic,
T-Gesic, Zydone

Vicodin is an analgesic combination. It acts on the central nervous system to relieve pain.

℞ QUICK FACTS

Purpose

℞ Used to treat moderate to moderately severe pain.

Dosage

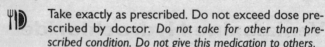 Take exactly as prescribed. Do not exceed dose prescribed by doctor. *Do not take for other than prescribed condition. Do not give this medication to others.*

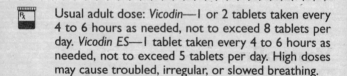 Usual adult dose: *Vicodin*—1 or 2 tablets taken every 4 to 6 hours as needed, not to exceed 8 tablets per day. *Vicodin ES*—1 tablet taken every 4 to 6 hours as needed, not to exceed 5 tablets per day. High doses may cause troubled, irregular, or slowed breathing.

Usual child dose: not generally prescribed for children.

Missed dose: *if taking on a regular basis*—take as soon as possible, unless almost time for next dose. In that case, do not take missed dose; go back to regular schedule. *Do not double doses.*

Side Effects

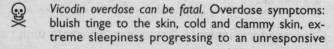 *Vicodin overdose can be fatal.* Overdose symptoms: bluish tinge to the skin, cold and clammy skin, extreme sleepiness progressing to an unresponsive

state, general feeling of bodily discomfort, heavy perspiration, limp muscles, liver failure, low blood pressure, nausea, slow heartbeat, troubled or slowed breathing, vomiting. If you suspect an overdose, immediately seek medical attention.

 More common side effects: dizziness, light-headedness, nausea, sedation, vomiting.

 Less common or rare side effects: anxiety; constipation; decreased mental and physical ability; difficulty urinating; drowsiness; fear; feeling of discomfort; mental clouding; mood changes; sluggishness; troubled, irregular, or slowed breathing.

Interactions

 Inform your doctor before combining Vicodin with: anti-anxiety medications such as Valium and Librium, MAO inhibitors such as Nardil and Parnate, medications to control muscle spasms such as Cogentin, major tranquilizers such as Thorazine and Haldol, other narcotic analgesics such as Demerol, tricyclic antidepressants such as Elavil and Tofranil.

 Avoid alcohol when taking Vicodin.

Special Cautions

 Do not take if pregnant or planning to become pregnant. Drug dependence occurs in newborns if the mother has taken Vicodin regularly before delivery. May appear in breast milk; could affect a nursing infant.

 No special precautions apply to seniors.

 Not generally prescribed for children.

May cause drowsiness and impair your ability to drive a car or operate machinery. *Do not take part in any activity that requires alertness.*

Avoid if sensitive to or allergic to any ingredients of Vicodin.

Use with caution if you have: head injury, severe liver or kidney disorder, underactive thyroid gland, Addison's disease (adrenal gland disease), enlarged prostate, or urethral stricture (narrowing of tube carrying urine from the bladder).

May interfere with diagnosing and treating abdominal conditions.

Use carefully if you have had surgery or lung disease; Vicodin suppresses the cough reflex.

Vi-Daylin/F

see POLY-VI-FLOR

Visken

Generic name: Pindolol

Visken is a beta-adrenergic blocking agent (beta-blocker). Beta-blockers decrease the workload of the heart and help regulate the heartbeat.

℞ QUICK FACTS

Purpose

 Used to treat high blood pressure.

Dosage

 Take exactly as prescribed, and on a regular basis for it to be effective. May take several weeks to observe effects. Once symptoms disappear, continue to take. May take with or without food. If not taken regularly, symptoms may worsen, or may cause chest pain or heart attack.

 Usual adult dose: 5 milligrams taken 2 times per day, either alone or with other high blood pressure medications. If blood pressure not reduced within 3 to 4 weeks, doctor may increase total daily dose by 10 milligrams at a time, at 3 to 4 week intervals, up to 60 milligrams per day. *Seniors*—doses are individualized.

 Usual child dose: not generally prescribed for children.

 Missed dose: take as soon as possible, unless within 4 hours of next dose. In that case, do not take missed dose; go back to regular schedule. *Do not double doses.*

Side Effects

 Overdose symptoms: bronchospasm (spasm of air passages), excessively slow heartbeat, heart failure, low blood pressure. If you suspect an overdose, immediately seek medical attention.

 More common side effects: abdominal discomfort, chest pain, difficult or labored breathing, dizziness, fatigue, joint pain, muscle pain or cramps, nausea, nervousness, strange dreams, swelling due to fluid retention, tingling or pins and needles, trouble sleeping, weakness.

 Less common or rare side effects: hallucinations, heart failure, itching, palpitations, rapid heartbeat, rash.

Interactions

 Inform your doctor before combining Visken with: airway-opening medications such as Proventil and Ventolin; blood pressure medications such as reserpine; digoxin (Lanoxin); epinephrine (EpiPen); hydrochlorothiazide (HydroDIURIL); insulin or oral antidiabetic medications such as Micronase; nonsteroidal anti-inflammatory medications such as Motrin; ritodrine (Yutopar); theophylline (Theo-Dur); thioridazine (Mellaril); verapamil (Calan or Verelan).

 No known food/other substance interactions.

Special Cautions

 If pregnant or planning to become pregnant, inform your doctor immediately. Appears in breast milk; could affect a nursing infant.

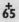 Seniors are prescribed individualized doses.

 Not generally prescribed for children.

 May cause disorientation and impair your ability to drive a car or operate machinery. *Do not take part in any activity that requires alertness.*

Should not take if you have: bronchial asthma, severe congestive heart failure, inadequate blood supply to the circulatory system (cardiogenic shock), heart block (heart irregularity), or severely slow heart-beat.

Tell your doctor *before* taking Visken if you have a history of severe allergic reactions.

Use with caution if you have: asthma, chronic bronchitis, emphysema, seasonal allergies or other bronchial conditions, coronary artery disease, or kidney or liver disease.

Tell your doctor or dentist in a medical emergency or before surgery or treatment that you are taking Visken.

Doctor may monitor pulse rate; Visken may cause slow heartbeat.

Symptoms of low blood sugar or altered blood sugar levels may occur. If diabetic, discuss this with your doctor.

Vistaril
see ATARAX

Vitamin A Acid
see RETIN-A

Vitamins with Fluoride
see POLY-VI-FLOR

Voltaren

∿∿∿∿∿∿∿∿∿∿∿∿∿∿∿∿∿∿∿∿∿∿∿∿∿∿∿∿∿∿∿∿∿∿∿∿∿∿

Generic name: Diclofenac sodium

Other brand name: Cataflam (diclofenac potassium)

Voltaren is a nonsteroidal anti-inflammatory drug (NSAID). It works by blocking the production of prostaglandins, which may trigger pain.

℞ QUICK FACTS

Purpose

℞ Used to treat the inflammation, swelling, stiffness, and joint pain associated with rheumatoid arthritis, osteoarthritis, and ankylosing spondylitis (arthritis and spine stiffness). Also used to treat menstrual pain.

Dosage

 Take exactly as prescribed. May take with food, milk, or an antacid to avoid stomach upset, but may delay onset of relief. Take with a full glass of water, and do not lie down for 20 minutes after taking to prevent upper digestive tract irritation.

· ·

Usual adult dose: *for osteoarthritis and rheumatoid arthritis—Voltaren or Cataflam*—100 to 150 milligrams per day divided into smaller doses of 50 milligrams, and taken 2 or 3 times per day. *Voltaren*—75 milligrams taken 2 times per day. Individuals with rheumatoid arthritis should not exceed 225 milligrams per day. *For ankylosing spondylitis*—100 to 125 milligrams per day divided into smaller doses of 25 milligrams, and taken 4 times per day with another 25 milligrams at bedtime if necessary. *For menstrual pain*—50 milligrams taken 3 times per day to start, then not to exceed 150 milligrams per day. Some women may be prescribed 100 milligrams to start, followed by 50-milligram doses.

 Usual child dose: not generally prescribed for children.

 Missed dose: *if taking on a regular basis*—take as soon as possible, unless almost time for next dose. In that case, do not take missed dose; go back to regular schedule. *Do not double doses.*

Side Effects

 Overdose symptoms: acute kidney failure, drowsiness, loss of consciousness, lung inflammation, vomiting. If you suspect an overdose, immediately seek medical attention.

 More common side effects: abdominal pain, constipation, cramps, diarrhea, dizziness, headache, indigestion, nausea.

 Less common side effects: abdominal bleeding; abdominal swelling; fluid retention; gas; itching; peptic ulcers; rash; ringing in ears. Rare side effects: anaphylaxis (severe allergic reaction); anemia; anxiety; appetite change; asthma; black stools; blood disorders; bloody diarrhea; blurred vision; changes in taste; colitis; congestive heart failure; decrease in white blood cells; decreased urine production; depression; double vision; drowsiness; dry mouth; hair loss; hearing loss (temporary); hepatitis; high blood pressure; hives; inability to sleep; inflammation of the mouth; irritability; itching; kidney failure; low blood pressure; nosebleed; red or purple skin discoloration; rash; sensitivity to light; skin eruptions; inflammation; scaling or peeling; Stevens-Johnson syndrome (severe skin eruption); swelling of eyelids, lips, and tongue; swelling of the throat due to fluid retention; vague feeling of illness; vision changes; vomiting; yellow eyes and skin.

Interactions

Inform your doctor before combining Voltaren with: aspirin; blood thinners such as Coumadin; carteolol (Cartrol); cyclosporine (Sandimmune); digitalis (Lanoxin); diuretics such as Dyazide and Lasix; insulin; oral antidiabetes medications such as Micronase; lithium (Lithonate); methotrexate.

No known food/other substance interactions.

Special Cautions

If pregnant or planning to become pregnant, inform your doctor immediately. Appears in breast milk; could affect a nursing infant.

No special precautions apply to seniors.

Not generally prescribed for children.

Immediately notify your doctor if you experience: nausea, fatigue, lethargy, itching, yellowed eyes and skin, tenderness in upper right area of abdomen, or flu-like symptoms.

Ulcers or internal bleeding may occur without warning; doctor should perform regular check-ups.

Avoid if sensitive to or allergic to Voltaren or Cataflam, or if you have had asthma attacks, hives, or other allergic reactions caused by aspirin or other nonsteroidal anti-inflammatory medications.

. . . .

Use with caution if you have: heart failure, kidney problems, or liver inflammation; may cause inflamed liver.

. . . .

May increase water retention; individuals with high blood pressure should use with caution.

Warfarin Sodium

see COUMADIN

Wellbutrin

Generic name: Bupropion hydrochloride

Wellbutrin is an antidepressant. It is thought to relieve depression by increasing the concentration of the chemicals necessary for nerve transmission to the brain.

℞ QUICK FACTS

Purpose

 Used to treat certain kinds of major depression and their symptoms: severely depressed mood for more than 2 weeks; sleep and appetite disturbances; agitation or lack of energy; feelings of guilt or worthlessness; decreased sex drive; inability to concentrate; and suicidal thoughts.

Dosage

 Take exactly as prescribed. Doctor may continue therapy for several months if Wellbutrin is effective.

 Usual adult dose: 200 milligrams per day to start. After 3 days doctor may increase to 300 milligrams per day, divided in 3 equal doses, with at least 6 hours between doses. Maximum dose is 150 mil-

ligrams taken 3 times per day. *Seniors*—may be prescribed lower doses.

· ·

 Usual child dose: not generally prescribed for children.

· ·

 Missed dose: take as soon as possible, unless within
4 hours of next dose. In that case, do not take
missed dose; go back to regular schedule. *Do not
double doses.*

Side Effects

 Overdose symptoms: hallucinations, heart failure,
loss of consciousness, rapid heartbeat, seizures.
Overdose involving other medications in combination with Wellbutrin: breathing difficulties, coma,
fever, rigid muscles, stupor. If you suspect an overdose, immediately seek medical attention.

· ·

 Most worrisome side effect: seizure. More common
side effects: agitation, constipation, dizziness, dry
mouth, excessive sweating, headache, nausea and
vomiting, skin rash, sleep disturbances, tremor.

· ·

 Other side effects: acne; bedwetting; blisters in the
mouth and eyes (Stevens-Johnson syndrome);
blurred vision; breathing difficulty; chest pain; chills;
complete or almost complete loss of movement;
confusion; dry skin; episodes of overactivity, elation,
or irritability; extreme calmness; fatigue; fever; fluid
retention; flu-like symptoms; gum irritation and inflammation; hair color changes; hair loss; hives; impotence; incoordination and clumsiness; indigestion;
itching; increased libido; menstrual problems; mood
instability; muscle rigidity; painful ejaculation; painful
erection; retarded ejaculation; ringing in ears; sexual
dysfunction; suicidal ideas; thirst disturbances; toothache; urinary disturbances; weight gain or loss.

· ·

Interactions

Do not take Wellbutrin within 14 days of taking a MAO inhibitor such as Nardil or Parnate; may cause sudden and dangerous blood pressure elevation. Inform your doctor before combining Wellbutrin with: antipsychotics such as Thorazine; Dilantin; levodopa (Laradopa); phenobarbital; Tagamet; Tegretol; tricyclic antidepressants such as Elavil and Tofranil. *Antipsychotics or antidepressants may trigger seizures.* If taking Valium or similar medications, taper off use rather than abruptly stopping.

Do not drink alcohol while taking Wellbutrin; may cause seizures.

Special Cautions

If pregnant or planning to become pregnant, inform your doctor immediately. May appear in breast milk; could affect a nursing infant.

Due to sensitivity to antidepressant medications, seniors are prescribed lower doses.

Not generally prescribed for children.

Do not take if sensitive to or allergic to Wellbutrin, or if you have a seizure disorder.

May impair your coordination and judgment and affect your ability to drive a car or operate machinery. *Do not take part in any activity that requires alertness.*

At risk for seizures if you are taking too high a dose of Wellbutrin or if you have had seizures or brain damage in the past.

⸱ ⸱ ⸱ ⸱ ⸱ ⸱ ⸱

Should not take if you have or had an eating disorder such as anorexia nervosa or bulimia; at increased risk for seizures.

Usually causes weight loss, but may cause weight gain. Doctor may not prescribe if your depression has already caused weight loss.

Wytensin

Generic name: Guanabenz acetate

Wytensin is an antihypertensive. It works to reduce blood pressure by reducing nerve impulses to the heart and arteries.

℞ QUICK FACTS

Purpose

℞ Used to treat high blood pressure. Works 60 minutes after taking a single dose and may slightly slow heartbeat.

Dosage

 May take with or without food. Take exactly as prescribed, and on a regular basis for it to be effective. May take several weeks to observe effects. Once symptoms disappear, continue to take.

⸱ ⸱ ⸱ ⸱ ⸱ ⸱ ⸱

 Usual adult dose: 4 milligrams taken 2 times per day to start, whether prescribed alone or with a thiazide diuretic. Doctor may increase dose in increments of 4 to 8 milligrams per day every 1 to 2 weeks, up to 32 milligrams taken 2 times per day maximum. Seniors—use with caution.

⸱ ⸱ ⸱ ⸱ ⸱ ⸱ ⸱

Usual child dose: not generally prescribed for children.

 Missed dose: take as soon as possible, unless almost time for next dose. In that case, do not take missed dose; go back to regular schedule. *Do not double doses. Contact your doctor if you miss 2 or more doses in a row.*

Side Effects

 Overdose symptoms: excessive contraction of the pupils, irritability, low blood pressure, sleepiness, slow heartbeat, sluggishness. If you suspect an overdose, immediately seek medical attention.

 More common side effects: dizziness, drowsiness, dry mouth, headache, weakness.

 Less common or rare side effects: abdominal discomfort, aches in arms and legs, anxiety, blurred vision, breast development in males, changes in taste, chest pain, constipation, decreased sex drive, depression, diarrhea, fluid retention, frequent urination, impotence, irregular heartbeat, itching, lack of muscle coordination, muscle aches, nausea, pounding heartbeat, rash, shortness of breath, sleep disturbances, stomach pain, stuffy nose, vomiting. Rare side effect: heartbeat irregularities.

Interactions

 Inform your doctor before combining Wytensin with: antihistamines such as Benadryl or Tavist; medications that depress the central nervous system such as Halcion, Valium, and phenobarbital.

 Avoid alcohol during Wytensin therapy.

Special Cautions

 If pregnant or planning to become pregnant, inform your doctor immediately. May appear in breast milk; could affect a nursing infant.

 Seniors should use with caution.

 Not generally prescribed for children.

 Do not take if sensitive to or allergic to Wytensin.

May cause drowsiness and impair your ability to drive a car or operate machinery. *Do not take part in any activity that requires alertness.*

Use with caution if you have: severe heart disease, stroke, or related disorders; severe liver or kidney failure; or if you had a recent heart attack.

Doctor will do blood pressure monitoring if you have kidney or liver disease.

Xanax

Generic name: Alprazolam

Xanax is a benzodiazepine tranquilizer. It reduces the activity of certain chemicals in the brain.

℞ QUICK FACTS

Purpose

 Used to treat symptoms of anxiety and anxiety associated with depression. Also prescribed for irritable bowel syndrome, panic attacks, depression, premenstrual syndrome, alcohol withdrawal, fear of open spaces, and fear of people.

Dosage

 Take with food or full glass of water if stomach irritation occurs. With long-term use, dependence and tolerance can occur. You may experience withdrawal symptoms if you abruptly stop taking this medication. Only your doctor should discontinue or change your dosage.

Usual adult dose: *for anxiety disorder*—0.25 to 0.5 milligrams taken 3 times per day. Dose may be increased every 3 to 4 days to a maximum of 4 milligrams per day divided into smaller doses. *For panic disorder*—starting dose is 0.5 milligrams taken 3 times per day, increased by 1 milligram per day every 3 or 4 days. Most people are prescribed 5 to 6 milligrams per day. *For seniors*—0.25 milligram taken 2 or 3 times per day to start. Doctor may gradually increase if necessary. *For people with liver or kidney disease*—generally prescribed lower doses.

Usual child dose: not generally prescribed for children.

Missed dose: take as soon as possible, *unless within 1 hour of next dose. In that case, do not take missed dose; go back to regular schedule. Do not double doses.*

Side Effects

An overdose of Xanax, combined with or without alcohol, can be fatal. Overdose symptoms may include: confusion, coma, impaired coordination, sleepiness, slowed reaction time. If you suspect an overdose, immediately seek medical attention.

Most common side effect is mild drowsiness during the first few days of therapy. Other more common side effects: abdominal discomfort, abnormal involuntary movement, agitated state, allergies, anxiety, blurred vision, chest pain, confusion, constipation, decreased or increased sex drive, depression, diarrhea, difficult urination, dream abnormalities, dry mouth, fainting, fatigue, fluid retention, headache, hyperventilation, inability to fall asleep, increase or decrease in appetite, increased or decreased salivation, impaired memory, irritability, lack of coordination, light-headedness, low blood pressure, irregular menstrual cycle, muscular twitching, nausea and vomiting, nervousness, palpations, rapid heartbeat, rash, restlessness, ringing in the ears, sexual dysfunction, skin inflammation, speech difficulties, stiffness, stuffy nose, sweating, tiredness or sleepiness, tremors, upper respiratory infections, weakness, weight gain or loss. Side effects due to decreased dosage or withdrawal from Xanax: blurred vision, decreased concentration, decreased mental clarity, diarrhea, heightened awareness of noise or bright lights, impaired sense of smell, loss of appetite, loss of weight, muscle cramps, seizures, tingling sensation, twitching.

Less common side effects: abnormal muscle tone, concentration difficulties, decreased coordination, dizziness, double vision, dry mouth, fear, hallucinations, hiccups, inability to control urination or bowel movements, infection, itching, loss of appetite, muscle cramps, muscle spasticity, rage, sedation, seizures, sleep disturbances, slurred speech, stimulation, talkativeness, taste alterations, temporary memory loss, tingling or pins and needles, uninhibited behavior, urine retention, warm feeling, weakness in muscle and bone, weight gain or loss, yellow eyes and skin.

Interactions

Inform your doctor before combining Xanax with: antihistamines such as Benadryl and Tavist; Carbamazepine (Tegretol); certain antidepressant drugs including Elavil, Norpramin, and Tofranil; Cimetidine (Tagamet); Digoxin (Lanoxin); Disulfiram (Antabuse); major tranquilizers such as Mellaril and Thorazine; oral contraceptives; other central nervous system depressants such as Valium and Demerol.

Alcohol may increase sedative effects; *do not drink alcohol when taking this medication.*

Special Cautions

If pregnant or planning to become pregnant, do not take; may cause birth defects. Increased risk of respiratory problems and muscular weakness in your baby. Infants may experience withdrawal symptoms. May appear in breast milk; could affect a nursing infant.

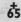 Seniors have heightened sensitivity and are prescribed lower doses.

 Not generally prescribed for children.

 If you have had an allergic reaction to this or other tranquilizers, you should not take Xanax.

Can aggravate narrow-angle glaucoma; however, if you have open-angle glaucoma, you may take it.

Should not be used for more than 3 to 4 months at a time.

Yocon

Generic name: Yohimbine hydrochloride

Yocon is an impotence agent. It is thought to work by stimulating the release of norepinephrine, a natural chemical regulator, resulting in increased blood flow to the penis.

℞ QUICK FACTS

Purpose

 Used to treat male impotence.

Dosage

 Take exactly as prescribed.

 Usual adult dose: one 5.4 milligram tablet, taken 3 times per day. Doctor may reduce dose to ½ tablet taken 3 times per day, and gradually increase if you experience nausea, dizziness, or nervousness. Doses are based on experimental research in the treatment of male impotence.

 Usual child dose: not prescribed for children.

 Missed dose: take as soon as possible, unless almost time for next dose. In that case, do not take missed dose; go back to regular schedule. *Do not double doses.*

Side Effects

 Overdose symptoms: no specific information available. If you suspect an overdose, immediately seek medical attention.

 Side effects: decreased urination, dizziness, flushing, headache, increase in blood pressure, increased heart rate, increased motor activity, irritability, nausea, nervousness, tremor.

 No known less common or rare side effects.

Interactions

 Inform your doctor before combining Yocon with antidepression medications such as Elavil or other medications that change mood.

 No known food/other substance interactions.

Special Cautions

 Not recommended for use in women. *Must not be used during pregnancy.*

 Not recommended for use in seniors.

 Not prescribed for children.

 Avoid if sensitive to or allergic to Yocon.

Should not be used by men with: kidney disease, heart disease, history of stomach or duodenal ulcer; or if being treated for a psychiatric disorder.

Yohimbine Hydrochloride
see YOCON

Zantac

Generic name: Ranitidine hydrochloride

Zantac is an antiulcer medication. It blocks the effects of histamine in the stomach, which reduces stomach acid secretion.

℞ QUICK FACTS

Purpose

℞ Used for short-term therapy (4 to 8 weeks) to treat active duodenal (upper intestinal) ulcers, active benign stomach ulcers, and maintenance therapy for duodenal ulcers. Also used to treat Zollinger-Ellison syndrome (peptic ulcer with too much acid), mastocytosis, and gastroesophageal reflux disease (GERD). Also prescribed to prevent stomach and duodenum damage from long-term use of nonsteroidal anti-inflammatory medications, to treat bleeding of the stomach and intestine, and stress-induced ulcers.

Dosage

 Take exactly as prescribed. Follow your doctor's diet program.

 Usual adult dose: *for active duodenal ulcer*—150 milligrams taken 2 times per day or 10 milliliters (2 teaspoonfuls) taken 2 times per day for 4 to 8 weeks. Or doctor may suggest 300 milligrams or 20 milliliters (4 teaspoonfuls) at bedtime. Long-term use dosage is 150 milligrams per day or 10 milliliters

(2 teaspoonfuls) per day, taken at bedtime. *For Zollinger-Ellison syndrome and mastocytosis*—150 milligrams or 10 milliliters (2 teaspoonfuls) taken 2 times per day. *For benign gastric ulcer and GERD*—150 milligrams or 10 milliliters (2 teaspoonfuls) taken 2 times per day for 6 to 8 weeks. *For individuals with reduced kidney function*—dose is adjusted by your doctor. *Seniors*—dose is individualized.

 Usual child dose: not generally prescribed for children.

 Missed dose: take as soon as possible, unless it is the next day. In that case, do not take the missed dose; go back to regular schedule. *Do not double doses.*

Side Effects

 Overdose symptoms: abnormal walking, low blood pressure, and exaggerated side effects. If you suspect an overdose, immediately seek medical attention.

 Most common side effect: headache (sometimes severe).

 Less common or rare side effects: abdominal discomfort and pain, agitation, changes in blood count (anemia), changes in liver function, constipation, depression, diarrhea, difficulty sleeping, dizziness, hair loss, hallucinations, heart block, hepatitis, hypersensitivity reactions, inflammation of the pancreas, involuntary movements, irregular heartbeat, joint pain, muscle pain, nausea and vomiting, rapid heartbeat, rash, reduced white blood cells, reversible mental confusion, sleepiness, slow heartbeat, vague feeling of bodily discomfort, vertigo, yellow eyes and skin.

Interactions

 Inform your doctor before combining Zantac with: enoxacin (Penetrex), glipizide (Glucotrol), itraconazole (Sporanox), ketoconazole (Nizoral), midazolam (Versed), theophylline (Theo-Dur), triamterene (Dyrenium), warfarin (Coumadin).

 Avoid alcohol when taking Zantac.

Special Cautions

 If pregnant or plan to become pregnant, inform your doctor immediately. Appears in breast milk; could affect a nursing infant.

 Seniors are prescribed Zantac according to individual needs.

 Not generally prescribed for children.

 Zantac assists in reducing the risk of duodenal ulcers recurring, and aids in the rapid healing of ulcers that occur during maintenance therapy.

Avoid if sensitive to or allergic to Zantac or similar medications.

Use with caution if you have kidney or liver disease.

Zaroxolyn

Generic name: Metolazone

Other brand name: Mykrox

Zaroxolyn is a thiazide diuretic. It reduces fluid accumulation in the body.

℞ QUICK FACTS

Purpose

Used to treat high blood pressure and other conditions requiring elimination of excess fluid from the body, including congestive heart failure and kidney disease. May be prescribed with or without other high blood pressure medications. Sometimes prescribed for kidney stones.

Dosage

If taking for high blood pressure, must take regularly for it to be effective. May take several weeks to observe the effects of Zaroxolyn. Continue to take even when symptoms disappear.

Usual adult dose: *for heart or kidney disease*—5 to 20 milligrams taken once per day. *For mild to moderate high blood pressure*—2.5 to 5 milligrams taken once per day. Doctor will prescribe lowest dose possible.

Usual child dose: not generally prescribed for children.

Missed dose: take as soon as possible, unless it is the next day. In that case, do not take the missed dose; go back to regular schedule. *Do not double doses.*

Side Effects

Overdose symptoms: difficulty breathing, dizziness, drowsiness, fainting, irritation of stomach and intestines, lethargy leading to coma. If you suspect an overdose, immediately seek medical attention.

Side effects: abdominal bloating, anemia, blood clots, blurred vision, chest pain, chills, constipation, depression, diarrhea, dizziness, drowsiness, fainting, fatigue, gout, headache, hepatitis, high blood sugar, hives, impotence, inflammation of the skin, inflammation of the pancreas, joint pain, loss of appetite, low potassium levels, muscle spasms or cramps, nausea, rapid or pounding heartbeat, rash, reddish or purplish skin spots, restlessness, sensitivity to light, sugar in the urine, tingling or pins and needles, upset stomach, vertigo, vomiting, weakness, yellow eyes and skin.

 No known less common or rare side effects.

Interactions

 Inform your doctor before combining Zaroxolyn with: ACTH; antidiabetic medications such as Micronase; barbiturates such as phenobarbital; corticosteroids such as prednisone (Deltasone); digitalis (Lanoxin); lithium (Lithonate); loop diuretics such as furosemide (Lasix); methenamine (Mandelamine); narcotics such as Percocet; nonsteroidal anti-inflammatory medications such as Advil; norepinephrine (Levophed); other high blood pressure medications such as Aldomet.

 Avoid alcohol during Zaroxolyn therapy.

Special Cautions

 If pregnant or plan to become pregnant, inform your doctor immediately. Appears in breast milk; could affect a nursing infant.

 No special precautions apply to seniors.

 Not generally prescribed for children.

 Should not take if you are unable to urinate or have severe kidney disease.

Avoid if sensitive to or allergic to Zaroxolyn or similar medications. If allergic to sulfa medications or quinethazone, at increased risk for allergic reaction.

Diuretics may cause potassium loss. Symptoms include muscle weakness and rapid or irregular heartbeat. Doctor may advise a potassium supplement or eating potassium-rich foods.

Doctor should monitor kidney function during Zaroxolyn therapy.

Use with caution if you have liver disease, diabetes, gout, or lupus erythematosus.

Fluid depletion (caused by dehydration, excessive sweating, severe diarrhea, or vomiting) may cause low blood pressure. Use care when exercising in hot weather.

Notify your doctor or dentist during a medical emergency or prior to surgery that you are taking Zaroxolyn.

Zestoretic

Generic name: Lisinopril with hydrochlorothiazide

Other brand name: Prinzide

Zestoretic is an angiotensin-converting enzyme (ACE) inhibitor/antihypertensive and a diuretic. It works to reduce blood pressure by preventing angiotensin I from converting into a more potent enzyme that increases salt and water retention; and it reduces fluid accumulation in the body.

℞ QUICK FACTS

Purpose

℞ Used to treat high blood pressure.

Dosage

 May take with or without food. Must take regularly for it to be effective. May take several weeks to observe the effects of Zestoretic. Continue to take even when symptoms disappear.

 Usual adult dose: 1 or 2 tablets taken once per day, once blood pressure is stable. If possible, discontinue diuretics before taking Zestoretic, or if it is not possible, doctor may give initial dose and supervise further doses. Doses are individualized.

 Usual child dose: not generally prescribed for children.

 Missed dose: take as soon as possible, unless it is the next day. In that case, do not take the missed dose; go back to regular schedule. *Do not double doses.*

Side Effects

 Overdose symptoms: dehydration, low blood pressure. If you suspect an overdose, immediately seek medical attention.

 More common side effects: cough, dizziness, fatigue, headache.

 Less common side effects: diarrhea; impotence; indigestion; low blood pressure; muscle cramps; nausea; rash; tingling or pins and needles; upper respiratory infection; vomiting; weakness. Rare side effects: abdominal pain; anemia; arthritis; back pain; back strain; blurred vision; bronchitis; bruising; chest discomfort; chest pain; common cold; confusion; constipation; decreased sex drive; depression; difficulty breathing; difficulty falling or staying asleep; dry mouth; earache; excessive perspiration; fainting; fever; flu; flushing; foot pain; gas; general feeling of illness; gout; hay fever; heart attack; heartburn; heart rhythm disturbances; hepatitis; hives; itching; joint pain; kidney failure; knee pain; loss of appetite; low blood pressure; lung congestion; muscle pain; muscle spasm; nervousness; palpitations; rapid heartbeat; red or purple skin spots; reduced urine output; restlessness; ringing in ears; sensitivity to light; shortness of breath; severe allergic reaction; shoulder pain; sinus inflammation; skin inflammation; sleepiness; sore throat; stomach and intestinal cramps; stroke; stuffy nose; swelling of the face, lips, tongue, throat, or arms and legs; trauma; urinary tract infection; vertigo; virus infection; vision abnormality in which objects have yellowish hue; yellow eyes and skin.

Interactions

Inform your doctor before combining Zestoretic with: barbiturates such as Nembutal and Seconal, corticosteroids such as prednisone, high blood pressure medications such as Procardia and Aldomet, indomethacin (Indocin), insulin, lithium (Lithonate), muscle relaxants such as Tubocurarine, narcotics such as Darvon and Dilaudid, nonsteroidal anti-inflammatory medications such as Naprosyn, oral antidiabetic medications such as Micronase, potassium supplements such as Slow-K, potassium-sparing diuretics such as Midamor.

Avoid alcohol while taking Zestoretic. *Do not use potassium-containing salt substitutes unless directed by your doctor.*

Special Cautions

 Can cause birth defects, premature births, or death in the fetus and newborn if taken during the second and third trimesters. If pregnant or plan to become pregnant, inform your doctor immediately. May appear in breast milk; could affect a nursing infant.

 No special precautions apply to seniors.

 Not generally prescribed for children.

 Inform your doctor *before* starting Zestoretic if you have: congestive heart failure, diabetes, liver disease, history of allergy or bronchial asthma, or lupus erythematosus.

Not recommended for individuals on dialysis.

Avoid if sensitive to or allergic to any of the ingredients in Zestoretic or other ACE inhibitor or sulfonamide-derived medications; if previous ACE inhibitor treatment resulted in angioedema (swelling of face, lips, tongue, throat, arms, or legs); or if you are unable to urinate. If you experience angioedema, it may require emergency treatment.

If you experience light-headedness or faint, stop taking and contact your doctor.

Fluid depletion (caused by dehydration, excessive sweating, severe diarrhea, or vomiting) may cause dangerously low blood pressure.

Immediately notify your doctor if you experience chest pain, sore throat, or fever and chills.

Doctor will monitor blood sugar levels if you are diabetic.

. . . . . .

Notify your doctor or dentist prior to surgery that you are taking Zestoretic.

Zestril

∿∿∿∿∿∿∿∿∿∿∿∿∿∿∿∿∿∿∿∿∿∿∿∿∿∿∿∿

Generic name: Lisinopril

Other brand name: Prinivil

Zestril is an angiotensin-converting enzyme (ACE) inhibitor. It works to reduce blood pressure by preventing angiotensin I from converting into a more potent enzyme that increases salt and water retention.

℞ QUICK FACTS

Purpose

℞ Used to treat high blood pressure.

Dosage

🍴🅓 May take with or without food. Must take regularly for it to be effective. May take several weeks to observe the effects of Zestril. Continue to take even when symptoms disappear. Abruptly stopping medication may cause rise in blood pressure.

. . . .

 Usual adult dose: *for hypertension*—if not taking diuretics—10 milligrams taken once per day. Once blood pressure is stabilized—20 to 40 milligrams per day in a single dose. May be used alone or with other high blood pressure medications. If taking diuretics—initial dose of 5 milligrams, and doctor will supervise additional doses. If you have kidney disorder, dosage is individualized. *For heart failure*—5 milligrams per day, taken with diuretics and Digitalis. Starting dose should be supervised by your doctor.

Ongoing dose range is 5 to 20 milligrams taken once per day. *Seniors*—doses are individualized.

 Usual child dose: not generally prescribed for children.

 Missed dose: take as soon as possible, unless it is the next day. In that case, do not take the missed dose; go back to regular schedule. *Do not double doses.*

Side Effects

 Overdose symptom: drop in blood pressure. If you suspect an overdose, immediately seek medical attention.

 More common side effects: abdominal pain, chest pain, common cold, cough, diarrhea, difficulty in breathing, dizziness, fatigue, headache, itching, low blood pressure, nausea, rash, respiratory infection, vomiting, weakness.

 Less common or rare side effects: arm pain, arthritis, asthma, back pain, blurred vision, breast pain, bronchitis, burning sensation, changes in heart rhythm, chills, confusion, constipation, coughing up blood, cramps in stomach or intestines, decreased sex drive, difficulty breathing at night, dizziness on standing, double vision, dry mouth, excessive sweating, fainting, feeling of illness, fever, flu, fluid retention, flushing, gas, gout, hair loss, heart attack, heartburn, hepatitis, hip pain, hives, impotence, inability to sleep or sleeping too much, incoordination, indigestion, inflamed stomach, intolerance of light, irregular heartbeat, irritability, joint pain, kidney failure, knee pain, leg pain, little or no urine, "little strokes," loss of appetite, lung cancer, memory impairment, muscle cramps, nasal congestion, neck pain, nervousness, nosebleed, painful breathing, painful urination, pelvic pain, pneumonia, prickling or burning sensation, rapid or fluttery heartbeat, rash, reddening of skin, ringing in ears, runny nose, sensitivity to light, severe allergic reactions, skin eruptions, shoulder pain, sinus inflammation, sore throat, spasm, stroke, sweating, swelling of face or arms and legs, thigh pain, tremor, upset stomach, urinary tract infection, vertigo, viral infection, vision changes, weight loss or gain, wheezing, yellow eyes and skin.

Interactions

 Inform your doctor before combining Zestril with: aspirin, diuretics such as Lasix, indomethacin (Indocin), lithium (Lithonate), potassium preparations such as K-Phos, potassium-sparing diuretics such as Midamor. If taking high doses of a diuretic, may cause extremely low blood pressure.

 Limit intake of potassium-rich foods such as bananas, prunes, raisins, orange juice, whole milk, and skim milk. Avoid salt substitutes that contain potassium.

Special Cautions

 Can cause birth defects, premature births, or death in the fetus and newborn if taken during the second and third trimesters. If pregnant or plan to become pregnant, inform your doctor immediately. May appear in breast milk; could affect a nursing infant.

 No special precautions apply to seniors.

 Not generally prescribed for children.

 May cause dizziness or fainting and impair your ability to drive a car or operate machinery. *Do not take*

part in any activity that requires alertness.

Avoid if sensitive to or allergic to any of the ingredients in Zestril or other ACE inhibitor or sulfonamide-derived medications; if previous ACE inhibitor
treatment resulted in angioedema (swelling of face,
lips, tongue, throat, arms, or legs); or if you are unable to urinate. If you experience angioedema, it may
require emergency treatment.

Doctor may perform blood tests periodically if you
have kidney disorder or connective tissue disease,
and may monitor kidney function.

Not recommended for individuals on dialysis.

Immediately notify your doctor if you experience
chest pain, sore throat, or fever and chills.

Fluid depletion (caused by dehydration, excessive sweating, severe diarrhea, or vomiting) may cause dangerously low blood pressure.

Zidovudine

see RETROVIR

Zithromax

Generic name: Azithromycin

Zithromax is a macrolide antibiotic. It prevents bacteria from multiplying and growing.

℞ QUICK FACTS

Purpose

 Used to treat a wide variety of bacterial infections, including skin infections; upper and lower respiratory tract infections such as strep throat, tonsillitis, and pneumonia; and sexually transmitted infections of the cervix or urinary tract.

Dosage

 Take on an empty stomach, at least 1 hour before or 2 hours after a meal. *Do not take with food or antacids containing aluminum or magnesium, such as Di-Gel, Gelusil, Maalox, and others.* Finish the entire prescription.

. . . .

 Usual adult dose: 500 milligrams in a single dose on day 1 of treatment, followed by 250 milligrams in a single dose each day for 4 days. Maximum amount taken should be 1.5 grams. *For nongonococcal urethritis and cervitis due to chlamydia*—a single gram (1,000 milligrams) taken one time only.

. . . .

 Usual child dose: *for children 16 and over*—prescribed adult dose. Not generally prescribed for children under 16 years.

. . . .

 Missed dose: take as soon as possible, unless it is the next day. In that case, do not take the missed dose; go back to regular schedule. *Do not double doses.*

Side Effects

 Overdose symptoms: no specific information available. If you suspect an overdose, immediately seek medical attention.

. . . .

⊕ More common side effects: abdominal pain, diarrhea or loose stools, nausea, vomiting.

. . . .

Less common side effects: blood in the stools, chest pain, dizziness, drowsiness, fatigue, gas, headache, heart palpitations, indigestion, jaundice (yellowing of the skin and whites of the eyes), kidney infection, light sensitivity, rash, severe allergic reaction including swelling (as in hives), sleepiness, vaginal inflammation, vertigo, yeast infection.

Interactions

Important to check with your doctor before using antacids containing aluminum or magnesium, such as Maalox and Mylanta. Inform your doctor before combining Zithromax with: carbamazepine (Tegretol); certain antihistamines such as Hismanal and Seldane; cyclosporine (Sandimmune); digoxin (Lanoxin or Lanoxicaps); ergot-containing drugs such as Cafergot or D.H.E.; hexobarbital; lovastatin (Mevacor); phenytoin (Dilantin); theophylline drugs such as Bronkodyl, Slo-Phyllin, and Theo-Dur; triazolam (Halcion); warfarin (Coumadin).

No known food/other substance interactions.

Special Cautions

If pregnant or planning to become pregnant, inform your doctor immediately. Not known if Zithromax appears in breast milk.

No special precautions apply to seniors.

Not generally prescribed for children under 16 years. Follow doctor's instructions carefully for children 16 and older.

Possibility of rare, serious reactions, including angioedema (swelling of face, lips, and neck that impedes

speaking, swallowing, and breathing) and anaphylaxis (violent, even fatal allergic reaction).

. . . .

May cause pseudomembranous colitis, a potentially life-threatening form of diarrhea.

. . . .

If a liver problem is present, should be monitored closely.

Zocor

Generic name: Simvastatin

Zocor is an antihyperlipidemic (lipid-lowering medication). It is thought to work by reducing the body's production of certain fats.

℞ QUICK FACTS

Purpose

℞   Used to lower cholesterol levels when diet alone does not sufficiently lower cholesterol levels.

Dosage

 Doctor will have you follow a cholesterol-lowering diet for 3 to 6 months before prescribing Zocor. Follow exercise program prescribed by your doctor. Zocor is a supplement, not a substitute for lowering cholesterol. Take Zocor exactly as prescribed.

. . . .

 Usual adult dose: initially—5 to 10 milligrams per day taken as a single dose in the evening. Doctor may increase up to 40 milligrams per day. Doctor may adjust dose every 4 weeks, reducing as cholesterol levels come down. *If you have severe kidney dis-*

ease—5 milligrams per day is prescribed, and use
with caution. *Seniors*—20 milligrams per day or less.

 Usual child dose: not generally prescribed for children.

 Missed dose: take as soon as possible, unless it is
the next day. In that case, do not take the missed
dose; go back to regular schedule. *Do not double
doses.*

Side Effects

 Overdose symptoms: no specific information available. If you suspect an overdose, immediately seek
medical attention.

 More common side effects: abdominal pain, constipation, diarrhea, gas, headache, muscle pain, nausea,
upper respiratory infection, upset stomach, weakness. Other potential side effects: aching joints and
muscles, altered sense of taste, anxiety, appetite
loss, breast enlargement in men, depression, difficulty moving eyes or facial muscles, diminished sex
drive or sexual performance, dizziness, hepatitis, insomnia, itching, loss of hair, memory loss, nerve pain
or palsy, numbness or tingling, pancreatitis, progression of cataracts, tremor, vomiting.

 No known less common or rare side effects.

Interactions

 Inform your doctor before combining Zocor with:
blood thinners such as Coumadin, cimetidine (Tagamet), clofibrate (Atromid-S), cyclosporine (Sandimmune), digoxin (Lanoxin), erythromycin (PCE), gemfibrozil (Lopid), nicotinic acid, spironolactone
(Aldactone).

No known food/other substance interactions.

Special Cautions

 May cause birth defects; doctor will prescribe only if you understand risks and are highly unlikely to become pregnant while taking Zocor. If pregnant or planning to become pregnant, inform your doctor immediately. Appears in breast milk and can cause serious adverse effects on a nursing baby.

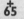 Seniors should use with caution.

 Not generally prescribed for children.

 Do not take if sensitive to or allergic to Zocor.

Do not take if you have active liver disease.

Doctor may advise checking liver enzyme levels (blood test) prior to starting Zocor, and every 6 weeks for the first 3 months of treatment, every 8 weeks for the rest of year 1, and every 6 months thereafter.

Inform your doctor if you experience unexplained muscle tenderness or weakness right away, especially if accompanied with a fever or sick feeling. May indicate muscle tissue damage. To minimize this risk, do not take Zocor at the same time you are taking other cholesterol-lowering medications such as Lopid.

Doctor may discontinue Zocor if risk of muscle or kidney damage increases, or you experience severe infection or seizures.

Zofran

Generic name: Ondansetron hydrochloride

Zofran is an anti-emetic. It is thought to act by inhibiting impulses to the vomiting center in the brain.

℞ QUICK FACTS

Purpose

℞ Used to control nausea and vomiting caused by cancer therapy.

Dosage

 Should not miss doses. To get maximum benefit, take all doses prescribed by your doctor.

 Usual adult dose: one 8-milligram tablet taken 3 times per day. Take first dose ½ hour before chemotherapy, and the other two doses 4 and 8 hours after the first dose. Doctor will suggest taking for 1 to 2 days after completing chemotherapy.

 Usual child dose: *children 12 years and older—are* prescribed adult dose. *Children 4 to 12 years—*one 4-milligram tablet taken 3 times per day. Take first dose ½ hour before chemotherapy, and the other 2 doses 4 and 8 hours after the first dose. Doctor will suggest taking for 1 to 2 days after completing chemotherapy.

 Missed dose: take as soon as possible.

Side Effects

 Overdose symptoms: no specific information available. If you suspect an overdose, immediately seek medical attention.

More common side effects: abdominal pain, constipation, headache, weakness.

 Less common or rare side effects: anaphylaxis (severe allergic reaction), dry mouth, rash, wheezing.

Interactions

 No drug interactions reported.

 No known food/other substance interactions.

Special Cautions

 If pregnant or plan to become pregnant, inform your doctor immediately. May appear in breast milk; could affect a nursing infant.

 No special precautions apply to seniors.

 Follow doctor's instructions carefully for children.

 Avoid if sensitive to or allergic to any of the ingredients in Zofran.

Zoloft

Generic name: Sertraline

Zoloft is a cyclic antidepressant. It increases the concentration of certain chemicals necessary for nerve transmission in the brain.

℞ QUICK FACTS

Purpose

 Used to treat major depression—a low mood that persistently interferes with everyday life. Symptoms include: loss of interest in usual activities, disturbed sleep, change in appetite, constant fidgeting or lethargic movement, fatigue, feelings of worthlessness or guilt, difficulty thinking or concentrating, recurring suicidal thoughts. Also used to treat obsessive-compulsive disorders.

Dosage

 Take exactly as prescribed. May take several days to a few weeks to observe improvement.

 Usual adult dose: 50 milligrams taken once per day either in the morning or evening. Doctor may increase dose up to 200 milligrams per day maximum.

 Usual child dose: not generally prescribed for children.

 Missed dose: take as soon as possible unless several hours have passed. In that case, do not take missed dose; go back to regular schedule. *Do not double doses.*

Side Effects

 Overdose symptoms: anxiety, dilated pupils, nausea, rapid heartbeat, sleepiness, vomiting. If you suspect an overdose, immediately seek medical attention.

 More common side effects: agitation, confusion, constipation, diarrhea or loose stools, difficulty with ejaculation, dizziness, dry mouth, fatigue, fluttery or throbbing heartbeat, gas, headache, increased sweating, indigestion, insomnia, nausea, nervousness, sleepiness, tremor, vomiting.

 Less common or rare side effects: abdominal pain, abnormal hair growth, abnormal skin odor, acne, altered taste, anxiety, back pain, bad breath, breast development in males, breast pain or enlargement, bruise-like marks on the skin, changeable emotions, chest pain, cold or clammy skin, conjunctivitis (pink eye), coughing, difficulty breathing, difficulty concentrating, difficulty swallowing, double vision, dry eyes, enlarged abdomen, excessive menstrual bleeding, eye pain, fainting, feeling faint upon arising, female sexual problems, fever, fluid retention, flushing, frequent urination, hair loss, heart attack, hemorrhoids, hiccups, high blood pressure, hot flushes, increased appetite, increased salivation, inflammation of nose or throat, inflammation of the penis, intolerance to light, itching, joint pain, lack of coordination, lack of menstruation, lack of sensation, loss of appetite, low blood pressure, menstrual problems, middle ear infection, migraine, movement problems, muscle cramps or weakness, muscle pain, need to urinate during the night, nosebleed, pain upon urination, painful menstruation, purple or red skin spots, racing heartbeat, rash, ringing in the ears, sensitivity to light, sinus inflammation, skin eruptions, sleepwalking, sores on tongue, speech problems, stomach and intestinal inflammation, swelling of the face, swollen wrists and ankles, thirst, tingling or pins and needles, twitching, urinary trouble, vaginal inflammation or discharge, varicose veins, vision problems, weight loss or gain, yawning. Other mental or emotional symptoms: abnormal dreams or thoughts, exaggerated feeling of well-being, depersonalization ("unreal" feeling), hallucinations, memory loss, paranoia, rapid mood shifts, suicidal thoughts, toothgrinding, worsened depression.

Interactions

 Inform your doctor before combining Zoloft with: cimetidine (Tagamet), diazepam (Valium), digitoxin (Crystodigin), lithium (Lithonate), MAO inhibitors such as Nardil and Parnate, other psychiatric medications such as Elavil and Mellaril, over-the-counter medications such as cold remedies, tolbutamide (Orinase), warfarin (Coumadin).

 Avoid alcohol while taking Zoloft.

Special Cautions

 If pregnant or plan to become pregnant, inform your doctor immediately. Not known if Zoloft appears in breast milk.

 No special precautions apply to seniors.

 Not generally prescribed for children.

 May experience weight loss.

May trigger mania (grandiose, inappropriate, out-of-control behavior) or hyper behavior (hypomania).

Doctor will closely monitor if you have kidney or liver disorder.

Zolpidem Tartrate

see AMBIEN

Zovirax

Generic name: Acyclovir

Zovirax is an antiviral. It is the only orally administered drug that can reduce the rate of growth of the herpes virus and its relatives.

℞ QUICK FACTS

Purpose

℞ Used to treat certain infections with herpes viruses including genital herpes, shingles, and chicken pox. Zovirax ointment is used to treat initial episodes of genital herpes and certain herpes simplex infections of the skin and mucous membranes.

Dosage

 Should not exceed prescribed dose, nor share medication with others. Avoid eye exposure to ointment. Use rubber glove or finger cot to protect against spreading infection.

 Usual adult dose: *for genital herpes*—one 200-milligram capsule or 1 teaspoonful of liquid every 4 hours, taken 5 times per day for 10 days. If herpes is recurrent, dose is 400 milligrams (two 200-milligram capsules or 2 teaspoonfuls) taken 2 times per day for up to 12 months. If herpes is intermittent, dose is one 200-milligram capsule or 1 teaspoonful of liquid every 4 hours, taken 5 times per day for 5 days. *Ointment*—apply to affected area every 3 hours, 6 times per day, for 7 days. *For herpes shingles*—800 milligrams (four 200-milligram capsules, two 400-milligram tablets, or 4 teaspoonfuls of liquid) every 4 hours, 5 times per day for 7 to 10 days. *If you have kidney disorder*—doctor will adjust dose.

 Usual child dose: 20 milligrams per 2.2 pounds of body weight, taken orally 4 times per day for 5 days. Maximum dose is 800 milligrams per day. Not generally prescribed for children under 2 years.

 Missed dose: take as soon as possible, unless almost time for next dose. In that case, do not take missed dose; go back to regular schedule. *Do not double doses.*

Apply missed ointment dose as soon as you remember, then continue your regular schedule.

Side Effects

 Overdose symptoms: Zovirax is generally safe; however, overdose may lead to kidney damage. If you suspect an overdose, immediately seek medical attention.

 More common side effects: confusion, constipation, diarrhea, dizziness, fever, fluid retention, general feeling of bodily discomfort, gland enlargement in the groin, hair loss, hallucinations, headache, hives, itching, muscle pain, nausea, pain, skin rash, sleepiness, stomach and intestinal problems, visual abnormalities, vomiting. Common side effects of Zovirax ointment: burning, itching, mild pain, skin rash, stinging, vaginal inflammation.

 Less common or rare side effects: abdominal pain, anaphylaxis (severe allergic reaction), diarrhea, dizziness, fatigue, gas, headache, inability to sleep, leg pain, loss of appetite, medicinal taste, rash, retention of fluid, sore throat, tingling or pins and needles, vomiting, weakness.

Interactions

 Inform your doctor before combining Zovirax with: cyclosporine (Sandimmune), interferon (Roferon), probenecid (Benemid), zidovudine (AZT/Retrovir).

 No known food/other substance interactions.

Special Cautions

 If pregnant or plan to become pregnant, inform your doctor immediately. May appear in breast milk; could affect a nursing infant.

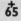 Seniors with reduced kidney function should take a lower oral dosage.

 Not generally prescribed for children under 2 years. Follow doctor's instructions for children 2 years and older.

 This medication should not be taken if you have experienced an allergic reaction to it or similar drugs.

If you are being treated for a kidney disorder, consult with your doctor before taking Zovirax.

Decreased sperm count has been observed in animals given high doses of Zovirax; however, this effect has not been documented in humans.

Zyloprim

Generic name: Allopurinol

Other brand names: Lopurin, Zurinol

Zyloprim is an antigout medication. It blocks the production of uric acid in the body.

℞ QUICK FACTS

Purpose

 Used to treat gout. Also used to treat cancer and other conditions associated with too much uric acid in the body, and to manage some types of kidney stones.

Dosage

 To avoid stomach irritation, take with food, a full glass of water or milk. May take 2 to 6 weeks before full effects are observed. To prevent kidney stones, drink 10 to 12 glasses of fluids per day, unless otherwise prescribed by your doctor.

Usual adult dose: *for gout*—100 milligrams taken once per day. Doctor may increase by 100 milligrams per day at 1 week intervals. Average dose for mild gout—200 to 300 milligrams. For moderate to severe gout—400 to 600 milligrams. Maximum daily dose—800 milligrams. *For recurrent kidney stones*—200 to 300 milligrams per day divided into smaller doses or taken as a single dose. *For management of uric acid levels in certain cancers*—600 to 800 milligrams per day for 2 to 3 days, with a high fluid intake.

Usual child dose: *for children 6 to 10 years*—300 milligrams per day to manage uric acid levels in certain types of cancer. *For children under 6 years*—150 milligrams per day.

Missed dose: take as soon as possible, unless almost time for next dose. In that case, do not take missed dose; go back to regular schedule. *Do not double doses.*

Side Effects

Overdose symptoms: no specific information available. If you suspect an overdose, immediately seek medical attention.

Most common side effect is skin rash. If you develop a rash, stop taking Zyloprim and call your doctor. Rash may be itchy or scaly, or skin may peel off in sheets; rash may be accompanied by chills and fever, aching joints, or jaundice. More common side effects: acute attack of gout, diarrhea, nausea, rash.

Less common side effects: abdominal pain; bruising; chills; fever; hair loss; headache; hepatitis; hives; indigestion; itching; joint pain; kidney failure; lack of ability to concentrate; loosening of nails; muscle disease; nosebleed; numbness; rare skin condition characterized by severe blisters and bleeding on the lips, eyes or nose; reddish-brown or purplish spots on the skin; skin inflammation or peeling; sleepiness; stomach inflammation; taste loss or change; tingling or pins and needles; unusual bleeding; vomiting; yellowing of skin and eyes.

Interactions

 Inform your doctor before combining Zyloprim with: amoxicillin (Amoxil or Polymox); ampicillin (Omnipen or Polycillin); azathioprine (Imuran); blood thinners such as Coumadin; drugs for diabetes such as Diabinese and Orinase; mercaptopurine (Purinethol); probenecid (Benemid or ColBEN-EMID); sulfinpyrazone (Anturane); theophylline (Theo-Dur or Slo-Phyllin); thiazide diuretics such as HydroDIURIL. Avoid taking large doses of Vitamin C.

 Avoid alcohol, beer, wine, and purine-rich foods such as anchovies, sardines, liver, kidneys, lentils, and sweetbreads when taking Zyloprim.

Special Cautions

 If pregnant or planning to become pregnant, notify your doctor immediately. May cause birth defects or interfere with baby's development. Caution—Zyloprim appears in breast milk.

 No special precautions apply to seniors.

 Follow doctor's instructions carefully for children.

If you develop a skin rash or other allergic reactions, stop taking Zyloprim and immediately contact your doctor. In some people, a Zyloprim-induced rash may lead to serious skin disease, generalized inflammation of a blood or lymph vessel, irreversible liver damage, or death.

May cause drowsiness and impair your ability to drive a car or operate machinery. *Do not take part in any activity that requires alertness.*

In the early stages of taking Zyloprim, you may experience attacks of gout. Attacks will decrease after several months of therapy.

If you have a kidney problem, high blood pressure or diabetes, your doctor should prescribe Zyloprim carefully and periodically monitor your kidney function.

WHY YOU NEED VITAMINS & MINERALS

The value of certain foods in maintaining health was recognized long before the first vitamins or minerals were actually identified. In the 18th century, for example, it had been demonstrated that the addition of citrus fruits to the diet would prevent the development of scurvy. And in the 19th century, it was shown that substituting unpolished for polished rice in a rice-based diet would prevent the development of beriberi.

The Dietary Guidelines for Americans established by the Food and Nutrition Board of the National Research Council, National Academy of Sciences, in Washington, D.C., include the basic food groups that supply people with an adequate diet of minerals, proteins, vitamins, and energy. While no guideline can guarantee perfect health, people who follow these recommendations will give themselves a good foundation for health. In general, people should:

- eat a variety of foods;
- maintain a desirable weight;
- avoid fried and fatty foods to cut down intakes of fat, saturated fat, and cholesterol;
- eat an adequate amount of fiber-rich foods;
- avoid too much sugar and starch; and
- drink alcohol only in moderation.

If you want to improve your health by increasing your intake of vitamins and minerals, there is one approach that health experts and nutritionists agree upon: *Eat more fruits and vegetables!* Fruits and vegetables contain hundreds of substances that have the potential to improve health, not just the few specific compounds that are available in pill form. In addition, a diet that includes lots of fruits and vegetables tends to be high in fiber and low in fat.

Of course, some people will choose to take one or more vitamin or mineral supplements to boost their dietary intake of these important substances. Others may choose a multivitamin/mineral supplement to get overall "nutritional insurance." If you decide to take supplements, you should know that the vitamin industry has not been effectively regulated by either the FDA or the USP, an independent group that sets standards for drugs.

About the Vitamin & Mineral Charts

The following charts provide a summary of basic information about the most commonly used vitamins and minerals. The recommended daily allowance (RDA) and other guidelines are established dosage levels for normal growth and development in healthy children, and to prevent nutrient depletion in healthy adults.

VITAMIN CHART

Vitamin Legend

RDA = Recommended Daily Allowance. Estimated levels of intake for essential nutritionals developed by the Food and Nutrition Board and the National Research Council of the National Academy of Sciences.

IU. = International Units
Mcg. = Micrograms
Mg. = Milligrams

Vitamin	What Vitamin Does	RDA (Recommended Daily Allowance)	Food Sources
Vitamin A	Fat soluble. Dietary supplement for normal growth, and decreases severity of sun exposure in people with porphyria. Helps with supple skin, nightblindness, bone formation, infection resistance, pregnancy and breastfeeding. Strengthens weak eyes and builds strong teeth. Aids in removing age spots. Acts as an anti-cancer agent. When applied externally, helps treat acne, superficial wrin-	*Women and girls 11+:* 4,000 IU. *Men and boys 11+:* 5,000 IU. *Nursing (months 1–6):* 6,500 IU; *(months 6–12):* 6,000 IU. *Infants 0 to 12 months:* 1,875 IU. *Children 1 to 10 years:* 2,000 to 3,300 IU.	Liver, kidney, eggs, cheese made with whole milk or cream, fortified non-fat milk, yellow-or-ange fruits and vegetables, dark-green leafy vegetables, milk, butter, margarine, cod liver oil.

Vitamin	What Vitamin Does	RDA (Recommended Daily Allowance)	Food Sources
Vitamin A (cont.)	kles, impetigo, boils, carbuncles, and open ulcers.		
Vitamin B-1 (Thiamine)	Water soluble. Essential for normal release of energy from carbohydrate, protein, and fat in food. Assists normal functioning of all body cells, especially nerves. Treats vitamin B-1 deficiency in persons with absorption disease, beriberi, and myocardial failure. Helps in energy production. Promotes growth. Aids in digestion. Helps fight air or sea sickness. Aids in treating herpes zoster.	*Adults:* 1.0 to 1.5 mg. *Pregnancy & nursing:* 1.5 to 1.6 mg.	Pork, liver, oysters, green peas, collard greens, oranges, dried peas and beans, wheat germ, fish, peanuts, Brewer's yeast, whole grain bread and enriched cereals, avocados, lean meat, milk, spinach, cauliflower, dried fruit.
Vitamin B-2 (Riboflavin)	Water soluble. Essential for normal release of energy from carbohydrate, protein, and fat in food. Dietary supplement for normal growth and development,	*Females 11 to 50 years:* 1.3 mg. *Females 51+:* 1.4 mg. *Males 11 to 50:* 1.5 to 1.7 mg. *Males 51+:* 1.4 mg. *Pregnancy:* 1.6 mg.	Liver, milk, oysters, lean meat, green leafy vegetables, mushrooms, asparagus, broccoli, avocados, brussels sprouts, salmon, eggs, kidneys.

Vitamin	What Vitamin Does	RDA (Recommended Daily Allowance)	Food Sources
Vitamin B-2 (Riboflavin) (cont.)	production and regulation of certain hormones, and formation of red blood cells. Treats anemia. Benefits vision and alleviates eye fatigue. May aid prevention of prostate cancer.	*Nursing (months 1 to 6):* 1.8 mg; *(months 6 to 12):* 1.7 mg. *Infants 0 to 12 months:* 0.4 to 0.5 mg. *Children 1 to 10 years:* 0.8 to 1.2 mg.	
Vitamin B-3 (Niacin)	Water soluble. Helps in energy production and cell function. Alleviates gastrointestinal disturbances. Helps prevent and eases severity of migraines. Used to regulate blood cholesterol levels and treat schizophrenia. Reduces toxic effect of cancer medication. Enhances effectiveness of epilepsy medications.	*Adults:* 13 to 19 mg. *Nursing:* 20 mg. *Infants 0 to 12 months:* 5 to 6 mg. *Children 1 to 10 years:* 9 to 13 mg. *Females 11 to 18 years:* 15 mg. *Females 11 to 18 years:* 17 to 20 mg. *Males 11 to 18 years:*	Lean meat, poultry, fish, cooked dried peas and beans, Brewer's (nutritional) yeast, peanut butter, non-fat or low-fat milk and cheese, soybeans, nuts, orange juice.

Vitamin	What Vitamin Does	RDA (Recommended Daily Allowance)	Food Sources
Vitamin B-5 (Pantothenic Acid— Calcium Pantothenate and Vitamin B-3)	Water soluble. Essential catalyst in the breakdown of fats, carbohydrates, and protein for energy. Involved in production of fats, cholesterol, bile, vitamin D, red blood cells, and some hormones and neurotransmitters. Stimulates wound healing. Builds antibodies. Prevents fatigue. Reduces effects of some antibiotics.	*Adults and children 11+:* 4 to 10 mg. *Infants 0 to 12 months:* 2 to 3 mg. *Children 4 to 10 years:* 3 to 5 mg.	Liver, fish, chicken, cheese, whole grain breads and cereals, avocados, cauliflower, green peas, cooked dried beans and peas, nuts, dates, potatoes, cooked soybeans, peanut butter, bananas, collard greens, oranges.
Vitamin B-6 (Pyridoxine)	Water soluble. Helps in energy production, red blood cell formation, and in forming prostaglandins. May aid in treating asthma, behavior disorders, carpal tunnel syndrome, toxicity of some cancer drugs, heart disease, immune system, and kidney disorders, and premenstrual syndrome. Aids in formation and	*Adult women:* 1.5 to 1.6 mg. *Adult men:* 2.0 mg. *Pregnancy:* 2.2 mg. *Nursing:* 2.1 mg. *Infants 0 to 6 months:* 0.3 to 0.6 mg. *Female children 1 to 14 years:* 1.0 to 1.4 mg. *Male children 1 to 14 years:* 1.0 to 1.7 mg.	Lean meat, whole grain cereals and breads, wheat germ, Brewer's (nutritional) yeast, poultry, fish, soybeans, cooked dried peas and beans, peanuts, avocados, bananas, cabbage, cauliflower, potatoes, dried fruit.

Vitamin	What Vitamin Does	RDA (Recommended Daily Allowance)	Food Sources
Vitamin B-6 (Pyridoxine) (cont.)	maintenance of nervous system. Aids with drug-induced deficiencies. Reduces night muscle spasms, leg cramps, hand numbness. Natural diuretic. Alleviates nausea.		
Vitamin B-7 (Biotin)	Water soluble. Necessary for body processes involving manufacturing and breaking down fats, amino acids, and carbohydrates. Aids in keeping hair from turning gray. Alleviates eczema and dermatitis. Eases muscle pains. Preventative aid for baldness.	*Adults:* 30 to 300 mcg. *Infants 0 to 12 months:* 10 to 15 mcg. *Children 1 to 10 years:* 20 to 30 mcg.	Kidneys, liver, oatmeal, egg yolk, soybeans, clams, mushrooms, bananas, peanuts, Brewer's yeast, peanut butter, salmon, milk, cooked brown rice.
Vitamin B-12 (Cyanocobalamin)	Water soluble. Dietary supplement. Necessary for normal processing of carbohydrate, protein, and fat in the body. Treats nerve damage, pernicious anemia. Treats and prevents vitamin B-12 deficiencies when stomach or intestines are removed. Prevents vi-	*Adults and children 11+:* 2 mcg. *Pregnancy:* 2.2 mcg. *Nursing:* 2.6 mcg. *Infants 0 to 12 months:* 0.3 to 0.5 mcg. *Children 1 to 10 years:* 0.7 to 1.4 mcg.	Lean meat, poultry, fish, shellfish, milk, liver, kidneys, cheese, eggs, oysters, clams, yogurt.

Vitamin	What Vitamin Does	RDA (Recommended Daily Allowance)	Food Sources
Vitamin B-12 (Cyanocobalamin) (cont.)	tamin B-12 deficiency in strict vegetarians and in persons with absorption disease. Helps build genetic material. Promotes growth and appetite stimulant in children. Increases energy.		
Vitamin C (Ascorbic Acid)	Water soluble. Prevents and treats scurvy and other vitamin C deficiencies. Treats anemia. Maintains acid urine. Necessary in the formation and maintenance of collagen, which promotes healing of wounds, bone fractures, bruises, hemorrhages, and bleeding gums; and forms a protective barrier around healthy tissue. Aids in decreasing blood cholesterol levels. Helps in bone formation and blood circulation, and builds strong teeth. Natural laxative.	Adults and children 15+: 60 mg. Pregnancy & nursing: 70 to 95 mg. Infants 0 to 12 months: 30 to 35 mg. Children 1 to 14 years: 40 to 50 mg.	Fresh fruits—oranges and orange juice, strawberries, cantaloupes, pineapples, bananas; fresh vegetables—brussels sprouts, broccoli, collard greens, tomato juice, cabbage, asparagus, green peas, potatoes, lima beans, mashed potatoes, corn on the cob, carrots.

Vitamin	What Vitamin Does	RDA (Recommended Daily Allowance)	Food Sources
Vitamin D	Fat soluble. Dietary supplement. Prevents rickets (bone disease). Treats hypocalcemia (low blood calcium) in kidney disease. Treats post-operative muscle contractions. Daily supplement for people who must use sunscreen daily. Helps in formation of normal bones and teeth. Aids in treating conjunctivitis (pink eye).	*Adults:* 200 to 400 IU or 5 to 10 mcg. *Infants 0 to 6 months:* 300 IU or 7.5 mcg.	Vitamin D-fortified milk, bread, cod liver and other fish oils, salmon, herring, mackerel, sardines, liver, egg yolk, butter.
Vitamin E (Tocopherol)	Fat soluble. An antioxidant—protects fats and vitamin A from destruction by oxygen fragments or free radicals. Protects tissues of the eyes, skin, liver, breast, and calf muscles. Regulates use and storage of vitamin A. Protects red blood cells from damage. Retards cellular aging due to oxidation. Increases endurance. Accel-	*Women and female children 11+:* 12 IU or 8 mg. *Men and male children 11+:* 15 IU or 10 mg. *Infants 0 to 12 months:* 4.5 to 6 IU, or 3 to 4 mg. *Children 1 to 10 years:* 9.0 to 10.5 IU or 6 to 7 mg.	Vegetable oils, seeds, wheat germ, nuts, avocados, peaches, whole grain breads and cereals, spinach, broccoli, asparagus, dried prunes.

Vitamin	What Vitamin Does	RDA (Recommended Daily Allowance)	Food Sources
Vitamin K	erates healing of burns. Alleviates leg cramps. Fat soluble. Regulates blood clotting. Treats bleeding disorders and malabsorption diseases due to vitamin K deficiency. Treats hemorrhagic disease of newborns, and bleeding due to overdose of oral anticoagulants. Aids in reducing excessive menstrual flow.	*Adults: 65 to 80 mcg. Pregnancy & nursing: 65 mcg. Infants 0 to 12 months: 5 to 10 mcg. Children 1 to 10 years: 15 to 30 mcg. Females 11 to 24 years: 45 to 60 mcg. Males 11 to 24 years: 45 to 70 mcg.*	Green leafy vegetables such as broccoli, turnip greens, romaine lettuce, and cabbage; cheese, egg yolk, liver.
Folic Acid (Folacin, Folate)	Water soluble. Maintains genetic code of cells, regulates cell division and transfer of inherited traits from one cell to another. Necessary for normal cell growth and maintenance. Improves lactation. Acts as an analgesic for pain. Protects against intestinal parasites and food poisoning. Aids in preventing canker sores.	*Adults and children 15+: 180 to 200 mcg. Pregnancy: 360 to 400 mcg. Nursing 1 to 6 months: 280 mcg. 6 to 12 months: 260 mcg. Infants 0 to 12 months: 25 to 35 mcg. Children 1 to 14 years: 50 to 150 mcg.*	Brewer's (nutritional) yeast, dark green leafy vegetables, liver, orange juice, avocados, beets, broccoli, romaine lettuce.

MINERAL CHART

Mineral Legend

RDA = Recommended Daily Allowance. Estimated levels of intake for essential nutritionals developed by the Food and Nutrition Board and the National Research Council of the National Academy of Sciences.

IU = International Units

Mcg. = Micrograms

Mg. = Milligrams

GRAS = Generally Recommended as Safe/Safe and Adequate Range established by the federal government.

EMRHP = Estimated Minimum Requirements of Healthy People. Used when no RDA has been established. Developed by the Senate Select Committee on Nutrition and Human Needs and the U.S. Dietary Goals.

Mineral	What Mineral Does	RDA (Recommended Daily Allowance)	Food Sources
Calcium	Develops and maintains healthy bones and teeth. Especially important during childhood, pregnancy and breastfeeding. Also aids in blood clotting, maintaining normal blood pressure, protection against colon cancer, produc-	Adults: 800 to 1,200 mg. Pregnancy & nursing: 1,200 mg. Infants 0 to 12 months: 400 to 600 mg. Children 1 to 10 years: 800 mg. Children 11 to 24 years:1,200 mg.	Low-fat and non-fat milk, low-fat cheese, low-fat yogurt, dark green leafy vegetables, broccoli, canned fish with the bones, cottage cheese, cooked dried

Vitamin	What Vitamin Does	RDA (Recommended Daily Allowance)	Food Sources
Calcium (cont.)	tion and activity of certain enzymes and hormones. Helps with maintaining all cell membranes and connective tissue, muscle contraction, and nerve transmission. May reduce occurrence and progression of periodontal disease. Alleviates insomnia.		beans and peas, tofu, soybeans, cheddar cheese, oysters, peanuts, walnuts, sunflower seeds, oranges, dried apricots, hard tap water.
Chromium	A component of glucose tolerance factor (GTF) that works with insulin to regulate blood sugar levels. Aids in growth. Helps prevent and lower high blood pressure.	No RDA GRAS Range for adults and children 7+: 50 to 200 mcg. Infants 0 to 12 months: 10 to 60 mcg. Children 1 to 6 years: 20 to 120 mcg.	Brewer's (nutritional) yeast, whole grain breads and cereals, pork, kidneys, molasses, lean meat, cheese, calf's liver, wheat germ, chicken, corn oil, clams.

Vitamin	What Vitamin Does	RDA (Recommended Daily Allowance)	Food Sources
Fluoride	Protects developing and mature teeth from decay. May aid in wound healing and enhancing absorption of iron.	*No RDA* *GRAS Range for adults:* fortified water yielding 1.5 to 4.0 mg. daily. *Infants 0 to 12 months:* 0.1 to 1.0 mg. *Children 1+:* 0.5 to 2.5 mg.	Fluoridated water, unintentional ingestion of fluoridated toothpaste, use of fluoridated water in food processing.
Iodine	Component of the thyroid hormones that regulate rate of metabolism and growth; reproduction; nerve and muscle function; protein synthesis; hair and skin growth; use of oxygen by cells; and body weight. Helps burn excess fat. Provides energy.	*Adults and children 11+:* 150 mcg. *Pregnancy:* 175 mcg. *Nursing:* 200 mcg. *Infants 0 to 12 months:* 40 to 50 mcg. *Children 1 to 10 years:* 70 to 120 mcg.	Fresh saltwater shellfish and seafood, kelp, iodized salt, foods grown on iodine-rich soil, milk processed in equipment cleaned with iodates and milk from cows with iodine-rich diet.
Iron	Carries oxygen in the blood. Determines how much oxygen reaches and is used by all body tissues including the brain, mus-	*Women up to 50 years:* 15 mg. *Women over 50 years:* 10 mg. *Men 19+:* 10 mg. *Pregnancy:* 30 mg.	Organ meats (liver and heart), lean red meat, dried fruits, cooked dried beans and peas,

Vitamin	What Vitamin Does	RDA (Recommended Daily Allowance)	Food Sources
Iron (cont.)	cles, heart, and liver: Strengthens immune system and increases resistance to colds, infections, and disease. Aids in growth. Cures and prevents iron-deficiency anemia.	*Nursing:* 15 mg. *Infants 0 to 12 months:* 6 to 10 mg. *Children 1 to 10 years:* 10 mg. *Young adult women 11+:* 15 mg. *Young adult men 11 to 18 years:* 12 mg.	dark green leafy vegetables, fish, poultry, prune juice, oysters, whole grain breads and cereals, green peas, strawberries, tomato juice, brussels sprouts, blackberries, nuts, broccoli, asparagus, molasses, oatmeal.
Magnesium	Helps convert carbohydrates, protein, and fats to energy; manufacture proteins; synthesize genetic material within each cell; and remove excess toxic substances such as ammonia. Aids in muscle relaxation and contraction, nerve transmission, and fighting depression. Prevents tooth decay, heart disease, and irregular heartbeat. Provides indigestion relief.	*Adults:* 280 to 350 mg. *Pregnancy & nursing:* 260 to 350 mg. *Infants 0 to 12 months:* 40 to 60 mg. *Children 1 to 10 years:* 80 to 170 mg. *Children 11 to 18 years:* 280 to 300 mg.	Nuts, cooked dried beans and peas, whole grain breads and cereals, soybeans, dark green leafy vegetables, seafood, low-fat milk, bananas, avocados, peanut butter, wheat germ, Brewer's yeast, oysters, figs, almonds, nuts, seeds.

Vitamin	What Vitamin Does	RDA (Recommended Daily Allowance)	Food Sources
Phosphorus	Contributes to structure and function of bones and teeth. Component of all soft tissues including kidney, heart, brain, and muscles. Fundamental to grow, maintain, and repair all body tissues. Helps maintain blood pH balance and activate the B vitamins. Provides energy. Aids in growth and body repair.	*Adults: 800 to 1,200 mg. Pregnancy & nursing: 1,200 mg. Infants 0 to 12 months: 300 to 500 mg. Children 1 to 10 years: 800 mg. Children and adults 10 to 24 years: 1,200 mg.*	Protein-rich foods such as meat, organ meats, fish, poultry, eggs. Also non-fat milk, low-fat yogurt, cooked soybeans, peanut butter, whole wheat breads, cooked broccoli, oranges, bananas, cooked carrots, nuts, seeds.
Potassium	Maintains normal balance and fluid distribution throughout the body. Important in regulating heartbeat. May aid in maintaining normal blood pressure and preventing hypertension. Aids in allergy treatment.	*No RDA EMRHP for adults and children 10+: 1,600 to 2,000 mg. Infants 0 to 12 months: 500 to 700 mg. Children 1 to 9 years: 1,000 to 1,600 mg.*	Lean meats, potatoes, avocados, bananas, apricots, orange juice, dried fruits, cooked dried beans and peas, citrus fruits, cantaloupes, tomatoes, sunflower seeds, mint leaves, green leafy vegetables.

Vitamin	What Vitamin Does	RDA (Recommended Daily Allowance)	Food Sources
Selenium	Component of the antioxidant enzyme glutathione peroxidase. Protects red blood cells and cell membranes from damage. Works with and can replace the antioxidant vitamin E. Anticancer effects for colon, rectum, breast, ovaries, and lung. Helps treat and prevent dandruff. Helps alleviate hot flashes and menopausal distress.	*Women 19+: 55 mcg.* *Men 19+: 70 mcg.* *Pregnancy: 65 mcg.* *Nursing: 75 mcg.* *Infants 0 to 12 months: 10 to 115 mcg.* *Children 1 to 10 years: 20 to 30 mcg.* *Female children 11 to 18 years: 45 to 50 mcg.* *Male children 11 to 18 years: 40 to 50 mcg.*	Whole wheat, brown rice, oatmeal if grain was grown on selenium-rich soil, poultry, low-fat dairy products, lean meat, organ meats, fish, onions, tomatoes, broccoli.
Sodium	Maintains normal balance and fluid distribution throughout the body. Aids in preventing sunstroke. Helps nerves and muscles function properly.	*No RDA* *EMRHP for adults and children 10+: 500 mg. or 1 teaspoonful of salt.* *Infants 0 to 12 months: 120 to 200 mg.* *Children 1 to 9 years: 225 to 400 mg.*	Diet of unprocessed, natural foods with no added salt provides more than daily recommendation for sodium.

Vitamin	What Vitamin Does	RDA (Recommended Daily Allowance)	Food Sources
Sulfur	Gives characteristic shape differences to proteins. Involved in forming bile acids important for fat digestion and absorption. Helps regulate blood clotting. Aids conversion of proteins, carbohydrates, and fats to energy. Assists in regulating blood sugar. Helps fight bacterial infections. Contributes to healthy hair, skin, and nails.	No RDA; the American diet supplies adequate amounts of sulfur.	Meat, organ meats, poultry, fish, eggs, cooked dried beans and peas, cabbage, milk milk products.
Zinc	Functions in detoxification of alcohol in the liver, bone mineralization, protein digestion, conversion of calorie-containing nutrients to energy, production of proteins, proper functioning of insulin in regulating blood sugar. Maintains genetic code, normal taste. Heals wounds. Involved in production of prostaglandins. Gets rid of white spots on fingernails. Aids in treating fertility and prostate problems.	*Women and children 11+:* 12 mg. *Men and boys 11+:* 15 mg. *Pregnancy in months 1 to 6:* 19 mg. *Pregnancy in months 6 to 12:* 16 mg. *Infants 0 to 12 months:* 5 mg. *Children 1 to 10 years:* 10 mg.	Oysters, lean meat, poultry, fish, organ meats, whole grain breads and cereal, Brewer's yeast, pumpkin seeds, eggs, non-fat dry milk, ground mustard.

Appendix A

DRUGS APPROVED IN 1995 BY THE FOOD AND DRUG ADMINISTRATION

Amaryl
Generic name: Glimepiride
Drug form: tablet—1, 2, and 4-milligram
Drug use: prescribed to lower blood sugar levels in the treatment of Type II diabetes.

Arimidex
Generic name: Anastrozole
Drug form: tablet—1-milligram
Drug use: treatment of advanced breast cancer in post-menopausal women when the disease has progressed following Tamoxifen therapy.

Azelex
Generic name: Azelaic acid 20% cream
Drug form: topical cream
Drug use: treatment for vulgaris.

Cedax
Generic name: Ceftibuten dihydrate
Drug form: capsule—400 milligram; oral suspension—18 milligrams/milliliters
Drug use: children—otitis media due to bacteria, pharyngitil, and tonsilitis; adults—previous indications plus chronic bronchitis

CellCept
Generic name: Mycophenolate mofetil
Drug form: capsule—250-milligram
Drug use: for use in preventing organ rejection in patients receiving allogeneic (similar) genetic background renal transplants.

Coreg
Generic name: Carvedilol
Drug form: tablet—6.25, 12.5 & 25-milligram
Drug use: for management of essential hypertension.

Cozaar
Generic name: Losartan potassium
Drug form: tablet—25 & 50-milligram

Drug use: for treatment of hypertension.

Epivir
See Appendix B.

Flolan
Generic name: Epoprostenol sodium
Drug form: injection—0.5 & 1.5-milligram per vial
Drug use: for the long-term intravenous treatment of nyha class iii and class iv patients with primary pulmonary hypertension.

Fosamax
Generic name: Alendronate sodium
Drug form: tablets—10 & 40-milligram
Drug use: primary indications: for osteoporosis in post-menopausal women and Paget's disease; secondary indication: temporary relief of headache; backache; muscular ache; toothache; minor pain of arthritis; pain of menstrual cramps; minor aches and pain.

Invirase
See Appendix B.

Nisocor
Generic name: Nisoldipine
Drug form: extended release tablet—10, 20, 30, 40, & 60-milligram
Drug use: for treatment of hypertension and angina.

Precose
Generic name: Acarbose
Drug form: tablet—50, 100 & 200-milligram
Drug use: an adjunct to diet to lower blood glucose and hemoglobin in patients with non-insulin dependent diabetes mellitus, Type II diabetes.

Prevacid
Generic name: Lansoprazole
Drug form: capsule—15 & 30-milligram
Drug use: for short-term treatment of active duodenal ulcer and erosive reflux esophagitis; and for long-term treatment of chronic hypersecretory conditions, including Zollinger-Ellison syndrome.

Revex
Generic name: Nalmefene with hydrochloride
Drug form: injection—0.1-milligram & 1.0-milligram/

milliliter (Nalmefene)

Drug use: for complete or partial reversal of opiod drug effects; management of known or suspected opiod overdose.

Rilutek

Generic name: Riluzole

Drug form: tablet—50-milligram

Drug use: to treat amyotrophic lateral sclerosis (ALS), more commonly known as Lou Gehrig's disease.

Ultane

Generic name: Sevoflurane

Drug form: inhalation liquid (volatile)—100% Sevoflurane

Drug use: general anesthetic for inpatient and outpatient surgery.

Ultram

Generic name: Tramadol hydrochloride

Drug form: tablets—50 & 100-milligram

Drug use: for treatment of acute or chronic moderate to moderately severe pain.

Ultravist

Generic name: Iopromide

Drug form: injection—370-milligram/milliliter as iodine

Drug use: radiopaque agent.

Univasc

Generic name: Moexipril hydrochloride

Drug form: 7.5 & 15-milligram

Drug use: an angiotensin-converting enzyme (ACE) inhibitor for treatment of hypertension.

Valtrex

Generic name: Valacyclovir hydrochloride

Drug form: tablet—500-milligram (Valacyclovir)

Drug use: antiviral, oral treatment for herpes zoster (shingles) in immunocompetent adults.

Zinecard

Generic name: Dexrazoxane

Drug form: powder for injection—250 and 500-milligram single dose vial packs

Drug use: to reduce incidence and severity of cardiomyopathy associated in women with metastatic breast cancer who have received Doxorubicin and who would benefit from continuing Doxorubicin therapy

Zyrtec
Generic name: Cetirizine
Drug form: tablet—5-milligram
Drug use: to treat seasonal and perennial allergic rhinitis and chronic hives.

DRUGS APPROVED IN 1996

. . . .

New Drug Combination

Prilosec and Biaxin

Generic name: Omeprazole (Prilosec); Clarithromycin (Biaxin)
Drug form: Prilosec—20-milligram capsule; Biaxin—250 and 500-milligram tablets
Drug use: the two drugs are prescribed together to treat gastric ulcers (both drugs are currently on the market)

See pages 741–743 for additional information on Prilosec; and pages 105–107 for additional information on Biaxin.

Appendix B

ACQUIRED IMMUNODEFICIENCY SYNDROME
(AIDS) DRUGS

Drugs approved by the FDA for the treatment of AIDS:

Crixivan**
Generic name: Indinavir sulfate
Drug form: capsule—200 and 400-milligram

Epivir*
Generic name: Lamivudine
Drug form: tablet—150-milligram; oral solution—
10 milliliters (Recommended for use with Retrovir.)

Hivid
Generic names: ddC, Zalcitabine
Drug form: tablet—0.375 and 0.75 milligram (May be pre-
scribed with or without Retrovir.)

Invirase**
Generic name: Saquinavir
Drug form: capsule—600-milligram (Most effective when
prescribed with Retrovir or Hivid.)

Norvir**
Generic name: Ritonavir
Drug form: oral solution—80 milligrams/milliliter; cap-
sules—100-milligram

Retrovir
Generic names: AZT, Zidovudine
Drug form: capsule—100-milligram; syrup—50 milligrams/5
milliliters; injection—10 milligrams/milliliter

Videx
Generic names: ddI, Didanosine
Drug form: tablet, buffered, chewable/dispersible—25, 50,
100, 150 milligrams; powder for oral solution,
buffered—100, 167, 250, 375 milligrams; powder for
oral solution, pediatric—2 and 4 grams. (May be prescribed with or without Retrovir.)

Zerit
Generic names: d4T, Stavudine

Drug form: capsule—15, 20, 30, and 40 milligrams (Recommended when intolerance of other therapies develops or when other therapies are contraindicated.)

Zovirax
Generic name: Acyclovir
Drug form: tablets—400 and 800 milligrams; capsules—200 milligrams; suspension—200 milligrams/5 milliliters; powder for injection—500 and 1,000 milligrams/vial

. . . .

Drugs used to prevent or delay life-threatening infections such as pneumocycstis carinii (also used for indications other than HIV):

Bactrim, Cotrim, Septra
Generic name: Trimethoprim and Sulfamethoxazole (oral)
Drug form: tablets—80 milligrams trimethoprim and 400 milligrams sulfamethoxazole; double strength tablets (Bactrim DS, Cotrim DS, Septra DS)—160 milligrams trimethoprim and 800 milligrams sulfamethoxazole; oral suspension (Bactrim Pediatric, Cotrim Pediatric, Septra, Sulfatrim)—40 milligrams trimethoprim and 200 milligrams sulfamethoxazole per 5 milliliters; injection (Bactrim IV, Septra IV)—80 milligrams trimethoprim and 400 milligrams sulfamethoxazole per 5 milliliters. (May interact with AZT.)

Cytovene
Generic name: Ganciclovir
Drug form: capsules—250 milligrams; powder for injection, lyophilized—500 milligrams/vial (as sodium) (May interact with AZT.)

Foscavir
Generic name: Foscarnet sodium
Drug form: injection—24 milligrams/milliliter

NebuPent, Pentam 300
Generic name: Pentamidine isethionate
Drug form: NebuPent (aerosol)—300 milligrams; Pentam 300 (injection)—300 milligrams per vial

. . . .

Drugs to raise red blood cell levels:

Epoetin Alfa, Procrit
Generic name: Erythropoietin
Drug form (Epoetin Alfa and Procrit): injection—2000, 3000, 4000, and 10,000 units/milliliter

. . . .

Drugs used to raise white blood cell levels (known as colony stimulating factors):

Neupogen
Generic name: Filgrastim or G-CSF (granulocyte colony stimulating factor)
Drug form: injection—300 micrograms/milliliter

Leukine
Generic name: Sargramostim or GM-CSF (granulocyte macrophage colony stimulating factor)
Drug form: powder for injection, lyophilized—250 and 500 micrograms

* Approved 1995
** Approved 1996

Drugs to raise red blood cell levels

Epoetin Alfa, Procrit
Generic name: Erythropoietin
Drug form (Epoetin Alfa and Procrit) injection—2000, 3000, 4000, and 10,000 units/milliliter

Drugs used to raise white blood cell levels (known as colony stimulating factors)

Neupogen
Generic name: Filgrastim or G-CSF (granulocyte colony stimulating factor)
Drug form injection—300 micrograms/milliliter

Leukine
Generic name: Sargramostim or GM-CSF (granulocyte macrophage colony stimulating factor)
Drug form powder for injection, lyophilized—250 and 500 micrograms

*Approved 1945
**Approved 1956

Index

ABOUT THE AUTHOR

Brenda D. Adderly, M.H.S.A., is a health care consultant, and holds a master's degree in Health Services Administration from The George Washington University in Washington, D.C. For the past 10 years, Ms. Adderly's health care career has covered federal, not-for-profit, and for-profit sectors of health care. Her work assignments have included: the Department of Health and Human Services; hospitals; managed care organizations, including a national health maintenance organization and a statewide (California) managed care organization; benefits consulting; and most recently, managed care consulting. Ms. Adderly is a founding partner of The Healthcare Redesign Group, a national managed care consulting practice based in the San Francisco Bay area. She resides in Los Angeles where she consults and writes on various health care and managed care topics.

EMERGENCY AND MEDICATION OVERDOSE HELP

Emergency

In the event of an emergency call 9-1-1 immediately.

Medication Overdose or Allergic Reaction

In the event of a medication overdose:

- Call 9-1-1 immediately.
- Call the Poison Control Center (phone numbers are listed in the front of the local White Pages telephone book).
- Call your doctor.

The American Association of Poison Control Centers now advises that in the event of a medication overdose, you should **IMMEDIATELY CALL FOR MEDICAL ASSISTANCE.**